PHYSICAL MEDICINE AND REHABILITATION SECRETS
Second Edition

PHYSICAL MEDICINE AND REHABILITATION SECRETS
Second Edition

BRYAN J. O'YOUNG, MD

Clinical Associate Professor
Department of Rehabilitation Medicine
New York University School of Medicine
Attending Physician
Rusk Institute of Rehabilitation Medicine
New York, New York

MARK A. YOUNG, MD, MBA, FACP

Chair, Department of Physical Medicine and Rehabilitation
The Maryland Rehabilitation Center
State of Maryland Department of Education
Faculty, Johns Hopkins University School of Medicine
Faculty, University of Maryland School of Medicine
Baltimore, Maryland

STEVEN A. STIENS, MD, MS

Associate Professor
Department of Rehabilitation Medicine
University of Washington School of Medicine
Attending Physician, Spinal Cord Injury Unit
Veterans Affairs Puget Sound Health Care System
Seattle, Washington

HANLEY & BELFUS, INC./Philadelphia

Publisher: HANLEY & BELFUS, INC.
               Medical Publishers
               210 South 13th Street
               Philadelphia, PA 19107
               (215) 546-7293; 800-962-1892
               FAX (215) 790-9330
               Web site: http://www.hanleyandbelfus.com

Note to the reader: Although the information in this book has been carefully reviewed for correctness of dosage and indications, neither the authors nor the editor nor the publisher can accept any legal responsibility for any errors or omissions that may be made. Neither the publisher nor the editor makes any warranty, expressed or implied, with respect to the material contained herein. Before prescribing any drug, the reader must review the manufacturer's current product information (package inserts) for accepted indications, absolute dosage recommendations, and other information pertinent to the safe and effective use of the product described.

Library of Congress Cataloging-in-Publication Data

Physical medicine and rehabilitation secrets / edited by Bryan O'Young, Mark A. Young, Steven A. Stiens.—2nd ed.
    p. ; cm.—(The Secrets Series®)
  Rev. ed. of: PM&R secrets, c1997.
  Includes bibliographical references and index.
  ISBN 1-56053-437-0 (alk. paper)
    1. Physical therapy—Miscellanea. 2. Medical rehabilitation—Miscellanea. I. O'Young, Bryan, 1962- II. Young, Mark A., 1960- III. Stiens, Steven A., 1959- IV. PM&R secrets. V. Series
    [DNLM: 1. Physical Medicine—Examination Questions. 2. Rehabilitation—Examination Questions. WB 18.2 P57786 2001]
  RM701 .P4746 2001.
  615.8'2'076—dc21

                                                                           2001039690

**PHYSICAL MEDICINE AND
REHABILITATION SECRETS, 2ND EDITION**   ISBN 1-56053-437-0

Last digit is the print number: 9   8   7   6   5   4   3   2   1

DEDICATION

To my beloved parents, Te See and Merla, for their lifelong love and inspiration

To my siblings, Andrew, Crosby, Dorene, and Eldred, for their support and encouragement

To my mentor, Keith Sperling, M.D., who instilled in me a valuable ethic: "Treat each patient as though he or she is the most important person in the world."

To my department chairman, Mathew Lee, M.D., who cultivated my resilience, creativity, and adaptivity to embrace life's challenges

BJO

To my dedicated and loving wife, Marlene Malka; my kids, Michelle, Michael, and Jennifer; and my brother, Evan

To my colleagues in PM&R who have provided invaluable friendship, mentorship, and motivation

In fond memory of my late parents, Michael and Rowena, whose shining example has instilled in me an unwavering commitment to quality, compassionate patient care, education, and leadership

MAY

To my wife, Beth, and children, Hanna, Duffy, Luke, and Olivia, for the love they keep in our "nest"

To my beloved and respected parents, Jean and Bill, for their devotion to meaningful work and their lifelong nurturing of my personhood

To my brothers, Scott and Doug, for their humor and creativity

To my first mentor, Gustav Eckstein, M.D., from the University of Cincinnati College of Medicine, who taught me that "the body does have a head!"

Reference: Eckstein G: The Body Has a Head. New York, Harper & Row, 1970.

SAS

DEDICATION

Howard A. Rusk, M.D., the founder of the institute that bears his name, is considered the father of comprehensive rehabilitation medicine. His innovative techniques, developed to help injured Air Force personnel during World War II, became the basis for rehabilitation medicine as it is now practiced. After the war, Dr. Rusk joined the faculty of the New York University School of Medicine and formed what has become a world-renowned facility for the rehabilitation of individuals with disabilities.

Dr. Rusk's philosophy of rehabilitation medicine emphasized treating the entire person—an individual with emotional, psychological, and social needs—not just the illness or disability. A compassionate and tireless advocate, he championed the idea that people with disabilities could contribute meaningfully to society.

Dr. Rusk's timeless efforts in Washington, DC, led to the establishment of dozens of research and training centers throughout our nation's academic institutions, which made possible the exponential growth of our discipline. He founded the World Rehabilitation Fund and the Korean-American Foundation and served as an advisor to presidents and world leaders. Recipient of two Lasker Awards, he was also a nominee for the Nobel Peace Prize. He established the first facility devoted entirely to rehabilitation medicine. He and Dr. Donald Covalt with the support of General Arnold were instrumental in the development of rehabilitation medicine in the Air Force and the Veterans' Administration.

Dr. Rusk enhanced the lives of countless men, women, and children by helping them achieve their maximum potential while helping to change society's attitudes toward people with disabilities.

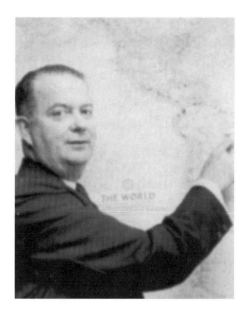

CONTENTS

I. PM&R ESSENTIALS

1. What is Physiatry? 1
   Mark A. Young, M.D., Bryan O'Young, M.D., and Steven A. Stiens, M.D., M.S.

2. Person-Centered Rehabilitation: Interdisciplinary Intervention to Enhance
   Patient Enablement 4
   Steven A. Stiens, M.D., M.S., Bryan O'Young, M.D., and Mark A. Young, M.D.

3. Functional Assessment for Outcome Analysis 9
   Gary S. Clark, M.D., and Carl V. Granger, M.D.

4. Research Concepts in PM&R 14
   *John E. Hewett, Ph.D., David G. McDonald, Ph.D., Richard Salcido, M.D.,
   and Jerry C. Parker, M.D.*

5. Nervous System Anatomy 20
   Stephen Goldberg, M.D.

6. Physiology of the Peripheral and Central Nervous Systems 30
   Gary Goldberg, M.D.

7. Anatomy and Kinesiology of the Musculoskeletal System 44
   Carson D. Schneck, M.D., Ph.D.

II. CARING FOR PERSONS WITH DISABILITIES

8. Communication Strategies for Rehabilitation Professionals:
   Disability Etiquette and Empowerment 53
   *Margaret G. Stineman, M.D., Susan M. Miller, M.D., Harlan Hahn, Ph.D.,
   and Steven A. Stiens, M.D., M.S.*

9. Rehabilitation of Patients with Severe Visual Impairments or Blindness......... 65
   Stanley F. Wainapel, M.D., M.P.H.

10. Rehabilitation Strategies in the Hearing Impaired 68
    *J. Michael Anderson, M.D., Denise W. Thrope, M.S., CCC-A,
    and Linda J. Anderson, O.T.R.*

11. Sexual Satisfaction Despite Disablement 75
    Steven A. Stiens, M.D., M.S., Ruth K. Westheimer, Ed.D., and Mark A. Young, M.D.

12. Environmental Adaptations.. 81
    *Shoshana Shamberg, OTR/L, Steven A. Stiens, M.D., M.S.,
    and Aaron Shamberg, OTR/L, M.S.*

13. Legislative Issues in the Field of Physical Medicine and Rehabilitation 90
    *Leighton Chan, M.D., M.P.H., Mary Richardson, Ph.D., M.H.A.,
    and Richard Verville, J.D.*

III. THE REHABILITATION EVALUATION

14. The Physiatric Consultation: Interdisciplinary Intervention
    and Functional Restoration.. 97
    Steven A. Stiens, M.D., M.S.

15. Neurologic Evaluation of the Rehabilitation Patient 102
    Rajiv R. Ratan, M.D., Ph.D., and Adriana Conforto, M.D.

16. Manual Muscle Testing and Range of Motion Measurement 109
   John J. Nicholas, M.D., and Ian B. Maitin, M.D.

17. Analysis of Gait and Kinesiology 111
   D. Casey Kerrigan, M.D., Susan Ehrenthal, M.D., and Richard Mazzaferro, D.O.

18. Evaluation of the Geriatric Patient 116
   Susan J. Garrison, M.D., and Gerald Felsenthal, M.D.

19. Impairment Evaluation and Disability Rating 121
   Richard T. Katz, M.D., and Robert D. Rondinelli, M.D., Ph.D.

IV. ELECTRODIAGNOSTIC FUNDAMENTALS

20. General Principles of Electrodiagnosis 125
   Mooyeon Oh-Park, M.D., and Dennis D. J. Kim, M.D.

21. Radiculopathies 132
   Timothy R. Dillingham, M.D.

22. Carpal Tunnel Syndrome and/or Median Neuropathy at the Wrist 137
   Janet C. Limke, M.D., Steven A. Stiens, M.D., M.S., and Larry Robinson, M.D.

23. Entrapment Neuropathy 144
   Jaywant J. P. Patil, MBBS, FRCPC

24. Peripheral Neuropathy 150
   Peter D. Donofrio, M.D., and Yadollah Harati, M.D.

25. Electrophysiology of Disorders of Neuromuscular Transmission 156
   Thomas E. McGunigal, Jr., M.D.

26. Sensory and Motor Evoked Potentials 160
   Gary Goldberg, M.D., Jeffrey L. Cole, M.D., and Mark A. Lissens, M.D., Ph.D.

V. REHABILITATION OF ORGAN-BASED SYSTEMS

27. Stroke 167
   Elliot J. Roth, M.D.

28. Multiple Sclerosis 177
   Brian D. Greenwald, M.D., Jan Lexell, M.D., Ph.D., and Allison Averill, M.D.

29. Movement Disorders 182
   *Kenneth H. Silver, M.D., Paul Fishman, M.D., Ph.D.,
   and John Speed, MBBS*

30. Traumatic Brain Injury 194
   Robert L. Harmon, M.D., M.S., and Lawrence J. Horn, M.D., M.R.M.

31. Spinal Cord Injury Medicine 203
   *Steven A. Stiens, M.D., M.S., Barry Goldstein, M.D., Ph.D.,
   Margaret Hammond, M.D., and James Little, M.D., Ph.D.*

32. Motor Neuron Disease 211
   *Michael Hatzakis, Jr., M.D., James C. Agre, M.D., Ph.D.,
   and Arthur A. Rodriquez, M.D.*

33. Frontiers and Fundamentals in Neurorehabilitation 220
   *Charles E. Levy, M.D., Andrea Behrman, Ph.D., Leslie Gonzalez Rothi, Ph.D.,
   Haim Ring, M.D., and Kenneth Heilman, M.D.*

34. Pulmonary Rehabilitation 233
   John R. Bach, M.D.

35. Cardiac Rehabilitation 241
    Yehoshua A. Lehman, M.D., Steven A. Stiens, M.D., M.S.,
    and Eugen M. Halar, M.D.

36. Peripheral Vascular Disease Rehabilitation 247
    Marvin M. Brooke, M.D., M.S.

VI. MUSCULOSKELETAL REHABILITATION

37. Neck Pain 251
    Rene Cailliet, M.D.

38. Low Back Pain 254
    Maury Ellenberg, M.D., and Joseph C. Honet, M.D., M.S.

39. The Shoulder: Anatomy, Pathology, and Diagnosis 258
    Rene Cailliet, M.D.

40. Rehabilitation of Shoulder Disorders 261
    Edward G. McFarland, M.D., Timothy C. Shen, M.D.,
    Tae Kyun Kim, M.D., Ph.D., and Gregory E. Lutz, M.D.

41. The Elbow: Anatomy, Pathology, and Diagnosis 265
    Edward Magaziner, M.D., and Francisco Santiago, M.D.

42. Rehabilitation of the Elbow 269
    Douglas Sheppard, M.D., Howard Choi, M.D.,
    Matthew Shatzer, D.O., Harry Brafman, P.T.,
    Mark A. Young, M.D., and Henk J. Stam, M.D., Ph.D.

43. The Wrist and Hand: Anatomy, Pathology, and Diagnosis 272
    Francisco H. Santiago, M.D., and Jaywant J. P. Patil, MBBS, FRCPC

44. Rehabilitation of Wrist and Hand Disorders 276
    Richard A. Rogachefsky, M.D., and Barry D. Stein, M.D.

45. The Hip: Anatomy, Pathology, and Diagnosis 280
    Howard Choi, M.D., David Fish, M.D., Mark A. Young, M.D.,
    and Peter Disler, Ph.D., MBBCh

46. Rehabilitation of Hip Disorders 283
    Gracia Etienne, M.D., Ph.D., Amar D. Rajadhyaksha, M.D.,
    Harpal Khanuja, M.D., and Michael A. Mont, M.D.

47. The Knee: Anatomy, Pathology, and Diagnosis 289
    Michael E. Frey, M.D., and Warren Slaten, M.D.

48. Rehabilitation of Knee Disorders 293
    Harpal Khanuja, M.D., Oliver Perez, B.S., Gracia Etienne, M.D., Ph.D.,
    Amar D. Rajadhyaksha, M.D., and Michael A. Mont, M.D.

49. The Ankle and Foot: Anatomy, Pathology, and Diagnosis 297
    C. Christopher Stroud, M.D., and Lew C. Schon, M.D.

50. Rehabilitation of Foot and Ankle Disorders 300
    Mooyeon Oh-Park, M.D., and Dennis D. J. Kim, M.D.

51. Management of Fractures 305
    Arun J. Mehta, M.B., FRCPC

52. Rehabilitation of Soft Tissue and Musculoskeletal Injury 312
    Howard J. Hoffberg, M.D.

VII. REHABILITATION AFTER SYSTEMIC DISEASE AND INJURY

  53. Rehabilitation of the Transplant Patient 317
        Mark A. Young, M.D., and Steven A. Stiens, M.D., M.S.

  54. Rehabilitation in Chronic Renal Failure and End-Stage Renal Disease 321
        Sally Sizer Fitts, Ph.D., Christopher R. Blagg, M.D.,
        and Diana D. Cardenas, M.D.

  55. Cancer Rehabilitation: General Principles 325
        Ki Y. Shin, M.D., Theresa A. Gillis, M.D., and Fae Garden, M.D.

  56. Rehabilitation of the Individual with HIV and AIDS 333
        Stephen F. Levinson, M.D., Ph.D., and Steven M. Fine, M.D., Ph.D.

  57. Rehabilitative Management of Rheumatic Diseases 337
        Jeanne E. Hicks, M.D., Galen O. Joe, M.D., and Jay P. Shah, M.D.

  58. Burn Rehabilitation 352
        W. Nicholas Sorensen, O.T.R., Steven V. Fisher, M.D.,
        and Elizabeth A. Rivers, O.T.R., R.N.

VIII. CHRONIC PAIN

  59. Pain Management 363
        Jaywant J. P. Patil, MBBS, FRCPC, Anthony Guarino, M.D.,
        and Peter Staats, M.D.

  60. Myofascial Pain and Fibromyalgia 369
        Andrew A. Fischer, M.D., Ph.D., David A. Cassius, M.D.,
        and Marta Imamura, M.D., Ph.D.

  61. Complex Regional Pain Syndromes 379
        Bryan O'Young, M.D., and Warren Slaten, M.D.

 IX. REHABILITATION IN SPORTS AND THE ARTS

  62. Sports Medicine 385
        Joel M. Press, M.D., and Jeffrey L. Young, M.D., M.A.

  63. Rehabilitation of the Performing Artist 391
        Scott E. Brown, M.D.

  X. REHABILITATION AND INDUSTRY

  64. Vocational Rehabilitation Counseling 397
        Ruth Torkelson Lynch, Ph.D., Rochelle Habeck, Ph.D.,
        and Rhodora C. Tumanon, M.D.

  65. Occupational Medicine and Rehabilitation of the Injured Worker 403
        Norman B. Rosen, M.D.

 XI. PEDIATRIC REHABILITATION

  66. General Pediatric Rehabilitation 409
        Frank S. Pidcock, M.D., and James R. Christensen, M.D.

  67. Developmental Milestones 415
        Scott Benjamin, M.D., Melissa Trovato, M.D., Edward A. Hurvitz, M.D.,
        Lisa Daley, M.D., and Mark G. Greenbaum, M.D.

68. Cerebral Palsy... 418
    Edward A. Hurvitz, M.D., and Rita N. Ayyangar, M.D.

69. Neural Tube Defects.. 424
    Sam S. H. Wu, M.D., M.P.H., M.B.A., Jeffrey M. Cohen, M.D.,
    and Steven A. Stiens, M.D., M.S.

XII. MEDICAL COMPLICATIONS IN REHABILITATION

70. Common Medical Problems on the Inpatient Rehabilitation Unit............. 429
    James K. Richardson, M.D., Paul T. Diamond, M.D., Steven A. Stiens, M.D., M.S.,
    Isabel C. Borras, M.D., and Michael Freedman, M.D.

71. Hazards of Immobilization: Preventing the Adverse Effects of Bed Rest....... 438
    Paul Corcoran, M.D., Eugen M. Halar, M.D., Kathleen R. Bell, M.D.,
    and Steven A. Stiens, M.D., M.S.

72. Spasticity.. 442
    Richard T. Katz, M.D.

73. Metabolic Bone Disease.. 447
    Charles E. Levy, M.D., Jeffrey Rosenbuth, M.D., Valery F. Lanyi, M.D.,
    and Bryan O'Young, M.D.

74. Heterotopic Ossification.. 456
    Jay V. Subbarao, M.D., M.S.

75. Pressure Ulcers... 460
    Michael M. Priebe, M.D.

76. Neurogenic Bowel Dysfunction: Evaluation and Adaptive Management....... 465
    Steven A. Stiens, M.D., M.S., and Lance L. Goetz, M.D.

77. Urologic Disorders in Rehabilitation................................. 471
    Inder Perkash, M.D.

78. Communication and Swallowing Impairments.......................... 478
    Donna C. Tippett, M.P.H., M.A., CCC-SLP

XIII. GENERAL THERAPEUTICS

79. Therapeutic Exercise... 487
    Ralph M. Buschbacher, M.D., and Mark Randall, Psy.D., Dr.P.H., M.A.

80. Nutrition and Dietary Issues in Rehabilitation......................... 494
    Marlene M. Young, B.A., Eli D. Ehrenpreis, M.D., and Mark A. Young, M.D.

81. Pharmacologic Agents in Rehabilitation Medicine...................... 496
    Jennifer J. James, M.D., Steven A. Stiens, M.D., M.S., Karen Lew, PharmD,
    Stephen P. Burns, M.D., and Mark A. Young, M.D.

82. Assistive Technology... 504
    Mark A. Young, M.D., Howard Choi, M.D., and Mary Macy, M.D.

83. Community Reintegration... 508
    David Tostenrude, M.P.A., CTRS, Carrie Booker, CTRS,
    and Steven A. Stiens, M.D., M.S.

XIV. PHYSICAL MODALITIES

84. The Physical Agents.. 513
    Jeffrey R. Basford, M.D., Ph.D., and Veronika Fialka-Moser, M.D.

85. Electrotherapy. 523
Peter H. Gorman, M.D., M.S., Norman Shealy, M.D., Ph.D., Saul Liss, Ph.D.,
Stanley H. Kornhauser, Ph.D., and Charles Cannizzaro, M.D., P.T.

86. Traction, Manipulation, and Massage. 528
Steven R. Hinderer, M.D., M.S., P.T., and Peter E. Biglin, D.O.

XV. INTERVENTIONAL PHYSIATRY

87. Epidural Blocks, Facet Injections, and Spinal Therapeutics. 533
Frank J. E. Falco, M.D., Charles M. Narrow, M.D.,
John R. Carbon, D.O., M.S., Gabriel Martinez, M.D.,
and Michael E. Frey, M.D.

88. Local Injections for Muscle Spasticity (Nerve Blocks) 537
Thomas J. Cava, M.D., and Christopher O'Brien, M.D.

89. Acupuncture 541
John Giusto, M.D., and Joseph M. Helms, M.D.

90. Injections of Peripheral Joints, Bursae, and Tendon Sheaths 547
Mark G. Greenbaum, M.D., and Stuart A. Rubin, M.D.

XVI. ORTHOTICS, PROSTHETICS, AND WHEELCHAIRS

91. Amputation Rehabilitation 553
Nasser Eftekhari, M.D.

92. Upper-Limb Orthoses. 562
John B. Redford, M.D., Abna A. Ogle, M.D.,
and Richard C. Robinson, M.D.

93. Upper-Limb Prostheses. 567
Atul T. Patel, M.D., Anthony S. Salzano, M.D.,
and Subhadra Lakshmi Nori, M.D.

94. Lower-Limb Orthoses. 572
Kristjan T. Ragnarsson, M.D., Jay Schechtman, M.D.,
and Richard A. Frieden, M.D.

95. Lower-Limb Prosthetics and Gait Deviations. 577
Joan E. Edelstein, M.A., P.T., FISPO, and Norman Berger, M.S.

96. Spinal Orthoses. 584
John B. Redford, M.D., Abna A. Ogle, M.D., and Richard C. Robinson, M.D.

97. Manual Wheelchairs 589
R. Lee Kirby, M.D.

Epilogue. 594
Martin Grabois, M.D., and Thomas E. Strax, M.D.

INDEX. 597

CONTRIBUTORS

James C. Agre, M.D., Ph.D.
Physiatrist, Department of Physical Medicine and Rehabilitation, Howard Young Clinics, Woodruff, Wisconsin

J. Michael Anderson, M.D.
Associate Professor, Department of Physical Medicine and Rehabilitation, Johns Hopkins University School of Medicine; Associate Professor, Division of Rehabilitation Medicine, Department of Neurology, University of Maryland School of Medicine; Sinai Hospital, Baltimore, Maryland

Linda J. Anderson, O.T.R.
Occupational Therapist in Private Practice, Owings Mills, Maryland

Allison Averill, M.D.
Assistant Professor and Associate Medical Director, Department of Physical Medicine and Rehabilitation, University of Medicine and Dentistry of New Jersey, New Jersey Medical School, Newark, New Jersey; Kessler Institute for Rehabilitation, East Orange, New Jersey

Rita N. Ayyangar, M.D.
Assistant Professor, Department of Physical Medicine and Rehabilitation, University of Michigan Health Systems, Mott Children's Hospital, Ann Arbor, Michigan

John R. Bach, M.D.
Professor of Physical Medicine and Rehabilitation, Professor of Neurosciences, University of Medicine and Dentistry of New Jersey, New Jersey Medical School; University Hospital, Newark, New Jersey

Jeffrey R. Basford, M.D., Ph.D.
Associate Professor, Department of Physical Medicine and Rehabilitation, Mayo Medical School, Mayo Clinic, Rochester, Minnesota

Andrea L. Behrman, Ph.D., P.T.
Associate Professor, Department of Physical Therapy, University of Florida; Shands Hospital, Gainesville, Florida

Kathleen R. Bell, M.D.
Associate Professor, Department of Rehabilitation Medicine, University of Washington School of Medicine; University of Washington Medical Center, Seattle, Washington

Scott E. Benjamin, M.D.
Fellow, Department of Pediatric Rehabilitation Medicine, Johns Hopkins University School of Medicine; Kennedy Krieger Institute, Baltimore, Maryland

Norman Berger, M.D.
Clinical Professor (retired), Department of Orthopadic Surgery, New York University Medical Center, New York, New York

Peter E. Biglin, D.O.
Department of Physical Medicine and Rehabilitation, Wayne State University Detroit Medical Center; Rehabilitation Institute of Michigan, Detroit, Michigan

Christopher R. Blagg, M.D.
Professor Emeritus of Medicine, University of Washington School of Medicine; Executive Director Emeritus, Northwest Kidney Centers, Seattle, Washington

Carrie L. Booker, CTRS
Recreation Therapist, Spinal Cord Injury Service, Veterans Affairs Puget Sound Health Care Systems, Seattle, Washington

Isabel C. Borras, M.D.
Attending Physician, Sinai Hospital, Baltimore, Maryland

Harry Brafman, P.T.
Physical Therapist, Baltimore, Maryland

Marvin M. Brooke, M.D., M.S.
Clinical Associate Professor, Department of Rehabilitation Medicine, University of Washington School of Medicine, Seattle, Washington; Medical Director, Department of Physical Medicine and Rehabilitation, Good Samaritan Hospital, Puyallup, Washington

Scott E. Brown, M.D.
Assistant Professor, Department of Neurology, University of Maryland School of Medicine; Chief, Department of Rehabilitation Medicine, Sinai Hospital of Baltimore, Baltimore, Maryland

Stephen P. Burns, M.D.
Assistant Professor, Department of Rehabilitation Medicine, University of Washington School of Medicine; Staff Physician, Spinal Cord Injury Service, Veterans Affairs Puget Sound Health Care System, Seattle, Washington

Ralph M. Buschbacher, M.D.
Clinical Associate Professor, Department of Physical Medicine and Rehabilitation, Indiana University School of Medicine; Indiana University Hospital; Community Hospital, Indianapolis, Indiana

Rene Cailliet, M.D.
Professor Emeritus, University of Southern California School of Medicine; Clinical Professor, University of California, Los Angeles, UCLA School of Medicine, Los Angeles, California

Charles Cannizzaro, M.D., P.T.
Orthopaedic, Sports, and Industrial Medicine Center of Dublin, Dublin, Georgia

John R. Carbon, D.O., M.S.
Physiatrist in Private Practice, Mid-Atlantic Spine and Sports Center, Baltimore, Maryland; Upper Chesapeake Health, Bel Air, Maryland

Diana D. Cardenas, M.D., M.H.A.
Professor, Department of Rehabilitation Medicine, University of Washington School of Medicine; University of Washington Medical Center, Seattle, Washington

David A. Cassius, M.D.
Attending Physician, Moss Bay Center, Seattle, Washington; Guest Faculty, University of Sao Paulo, Sao Paulo, Brazil

Thomas J. Cava, M.D.
Director of Physical Medicine and Rehabilitation, PC Rehabilitation Medicine, West Orange, New Jersey; Attending Physician, Saint Barnabas Medical Center, Mountainside Hospital, Livingston, New Jersey

Leighton Chan, M.D., M.P.H.
Assistant Professor, Department of Rehabilitation Medicine, University of Washington School of Medicine; Medical Epidemiologist, Division of Clinical Standards and Quality, Health Care Financing Administration, Seattle, Washington

Howard Choi, M.D.
Fellow, Spinal Cord Injury Medicine, Harvard Medical School, Boston, Massachusetts

James R. Christensen, M.D.
Assistant Professor, Departments of Physical Medicine and Rehabilitation and Pediatrics, Johns Hopkins University School of Medicine; Kennedy Krieger Institute; Johns Hopkins Hospital, Baltimore, Maryland

Gary S. Clark, M.D., C.P.E.
Chairman, Department of Physical Medicine and Rehabilitation, Case Western Reserve University School of Medicine; MetroHealth Medical Center, Cleveland, Ohio

Jeffrey M. Cohen, M.D.
Clinical Assistant Professor, Department of Rehabilitation Medicine, New York University School of Medicine; Rusk Institute of Rehabilitation Medicine, New York University Medical Center, New York, New York

Jeffrey L. Cole, M.D.
Clinical Associate Professor of Rehabilitation Medicine, Department of Surgery, Weill Medical College of Cornell University, New York, New York; New York Hospital Center of Queens, Flushing, New York

Adriana B. Conforto, M.D.
Fellow, National Institute of Neurological Disorders and Stroke, National Institutes of Health, Bethesda, Maryland

Paul J. Corcoran, M.D., M.S.
Department of Physical Medicine and Rehabilitation, Harvard Medical School; Staff Physiatrist, Spaulding Rehabilitation Hospital, Boston, Massachusetts

Lisa M. Daley, M.D.
Medical Director, Allied Medical and Rehabilitation, P.C., Bellmore, New York, and Massapequa, New York

Paul T. Diamond, M.D.
Associate Professor, Department of Physical Medicine and Rehabilitation, University of Virginia Health System, Charlottesville, Virginia

Timothy R. Dillingham, M.D.
Associate Professor, Department of Physical Medicine and Rehabilitation, Johns Hopkins University School of Medicine; Johns Hopkins Hospital, Baltimore, Maryland

Peter Disler, Ph.D., MBBCh, FRACP, FAFRM
Professor of Rehabilitation, University of Melbourne; Clinical Director, Rehabilitation Programme, Royal Melbourne Hospital; Director, Victorian Rehabilitation Research Institute, Cedar Court Health South Rehabilitation Hospital, Melbourne, Australia

Peter D. Donofrio, M.D.
Professor, Department of Neurology, Wake Forest University School of Medicine; North Carolina Baptist Hospital, Winston-Salem, North Carolina

Joan E. Edelstein, M.A., P.T., FISPO
Associate Professor of Clinical Physical Therapy and Director, Program in Physical Therapy, Department of Rehabilitation Medicine, Columbia University, New York, New York

Nasser Eftekhari, M.D.
Clinical Assistant Professor, Department of Orthopaedics and Rehabilitation, University of Miami School of Medicine; Physical Medicine and Rehabilitation Service, Veterans Affairs Hospital, Miami, Florida

Eli D. Ehrenpreis, M.D.
Faculty, Department of Gastroenterology, University of Chicago Hospital, Chicago, Illinois

Susan Ehrenthal, M.D.
Co-Director, Ortho-Med Program, Rehabilitation Hospital of the Cape and Islands, Sandwich, Massachusetts

Maury Ellenberg, M.D., FACP
Clinical Associate Professor and Residency Program Director, Department of Physical Medicine and Rehabilitation, Wayne State University School of Medicine; Sinai-Grace Hospital, Detroit Michigan; Providence Hospital, Smithfield, Michigan

Gracia Etienne, M.D., Ph.D.
Faculty, Department of Orthopaedics, Johns Hopkins University School of Medicine; Good Samaritan Hospital, Baltimore, Maryland

Frank J. E. Falco, M.D.
Department of Physical Medicine and Rehabilitation, Temple University School of Medicine, Philadelphia, Pennsylvania

Gerald Felsenthal, M.D.
Clinical Professor, Department of Epidemiology and Preventive Medicine, University of Maryland School of Medicine; Chairman Emeritus, Department of Rehabilitation Medicine, Sinai Hospital of Baltimore, Baltimore, Maryland

Veronika Fialka-Moser, M.D.
Chair, Department of Physical Medicine and Rehabilitation, University of Vienna, Vienna, Austria

Steven M. Fine, M.D., Ph.D.
Assistant Professor, Department of Medicine, Infectious Diseases Unit, University of Rochester Medical Center; Attending Physician, Strong Memorial Hospital; Highland Hospital, Rochester, New York

Andrew A. Fischer, M.D., Ph.D.
Associate Clinical Professor, Department of Rehabilitation Medicine, Mount Sinai School of Medicine, City University of New York; Mount Sinai Hospital; Elmhurst Hospital, New York, New York

David E. Fish, M.D., M.P.H.
Department of Physical Medicine and Rehabilitation, Johns Hopkins University School of Medicine, Baltimore, Maryland

Steven V. Fisher, M.D., M.S.
Associate Professor, Department of Physical Medicine and Rehabilitation, University of Minnesota School of Medicine; Chief of Physical Medicine, Hennepin County Medical Center, Minneapolis, Minnesota

Paul Fishman, M.D., Ph.D.
Associate Professor, Department of Neurology, University of Maryland School of Medicine; University of Maryland Hospital; Veterans Affairs Medical Center, Baltimore, Maryland

Sally Sizer Fitts, Ph.D.
Professional Staff, Department of Psychosocial and Community Health, University of Washington School of Nursing, Seattle, Washington

Michael Freedman, M.D.
Faculty, Johns Hopkins University School of Medicine; Attending Physician, Sinai Hospital, Baltimore, Maryland

Michael E. Frey, M.D.
Chief Resident and Clinical Instructor, Department of Physical Medicine and Rehabilitation, Temple University School of Medicine; Temple University Hospital, Philadelphia, Pennsylvania

Richard A. Frieden, M.D.
Assistant Professor, Department of Rehabilitation of Medicine, Mount Sinai School of Medicine, City University of New York; Assistant Attending, Mount Sinai Hospital, New York, New York

Fae H. Garden, M.D.
Associate Professor, Department of Physical Medicine and Rehabilitation, Baylor College of Medicine; St. Luke's Episcopal Hospital, Houston, Texas

Susan J. Garrison, M.D.
Associate Professor, Department of Physical Medicine and Rehabilitation, Baylor College of Medicine; Medical Director, Rehabilitation Center, The Methodist Hospital, Houston, Texas

Theresa A. Gillis, M.D.
Assistant Professor, Department of Physical Medicine and Rehabilitation, Baylor College of Medicine; Medical Director, Rehabilitation Services, and Chief of Physical Medicine and Rehabilitation Section, University of Texas M.D. Anderson Cancer Center, Houston, Texas

John Giusto, M.D.
Attending Physiatrist, Triangle Orthopaedic Associates, Durham, North Carolina

Lance L. Goetz, M.D.
Assistant Professor, Department of Physical Medicine and Rehabilitation, University of Texas Southwestern Medical Center; Staff, Dallas Veterans Affairs Spinal Cord Injury Center, Dallas, Texas

Gary Goldberg, M.D.
Professor, Department of Physical Medicine and Rehabilitation, University of Pittsburgh School of Medicine; Director, Brain Injury Rehabilitation, UPMC Rehabilitation Hospital, Pittsburgh, Pennsylvania

Stephen Goldberg, M.D.
Professor Emeritus, Department of Cell Biology and Anatomy, University of Miami School of Medicine, Miami, Florida

Barry Goldstein, M.D., Ph.D.
Associate Professor, Department of Rehabilitation Medicine; Associate Chief Consultant, Spinal Cord Injury Healthcare Group, University of Washington School of Medicine; Veterans Affairs Puget Sound Health Care System; Attending Physician, Harborview Medical Center, Seattle, Washington

Peter H. Gorman, M.D., M.S.
Associate Professor, Departments of Neurology and Rehabilitation Medicine, University of Maryland School of Medicine; Director, Spinal Cord Injury Service, Kernan Hospital; Attending Physician, Physical Medicine and Rehabilitation Service, Veterans Affairs Maryland Healthcare System, Baltimore, Maryland

Martin Grabois, M.D.
Professor and Chairman, Department of Physical Medicine and Rehabilitation, Baylor College of Medicine, Houston, Texas

Carl V. Granger, M.D.
Professor and Chairman, Department of Rehabilitation Medicine, University of Buffalo School of Medicine; Erie County Medical Center; Kaleida Health System, Buffalo, New York

Mark G. Greenbaum, M.D.
Clinical Assistant Professor, Department of Rehabilitation Medicine, Albert Einstein College of Medicine of Yeshiva University; Voluntary Attending, Montefiore Medical Center, Bronx, New York

Brian D. Greenwald, M.D.
Assistant Professor, Department of Physical Medicine and Rehabilitation, University of Medicine and Dentistry of New Jersey, New Jersey Medical School; Director of Trauma Rehabilitation, University Hospital, Newark, New Jersey

Anthony Guarino, M.D.
Chief of Pain Management, Department of Anesthesiology, Washington University School of Medicine, St. Louis, Missouri

Rochelle V. Habeck, Ph.D.
Adjunct Professor, Office of Rehabilitation and Disability Studies, Michigan State University, East Lansing, Michigan

Harlan Hahn, Ph.D.
Private Practice, Santa Monica, California

Eugen M. Halar, M.D.
Professor Emeritus, Department of Rehabilitation Medicine, University of Washington School of Medicine; University of Washington Medical Center, Seattle, Washington

Margaret C. Hammond, M.D.
Associate Professor, Department of Rehabilitation Medicine, University of Washington School of Medicine; Chief, Spinal Cord Injury Service, Veterans Affairs Puget Sound Health Care System, Seattle, Washington

Yadollah Harati, M.D., FACP
Professor of Neuromuscular Diseases, Department of Neurology, Baylor College of Medicine; Executive, Neurology Care Line, Veterans Affairs Medical Center, Houston, Texas

Robert L. Harmon, M.D., M.S.
Associate Clinical Professor, Departments of Medicine and Neurology, Medical College of Georgia; Medical Director of Neurological Rehabilitation, Walton Rehabilitation Hospital, Augusta, Georgia

Michael Hatzakis, Jr., M.D.
Assistant Professor, Department of Rehabilitation Medicine, University of Washington School of Medicine; Veterans Affairs Puget Sound Health Care System, Seattle, Washington

Kenneth M. Heilman, M.D.
James S. Rooks, Jr., Distinguished Professor, Department of Neurology, University of Florida College of Medicine; Shands Teaching Hospital of University of Florida; Veterans Affairs Medical Center, Gainesville, Florida

Joseph M. Helms, M.D.
Chairman, Physician Acupuncture Education, Office of Continuing Medical Education, University of California, Los Angeles, UCLA School of Medicine, Los Angeles, California; Director, Helms Medical Institute, Berkeley, California

John E. Hewett, Ph.D.
Emeritus Professor, Department of Statistics, University of Missouri; University of Missouri Health Sciences Center, Columbia, Missouri

Jeanne E. Hicks, M.D.
Adjunct Associate Professor, Department of Internal Medicine, George Washington University Medical Center; Adjunct Associate Professor of Rehabilitation, Department of Orthopedics, Georgetown University Medical Center, Washington, DC; Deputy Chief, Department of Rehabilitation Medicine, National Institutes of Health, Bethesda, Maryland

Steven R. Hinderer, M.D., M.S., P.T.
Associate Professor and Interim Chairman, Department of Physical Medicine and Rehabilitation, Wayne State University School of Medicine; Rehabilitation Institute of Michigan; Specialist-in-Chief, Department of Physical Medicine and Rehabilitation, Detroit Medical Center, Detroit, Michigan

Howard J. Hoffberg, M.D.
Associate Medical Director, Rehabilitation and Pain Management Associates, Baltimore, Maryland

Joseph C. Honet, M.D.
Professor, F.T.A., Department of Physical Medicine and Rehabilitation, Wayne State University School of Medicine; Chief, Department of Physical Medicine and Rehabilitation, Sinai Grace Hospital of Detroit Medical Center, Detroit, Michigan

Lawrence J. Horn, M.D., M.R.M.
Professor and Chairman, Department of Physical Medicine and Rehabilitation, Medical College of Ohio; St. Vincent's-Mercy Medical Center, Toledo, Ohio

Edward A. Hurvitz, M.D.
Assistant Professor, Department of Physical Medicine and Rehabilitation, University of Michigan Health Systems, Mott Children's Hospital, Ann Arbor, Michigan

Marta Imamura, M.D., Ph.D.
Division of Physical Medicine, Department of Orthopaedics and Traumatology, University of Sao Paulo School of Medicine; Hospital Das Clinicas, Sao Paulo, Brazil

Jennifer J. James, M.D.
Clinical Assistant Professor, Department of Physical Medicine and Rehabilitation, University of Washington School of Medicine; Attending Physician, Spinal Cord Injury Unit, Seattle Veterans Affairs Medical Center, Seattle, Washington

Galen O. Joe, M.D.
Clinical Staff Physiatrist, Department of Rehabilitation Medicine, National Institutes of Health, Bethesda, Maryland

Richard T. Katz, M.D.
Associate Professor, Department of Occupational Medicine, St. Louis University School of Medicine, St. Louis, Missouri

D. Casey Kerrigan, M.D.
Associate Professor and Director of Research, Department of Physical Medicine and Rehabilitation, Harvard Medical School; Director, Center for Rehabilitation Science, Spaulding Rehabilitation Hospital, Boston, Massachusetts

Harpal S. Khanuja, M.D.
Department of Orthopaedic Surgery, Johns Hopkins University School of Medicine; Good Samaritan Hospital, Baltimore, Maryland

Dennis D. J. Kim, M.D.
Associate Professor, Department of Rehabilitation Medicine, Albert Einstein College of Medicine of Yeshiva University; Director of Electrodiagnostic Service and Chief, Montefiore Medical Center, East Campus, Bronx, New York

Tae Kyun Kim, M.D., Ph.D.
Division of Sports Medicine and Shoulder Surgery, Department of Orthopaedics, Johns Hopkins University School of Medicine; Johns Hopkins Hospital, Baltimore, Maryland

R. Lee Kirby, M.D., FRCPC
Professor, Division of Physical Medicine and Rehabilitation, Department of Medicine, Dalhousie University Faculty of Medicine; Queen Elizabeth II Health Sciences Centre, Halifax, Nova Scotia, Canada

Stanley H. Kornhauser, Ph.D.
Chief Operating Officer, Queens Surgi-Center, Queens, New York

Valery F. Lanyi, M.D.
Professor, Department of Rehabilitation Medicine, New York University Medical Center; Attending, Rusk Institute of Rehabilitation Medicine, NYU Downtown Hospital, New York, New York

Mathew H. M. Lee, M.D., M.P.H., FACP
Professor and Chairman, Department of Rehabilitation Medicine, New York University School of Medicine; Medical Director, Rusk Institute of Rehabilitation Medicine, New York University Medical Center, New York, New York

Yehoshua A. Lehman, M.D.
Attending Physician, Rehabilitation Unit, Geriatric Center of Netanya, State of Israel, Ministry of Health, Netanya, Israel

Stephen F. Levinson, M.D., Ph.D.
Associate Professor and Chair, Department of Physical Medicine and Rehabilitation, University of Rochester School of Medicine; Strong Memorial Hospital, Rochester, New York

Charles E. Levy, M.D.
Associate Professor, Department of Orthopaedics and Rehabilitation, University of Florida College of Medicine; Chief, Physical Medicine and Rehabilitation Service, North Florida–South Georgia Veterans Health System, Gainesville, Florida

Karen Lew, PharmD
Clinical Pharmacist, Veterans Affairs Puget Sound Health Care System, Seattle, Washington

Jan Lexell, M.D., Ph.D.
Professor and Medical Director, Department of Health Sciences, Luleå University of Technology, Luleå, Sweden; Department of Rehabilitation, Lund University Hospital, Lund Sweden

Janet C. Limke, M.D.
Spine Center, New England Baptist Bone and Joint Institute, Boston, Massachusetts

Saul Liss, Ph.D.
President and Chief Executive Officer, MEDI Consultants, Inc., Paterson, New Jersey

Mark A. Lissens, M.D., Ph.D.
Associate Professor of Physical Medicine and Rehabilitation, Department of Health Sciences and Chemistry, KHK University, Geel, Belgium

James W. Little, M.D., Ph.D.
Professor, Department of Rehabilitation Medicine, University of Washington School of Medicine; Veterans Affairs Medical Center, Seattle, Washington

Gregory E. Lutz, M.D.
Assistant Professor, Department of Rehabilitation Medicine, Weill Medical College of Cornell University; Chief of Physiatry, Hospital for Special Surgery, New York, New York

Ruth Torkelson Lynch, Ph.D.
Professor and Department Chairperson, Department of Rehabilitation Psychology and Special Education; Affiliate Faculty, Department of Rehabilitation Medicine, University of Wisconsin–Madison, Madison, Wisconsin

Mary Macy, M.D.
Chief Resident, Sinai-Johns Hopkins Residency Program, Baltimore, Maryland

Edward Magaziner, P.T., M.D.
Assistant Professor, Department of Physical Medicine and Rehabilitation, New York Medical College, Valhalla, New York; Clinical Professor, Department of Physical Medicine and Rehabilitation, University of Medicine and Dentistry of New Jersey, Robert Wood Johnson School of Medicine; Robert Wood Johnson Hospital; St. Peter's University Hospital, New Brunswick, New Jersey

Ian B. Maitin, M.D.
Assistant Professor and Residency Program Director, Department of Physical Medicine and Rehabilitation, Temple University School of Medicine; Temple University Hospital, Philadelphia, Pennsylvania

Gabriel Martinez, M.D.
Staff Physician, Mercy Medical Center; Union Memorial Hospital; Franklin Square Medical Center; Kernan Hospital, Baltimore, Maryland

Richard Mazzaferro, D.O.
Department of Physical Medicine and Rehabilitation, Harvard Medical School; Spaulding Rehabilitation Hospital, Boston, Massachusetts

David G. McDonald, Ph.D.
Professor, Department of Psychology, University of Missouri–Columbia, Columbia, Missouri

Edward G. McFarland, M.D.
Associate Professor, Director, Division of Sports Medicine and Shoulder Surgery, Department of Orthopaedic Surgery, Johns Hopkins School of Medicine, Baltimore, Maryland

Thomas E. McGunigal, Jr., M.D.
Staff Physiatrist, Rehabilitation Hospital of Rhode Island, North Smithfield, Rhode Island

Arun J. Mehta, M.B., FRCPC
Associate Clinical Professor, Department of Medicine, University of California, Los Angeles, UCLA School of Medicine, Los Angeles, California

Susan M. Miller, M.D.
Director, Residency Training Program, National Rehabilitation Hospital; Georgetown University Hospital, Washington, DC

Michael A. Mont, M.D.
Associate Professor and Part-time Staff, Department of Orthopaedics, Johns Hopkins University School of Medicine; Institute for Advanced Orthopaedics, Sinai Hospital of Baltimore, Baltimore, Maryland

Charles M. Narrow, M.D.
Staff Physician, St. Agnes Health Care, Baltimore, Maryland

John J. Nicholas, M.D.
Professor and Chairman, Department of Physical Medicine and Rehabilitation, Temple University School of Medicine; Temple University Hospital, Philadelphia, Pennsylvania

Subhadra Lakshmi Nori, M.D.
Department of Rehabilitation Medicine, Albert Einstein College of Medicine of Yeshiva University; Montefiore Medical Center, Bronx, New York

Christopher O'Brien, M.D.
Vice President of Medical Affairs, Elan Biopharmaceuticals, San Diego, California

Abna A. Ogle, M.D.
Clinical Associate Professor, Department of Rehabilitation Medicine, University of Kansas Medical Center; Staff Physician, Research Medical Center; Staff Physician, Baptist Medical Center; Kansas City Veterans Affairs Medical Center, Kansas City, Kansas

Mooyeon Oh-Park, M.D.
Assistant Professor, Department of Rehabilitation Medicine, Albert Einstein College of Medicine of Yeshiva University; Montefiore Medical Center, Bronx, New York

Bryan J. O'Young, M.D.
Clinical Associate Professor, Department of Rehabilitation Medicine, New York University School of Medicine; Attending Physician, Rusk Institute of Rehabilitation Medicine, NYU Downtown Hospital, New York, New York

Jerry C. Parker, Ph.D.
Clinical Professor, Department of Physical Medicine and Rehabilitation, University of Missouri–Columbia School of Medicine; Director, Mental Health Service, Harry S. Truman Memorial Veterans' Hospital, Columbia, Missouri

Atul T. Patel, M.D.
Associate Professor, Department of Rehabilitation Medicine, University of Kansas Medical Center, Kansas City, Kansas; Research Medical Center, Kansas City, Missouri

Jaywant J. P. Patil, MBBS, FRCPC
Associate Professor, Division of Physical Medicine, Department of Medicine, Dalhousie University Faculty of Medicine; Queen Elizabeth II Health Sciences Centre, Halifax, Nova Scotia, Canada

Oliver Perez, B.S.
Johns Hopkins University School of Medicine, Baltimore, Maryland

Inder Perkash, M.D., M.S., FRCS, FACS
Professor of Urology and Functional Restoration (PM&R); Paralyzed Veterans of America Professor of Spinal Cord Injury Medicine, Departments of Urology and Functional Restoration, Stanford University School of Medicine; Veterans Affairs Palo Alto Health Care System, Palo Alto, California

Frank S. Pidcock, M.D.
Assistant Professor, Departments of Physical Medicine and Rehabilitation and Pediatrics, Johns Hopkins University School of Medicine; Kennedy Krieger Institute, Baltimore, Maryland

Joel M. Press, M.D.
Assistant Professor, Department of Physical Medicine and Rehabilitation, Northwestern University Medical School; Rehabilitation Institute of Chicago, Chicago, Illinois

Michael M. Priebe, M.D.
Associate Professor, Department of Physical Medicine and Rehabilitation, University of Texas Southwestern Medical Center; Chief, Spinal Cord Injury Service, Veterans Affairs North Texas Health Care System, Dallas, Texas

Kristjan T. Ragnarsson, M.D.
Lucy G. Moses Professor of Rehabilitation Medicine, Mount Sinai School of Medicine of the City University of New York; Director, Department of Rehabilitation Medicine, Mount Sinai Hospital, New York, New York

Amar D. Rajadhyaksha, M.D.
Research Associate, Department of Orthopaedics, Johns Hopkins University Medical Institutions, Baltimore, Maryland

Mark Randall, Psy.D., Dr.P.H., M.A.
Adjunct Faculty, Indiana University School of Medicine; Community Hospital, Indianapolis, Indiana

Rajiv R. Ratan, M.D., Ph.D.
Associate Professor, Department of Neurology, Harvard Medical School; Beth Israel Deaconess Hospital, Boston, Massachusetts

John B. Redford, M.D.
Professor Emeritus, Department of Rehabilitation Medicine, University of Kansas Medical Center, Kansas City, Kansas

James K. Richardson, M.D.
Department of Physical Medicine and Rehabilitation, University of Michigan Medical School; Medical Director, Inpatient Rehabilitation Unit, University of Michigan Medical Center, Ann Arbor, Michigan

Mary Richardson, Ph.D., M.H.A.
Associate Professor, Department of Health Services, University of Washington, Seattle, Washington

Haim Ring, M.D., MSc
Professor and Chairman, Department of Neurological Rehabilitation, Sackler School of Medicine, Tel Aviv University; Institute for Functional Evaluation, Loewenstein Hospital, Ramat Aviv, Israel

Elizabeth A. Rivers, O.T.R., R.N.
Clinical Instructor in Rehabilitation (retired), University of Minnesota Medical School, Minneapolis, Minnesota; Burn Rehabilitation Specialist, St. Paul-Ramsey Burn Center, St. Paul, Minnesota

Lawrence R. Robinson, M.D.
Professor and Chair, Department of Rehabilitation Medicine, University of Washington School of Medicine; Harborview Medical Center; University of Washington Medical Center, Seattle, Washington

Richard C. Robinson, M.D.
Assistant Professor, Department of Rehabilitation Medicine, University of Kansas Medical Center; Dwight D. Eisenhower Veterans Affairs Medical Center, Kansas City, Kansas

Arthur A. Rodriguez, M.D., M.S.
Associate Professor, Department of Rehabilitation Medicine, University of Washington School of Medicine; Director of Rehabilitation Care Services, Veterans Affairs Puget Sound Health Care System, Seattle, Washington

Richard A. Rogachefsky, M.D.
Assistant Professor, Department of Orthopedics, University of Miami School of Medicine; Jackson Memorial Medical Center, Miami, Florida

Robert D. Rondinelli, M.D., Ph.D.
Professor and Chair, Department of Rehabilitation Medicine, University of Kansas Medical Center, Kansas City, Kansas

Norman B. Rosen, M.D.
Medical Director, Rehabilitation and Pain Management Associates of Baltimore, Baltimore, Maryland

Jeffrey Rosenbuth, M.D.
Clinical Instructor, Department of Physical Medicine and Rehabilitation, University of Utah School of Medicine; Attending Physician, Rehabilitation Unit, University Hospital, Salt Lake City, Utah

Elliot J. Roth, M.D.
Paul B. Magnuson Professor and Chairman, Department of Physical Medicine and Rehabilitation, Northwestern University Medical School; Donnelley Senior Vice President and Medical Director, Rehabilitation Institute of Chicago, Chicago, Illinois

Leslie J. Gonzalez Rothi, Ph.D.
Professor, Department of Neurology, University of Florida College of Medicine; Director, Brain Rehabilitation Research Center, Gainesville Veterans Affairs Medical Center, Gainesville, Florida

Stuart A. Rubin, M.D.
Medical Director, Comprehensive Pain and Rehabilitation Center; Bethesda Memorial Hospital, Boynton Beach, Florida; Joseph L. Morse Geriatric Center, West Palm Beach, Florida

Richard Salcido, M.D.
William Erdman Professor and Director, Department of Rehabilitation Medicine; Associate, Institute for Medical Bioengineering; Senior Fellow, Institute on Aging, University of Pennsylvania School of Medicine, Philadelphia, Pennsylvania

Anthony S. Salzano, M.D.
Assistant Professor, Department of Rehabilitation Medicine, Albert Einstein College of Medicine of Yeshiva University; Chief, Department of Physical Medicine, New York Westchester Square Medical Center, Bronx, New York

Francisco H. Santiago, M.D.
Attending, Department of Physical Medicine and Rehabilitation, Bronx-Lebanon Hospital, Bronx, New York

Jay Schechtman, M.D., M.B.A.
Assistant Clinical Professor, Department of Rehabilitation Medicine, Mount Sinai Medical School of the City University of New York; Mount Sinai Hospital, New York, New York

Carson D. Schneck, M.D., Ph.D.
Professor of Anatomy and Diagnostic Imaging, Department of Anatomy and Cell Biology, Temple University School of Medicine, Philadelphia, Pennsylvania

Lew C. Schon, M.D.
Department of Orthopaedics, Union Memorial Hospital, Baltimore, Maryland

Jay P. Shah, M.D.
Clinical Staff Physiatrist, Department of Rehabilitation Medicine, National Institutes of Health, Bethesda, Maryland

Aaron Shamberg, OTR/L, M.S.
President, Landcare, Baltimore, Maryland

Shoshana Shamberg, OTR/L, M.S.
President and Clinical Director, Abilities O.T. Services, Inc., Baltimore, Maryland

Matthew M. Shatzer, D.O.
Department of Physical Medicine and Rehabilitation, Johns Hopkins University School of Medicine; Sinai Hospital, Baltimore, Maryland

C. Norman Shealy, M.D., Ph.D.
Professor, Department of Psychology, Forest Institute of Professional Psychology; Director, Shealy Institute, Springfield, Missouri

Timothy C. Shen, M.D.
Department of Physical Medicine and Rehabilitation, Hospital for Special Surgery, New York, New York

Douglas Sheppard, M.D.
Physiatrist, Mercy Hospital, Baltimore, Maryland

Ki Y. Shin, M.D.
Baylor College of Medicine, Houston, Texas

Kenneth H. Silver, M.D.
Associate Professor, Division of Rehabilitation Medicine, Department of Neurology, University of Maryland School of Medicine; Chief, Division of Rehabilitation, Kernan Hospital, Baltimore, Maryland

Warren K. Slaten, M.D.
Staff Physiatrist, Medical Rehabilitation Associates, Milwaukee, Wisconsin

W. Nicholas Sorensen, O.T.R.
Regions Hospital, Saint Paul, Minnesota

John Speed, MBBS
Associate Professor and Interim Chair, Division of Physical Medicine and Rehabilitation, University of Utah School of Medicine; University of Utah Hospitals and Clinics, Salt Lake City, Utah

Peter Staats, M.D.
Director, Pain Management and Anesthesiology, Johns Hopkins Hospital, Baltimore, Maryland

Henk J. Stam, M.D., Ph.D.
Professor, Department of Rehabilitation Medicine, Erasmus University Rotterdam; University Hospital, Rotterdam, The Netherlands

Barry D. Stein, M.D.
Clinical Assistant Professor, Department of Epidemiology and Preventive Medicine, University of Maryland School of Medicine, Baltimore, Maryland

Neil D. Stern, D.O.
Department of Emergency Medicine, University of Florida Health Sciences Center–Jacksonville; Shands Hospital, Jacksonville, Florida

Steven A. Stiens, M.D., M.S.
Associate Professor, Department of Rehabilitation Medicine, University of Washington School of Medicine; Attending Physician, Spinal Cord Injury Unit, Veterans Affairs Puget Sound Health Care System; University Hospital; Harborview Medical Center, Seattle, Washington

Margaret G. Stineman, M.D.
Associate Professor, Department of Rehabilitation Medicine, University of Pennsylvania School of Medicine; Hospital of the University of Pennsylvania, Philadelphia, Pennsylvania

Thomas E. Strax, M.D.
Professor and Chairman, Department of Physical Medicine and Rehabilitation, University of Medicine and Dentistry of New Jersey, Robert Wood Johnson Medical School, New Brunswick, New Jersey; Medical Director, JFK Rehabilitation Institute, Edison, New Jersey

C. Christopher Stroud, M.D.
Department of Orthopaedics, Union Memorial Hospital, Baltimore, Maryland

Jay V. Subbarao, M.D., M.S.
Clinical Professor, Division of Physical Medicine and Rehabilitation, Department of Orthopaedic Surgery, Loyola University Medical Center, Maywood, Illinois; Associate Chief of Staff for Rehabilitative Services, Hines Veterans Affairs Hospital, Hines, Illinois

Denise W. Thrope, M.S., CCC/A
Clinical Audiologist in Private Practice, Owings Mills, Maryland

Donna C. Tippett, M.P.H., M.A., CCC-SLP
Senior Speech-Language Pathologist, Department of Communication Sciences and Disorders, University of Maryland Medical System; Instructor, Department of Physical Medicine and Rehabilitation, Johns Hopkins University School of Medicine, Baltimore, Maryland

David A. Tostenrude, M.P.A., CTRS
Recreation Therapy Manager, Spinal Cord Injury Service, Veterans Affairs Puget Sound Health Care System, Seattle, Washington

Melissa K. Trovato, M.D.
Department of Pediatric Rehabilitation Medicine, Johns Hopkins University School of Medicine; Kennedy Krieger Institute, Baltimore, Maryland

Rhodora C. Tumanon, M.D.
Medical Director, Maryland Rehabilitation Center; Medical Advisor, Division of Rehabilitation Services, State of Maryland, Baltimore, Maryland

Richard Verville, J.D.
Attorney, Powers, Pyles, Sutter, and Verville, Washington, DC

Stanley F. Wainapel, M.D., M.P.H.
Professor of Clinical Rehabilitation Medicine, Department of Rehabilitation Medicine, Albert Einstein College of Medicine of Yeshiva University; Clinical Director, Rehabilitation Medicine, Montefiore Medical Center, Bronx, New York

Ruth K. Westheimer, Ed.D.
Professor, Department of Continuing Education, New York University, New York, New York

Sam S. H. Wu, M.D., M.P.H., M.B.A.
Clinical Assistant Professor, Department of Rehabilitation Medicine; Coordinator and Associate Director, Kathryn Walter Stein Chronic Pain Laboratory, New York University School of Medicine; Rusk Institute of Rehabilitation Medicine, New York University Medical Center, New York, New York

Jeffrey L. Young, M.D., M.A.
Department of Physical Medicine and Rehabilitation, Northwestern University Medical School, Chicago, Illinois

Mark A. Young, M.D., M.B.A., FACP
Chair, Department of Physical Medicine and Rehabilitation, Maryland Rehabilitation Center, State of Maryland Department of Education; Faculty, Johns Hopkins University School of Medicine; Faculty, University of Maryland School of Medicine, Baltimore, Maryland

Marlene M. Young, B.A.
University of Maryland, College Park, Maryland

FOREWORD

The art of patient care is in the caring!
—Sir William Osler

It is my pleasure to write this foreword to the 2nd edition of *Physical Medicine and Rehabilitation Secrets*. In the years since its debut, *PM&R Secrets* has earned a prominent place in the hearts and minds of students of rehabilitation, nationally and internationally. Edited by three visionary physiatrists, Bryan J. O'Young, Mark A. Young, and Steven A. Stiens, who share a deep and abiding dedication to physiatric education, leadership, and scholarship, *PM&R Secrets* has carved a well-deserved niche on the bookshelves of rehabilitation specialists.

Dr. Howard Rusk, the father of comprehensive rehabilitation medicine, championed the concept of helping people with disabilities achieve their maximum potential, through rehabilitation, education, and team effort. This noble philosophy has had an enduring impact on physiatry and has poignantly touched the lives of many. Almost a half a century later, the editors and contributing authors of the second edition of *PM&R Secrets* have reaffirmed their commitment to preserving the philosophy of Dr. Rusk and the mission and vision of rehabilitation medicine. Through the unique educational question-and-answer formula of the Secrets Series®, the editors, in collaboration with a talented domestic and international faculty of authors, have enabled students, residents, and fellow physiatrists to achieve their optimal academic potential.

Hardly a day passes that I don't see my own residents or faculty reading and discussing the book on the wards or in the clinics. This scene reminds me of the early days of rehabilitation medicine when Dr. Rusk would stand at the bedside, telling stories that would motivate patients and students to see the big picture and maximize their potential. The book has been translated into many languages and has earned the acclaim of rehabilitation physicians throughout the world from Australia to Zimbabwe.

The editors of *PM&R Secrets* and their distinguished panel of contributing experts have captured the altruistic spirit of Howard Rusk and his supreme commitment to education.

This book is truly a testament to the field of physiatry—a medical specialty that never ceases to care.

Mathew H. M. Lee, MD, MPH, FACP
Professor and Chairman
Department of Rehabilitation Medicine
New York University School of Medicine
New York, New York

ACKNOWLEDGMENTS

We want to thank our students, residents, colleagues, and 1st edition authors and readers who have inspired us to produce this 2nd edition. We are extremely grateful for the support that has been provided.

The Editors also wish to extend special thanks to the publishing staff at Hanley & Belfus, Cecelia Bayruns, William Lamsback, and Linda Belfus, for their guidance and expertise.

Gratitude is extended to our colleagues and residents at the New York University, University of Washington, Johns Hopkins University, University of Maryland, the Veterans Administration, and the Maryland Rehabilitation Center.

This book would not be in print without the creative, congenial, and diligent support of our editorial assistant, Nicole Royer; Laura Song, who provided hours of enthusiastic and dedicated support; and our staff, Joseph Powers, Debra Walters, and Jennifer Ryan. Thanks are also due to Booyeon Kim, who revised manuscripts; Mia Hannula and other VA library staff, who researched topics; Karna McKinney, who created figures; Eden Palmer, who generated photographs; and the staff of the VA Medical Media Department.

The authors wish to thank members of our academic and resident peer review editorial panel including Dr. Michael Frey and Dr. Howard Choi. Thanks to Dr. Mathew Lee, Dr. Justus Lehmann, Dr. Tsai Chung Chao, Dr. Stanley Kornhauser, Dr. Rhodora Tumanon, Dr. Margaret Hammond, and Dr. Lawrence Robinson for their support.

PREFACE

Learning is not attained by chance; it must be sought for with ardor and attended to with diligence.

—Abigail Adams, 1780

1. Why use a PM&R textbook filled with questions and answers?

Rehabilitation learning is made more accessible using the question-and-answer approach. *Physical Medicine and Rehabilitation Secrets* is all about simple, straightforward learning. For every topic, carefully selected, clinically relevant, thought-provoking questions are accompanied by straightforward answers. *PM&R Secrets* has been called a "bridge-text," because it strategically links vital information from the literature, textbooks, and research. Modeled after the "Socratic method" of medical education and the acclaimed Secrets Series®, *PM&R Secrets, 2nd Edition*, offers readers a valuable learning advantage.

2. How does *PM&R Secrets, 2nd Edition* differ from the 1st edition?

To keep things current, the editors have thoroughly revised the content. There are many new chapters, new topics, new authors, and new references. Although the backbone of *PM&R Secrets* continues to be chapters covering basic, "bread, butter, and board" topics, there are many new chapters addressing cutting-edge advances including "Interventional Physiatry" and "Transplantation Rehabilitation."

3. What is the major objective of *PM&R Secrets, 2nd Edition*?

To serve as a rehabilitation resource for residents, students, interns, faculty, and clinicians across all specialties and disciplines. Written in a straightforward fashion, the book covers all of the major topics in physiatry. It is intended to be a review text and can be effectively used as a learning tool and an adjunct to the classic textbooks in the field.

4. Any interesting trivia about *PM&R Secrets*?

The producers of the popular television show *ER* used the book to research an episode on brain injury and interviewed the chapter author.

5. Is there a way to provide feedback about *PM&R Secrets*?

The editors have created a feedback web site (www.pmrsecrets.com) and e-mail address (pmrsecrets@yahoo.com) where the authors can be contacted. Or contact the publisher, Hanley & Belfus, at www.hanleyandbelfus.com.

6. Any closing words about *PM&R Secrets*?

Questions and answers are a fun, quick and convenient way of learning. Review of questions and answers provides a springboard for group discussions and should spark curiosity and problem-based learning. This book is unique in that it offers the reader information suited to *all* stages of education and practice development. For the new student of rehabilitation, clear definitions and outlines of the rehabilitation process are offered. For the resident, specific practice pearls and pointers are generously provided. For the rehabilitation educator, tantalizing, thought-provoking questions are shared. Read on and carry on the Socratic tradition!

Bryan J. O'Young, MD
Mark A. Young, MD, MBA
Steven A. Stiens, MD, MS

INTRODUCTION: DEVELOPING YOUR KNOWLEDGE AND PRACTICE OF PM&R

A physician is obligated to consider more than a diseased organ, more even than the whole person; the physician must view patients in their world.
—Harvey Cushing

1. What is learning in context? How does *Physical Medicine and Rehabilitation Secrets* achieve that?

Learning in context is a method of placing yourself in the situation that you are studying and testing your ability to respond to problems. Learning tools such as PM&R Secrets will strengthen your problem-solving ability through this method. This book is designed to recreate common challenges that you will confront on clinical rounds, on oral board examinations, and during patient encounters.

2. What is the Socratic method of learning and how does it relate to the study of medicine and rehabilitation?

Socrates was a Greek philosopher and moralist who focused primarily on the thinker and methods for knowing rather than the knowledge itself. The Socratic method requires an engaging dialogue often prompted by problems at hand. The discussions between the mentor and the protégé "bring the learner from a state of complacent dogmatic slumber of an unexamined opinion to a state of humility and perplexity." It is a process of debunking pretensions and assumes that ignorance is a pedagogically useful device.

This form of engaging conversation produces an educational model that is particularly potent because it focuses on immediate patient problem solving and implicitly educates the audience by answering their questions. Furthermore, the exercise teaches students and staff members communication skills that enable them to discuss and resolve critical rehabilitation issues.

3. What is pimping? Is it legal?

Pimping is the ancient academic game played by a "teacher" who riddles the trainee with a series of difficult and obscure questions. Sir William Osler was reported to fire such questions at residents like a Gatling gun on the wards of Johns Hopkins Hospital.[1] The tradition is celebrated to this day in rehabilitation education when residents are asked to present the intricate details of physical findings, impairments, limitations to activity and barriers to participation, environmental characteristics, and patient's life goals while under the scrutiny of master clinicians. Favorite details requested include the number of steps into the patient's house, the location and pile height of carpets, car type, and manual versus automatic transmission. These events are educational, lively, and humorous if orchestrated sensitively and received without pretension. This Socratic exercise builds effective physiatrists, nurses, therapists, prosthetists/orthotists, and other members of allied rehabilitation fields.

4. How does one learn rehabilitation medicine?

The foundation of effective practice stems from a sound understanding of anatomy, physiology, kinesiology, and the social sciences. Prerequisites include a reflective awareness of one's own personal development and an empathic regard for others. The practice of physical medicine and rehabilitation extends beyond general diagnosis and treatment into improvement of the patient's function and quality of life. A firm understanding of the basic signs and symptoms is essential for the physiatrist because the diagnosis and treatment of all conditions that limit physical and mental health can only enhance the rehabilitation process.

The practice of rehabilitation is an extension of the medical model to the practice of person-centered enablement. As such, rehabilitation knowledge and skills are required. The foundations of rehabilitation come from the Biopsychosocial Model and the World Health Organization Model of disablement. Skills in rehabilitation arise from careful questioning of the patient for person-centered goals and intervention to meet those goals in a sequence with the most practical and effective method. To develop an understanding of the disabling effects of disease and injury, the exploration of the medical history must go beyond diagnosis to understand the patients' capabilities for activity and social participation. The overall clinical and functional condition can best be understood from microscopic to macroscopic biopsychosocial levels as outlined in the Hierarchy of Natural Systems. The Natural Systems categories include atoms, molecules, organelles, cells, tissues, organ systems, nervous system, one-person, two-person, family, community, culture-subculture, society, nation, and biosphere.[2]

Learning through the practice of rehabilitation requires an ongoing commitment to understanding each patient's personal goals and designing interventions to achieve these goals. Rehabilitation is therefore learned one patient at a time as unique combinations of interventions are orchestrated to produce unique solutions for particular persons. Thus, the practitioner becomes increasingly astute with the encounter and enablement of each and every patient.

Your patients are your teachers. Each success is a lesson to guide your future practice.

5. How does the rehabilitation problem list guide learning?

A *problem list* includes the diagnoses, findings, and various aspects of the patient's condition that are evaluated and treated by the interdisciplinary team. Because each patient has particular needs, a problem list should be as unique to the patient as his or her fingerprint. Reading the problem list should project a mental picture of the patient and his or her anticipated outcome. The list should be organized with the primary diagnosis at the top, followed by the secondary diagnoses that require intervention and surveillance. Next, all impairments, such as pain, contracture, and neurogenic bladder, are listed. Subsequently, all disabilities are listed including mobility deficits and activities of daily living. Thereafter, problems that address handicaps are listed: psychological adaptation, social role function, community reintegration, architectural accessibility, educational/vocational needs, and spirituality.

The problems list should be easily accessible upon seeing patients or discussing their care. The problem list serves as an agenda to ensure that all the varied aspects of the treatment plan are addressed.

6. How can this small textbook, *Physical Medicine and Rehabilitation Secrets*, guide my study and improve my practice?

The chapter titles are organized with sequential development of PM&R knowledge, but the book need not be read in order; rather, the clinical challenges should dictate which topics to peruse by the reader. Again, the book is designed to be used "in context." The book is meant to be kept close at hand while on the ward, in clinic, or on a home visit. Short periods that present themselves in the process of clinical care provide the opportunity to review a topic to address the pertinent issue at hand. To gain a more comprehensive and in-depth knowledge of the topic, it is recommended that one read the textbooks, search the literature, and explore websites. The text attempts to anticipate questions and provide answers. Reviewing these questions and answers provides a springboard for group discussions and stimulates new sets of questions.

7. What do you mean when you say this book is a developmental textbook?

Physical Medicine and Rehabilitation Secrets offers the learner information that meets his or her needs through all stages of rehabilitation medicine practice development. The book is as useful to a beginner as it is to an established practitioner and experienced educator in rehabilitation. For the novice student of rehabilitation, clear definitions and outlines of the rehabilitation process are provided. For the resident, specific evaluation techniques and questions are provided as a means to complement the resident's established medical knowledge and expand and integrate the functional approach to illness. For the rehabilitation educator, new questions are offered to carry on the Socratic tradition. Share it and enjoy!

REFERENCES

1. Albanese MA, Mitchell S: Problem-based learning: A review of literature on its outcomes and implementation issues. Acad Med 68:52–81, 1993.
2. American Academy of Physical Medicine and Rehabilitation: Self-directed physiatric education program [2001 study guide]. Arch Phys Med Rehabil 82(suppl 1):S3–S89, 2001.
3. Brancati FL: The art of pimping. JAMA 262:89–90, 1989.
4. Engel GL: The clinical application of the biopsychosocial model. Am J Psychiatry 137:535–544, 1980.
5. Pekarsky D: Socratic teaching: A critical assessment. J Moral Educ 23:119–134, 1994.
6. Sherman RS: Is it possible to teach socratically? Thinking 6:28–36, 1986.
7. Stolov WC, Hays RH: Evaluation of the patient. In Kottke FS, Lehmann JF (eds): Krussen's Handbook of Physical Medicine and Rehabilitation, 4th ed. Philadelphia, W.B. Saunders, 1990, pp 1–20.

Steven A. Stiens, M.D., M.S.
Bryan J. O'Young, M.D.
Mark A. Young, M.D., M.B.A.

I. PM&R Essentials

1. WHAT IS PHYSIATRY?

Mark A. Young, M.D., Bryan O'Young, M.D., and Steven A. Stiens, M.D., M.S.

Alone we can do so little, together we can do so much.
—Helen Keller

1. What is physiatry?

Physiatry, also known as physical medicine and rehabilitation (PM&R), is a medical specialty focused on prevention, diagnosis, and nonsurgical treatment of disorders associated with disability. PM&R specialists also care for patients with musculoskeletal disorders, with acute and chronic pain, and in need of rehabilitation services. Physiatry has been aptly branded the "quality of life medical specialty" because its goal is to restore optimal patient function in all spheres of life, including the medical, social, emotional, and vocational dimensions.

2. Does physiatry have a mission and a motto?

A team-oriented medical specialty, PM&R strives to promote a person's quality of life and functional outcomes. By blending the best of the traditional medical approach ("**adding years to life**") with the functional model ("**adding life to years**"), PM&R accomplishes its noble mission.

3. Is there any magic to the name physical medicine and rehabilitation?

The official name of the field reflects the two important parts of the specialty:

Physical medicine—Diagnosis and treatment of musculoskeletal disorders with the use of medications, modalities, procedures, and exercise.

Rehabilitation—The process of making the person with a disability "maximally able" again, through the application of rehabilitation principles and techniques.

4. What makes the practice of PM&R particularly satisfying?

Physicians choose PM&R for many reasons.

1. You seldom work alone. You practice as part of an interdisciplinary team. All team members have varied experience that complements one another in meeting patients' needs. The physiatrist is often the team leader working to orchestrate the collaborative effort.

2. Your work requires that you know your patients as persons and , each team member as a holistic professional, and you need to have intimate knowledge of the existing resources and pitfalls in your patients' environment. Supporting patients to enable them as they achieve their goals and sharing their ses successes with the treatment team is is really is what we truly relish.

3. Working individually with patients who have functional limitations, pain, or musculoskeletal complaints offers a variety of potentially satisfying life-enhancing solutions. You often follow patients for years and help them solve a variety of problems as they age and engage in new activities.

All of these aspects involve the continuing rediscovery of patients and team members and the existing options within their environments. You make possible the synergistic efforts by which the patient and the rehabilitation team, in working together, can maximize each other's potential.

5. Which medical conditions are treated by physiatrists?

While many physiatrists view themselves as primary care physicians for people with disabilities (and therefore offer comprehensive care for persons with diverse medical conditions), a growing number of physiatry specialists have elected to focus on specific rehabilitation areas. Common conditions treated by physiatrists include amputations, arthritis, brain injuries, burns, cancer, cardiac disorders, fibromyalgia, industrial injuries, multiple sclerosis, neuromuscular diseases, neuropathies, orthopaedic injuries, pain disorders, pediatric disorders, pulmonary disorders, spinal cord injuries, stroke, and trauma.

6. How did PM&R get started?

Around the middle of the 20th century, a major shift in thinking among health care providers began to take place. Holistic, comprehensive, team-oriented care for people with disabilities began to be recognized as an important societal obligation. This powerful philosophy sparked a burgeoning interest among health care providers to treat people with disabilities.

The year 1936 was a banner year for physiatry when **Dr. Frank Krusen** inaugurated the very first residency-training program at the Mayo Clinic. Dr. Krusen coined the term *physiatrist* and is credited as the author of the first comprehensive rehabilitation textbook. Dr. Krusen's monumental work has had a lasting imprint on the field.

During the latter part of the century when thousands of "disabled" veterans returned from the battlefields of World War II, the need for focused care for folks with disabilities became even more apparent and the field of rehabilitative medicine expanded greatly. Pioneer physicians in the field helped to plant the seeds for an exciting new specialty, which cared for the whole person, not just the disease.

7. When did PM&R become recognized as a specialty?

Although the American Academy of Physical Medicine and Rehabilitation traces its origins to 1938, the American Board of PM&R (ABPM&R) was established in 1947 by members of the academy in response to the dire need for a certifying authority. The ABPM&R was approved in 1947 by the Advisory Board of Medical Specialties as one of twenty-four "official" medical specialties.

8. How does one become a "card-carrying" physiatrist?

First, there is medical school (4 years). Then, there is internship (1 year of internal medicine, surgery, or the equivalent), followed by a 3-year residency. For some, there is fellowship (from 1 to 3 years). Like many medical specialization career paths, the road to becoming a PM&R diplomate is an exciting and challenging journey beginning with medical school and concluding with residency. At the conclusion of PM&R residency, qualified candidates take a written certification exam (part 1) given by the ABPM&R. When you have completed residency, another exam (oral; part 2) is administered after your first year of practice. Upon successful completion of parts 1 and 2, you can proudly display your hard-earned sheepskin.

9. What about recertification in physiatry?

You never stop learning. Recertification is required every 10 years.

10. What's the best way to prepare for certification?

1. Be good to your patients.
2. Always provide quality and compassionate care
3. Remember that your patients are good teachers, as well.
4. Fashion your practice after role model attending physiatrists.
5. Link your learning to your patients' problems.
6. Throughout training, read major contemporary texts (see Bibliography).
7. Complement your learning and practice knowledge by reading *PM&R Secrets, 2nd edition.*

11. How can I learn more about PM&R in medical school?

Some medical schools have established mandatory rotations in PM&R, whereas others offer it as an elective. A growing number of academic departments have created educational opportunities such as lectures, courses, seminars, and symposia for interested medical students. Some have even created "shadow experiences" for undergraduates interested in an early exposure to physiatry. As part of the physical diagnosis curriculum established in many medical schools, students may spend their time on the rehabilitation service where patients are medically stable and exhibit a broad array of pathologies, which lends itself to good learning.

12. Tell me about PM&R residency training programs.

With over 80 accredited residency programs in PM&R in the United States, there are ample opportunities for postgraduate education. All accredited programs adhere to program requirements written and administered by the Residency Review Committee for PM&R. This hopefully assures uniformity in quality training experience and exposure among the various programs. As an added "bonus," some programs offer opportunities for advanced degrees (M.B.A., M.S., Ph.D.), specialized electives, and research opportunities. A select group of senior residents who become chief residents may have the opportunity to develop additional administrative and leadership skills. There are even some institutions that offer combined programs such as PM&R/neurology, PM&R/pediatrics, and PM&R/internal medicine.

13. What about subspecialty training in physiatry?

For those who want to specialize in specific areas, subspecialty fellowships accredited by ABPM&R are currently available in spinal cord injury medicine, pain, and pediatrics (2002). Other nonaccredited fellowship opportunities exist in many areas.

14. What about accreditation of PM&R education?

The ACGME delegates authority to the Residency Review Committee for PM&R to confer *direct* certification of PM&R residency training programs. Accreditation is a voluntary process and confers a stamp of approval to a given program. The ACGME is an offspring of several important organizations, including the American Board of Medical Specialties (ABMS), Council on Medical Education (CME), American Medical Association (AMA), American Hospital Association (AHA), and Association of American Medical Colleges (AAMC).

15. What is the role of a practicing physiatrist?

Physiatrists treat patients with acute and chronic pain and neuromusculoskeletal disorders. They often practice in major rehabilitation centers, hospitals, and private settings as either a primary caregiver or a specialist. Often, a physiatrist coordinates a team of doctors and other health care professionals. A comprehensive rehabilitation program may include physical therapists, speech therapists, occupational therapists, recreational therapists, nurses, psychologists, social workers, and specialists in allied medical specialties.

16. What diagnostic tools are used in physiatry?

Diagnostic tools include those used by other physicians (medical history, physical examinations, x-rays, and laboratory tests), as well as special techniques in electrodiagnostic medicine such as electromyography (EMG), nerve conduction studies, and somatosensory and motor evoked potentials. EMG examinations and nerve conduction studies are the most common procedures used.

17. What treatments does a physiatrist offer?

Treatment options include the use of medications; modalities such as hot packs, cold packs, ultrasound, and electrotherapy; assistive devices, such as a brace or artificial limb; massage; biofeedback; traction; and therapeutic exercise. Surgery is not used. Physiatrists, with added training, also perform interventional procedures, including spinal blocks, botulinum toxin injections, and acupuncture.

18. How can I review the fundamentals of PM&R in an entertaining and engaging way?

Read on and find out.

BIBLIOGRAPHY

1. Braddom RL (ed): Physical Medicine and Rehabilitation, 2nd ed. Philadelphia, W.B. Saunders, 2001.
2. DeLisa JA, Gans BM (eds): Rehabilitation Medicine: Principles and Practice, 3rd ed. Philadelphia, Lippincott Williams & Wilkins, 1998.
3. Grabois M, Garrison SJ, Hart KA, Lehmkul LD (eds): Physical Medicine and Rehabilitation: The Complete Approach. Cambridge, MA, Blackwell Science, 2000.
4. Honet JC: PM&R education. In O'Young B, Young MA, Stiens SA (eds):PM&R Secrets. Philadelphia, Hanley & Belfus, 1997, pp 15–17, 1997.
5. Stiens SA, Berkin DI: A Clinical Rehabilitation Course for College Undergraduates provides an introduction to the biopsychosocial interventions that minimize disablement. Am J Phys Med Rehabil 76:462–470, 1998.
6. Young MA, Stiens SA, Hsu P: The PM&R chief resident: A balance between administration and education. Am J Phys Med Rehabil 75:257–262, 1996.

2. PERSON-CENTERED REHABILITATION: INTERDISCIPLINARY INTERVENTION TO ENHANCE PATIENT ENABLEMENT

Steven A. Stiens, M.D., M.S., Bryan O'Young, M.D., and Mark A. Young, M.D.

1. How are the person and personhood relevant to rehabilitation?

The **person** is a particular living human being with characteristic genetic, physical, mental, social, and spiritual dimensions. He or she is guided by past experience, changes through development, and is self-determining through life decisions made with free will.

The person therefore is the "real self," the subject of rehabilitation intervention. As such, **personhood** is the dynamic process of being and becoming the self. Awareness of the patient's self-understanding is critical to rehabilitation success. The person has the right of choice in problem-solving and is an essential contributor to health goal-setting.

2. Define health, illness, and disease.

Health is the optimum condition of a person's physical, mental, and social well-being. Health is not merely the absence of disease or infirmity. An **illness** is the patient's unique subjective experience of "unwellness," distress, or failed function. Illness not only is a biologic state but also can be an existential transformation that affects trust in the body and reliance on the future. Illness determines the psychological response of the patient and his or her perception of the functional capacity of the body. The illness experience contributes to the psychological state, which influences the perception of the body's ability to function in the present and future. A **disease** is a medical construct that diagnoses a disorder as characterized by a set of symptoms, signs, and pathology and attributable to infection, diet, heredity, or environment.

3. Define patient, case, client, and customer.

A **patient** is a person who is affected by injury, illness, or disease and is under active medical treatment to return to better health. Working with a person as a patient implies an active medical relationship with expectations beyond that of a case, client, or customer. A **case** is an instance of disease or injury with its attendant circumstances as abstracted from the person for scientific study or education. A **client** is one for whom services are rendered, a patron, and does not require the person's participation in the relationship. Things are done for clients. A **customer** merely buys goods or services.

4. What are the five responsibilities of the physician in the physician–patient relationship?

1. **Suspension of judgment** means respect for the patient's personal values and priorities without imposing your own. Through empathy, the physician seeks the patient's perspective.

2. **Evaluation** requires acquiring knowledge of the patient as a person, the manifestations of his or her disease or illness, and his or her unique experience of disablement.

3. **Diagnosis** requires an integration of many symptoms, signs, findings, and test results and deduction to a cause or syndrome.

4. In **reporting**, the physician interprets the diagnosis and prognosis of the condition for the patient and provides the education required for informed choices.

5. **Treatment** requires a formulation, prescription, or plan, which is then offered to the patient for informed consent.

5. What are the three responsibilities of the patient in the physician-patient relationship?

1. **Submission.** Patients reveal aspects of their experience through medical history and present their bodies, equipment, and home for examination. They participate in the evaluation process by demonstrating their physical and functional condition and by participating in the development of person-centered goals for the rehabilitation team. By submitting their whole selves to the evaluation process, patients provide the rehabilitation team with the optimal opportunity to understand their personality and unique needs. This leads to the formulation of the best patient-centered plan.

2. **Compliance.** Patients receive a report from the physician (and the interdisciplinary team) outlining the plan for intervention and expected outcome. The concept of compliance requires that patients understand the plan, accept it, and work toward its goals.

3. **Payment.** Patients are obligated to pay. They may be in an entitlement group that is paying, but they nonetheless need to recognize and support the value of the service.

6. How does the understanding of suffering contribute to patient care?

Suffering must be differentiated from pain: **pain** is the psychophysiologic process of perception in response to nociceptive stimuli, whereas **suffering** is the perception of a threat to the intactness of personhood (i.e., the person's perception of his or her past, present, and future, the family, culture and societal roles, and others). Suffering can include physical pain but is not limited to it. Suffering can be relieved when the perception of threat is reinterpreted into a positive meaning. For example, childbirth can be excruciatingly painful yet considered rewarding. The perceived meaning of pain influences the amount of medication required to control it. For example, a patient who believed that her pain was caused by sciatica could control it with small doses of codeine, but when she discovered that it was caused by malignant disease, a much greater amount of medication was required for relief. When evaluating pain, the clinician must remember that pain is a subjective phenomenon that is in the eyes of the beholder and is part of the patient's illness experience. Pain perception and behavior vary among different cultures and between genders. Suspension of judgment is essential.

7. How can the effects of the disease on the person be practically classified?

The World Health Organization originally published the *International Classification of Impairments, Disabilities, and Handicaps* (ICIDH) in 1980 as a conceptual scheme for the consequences of disease. The classification has recently been revised as ICIDH-2. These collective consequences of disease on the health of the person, or **disablement**, can be conceptualized within three related system domains: (1) the **organ** or system, (2) the **person**, and (3) **society**. Limitations or deficits within these domains lie in three respective dimensions: impairment (organ domain), disability/activity (person domain), or handicap/participation (societal domain). The new ICIDH-2 terms for these domains are *impairment*, *activity*, and *participation*.

8. Define impairment.

An **impairment** is any loss or abnormality of a psychological, physiologic, or anatomic structure, appearance, or function of an organ or system. Examples include loss of limb, weakness, sensory deficit, and facial disfigurement.

9. Define disability and activity.

A **task** is a purposeful activity that requires engagement of the whole person. A **disability** is any restriction or lack (resulting from an impairment) of a person's ability to perform a task or activity within the range considered normal for a human of a particular age. An example is an inability to perform activities of daily living, such as dressing, driving, shopping, or cooking. Disabilities reflect the consequences of impairment on activities of the individual. Activities are performance of personal-level tasks or activities undertaken by the person.

10. How is handicap defined in the relationship of the person to society?

Handicap results from the interaction of the person (including impairments and disabilities) with the environment. The environment is all that surrounds the patient and therefore has a profound impact on his or her self-perception and function. Specifically, the characteristics of the environment that need to be considered are physical, psychological, social, and political. The **physical environment** provides the conduit for travel through obstructive barriers that may limit access. Adaptations are modifications to the built or natural environment that enable the person with disabilities to fully participate in life activities. The **psychological environment** is all the stimuli uniquely experienced by the person living with disablement, including communicated attitudes and expectations of the person. The **social environment** includes the predominant cultural role with expectations for acceptance in family, work, and leisure acitivities. The **political environment** includes the laws, guaranteed rights of each person regardless of handicap. The resultant handicap is the disadvantage for a given individual, stemming from impairments or disabilities, in performing a role otherwise normal (age- or sex-appropriate) for an individual. Full subclassification of handicap circumstances would be impossible. Some subdivision has been written into ICIDH-2 by limiting the range of handicap circumstances to disadvantage in performance of social roles, the cultural expectations of others. **Disadvantage** is defined as socially perceived failure to conform to expected role behaviors either by deficit or excess behavior.

11. What is the relationship between handicap and participation?

The relationship is reciprocal. **Participation** is defined as the person's involvement in life situations. **Involvement** means inclusion in life activities in the context of the person's own community. As participation increases, handicap decreases. The restriction of participation or involvment in life activities by external factors (social roles) is termed **participation limitation/ restriction.**

12. What are contextual factors?

The context is the life situation within and around the person. ICIDH-2 describes environmental and personal contextual factors. Environmental factors can be considered in six categories: products and technology; natural environments; man-made changes to the environment; support and relationships; attitudes, values, and beliefs; services; and systems and policies. Personal factors refer to patient characteristics that may contribute to or limit adaptation. They include gender, age, diagnoses, fitness, lifestyle, upbringing, coping styles, social background, education, profession, past experiences, character style, and physical and psychological assets.

13. Has functional loss been addressed on a more universal or spiritual level? If so, how does this apply in the rehabilitation setting?

We propose that the term *suffering* be used to describe loss of function on a spiritual level. The term is useful because it addresses a spiritual dimension that is not specifically included in the three domains of disablement. It is essential that rehabilitation specialists identify and address a person's needs on different levels in order to maximize a person's potential. For many, the highest form of need to be addressed is the spiritual need. By instilling meaning into a patient's illness, this can empower a person to maximize his or her health to live with meaning. This serves as a seed that can be tended by a health care professional into a fruitful discussion with patient and others in the field of rehabilitation and beyond.

14. What is rehabilitation?

In contrast to classic medical therapeutics, which emphasizes diagnosis and treatment directed against the pathologic process, rehabilitation produces multiple simultaneous interventions addressing both the cause and secondary effects of injury and illness (**biopsychosocial model**). Traditionally, medical science has directed treatment at the cause of disease (**biomedical model**), neglecting the secondary effects of illness. The very nature of rehabilitation includes assessment of the individual's personal capacities, role performance, and life aspirations.

Rehabilitation has been defined as the development of a person to his or her fullest physical, psychological, social, vocational, avocational, and educational potential, consistent with his or her physiology or anatomic impairment and environmental limitations. **Comprehensive rehabilitation** can be further considered to require five necessary and sufficient subcomponents:

1. Unique, patient-centered plan formulated by the patient and rehabilitation team
2. Goals derived and prioritized through an interdisciplinary process
3. Patient participation required to achieve the goals
4. Results in improvement in the patient's personal potential
5. Outcomes demonstrate reduction in impairments, disabilities, and handicaps

15. What is patient-centered rehabilitation medicine?

It is a process of interaction and intervention that requires knowledge of the patient as a whole person, derivation of goals specifically to meet the patient's life plan, and interventions that maximize all of the patient's capabilities and potential. The process has six interactive components:

1. Exploration of both the illness experience and the disease
2. Understanding of the whole person
3. Defining common ground in team treatment planning and patient compliance
4. Incorporating prevention and health promotion
5. Enhancing the treatment relationships between the interdisciplinary team and the patient
6. Taking a realistic and practical perspective

16. What is the multidisciplinary practice of patient care? How does it differ from interdisciplinary practice?

Multidisciplinary teams consist of various professionals treating the patient separately, with discipline-specific goals. Patient progress with each discipline is communicated through documentation or at meetings for information exchange.

In the **interdisciplinary** collaborative practice model, each distinct profession evaluates the patient separately and then interacts together at team meetings, where they share assessments of short-term and long-term goals. Goals are initially derived from each interdisciplinary team member's interaction with the patient and are further refined through interdisciplinary process. The goals of each discipline are combined into a unified coordinated plan through the synergistic interaction of the team. The whole outcome therefore is more than the sum of the component parts. In addition, the team collaboratively participates in problem-solving and decision-making as the plan is executed.

17. What nine conditions maximize the success of interdisciplinary rehabilitation teams?

1. Allegiance to a mission statement (i.e., person-centered rehab in the least restrictive setting)
2. Specifically delineated roles for each discipline
3. Balance of participation by each professional
4. Agreement on and implementation of ground rules for interaction
5. Clear and effective communication and documentation

6. Scientific approach to patient problems
7. Clearly defined, measurable goals
8. Working knowledge of group process
9. Expedient procedures for coming to consensus and decision-making

18. How does a transdisciplinary team interact?

Transdisciplinary teams are designed through cross-training of members and procedure development to allow **overlap of responsibilities** between disciplines. This overlap allows flexibility in problem-solving and produces closer interdependence of team members. Leadership may differ for each patient served by the team. Disciplines with extensive involvement with the patient may become **case managers** and coordinate team efforts.

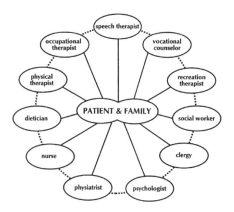

Interdisciplinary team interaction. (From Mumma CM, Nelson A: Models for theory-based practice of rehabilitation nursing. In Hoeman SD (ed): Rehabilitation Nursing: Process and Application. St. Louis, Mosby, 1995, with permission.)

19. Describe the phases in the rehabilitation process.

Phase I (evaluation) requires knowledge of the patient's personal life tasks, roles, and aspirations. The individual effects of disablement (impairment, disability, and handicap) of the person are quantified. The person's unique characteristics—mediators that allow for adaptive capacity—limiting disablement severity are identified and targeted as foci for therapy.

Phase II emphasizes treatment to arrest the pathophysiologic processes causing tissue injury.

Phase III (therapeutic exercise) focuses on enhancement of organ performance.

Phase IV (task reacquisition) emphasizes total person adaptive techniques.

Phase V (environmental modification) directs efforts toward environmental enhancement (physical, psychological, social, and political) to reduce handicap.

These phases approximate the emphasis of the team's interventions during a continuum that guides the patient out of acute treatment to reintegrate with the community. The rehabilitation problem list is a sequence of diagnoses, impairments, disabilities, and handicaps that guide goal setting. Members of the rehabilitation team derive goals from their encounters with the patient as a whole person. The patient drives the process by demonstrating his or her particular predicament with disablement. Adaptation is achieved by enhancing the patient's personal characteristics that mediate or limit the disablement. The overall goal is the fullest personal enablement and action toward fulfillment of life roles.

BIBLIOGRAPHY

1. Cassell EJ: The nature of suffering and the goals of medicine. N Engl J Med 306:639–645, 1982.
2. Emanuel EJ, Emanuel LL: Four models of the physician-patient relationship. JAMA 267:2221–2226, 1992.
3. Granger CV, Gresham GE: International classification of impairments, disabilities, and handicaps (ICIDH) as a conceptual basis for stroke outcome research. Stroke 21(suppl II):II66–II67, 1990.
4. Gray DB, Hendershot GE: The ICIDH-2: Development for a new era of outcomes research. Arch Phys Med Rehabil 81(suppl 2):S10–S14, 2000.

5. Ozer MN, Payton OD, Nelson CE: Treatment Planning for Rehabilitation: A Patient-Centered Approach. New York, McGraw-Hill, 2000.
6. Rogers CR: A theory of therapy, personality and interpersonal relationships as developed in the client-centered framework. In Koch S (ed): A Study of Science: Vol III. Formulation of the Person and the Social Context. New York, McGraw-Hill, 1959, p 184.
7. Stewart M, Brown JB, Weston WW, et al: Patient-Centered Medicine: Transforming the Clinical Method. Thousand Oaks, CA, Sage Publications, 1995.
8. Stiens SA, Haselkorn JK, Peters DJ, Goldstein B: Rehabilitation intervention for patients with upper extremity dysfunction: Challenges of outcome evaluation. Am J Ind Med 29:590–601, 1996.
9. World Health Organization: International Classification of Functioning and Disability, Beta-2 draft, short version (ICIDH-2). Geneva, WHO, 1999.
10. Young MA, Baar K: Women in Pain. New York, Hyperion Publishers, 2002.

3. FUNCTIONAL ASSESSMENT FOR OUTCOME ANALYSIS

Gary S. Clark, M.D., and Carl V. Granger, M.D.

Obviously, a man's judgment cannot be better than the information on which he has to base it.
—A.H. Sulzberger

1. What is so important about functional assessment and outcome?

Inpatient rehabilitation treatment programs are labor-intensive (involving many health professionals on the rehab team) and relatively expensive, at least in the short term. This makes rehabilitation a likely target for cost-cutting under a managed-care health system, unless the cost-effectiveness of these services is documented objectively. To accomplish this goal, we must be able to measure (**functional assessment**) improvement in function over time as a result of the rehabilitation intervention (**functional outcome**).

2. How can functional assessment help to establish cost-effectiveness of rehabilitation services?

The goal of rehabilitation intervention is to maximize functional independence such that an individual is able to function without needing assistance from others, or as little assistance as possible. That person's quality of daily living is thereby improved by enhancing personal independence and minimizing the need for physical or cognitive assistance from others. By reducing the "burden of care," which can be costly, the up-front investment in rehabilitation services proves to be cost-effective in the long run.

3. What exactly is functional assessment?

According to Lawton, functional assessment includes "any systematic attempt to measure objectively the level at which a person is functioning, in any of a variety of areas such as physical health, quality of self-maintenance, quality of role activity, intellectual status, social activity, attitude toward the world and self, and emotional status."

In the context of rehabilitation, functional assessment has typically been applied to measuring what an individual does do for himself or herself, most commonly in self-care (activities of daily living [ADLs]) and mobility. Other areas of function frequently assessed include homemaking skills (e.g., cooking, cleaning, laundry) and related instrumental ADL (IADL) skills, also referred to as community survival skills (e.g., using a telephone, managing a checkbook, shopping). Functional assessment enables accurate "diagnosis" and quantification of the functional loss, which leads to development of appropriate and effective rehabilitation.

4. What self-care skills are included in ADL?

Eating, grooming (e.g., brushing teeth, combing hair, shaving, applying makeup), bathing, dressing, and personal hygiene (e.g., toileting). Bathing and dressing can be divided into upper-body and lower-body management.

5. Aren't there different forms of mobility?

Several types of mobility can be assessed. **Bed mobility** includes sitting up and lying down in bed, as well as turning side-to-side. **Transfers** refer to moving between bed, chair (or wheelchair), toilet, and bathtub. **Stand-pivot-sit transfers** are most commonly used, but if an individual has lower-extremity weakness, a **side-slide transfer** technique may be used, with or without a sliding board. Other forms of mobility include propelling a wheelchair (**wheelchair mobility**), actual walking (**ambulation**), as well as negotiating stairs, curbs, and uneven surfaces (e.g., sidewalks, ramps, gravel, grass).

6. How is function measured if someone needs help in performing an activity?

Most functional assessment scales include an indicator of level of function, or degree of assistance needed to complete a particular task. Someone who is able to complete a task with no outside assistance is considered **independent**. Another individual may demonstrate **modified independence**, needing an assistive device (such as a cane or long-handled reacher) or needing to take two to three times longer than expected or because independent activity may involve some safety risk. An individual performs an activity **with supervision** if he or she needs verbal cueing, coaxing, or set-up, without physical contact. The need for **physical assistance** ranges from contact guard (touching for balance only), to minimal assist, moderate assist, maximal assist, or dependent (depending on the amount of assistance required). For cognitive functioning, the need for assistance may be in the form of prompting or providing direction.

7. Can other types of function, besides physical function, be measured?

Assessment strategies have been developed for a variety of other domains, including **mental functioning** (cognition, emotional, or affective state), **social functioning** (social contacts and relationships, social roles, activities), and **quality of daily living**. Attempts have also been made to combine multiple domains in global or multidimensional measures. By the same token, more focused (unidimensional) scales have also been developed (e.g., for aphasia).

8. Why do we need to measure function? Why not just describe it?

Standardized measurements of function improve on a clinician's observation and narrative description by providing objective, uniform data in a format useful for clinical decision-making. Functional assessment measurements can provide a baseline against which changes in function can be detected and monitored over time. These data may be useful in determining the effectiveness of a particular intervention (e.g., medication, bracing, therapy). Functional assessment instruments have been studied in different health care settings (inpatient rehab, outpatient, long-term care), demonstrating their ability to detect functional, cognitive, affective, and continence dysfunctions unrecognized on clinical examination.

9. If functional assessment is so helpful, why doesn't everyone use it?

There is no single assessment instrument that can measure everything that may be necessary or important clinically. Many measures were developed for a specific purpose or in a particular setting but may not be generalizable to other settings or purposes. The more comprehensive an instrument, the more cumbersome it is—i.e., more time is required for clinicians to learn to administer it properly, and it takes longer to complete (and analyze). All functional assessment scales have inherent limitations in their use and interpretation. It is important to decide first what it is you want to assess, and why. Functional assessment can be used to determine what type of treatment or intervention to prescribe, to evaluate the effectiveness and efficiency of treatment, to track patients through different levels of care for case management purposes, to determine what treatment resources are needed, as well as to assist in quality improvement and program evaluation purposes.

10. Discriminate between impairment, disability, and handicap. How are they pertinent to outcome?

An **impairment** is a physical (or psychological) abnormality, which is usually a manifestation of a disease process or injury (tissue or organ level). Examples include painful limited joint ROM due to arthritic inflammation or muscle weakness after a stroke.

Disability is the resulting loss of ability to perform a particular activity or function, such as buttoning a shirt for the arthritis patient or ambulating for the stroke patient (whole-person level). There is clearly neither a one-to-one nor fixed relationship between impairment and disability; for example, the arthritis patient's joint inflammation may improve with medication, enabling him or her to regain function, or else an adaptive device may be used to compensate for the impairment.

An individual who is unable to fulfill a usual role or life activity as a result of an impairment or disability now has a **handicap** (environmental level). This could occur for a stroke patient if he or she is unable to get out of a nonaccessible house because of stairs. The handicap might be reversed by installing a chair-glide or elevator, without necessarily changing the patient's underlying impairment or disability.

The more recent version of the International Classification of Impairment, Disability, and Handicap (ICIDH) suggests substitution of terms with more positive connotations, such as *activity* for disability and *participation* for handicap. The fullest assessment of outcome should include measures that sensitively quantify all these areas of disablement.

11. So how do you measure functional status?

A number of functional assessment "instruments" (or scales) have been developed over the last several decades, beginning with the PULSES profile and Rankin, both in 1957. These measurements vary in their purpose, scope, detail, and often the type of patient or patient care setting for which they were developed. Another variable is the method used to obtain information about patients. Self-report scales involve completion of a questionnaire by the patient. Observer-report scales are similar, but rely on a proxy to complete the questionnaire (usually a family member living with the patient or a health care professional working with the patient). Discrepancies may occur between these two measures, as patients frequently rate their function higher than observers do. Advantages of interviewer-administered scales include ensuring that a complete data set is obtained and the ability to explore identified problem areas further. Disadvantages involve the time and cost to conduct the interview and the potential for interviewer bias in recording responses. Finally, the direct observation method requires a trained examiner/observer who rates the ability of a patient to perform various functional tasks. While more precise and accurate, these instruments are time-consuming. Generally speaking, when the patient is in a more dependent state (i.e., needing daily help from another person), assessment performed by a trained professional will be more accurate. However, when the patient is living in the community and is not very dependent but may be limited by pain, physical causes or emotional distress, then responses from the patient answering standardized questionnaires are more useful.

12. What are the characteristics of an ideal functional assessment scale?

Validity, reliability, and sensitivity to change are probably the most important variables to consider first. **Validity** of an instrument refers to whether it actually measures what it is intended to measure. *Face validity* involves the appearance of measuring the desired characteristic, while *criterion validity* is determined by comparing the instrument to a commonly accepted "gold standard." Comparing two scales that purportedly measure the same characteristics provides *concurrent validity*, while *construct validity* is tested by comparing a scale's performance with other scales measuring similar but not identical functions.

Reliability relates to the reproducibility of findings from the instrument, including *interrater reliability* (same results when given by different raters) and *test-retest reliability* (consistency of findings on serial evaluation). Analysis of correlations between similar items on the scale and between individual items and the entire instrument yields *internal reliability*. The ideal measure is also reliable across differing educational, racial, and socioeconomic backgrounds.

Finally, the instrument must show **sensitivity to change**, such that clinically significant changes in functional ability can be detected, quantified, and monitored.

Newer issues involving *measurement* have been added to the functional assessment literature. These involve transformation of ordinal scales into equal interval measures and testing scales to determine if they are unidimensional, meaning consistently describing a *latent variable*.

13. What is the difference between the four types or levels of measurement scales?

The four basic levels of measurement data include nominal, ordinal, interval and ratio. Nominal and ordinal scales are used to classify discrete measures (because scores fall into discrete categories or levels), while interval and ratio scales classify continuous measures. A **nominal** scale is used to categorize data into different groups where there is no rank order. **Ordinal** scales have a logical hierarchy of categories that are mutually exclusive and discrete, but distances between categories are not equal. Ordinal scales, such as the FIM instrument, are the most commonly used level of measurement in the clinical setting. **Interval** scales are continuous, with equal distances between categories (e.g., degrees Celsius), while **ratio** scales feature a "zero point" which reflects total absence of the quantity being measured (e.g., quantitative muscle strength testing, where "zero" means absence of muscle function).

14. Why can't you just add up the (ordinal) scores and calculate a mean value?

Parametric statistics, such as mean, standard deviation, and analysis of variance, are based on the assumption that the data are measured with an interval scale, with equal distance between each pair of observations. Since functional assessment scores like the FIM instrument are ordinal based, statistical adjustments must be made (e.g., Rasch analysis) or nonparametric statistical calculations used.

15. What other problems can occur with functional assessment scales?

Several issues may affect the use and interpretation of functional assessment instruments. Depending on the method of test administration, the scale may reflect a patient's capacity to perform an activity, rather than his or her actual performance. Disparities between performance and capacity occur most often as a result of poor motivation, depression, cognitive impairment, or intercurrent illness. Scales may be limited in the range of potential scores due to ceiling or floor effects, which may affect appropriate interpretation.

Another pitfall is the tendency to use summary scores for overall function, which hides changes that could be significant in individual items. Furthermore, some scales weight certain variables more heavily than others, with proportionately greater impact on the summary score. A great deal of caution is advised when interpreting summary scores, particularly in regard to clinical decision-making based on functional assessment.

16. Name some of the older functional assessment scales.

PULSES Profile (1957 and 1979)—A global scale that provides a measure of general functional performance, including overall mobility and self-care ability, as well as medical status and psychosocial factors. The scale rates physical condition (**P**), upper limbs (**U**), lower limbs (**L**), sensory (sight, speech, and hearing) status (**S**), excretory management (**E**), and psychosocial status (**S**), with scoring ranging from 6 (fully independent, medically stable) to 24 (dependent, requiring extensive medical/nursing care).

Katz Index of ADL (1963)—Developed from studies of geriatric patients with various disabilities, it rates six ADLs: bathing, dressing, toileting, transfers, continence, and feeding. Each area is rated as independent or not, with functional status graded from A (totally independent) to G (totally dependent). The Katz Index has practical utility but is mainly a descriptive, not a quantitative, instrument.

Kenny Self-Care Evaluation (1965)—Rates patients from 0 (dependent) to 4 (independent) in six categories of self-care: bed activities, transfers, locomotion, dressing, personal hygiene, and feeding. With a score ranging from 0 to 24, this scale has proven to be one of the most sensitive to change in functional ability.

Barthel Index (1965)—Was one of the most frequently used functional assessment scales 5 or 10 years ago. It rates 10 aspects of function, using different relative weights for each variable based on the authors' clinical experience, with a score ranging from 0 (totally dependent) to 100 (totally independent). The original Barthel Index, as well as adapted versions, have been extensively studied, showing a high degree of validity and reliability, sensitivity to changes in function over time, and ability to use across many types of physical disability. It does not have a cognitive assessment component.

17. Which functional assessment instruments are used most commonly today?

In a continuing quest to improve sensitivity, validity, and reliability of functional assessment, a national task force sponsored by the American Academy of Physical Medicine & Rehabilitation and the American Congress of Rehabilitation Medicine used a professional consensus process to develop the **Functional Independence Measure** (FIM). The FIM instrument consists of 18 items of function (arranged under self-care, sphincter control, mobility, locomotion, communication, and social/cognition domains), with each item being scored on a scale from 1 (dependent) to 7 (independent). The FIM instrument incorporates components of the Barthel Index but is more sensitive and inclusive, and it is the most commonly used functional measure in medical rehabilitation for the past 5 years or so.

Another functional assessment instrument developed by a multidisciplinary team is the **Patient Evaluation and Conference System** (PECS), which tracks function (also using a 1 to 7 scoring range) among medical, physical, psychological, and social behaviors. PECS also tracks rehabilitation team goals, providing feedback on frequency of goal achievement by patients (program evaluation).

18. Why are inpatient medical rehabilitation units and hospitals "DRG exempt"?

Diagnosis-related groups (DRGs) form the basis of Medicare prospective payment for acute medical-surgical care, based on the correlation of intensity (and cost) of resource utilization (diagnostic tests, medications, staffing) associated with various diagnoses (diseases or conditions). However, there is no distinct or direct relationship between a particular disease (or diagnosis) and the degree of functional limitation that may result. In fact, a single disease (or diagnosis) may be associated with multiple functional limitations (e.g., a stroke may result in impairments in language, swallowing, self-care ability, mobility and continence). So, DRGs do not accurately predict the costs of rehabilitation treatment, and rehabilitation hospitals and hospital-based rehabilitation units were declared "DRG exempt." They continued to be paid on a *per diem* (daily rate) basis, however, with a maximum amount determined by the TEFRA system.

19. But isn't rehabilitation also supposed to come under a prospective payment system (PPS)?

Congress has mandated that rehabilitation hospitals and hospital-based rehabilitation units be reimbursed under a rehabilitation prospective payment system (RPPS), but there has been lack of agreement as to what payment strategy to use. For inpatient rehabilitation settings, functional status has been documented to be the best predictor of length of stay and resource utilization. The Health Care Financing Administration controls Medicare payments and has recently determined that a new case-mix measure shall be used to classify rehabilitation inpatients into FIM-based function-related groups (or FIM-FRGs), which will provide the basis for classifying patients into appropriate groups for prospective payment for inpatient rehabilitation.

BIBLIOGRAPHY

1. Applegate WB, Blass JP, Williams TF: Instruments for the functional assessment of older patients. N Engl J Med 322:1207–1214, 1990.
2. Clark GS, Granger CV: Functional evaluation and outcome measurement. In Grabois M, Garrison SJ, Hart KA, Lehmkul LD (eds): Physical Medicine and Rehabilitation: The Complete Approach. Cambridge, MA, Blackwell Science, 2000, pp 225–241.

3. Dijkers M: Measuring quality of life: Methodological issues. Am J Phys Med Rehabil 78:286–300, 1999.
4. Eastwood EA: Functional status and its uses in rehabilitation medicine. Mt Sinai J Med 66:179–187, 1999.
5. Granger CV, Albrecht GL, Hamilton BB: Outcome of comprehensive medical rehabilitation: Measurement by PULSES profile and Barthel index. Arch Phys Med Rehabil 60:145–154, 1979.
6. Granger CV, Cotter AC, Hamilton BB, Fiedler RC: Functional assessment scales:A study of persons after stroke. Arch Phys Med Rehabil 74:133–138, 1993.
7. Granger CV, Gresham GE (eds): Functional Assessment in Rehabilitation Medicine. Baltimore, Williams &Wilkins, 1984.
8. Granger CV, Gresham GE (eds): New developments in functional assessment. Physical Medicine and Rehabilitation Clinics of North America, vol. 4, no 3. Philadelphia, W.B. Saunders, 1993.
9. Guide for the Uniform Data Set for Medical Rehabilitation (Adult FIM), ver 4.0. Buffalo, NY, State University of New York at Buffalo, 1993.
10. Hamilton BB, Granger CV, et al: A uniform national data system for medical rehabilitation. In Fuhrer MJ (ed): Rehabilitation Outcomes: Analysis and Measurement. Baltimore, Brookes Publishers, 1987, pp 137–147.
11. Kane RA, Kane RL: Assessing the Elderly. Lexington, MA, Lexington Books, 1981.
12. Seltzer GB, Granger CV, Wineberg DE: Functional assessment: Bridge between family and rehabilitation medicine within an ambulatory practice. Arch Phys Med Rehabil 63:453–457, 1982.
13. Stiens SA, Haselkorn JK, Peters J, Goldstein B: Rehabilitation Intervention for patients with upper extremity dysfunction: Challenges of outcome evaluation. Am J Industr Med 29:590–601, 1996.
14. Stineman MG, Escarce JJ: Analysis of case mix and the prediction of resource use in medical rehabilitation. Phys Med Rehabil Clin North Am 4:451–461, 1993.
15. Wright BD, Linacre JM: Observations are always ordinal; measurements, however, must be interval. Arch Phys Med Rehabil 70:857–860, 1989.

4. RESEARCH CONCEPTS IN PM&R

John E. Hewett, Ph.D., David G. McDonald, Ph.D., Richard Salcido, M.D., and Jerry C. Parker, Ph.D.

Many scientists owe their greatness not to their skill in solving problems but to their wisdom in choosing them.

—E. Bright, 1952

1. What are the sources and characteristics of a good research hypothesis?

The sources of a hypothesis can be termed systematic and unsystematic. There are at least three **systematic** sources:(1) from existing theory; (2) based on an integration of research literature; and (3) in applied research, out of need for a solution to a problem. The **unsystematic** sources include, but are not limited to: (1) naturalistic observations; (2) listening to a colleague; and (3) the product of quiet reflection. A good idea is a good idea, regardless of its source.

What is a good hypothesis? It must be testable. The topic must be phrased in terms of variables that can be defined and measured, and it should be important rather than trivial or transient.

2. Why is the literature search important to the success of a research project?

The process of scientific discovery involves the combined efforts of many individual scientists. The hypotheses of a new investigator frequently were tested in the experiments of the past. Exploration of the experiments, data, and conclusions of the past provides a context for refinement of research questions.

3. What are the prerequisites for informed consent prior to conducting a research study?

Institutional Review Board regulations require four conditions for informed consent:

1. The participant must be **legally competent**; otherwise, consent from the guardian is required.

2. The consent must be **voluntary**; no pressures, even subtle, must be operating to sway a participant's choice.

3. Consent must be **truly informed**. The participant must receive and understand all necessary information prior to making a decision.

4. **Comprehension** of the consent information and awareness of the alternative choices must be assured. Complicated consent forms or technical jargon must be avoided.

4. How do basic and applied research differ?

Basic research is research in which the investigator seeks to discover fundamental laws of nature, without regard for their ultimate application in solving practical problems. It is also frequently described as **theory-driven**, since this form of research is generally based on hypotheses derived from existing theory.

Applied research is any investigation undertaken solely to solve some real-world problem, without regard for the theories or natural laws that may be relevant. The primary goal is to determine if a better solution can be found, and it is frequently described as **problem-solving** research. Examples of applied research would include a study of the relative comfort and maneuverability of several different wheelchair designs or a study of the relative effectiveness of two methods of using a cane in patients with knee injury.

In the field of rehab medicine, many research projects are both basic and applied. For example, a study of the Functional Independence Measure (FIM) scores of AIDS patients is basic research in that it tells us something new about AIDS, but it is also applied research in that it gives us more information on management of AIDS patients as well as the usefulness of the FIM scale.

5. Why is theory important in science?

A theory is a relatively general statement of mechanisms or relationships derived from partially verified cause-and-effect relationships in nature. Theories are a motivating logical force in most basic research, which is often described as theory-driven research.

Good theories have the following characteristics:

1. They can account for existing data.
2. They have explanatory relevance (the explanation makes sense).
3. They can be tested.
4. They predict novel events or new phenomena.
5. They are parsimonious (make few assumptions).

Good theories also perform several functions:

1. They promote understanding.
2. They can be used to predict outcomes in systems processes.
3. They provide a framework for organizing and interpreting research results.
4. They generate research if they have heuristic or seminal value.

6. What is a variable? What types are there?

A variable is any phenomenon that varies. Variables can be sorted into various categories:

1. **Behavioral, stimulus, and organismic/subject variables:** A behavioral variable is any observable response of the patient or subject. Stimulus variables are quantifiable aspects of the experimental context that have potential effects on the response of subjects. Organismic/subject variables are any relevant characteristics of the subjects, such as age, gender, or diagnosis.

2. **Independent versus dependent variables:** The independent variable is the intervention or treatment administered by the investigator to the experimental group (e.g., an analgesic) and withheld from the control group (e.g., placebo). The dependent variable is the outcome variable hypothesized to have a relationship to the independent variable in a study (e.g., measure of pain reduction produced by the analgesic).

3. **Extraneous variable or confound:** An extraneous variable is any variable (other than the independent variable) that can affect the dependent variable in a study. Extraneous variables can be especially troublesome if they mimic or cancel the effect of the independent variable. Examples include age, gender, drug effects, and diagnosis. Therefore, they must be controlled by

holding them constant across groups in a study (e.g., using groups of equal age, gender mix, drug treatment, and diagnosis). An uncontrolled extraneous variable is called a **confound**. It is best to deal with confounds at the design phase but when this is not possible, often the effect of a confound can be dealt with statistically.

4. **Latent versus manifest variables:** A latent variable is any theoretical concept or construct that is assumed to exist but cannot be measured directly. A manifest variable is any measured variable that is used as an observed indicator of a latent variable.

7. What is the difference between categorical, ordinal, interval, and ratio measurements?

The concepts of categorical, ordinal, interval, and ratio measurement reflect increasing degrees of precision (reliability and consistency) in measurement with whatever methods are available.

Categorical measurement: naming or labeling only. Examples include studies in which subjects are grouped by category, such as gender, ethnic, or cultural background. The dependent variable (outcome variable) in a study can also be a categorical measure, such as "recovered" versus "not recovered."

Ordinal measurement: measurement by ranking in order or along a scale of mutually exclusive categories, meaning that measurement is precise enough to determine if one of two observations is greater or lesser than the second. Use of rating scales, such as the FIM, is an example of ordinal measurement.

Interval measurement: similar to ordinal measurement, except that in addition, the units between successive steps on the scale are equal and constant. An example of interval measurement is temperature on the Fahrenheit scale; the difference between 30°F and 35°F is the same as the difference between 100°F and 105°F.

Ratio measurement: almost the same as interval measurement, except that there is a known true zero point. Examples might be age or elapsed time in performance tasks.

8. What are the four major types of research design? How do they differ?

1. **True experiments** have four primary characteristics: (1) there is an independent and dependent variable; (2) there is a high degree of control of extraneous variables; (3) experiments are repeatable (replication is feasible), which is a reason for publication of experiments in research journals; and (4) the experimental and control groups are formed by random assignment of subjects. This last characteristic is highly critical and unique to true experiments. True experiments are the leading scientific method for establishing cause-and-effect relationships, the primary long-range goal of most science.

2. **Quasi-experiments** are "almost" experiments, but not quite. The essential difference is that subjects are not allocated to groups by random assignment, but rather on the basis of some preexisting variable, which raises the question of some preexisting confound. Examples of quasi-experiments are common in medicine and include studies comparing almost any patient group with nonpatient controls, where a true experiment would not be ethical or legally permissible. Although quasi-experiments do not provide incontrovertible evidence of cause-and-effect relationships, the procedure still reveals relationships between variables.

3. In **correlational studies**, the investigator simply wishes to determine whether two variables are related, i.e., that they co-vary. The typical statistical procedure employed is the correlation coefficient. These studies do not establish causality, but the association demonstrated by this method can be further investigated.

4. **Descriptive studies** consist simply of collecting systematic observations and/or measurements of any real-world phenomenon, with no control of confounds or manipulation of independent variables. When conducted outside the laboratory, these studies are often called **naturalistic studies**. Surveys and clinical case studies are descriptive studies. Descriptive studies can be valuable in the early stages of any research area.

9. How do "between-subjects" and "within-subjects" designs differ?

In **between-subjects designs**, comparisons are made between groups of subjects, such as experimental and control groups. If there is more than one experimental group (common in drug studies), each group experiences only one level of the independent variable (e.g., high, medium, or low dose of the drug). In actual practice, most studies are, therefore, between-subject studies.

In **within-subjects designs**, there is only one group, but each subject experiences every value of the independent variable, usually in some counterbalanced order. The advantage of this procedure is that it may be preferable with small sample groups.

10. What is a randomized controlled trial?

A randomized controlled trial (RCT) is synonymous with a true experiment. Large-sample RCTs are sometimes described as gold standard studies, due to the fact that there is no more superior method of determining cause-and-effect relationships.

11. What do we need to know about statistics to be successful investigators in PM&R?

What is needed is a thorough understanding of the research question (significance, variables to validly answer, confounds). This type of information allows the investigator to interact successfully with a statistician. The statistician is then able to provide the statistical expertise to design the experiment and answer the question. A basic understanding of statistical techniques allows the investigator to effectively translate naturalistic observations and hypotheses into *answerable* questions.

12. What is meant by the term "descriptive statistics"?

Let $x_1 \ldots x_n$ denote a set of numbers. A descriptive statistic for this set of numbers is a number computed from the set that summarizes a particular type of information contained in the set. Examples of descriptive statistics are the mean ($\bar{x}$), median ($\tilde{x}$), standard deviation (SD), and percentiles (x_p). The median is the 50th percentile. The mean and median provide information about the middle of the set, and the standard deviation and various percentiles provide information about the spread of the data.

13. What is meant by inferential statistics?

Statistical inference is drawing conclusions about the population as a whole based on the information that is derived from a sample of that population. By population, we mean the totality of subjects who are of interest to us. By a sample, we simply mean a subset of all subjects of interest to us. There are three general types of statistical inference: point estimation, interval estimation, and hypothesis testing.

14. What is hypothesis testing?

A **statistical hypothesis** is a conjecture about a population. If the population is characterized in terms of parameters, then these hypotheses will be conjectures about the parameters of the population, such as the population mean and/or the population standard deviation (parametric statistical hypotheses). Suppose that we have a population of hemiplegic patients and would like to determine if the proportion of these patients who can complete a task differs from the proportion of control subjects who can complete the same task. Here, the **alternative hypothesis** is that the two proportions are not the same, and the **null hypothesis** is that the two proportions are the same.

If the population cannot be characterized relative to parameters, then our conjecture (hypothesis) will be about the population itself, and the procedures employed will be called **nonparametric procedures**. The most commonly used nonparametric methods are those based on ranks rather than on the raw data.

15. What are type I and type II errors?

The terms type I and type II errors are used in the context of hypothesis testing. A **type I error** is made when we conclude that a null hypothesis is false when, in fact, it is true. A **type II error** is made when the data lead us to conclude that the null is true when, in fact, it is not.

A test of a statistical hypothesis is a decision rule that tells us whether we should reject the null hypothesis in question. By the significance level (**alpha level**, denoted by α) of the test, we mean the probability of rejecting the null hypothesis when, in fact, it is true. By the **beta level** (β)

of the test, we mean the probability of not rejecting the null hypothesis when it is false. This depends on the actual magnitude of difference that exists. In a two-population study comparing means, this depends on the actual magnitude of the difference in means which actually exist. The **power** of the test is $1 - \beta$.

16. Define probability.

The classical definition of the probability of an event is the number of times the event occurs, divided by the number of chances the event has to occur.

17. Define p-value.

Suppose we are testing a null hypothesis H_0 versus an alternative hypothesis H_A, and large values of the test statistic T support H_A. If H_0 is really true, we would not expect t, the value of T obtained from the observed data, to be large. If H_0 is really true, how likely is it that the sample should produce a value of $T \geq t$, the value actually produced? The p-value is a measure of this. Thus, a small p-value (e.g., $p < 0.05$) is an indication that the truth of the null hypothesis is unlikely.

18. What is meant by effect size?

The effect size is the average magnitude of change in the dependent variable produced by the independent variable. It can be mathematically defined simply as the difference between group means (the experimental group mean minus the control group mean, which is the effect of the independent variable). This difference can be divided by the pooled standard deviation (SD) of the two groups combined or simply the control group to convert the effect size into SD units, a form of standard score similar to another familiar standard score, the **z score**. In this way, effect sizes obtained in different studies can be meaningfully compared.

Suppose we want to compare the means of two populations which have a common SD and where the difference in the means of the two populations would be attributed to the independent variable. The effect size is the absolute value of the difference between the population means. The standardized effect size is this absolute value divided by the common SD. Thus the standardized effect size is simply the number of SDs by which the means differ. This allows effect sizes from different studies to be compared. Cohen has provided a helpful definition of small, medium, and large standard effect sizes as those with values of about 0.20, 0.50, and 0.80, respectively. Effect size is an essential tool used in two important areas: statistical power analysis and meta-analysis.

19. How does one determine the optimal sample size in a study? How do you know if a given sample is large enough to answer the question?

The four variables—**sample size, statistical power, significance level (alpha)**, and **effect size**—are interrelated in such a way that knowing any three allows one to estimate the fourth. Thus, for a given alpha, effect size, and power, the necessary sample size can be estimated.

Consider a hypothetical two-independent group study in which the experimenter sets the alpha at 0.05, the desired power at 0.80, and expects a relatively moderate effect size of 0.50. Then, using these values in appropriate tables, it can be determined that a sample size of 64 subjects in each group will be required with these specified parameters to reach a statistically valid conclusion. However, if one expects a relatively small effect (say 0.20, instead of 0.50), then the required sample size is almost 400 subjects/group in order to maintain a statistical power of 0.80.

One dismaying consequence of this fact is that an unknown number of published reports in the journal literature suffer from the common problem of relying on a sample size that is too small. This means that the resulting statistical power is considerably less than 0.80, often less than 0.50, in which case their odds of finding the effect are less than 50-50! When the experimenters also fail to reject the null hypothesis, then one must seriously consider that their report may represent a type II error, rather than a true finding of no effect of the independent variable.

20. What is the analysis of variance (ANOVA)?

ANOVA refers to a set of statistical methods associated with testing the equality of two or more means. For example, it could be used to determine if three different methods of teaching stroke patients how to do a task result in different mean times to complete the task.

21. Define regression.

With regression, we are interested in building a model in which one or more variables are used to predict another variable. In the **simple regression** model, we have a variable, called the independent variable, that is used to provide information about another variable, called the dependent variable. In **multiple regression**, rather than using just one variable to predict the dependent variable, two or more independent variables are used. As an example of a multiple regression model, the dependent variable might be the length of time that it takes to complete a task and the independent variables would be duration of disease, age, and weight.

22. What is meant by analysis of covariance?

Analysis of covariance combines regression and ANOVA methods for the purpose of forming ANOVA models with reduced error variance. It does this by making use of quantitative variables that are related to the independent variable. For example, in a study designed to determine if two populations have different numbers of foot abnormalities, there may be some possible additional variables that could affect the outcome variable of interest. One specific example would be the age of the subjects in the study. Age would be a variable that could affect whether an individual has a foot abnormality or not. Thus, age could be built into the statistical analysis as a covariate.

23. How is meta-analysis done?

Meta-analysis is an objective (statistical) method of collectively analyzing the results of more than one study. The introduction of meta-analysis has provided exciting capabilities in synthesizing the results of diverse studies, and it promises to have an increasingly greater impact in the future. The essential elements in conducting a meta-analysis are:

1. Identify the hypothesis or research question, conduct a literature search, and then determine the criteria for including and excluding existing studies.

2. Calculate the effect size (see question 19) for each of the studies included. Studies with larger samples are weighted more heavily in the analysis.

3. Calculate whether the resulting overall effect size is or is not significantly greater than 0, a conclusion that is not always apparent to (subjective) narrative reviewers.

4. It can be determined at this point whether the overall effect of the independent variable was small, medium, or large, a finding that some would argue is even more important than knowing if the overall effect was significant or not.

24. What are the essential elements in the adminstrative and financial management of grants?

1. The investigator must realize that the grant monies that are awarded cover the **direct cost** of the grant (the actual cost of the grant activity) and **indirect cost** (the overhead cost for facilities and equipment). Federal grants usually allow the most indirect cost and private foundations limit the amount of indirect cost.

2. The salary support should fund sufficient protected time for the investigator to perform the functions outlined in the proposal. Any institutional negotiation of the allocation of monies derived from the grant should be accomplished at the time of grant submission. Thereafter, the budget and the proposal become the source document for further discussions about disbursements of grant monies.

3. The investigator should establish a good working relationship with all personnel who have the responsibility to carry out the administrative processing of all grants and contracts; these personnel can facilitate the project and allow the investigator to focus on conducting the proposed research. The investigator should appreciate and understand the institutional policy (written) and procedure (process) in applying for, conducting, and reporting grant activity.

25. What is the Instiutional Review Board (IRB) and what are their functions?

The IRB is the group of scientists, doctors, clergy, and consumers at each health care facility where a clinical trial takes place. This group is charged with protecting patients who take part in studies. IRBs review and must approve the protocols (procedures) for all research projects conducted in the institution. They check to see that the study is well designed, does not involve undue risks, and includes safeguards for the patients.

A major activity for the IRB is review and modification of the consent form. The consent form should be written in a manner that informs the subject about the risks and benefits of participating in the research (**informed consent**):

1. Informed consent is the process by which a person learns key facts about a clinical trial or research study and then agrees voluntarily to take part or decides against it. The process includes signing a form that describes the benefits and risks that may occur if the person decides to take part.

2. The consent must describe the technical aspects of the proposed protocol while at the same time be written in simple and direct language, understandable to the research subject.

BIBLIOGRAPHY

1. Campbell DT, Stanley JC: Experimental and Quasi-experimental Designs for Research. Chicago, Rand-McNally, 1966.
2. Cohen J: Statistical Power Analysis for the Behavioral Sciences, 2nd ed. Hillsdale, NJ, Lawrence Erlbaum Assoc., 1988.
3. Colton T: Statistics in Medicine. Boston, Little Brown, 1974.
4. Cooper HM:Integrating Research: A Guide for Literature Reviews, 2nd ed. Beverly Hills, CA, Sage, 1989.
5. Hulley SB, Cummings SR: Designing Clinical Research: An Epidemiological Approach. Baltimore, Williams & Wilkins, 1988.
6. Shott S: Statistics for Health Professionals. Philadelphia, W.B.Saunders, 1990.
7. Smith ML, Glass GV: Meta-analysis of pyschotherapy outcome studies. Am Psychol 32:752–760, 1977.
8. Zeiger M: Essentials of Writing Biomedical Research Papers. New York, McGraw-Hill, 1991.

5. NERVOUS SYSTEM ANATOMY

Stephen Goldberg, M.D.

1. What structures comprise the central nervous system (CNS)?

Spinal cord
Brain stem (medulla, pons, midbrain)
Cerebellum
Cerebrum
Diencephalon (everything that contains the name *thalamus*—thalamus, hypothalamus, epithalamus, subthalamus)
Basal ganglia (caudate nucleus, globus pallidus, putamen, claustrum, amygdala)

2. How many structures make up the peripheral nervous system?

31 pairs of spinal nerves
12 cranial nerves (although the optic nerve technically is an outgrowth of the CNS)

3. What is the autonomic nervous system?

The autonomic nervous system innervates smooth muscle, cardiac muscle, and glands. It includes the **sympathetic nerves**, which originate from spinal cord segments T1–L2, the **parasympathetic nerves**, which originate from spinal cord segments S2–S4, and four cranial nerves

(CN): CN3 (oculomotor nerve fibers to pupil and ciliary body), CN7 (facial nerve fibers to sub-lingual, submaxillary, and lacrimal glands), CN9 (glossopharyngeal nerve fibers to parotid glands), and CN10 (vagus nerve fibers to heart, lungs, and GI tract to the splenic flexure).

PERIPHERAL NERVES

4. What type of nerve fibers are found in anterior (ventral) nerve roots?
Mainly motor axons.

5. What type of nerve fibers are found in posterior (dorsal) nerve roots?
Mainly sensory axons.

6. What is found in posterior (dorsal) root ganglia?
Posterior root ganglia contain cell bodies of sensory axons, but no synapses. This has important implications for nerve conduction studies. If the lesion is proximal to the dorsal root ganglion, then sensory conduction will be normal in the peripheral nerve, since the cell bodies are intact.

7. What sensory features distinguish a peripheral nerve lesion from a CNS lesion?
Peripheral nerve lesions can be distinguished from CNS lesions by the different kinds of sensory and motor deficits that arise. Peripheral nerve lesions result in **dermatome**-type sensory deficits—i.e., there is a striplike loss of sensation along a particular area of the body, corresponding to the extension of individual peripheral nerves away from the spinal cord. L4–5 radiculopathies are particularly common, as are C6, C7, and C8 radiculopathies. However, the CNS is not organized by dermatomes. A CNS motor lesion will more likely result in a **general sensory loss** in an extremity rather than in the striplike dermatome deficit.

8. Which dermatomes are innervated by which nerves?
C1: no sensory distribution	C6: "thumb suckers suck C6"
C2: skull cap	T10: belly button
C3: collar around the neck	L1 = IL (region of inguinal ligament)
C4: cape around the shoulders	L4: knee jerk
T5: nipples	S1: ankle jerk

9. Can motor features distinguish a peripheral nerve lesion from a CNS lesion?
Peripheral nerve lesions produce lower motor neuron deficits. CNS lesions produce upper motor neuron deficits (see question 29).

10. Which roots comprise the brachial plexus?
The brachial plexus contains the ventral rami of C5, 6, 7, 8 and T1.

11. Which nerves arise from the anterior (ventral) rami of the roots prior to the formation of the brachial plexus?
The **dorsal scapular nerve**, from C5 to the rhomboid and levator scapula muscles, is responsible for elevating and stabilizing the scapula. The **long thoracic nerve**, from C5, 6, and 7 to the serratus anterior muscle, is responsible for abduction of the scapula.

12. Which roots form the trunks of the brachial plexus?
The superior trunk arises from C5 and 6. The suprascapular nerve (C5) comes off the upper trunk and supplies the supraspinatus (abduction) and infraspinatus (external rotation) muscles of the shoulder. The middle trunk comes from C7. The lower trunk comes from C8 and T1.

13. What nerve is commonly affected in shoulder dislocations or humerus fractures?
The axillary nerve is commonly affected, resulting in weakness of abduction of the shoulder and anesthesia over the lateral proximal arm.

14. What is the thoracic outlet syndrome?

This syndrome, usually caused by an extra cervical rib that compresses the medial cord of the brachial plexus and the axillary artery, results in tingling and numbness in the medial aspect of the arm, along with decreased upper extremity pulses.

15. Describe the anatomy of the peripheral nerves to the upper extremity.

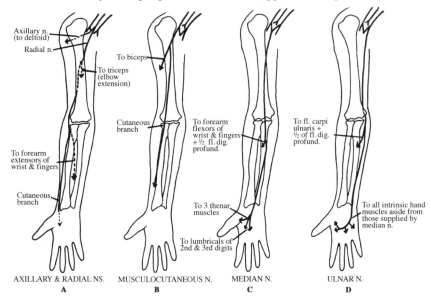

Anatomy of the nerves to the upper extremity. (From Goldberg S: Clinical Anatomy Made Ridiculously Simple. Miami, MedMaster, 2002; with permission.)

16. What motor functions are impaired by peripheral nerve injuries in the upper extremity?

Radial nerve (C5–8)—Elbow and wrist extension (patient has wrist drop); extension of fingers at MCP joints; triceps reflex

Median nerve (C8–T1)—Wrist, thumb, index, and middle finger flexion; thumb opposition; forearm pronation; ability of wrist to bend toward the radial (thumb) side; atrophy of thenar eminence (ball of thumb)

Ulnar nerve (C8–T1)—Flexion of wrist, ring and small fingers (claw hand); opposition of little finger; ability of wrist to bend toward ulnar (small finger) side; adduction and abduction of fingers; atrophy of hypothenar eminence in palm (at base of ring and small fingers)

Musculocutaneous nerve (C5–6)—Elbow flexion (biceps); forearm supination; biceps reflex

Axillary nerve (C5–6)—Ability to move upper arm outward, forward, or backward (deltoid atrophy)

Long thoracic nerve (C5–7)—Ability to elevate arm above horizontal (winging of scapula)

17. Describe the anatomy of the lumbosacral plexus.

The roots of L1 through S4 contribute to the lumbosacral plexus, which innervates the skin and skeletal muscles of the lower extremity and perineal area. As in the brachial plexus, its nerve fibers are extensions of anterior (ventral) rami. The inferior gluteal nerve supplies the gluteus maximus. The superior gluteal nerve supplies the gluteus medius and minimus. Injury to the superior gluteal nerve (e.g., direct trauma, polio) results in the "gluteus medius limp"—the abductor function of gluteus medius is lost, and the pelvis tilts to the unaffected side when the unaffected extremity is lifted on walking.

Overview of the lumbosacral plexus. (From Goldberg S: Clinical Anatomy Made Ridiculously Simple. Miami, MedMaster, 2002; with permission.)

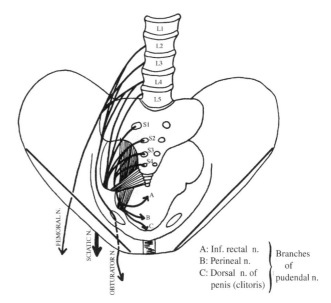

A: Inf. rectal n. ⎫ Branches
B: Perineal n.   ⎬ of
C: Dorsal n. of   ⎭ pudendal n.
   penis (clitoris)

18. Describe the route of the peripheral nerves to the lower extremity.

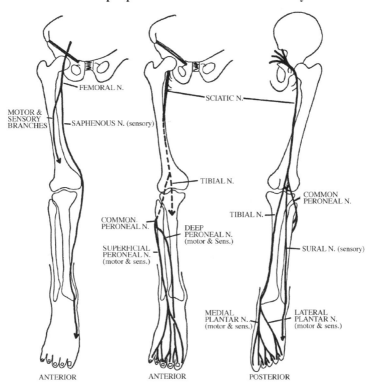

Anatomy of the nerves to the lower extremity. (From Goldberg S: Clinical Anatomy Made Ridiculously Simple. Miami, MedMaster, 2002; with permission.)

19. **What motor functions are impaired by peripheral nerve injuries in the lower extremity?**
    Femoral nerve (L2–4): Knee extension; hip flexion; knee jerk
    Obturator nerve (L2–4): Hip adduction (patient's leg swings outward when walking)
    Sciatic nerve (L4–S3): Knee flexion plus other functions along its branches, the tibial and common peroneal nerves
    Tibial nerve (L4–S3): Foot inversion; ankle plantar flexion; ankle jerk
    Common peroneal nerve (L4–S2): Foot eversion; ankle and toes dorsiflexion (patient has high-stepping gait due to foot-drop)

20. **Name the other branches of the lumbar plexus.**
    Iliohypogastric nerve (L1): supplies abdominal muscles and skin over the hypogastric and gluteal areas
    Ilioinguinal nerve (L1): innervates skin over the groin and scrotum/labia
    Genitofemoral nerve (L1, 2): runs in the inguinal canal to reach the skin at the base of the penis and scrotum/clitoris and labia majora

21. **What is meralgia paresthetica?**
    Commonly found in obese individuals, it is a numbness over the lateral thigh that results from compression of the lateral femoral cutaneous nerve where it runs under the inguinal ligament.

22. **Which nerve supplies the perineum?**
    The pudendal nerve (S2, 3, 4). Parasympathetic branches of S2, 3, 4 supply the bladder and are critical in bladder emptying. Sympathetic fibers to the bladder (from T11 to L2) promote retention of urine, but severing of sympathetic fibers to the bladder does not significantly affect bladder function.

SPINAL CORD

23. **Name the five major divisions of the spinal cord.**
    Cervical, thoracic, lumbar, sacral, and coccygeal.

24. **Where does the spinal cord end?**
    About the level of vertebrae L1–2.

25. **How many nerves exit the spinal cord?**
    There are 31 pairs of spinal nerves: 8 cervical, 12 thoracic, 5 lumbar, 5 sacral, and 1 coccygeal. Each spinal nerve is the fusion of a dorsal and ventral nerve root.

26. **What are the coverings (meninges) of the spinal cord?**
    The meninges surround the entire CNS and consist of the **pia**, which hugs the spinal cord and brain; the **arachnoid membrane**; and the **dura**, which is closely adherent to bone.

27. **Where do you find the cauda equina?**
    The cauda equina ("horse's tail") is the downward extension of spinal cord roots at the inferior end of the spinal cord.

MOTOR AND SENSORY PATHWAYS

28. **What are the major motor pathways to the extremities?**
    Corticospinal tract (pyramidal tract): extends from the motor area of the cerebral frontal cortex (Brodmann's areas 4, 6) through the internal capsule, brainstem, and spinal cord, crossing over at the junction between the brainstem and spinal cord at the level of the foramen magnum.

Therefore, lesions to the corticospinal tract above the level of the foramen magnum result in contralateral weakness, whereas lesions below the level of the foramen magnum result in ipsilateral weakness.

Rubrospinal tract: connects the red nucleus of the midbrain with the spinal cord
Tectospinal tract: connects the tectum of the midbrain with the spinal cord
Reticulospinal tract: connects the reticular formation of the brainstem with the spinal cord
Vestibulospinal tract: connects the vestibular nuclei of the brainstem with the spinal cord

29. What distinguishes an upper motor neuron lesion from a lower motor neuron lesion?

An *upper motor neuron* lesion generally refers to an injury to the corticospinal tract. The corticospinal pathway synapses in the anterior horn of the spinal cord just before leaving the cord. A *lower motor neuron* lesion is an injury to the peripheral motor nerves or their cell bodies in the gray matter of the anterior horn on which the corticospinal tract synapses.

Upper MN Defect	Lower MN Defect
Spastic paralysis	Flaccid paralysis
No significant muscle atrophy	Significant atrophy
No fasciculations or fibrillations	Fasciculations and fibrillations present
Hyperreflexia	Hyporeflexia
Babinski reflex may be present	Babinski reflex not present

30. How do the effects of corticospinal tract injuries differ from those of cerebellar and basal ganglia injuries?

All of the injuries produce motor problems. **Corticospinal tract** injuries cause paralysis. **Cerebellar** injuries are characterized by awkwardness of movement (**ataxia**), not paralysis. The awkwardness is on intention—i.e., at rest, the patient shows no problem, but ataxia becomes noticeable when the patient attempts a motor action. There may be awkwardness of posture and gait, poor coordination of movement, dysmetria, dysdiadochokinesia, scanning speech, decreased tendon reflexes on the affected side, asthenia, tremor, and nystagmus. **Basal ganglia** disorders, like cerebellar disorders, are characterized by awkward movements rather than paralysis. The movement disorder, however, is present at rest, including such problems as parkinsonian tremor, chorea, athetosis, and hemiballismus.

31. Name three major sensory pathways in the spinal cord.

1. Pain-temperature—spinothalamic tract
2. Proprioception-stereognosis*—posterior columns (*Proprioception is the ability to tell, with the eyes closed, if a joint is flexed or extended. Stereognosis is the ability to identify, with the eyes closed, an object placed in one's hand.)
3. Light touch—spinothalamic tract and posterior columns

BRAIN STEM AND CRANIAL NERVES

32. Name the three parts of the brain stem.

Midbrain (most superior), pons, and medulla (most inferior).

33. What are the functions of the cranial nerves?

CN1 (olfactory): smell
CN2 (optic): sight
CN3 (oculomotor): constricts pupils, accommodates, moves eyes
CN4 (trochlear), CN6 (abducens): move eyes
CN5 (trigeminal): chews, feels front of head
CN7 (facial): moves face, taste, salivation, crying
CN8 (vestibulocochlear): hearing, regulates balance
CN9 (glossopharyngeal): taste, salivation, swallowing, monitors carotid body and sinus

CN10 (vagus): taste, swallowing, lifts palate; communication to and from thoracoabdominal viscera to the splenic flexure of the colon

CN11 (accessory): turns head, lifts shoulders

CN12 (hypoglossal): moves tongue

34. What is Horner's syndrome?

Horner's syndrome is ptosis, miosis, and anhydrosis (lack of sweating) from a lesion of the sympathetic pathway to the face. The lesion may lie within the brainstem or the superior cervical ganglion or its sympathetic extensions to the head.

35. Which cranial nerves exit from the three parts of the brainstem?

Midbrain—CN3, CN4

Pons—CN5, CN6, CN7, CN8

Medulla—part of CN7 and CN8, CN9, CN10, CN12

CN11 exits from the upper cervical cord, goes through the foramen magnum, touches CNs 9 and 10, and then returns to the neck via the jugular foramen. The optic nerve lies superior to the brain stem. The olfactory nerve lies in the cribriform plate of the ethmoid bone.

36. What CNS areas connect with the brain stem?

The midbrain connects with the diencephalon above. The medulla connects with the spinal cord below. Each section of the brain stem has two major connections (right and left) with the cerebellum: two superior cerebellar peduncles connect with the midbrain, two middle cerebellar peduncles connect with the pons, and two inferior cerebellar peduncles connect with the medulla.

37. What are the two pigmented areas of the brain stem?

The substantia nigra, which lies in the midbrain, and the locus coeruleus, which lies in the pons.

38. What is the red nucleus?

The red nucleus lies in the midbrain. It receives major output from the cerebellum via the superior cerebellar peduncle. It has major connections to the cerebral cortex as well as to the spinal cord via the rubrospinal tract.

39. What is the medial longitudinal fasciculus (MLF)?

The MLF is a pathway that runs through the brain stem and interconnects the ocular nuclei of CNs 3, 4, and 6 and the vestibular nuclei. It plays an important role in coordinating eye movements with head and truncal posture.

40. What is the Edinger-Westphal nucleus?

It is the parasympathetic nucleus of the third cranial nerve in the midbrain. It supplies motor fibers responsible for pupillary constriction and lens accommodation.

41. What is an Argyll-Robertson pupil?

One of the classic signs of tertiary syphilis. The pupil constricts on accommodating but does not constrict to light. The lesion is believed to be in the midbrain.

42. Describe the pathway for vision.

Optic nerve fibers extend from the retina to the optic nerve, to the optic chiasm, to the optic tract, to the lateral geniculate body, and to the visual area of the brain via the optic radiation. Optic radiation fibers that extend through the parietal lobe end up superior to the calcarine fissure in the occipital lobe. Optic radiation fibers that extend through the temporal lobe end up inferior to the calcarine fissure in the occipital lobe.

43. What causes a left homonymous hemianopsia? Bitemporal hemianopsia? Superior quadrantanopsia?

Left homonymous hemianopsia: a lesion to the right optic tract, right lateral geniculate body, right optic radiation, or right occipital lobe.

Bitemporal hemianopsia: a lesion to the optic chiasm, generally from a pituitary tumor.

Superior quadrantanopsia: a lesion in the inferior aspect of the optic radiation.

44. What is most peculiar about the exit point of CN4 from the brain stem?

CN4 is the only cranial nerve to exit on the posterior side of the brain stem. In addition, it crosses over the midline before continuing on its course.

45. If a child has a head tilt, how do you know if it is due to a CN4 palsy or a stiff neck?

Cover one eye. If the head straightens out, then the tilt is due to a CN4 palsy. The child tilts the head in a CN4 palsy to avoid double vision. Covering one eye eliminates double vision, so the head straightens out.

46. Which CNs exit at the pontomedullary junction?

CN6 exits by the midline; CNs 7 and 8 exit laterally.

47. Where do the motor and sensory branches of CN5 exit the brain stem?

Both exit the brain stem at the same point, in the lateral aspect of the pons.

48. What are the sensory branches of CN5?

V1—ophthalmic
V2—maxillary
V3—mandibular

49. Which cranial nerve nucleus extends through all sections of the brain stem?

The trigeminal sensory nucleus. Its mesencephalic nucleus (facial proprioception) lies in the midbrain. Its main nucleus (facial light touch) lies in the pons. Its spinal nucleus (facial pain/temperature) lies in the medulla and upper spinal cord.

50. What is the function of CN 7?

CN7 innervates the muscles of facial expression; supplies parasympathetic fibers to the lacrimal, submandibular, and sublingual glands; receives taste information from the anterior two-thirds of the tongue; and receives a minor sensory input from the skin of the external ear.

51. How does the facial weakness that results from a CN7 lesion differ from that due to a lesion of the facial motor area of the cerebral cortex?

A CN7 lesion (as in Bell's palsy of CN7, which occurs in the facial nerve canal) results in ipsilateral facial paralysis, which includes the upper and lower face. A cerebral lesion results in contralateral facial paralysis, confined to the lower face.

52. What is Mobius syndrome?

A congenital absence of both facial nerve nuclei, resulting in bilateral facial paralysis. The abducens nuclei may also be absent.

53. What are the nucleus ambiguus, nucleus solitarius, and salivatory nucleus?

The **nucleus ambiguus**, which lies in the medulla, is a motor nucleus (CN 9 and 10) that innervates the deep throat, i.e., the muscles of swallowing (CN 9, 10) and speech (CN10).

The **nucleus solitarius** is a visceral sensory nucleus (CNs 7, 9, 10) that lies in the medulla. It receives input from the viscera as well as taste information. It is a relay in the gag reflex.

The **salivatory nucleus**, which contains superior and inferior divisions, innervates the salivary glands (CNs 7 and 9) and lacrimal glands (CN7).

54. What does CN9 do?

CN9, the glossopharyngeal nerve, innervates the stylopharyngeus muscle of the pharynx and the parotid gland. It receives taste information from the posterior one-third of the tongue, sensory tactile input from the posterior one-third of the tongue and the skin around the external ear canal, and sensory input from the carotid body and sinus.

55. Which side does the tongue deviate to if CN 12 (hypoglossal nerve) is injured?

The tongue deviates to the side of the lesion. Imagine you are riding a bicycle and your left hand becomes paralyzed. When you push on the handle bars, the wheel will turn to the left. The genioglossus muscle, which is innervated by CN12 and pushes out the tongue, operates on a similar principle.

CEREBRUM

56. What does the frontal lobe do?

Motor areas of the frontal lobe control **voluntary movement** on the opposite side of the body, including eye movement. The dominant hemisphere, usually the left, contains Broca's speech area, which when injured results in motor aphasia (**language** deficit). Areas of the frontal lobe anterior to the motor areas are involved in complex **behavioral** and **executive** activities. Lesions here result in changes in judgment, abstract thinking, tactfulness, and foresight.

57. What does the parietal lobe do?

It receives contralateral light touch, proprioceptive, and pain sensory input. Lesions to the dominant hemisphere result in tactile and proprioceptive agnosia (complex receptive disabilities). There may also be confusion in left-right discrimination, disturbances of body image, and apraxia (complex cerebral motor disabilities, caused by cutting off impulses to and from association tracts that interconnect with nearby regions).

58. What effects do temporal lobe lesions have? Occipital lobe lesions?

Temporal lobe lesions in the dominant hemisphere result in auditory aphasia. The patient hears but does not understand. He speaks but makes mistakes unknowingly, due to an inability to understand his own words. Lesions may result in alexia and agraphia (inability to read and write).

Destruction of an **occipital lobe** causes blindness in the contralateral visual field. Lesions that spare the most-posterior aspect of the occipital lobe do not cause blindness, but cause difficulty in recognizing and identifying objects (visual agnosia). A region of the occipital lobe also controls involuntary eye movements to the contralateral side of the body.

CEREBRAL CIRCULATION

59. Define the terms anterior and posterior cerebral circulation.

The **anterior** circulation is the distribution of the internal carotid artery to the cerebrum via the anterior and middle cerebral arteries. The **posterior** circulation is the distribution of the vertebral arteries to the brainstem, cerebellum, and cerebrum via the basilar artery and posterior cerebral artery.

60. Which brain region is supplied by the anterior cerebral artery?

The midline of the cerebrum, specifically the frontal and parietal lobes and the superior portions of the temporal and occipital lobes.

61. Which brain region is supplied by the middle cerebral artery?

The lateral surface of the cerebrum. Specifically, the frontal and parietal lobes and the superior portions of the temporal and occipital lobe (as is the case for the anterior cerebral artery).

62. Which region is supplied by the posterior cerebral artery?
The medial and lateral surface of the cerebrum. Specifically, the inferior portions of the temporal and occipital lobes.

63. What is the first branch of the internal carotid artery?
The ophthalmic artery.

64. Where does the brain stem get its blood supply?
From the posterior circulation—namely, branches from the vertebral arteries (to the medulla) and branches from the basilar artery (to the pons and midbrain).

65. What blood vessels supply the cerebellum?
The cerebellar blood supply comes from branches of the basilar artery: the superior cerebellar, the anterior inferior cerebellar, and the posterior inferior cerebellar arteries.

66. What is the blood supply of the thalamus and internal capsules?
From branches of the circle of Willis, including the lenticulostriate and choroidal arteries.

67. Which vessels comprise the circle of Willis?
The anterior communicating artery, the two anterior cerebral arteries, the two middle cerebral arteries, the two posterior communicating arteries, and the two posterior cerebral arteries.

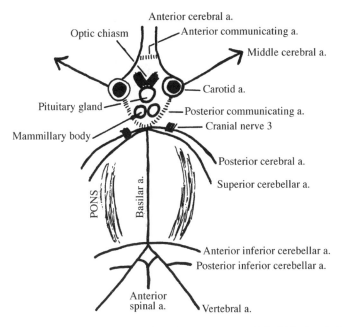

The circle of Willis. (From Goldberg S: Clinical Neuroanatomy Made Ridiculously Simple. Miami, MedMaster, 2000; with permission.)

68. Where does the spinal cord derive its blood supply?
The anterior spinal artery supplies the anterior two-thirds of the spinal cord. Two posterior spinal arteries supply the posterior third. Also, there are rich anastomoses from branches of the vertebral artery and aorta, so a stroke of the spinal cord is rare.

CEREBROSPINAL FLUID

69. Where is the CSF produced?
It is produced by the choroid plexus, which may be found in the four ventricles of the brain.

70. How much CSF is produced daily?
About 500 ml.

71. How does the CSF flow through the brain?
The CSF flows from the two lateral ventricles (in the cerebral hemispheres), to the single midline third ventricle (between the right and left thalamus and hypothalamus), to the single midline fourth ventricle (which overlies the pons and medulla), through the foramina of Magendie and Luschka (in the fourth ventricle), to the subarachnoid space (the space between the pia and arachnoid membranes), which lies outside the brain. CSF leaves the subarachnoid space by filtering through the arachnoid granulations of the superior sagittal sinus, where the CSF joins the venous circulation.

72. How do communicating and noncommunicating hydrocephalus differ?
In hydrocephalus, there is elevated CSF pressure and dilation of the ventricles secondary to obstruction to CSF flow. In **communicating** hydrocephalus, the obstruction lies outside the ventricular system, beyond the foramina of Magendie and Luschka. In **noncommunicating** hydrocephalus, obstruction occurs within the ventricular system before the foramina of Magendie and Luschka.

73. Where is spinal fluid extracted during a spinal tap?
From the subarachnoid space between vertebrae L2 and S2. Normally, the fluid is extracted about vertebra level L4–5.

BIBLIOGRAPHY

1. Carpenter MB, Sutin J: Human Neuroanatomy. Baltimore, Williams & Wilkins, 1983.
2. Goldberg S: Clinical Neuroanatomy Made Ridiculously Simple. Miami, MedMaster, 2000.
3. Haines DE: Neuroanatomy: An Atlas of Structures, Sections and Systems. Baltimore, Urban & Schwarzenberg, 1991.
4. Kandel ER, Schwartz JH, Jessell TM: Essentials of Neural Science and Behavior. Norwalk, CT, Appleton & Lange, 1995.
5. Martin JH: Neuroanatomy: Text and Atlas. Norwalk, CT, Appleton & Lange, 1996.

6. PHYSIOLOGY OF THE PERIPHERAL AND CENTRAL NERVOUS SYSTEMS

Gary Goldberg, M.D.

1. As a rehabilitation clinician, why do I need to know about basic neurophysiology?
Rehabilitation assesses function and treats disability. Because the lost function of many disabilities is a result of structural or physiologic impairment, all rehabilitation clinicians must have a basic understanding of normal anatomy and physiology. The more one understands about normal physiology and the pathophysiology of the nervous system, the better one can appreciate the neurophysiologic mechanisms of disability and adaptation and the better one can be prepared to develop strategies for treating the disability. In Mountcastle's famous words, "Physiology is what transforms structure into action."

2. Name the basic elements of the neuron.

A typical vertebrate neuron gives rise to tow types of processes: dendrites and axons. The **dendrite** receives stimulatory input from other nerve cells and carries that input to the cell body. The **axon** is the transmission process that carries action potentials to points distant from the cell body. The action potential that travels down the axon is initiated at the axon hillock. Each neuron may communicate with up to 1000 other neurons through contact via synapses.

(Figure reproduced from Kandel ER, Schwartz JH, Jessel TM (eds): Principles of Neural Science, 3rd ed. New York, Elsevier, 1991, p 19; with permission.)

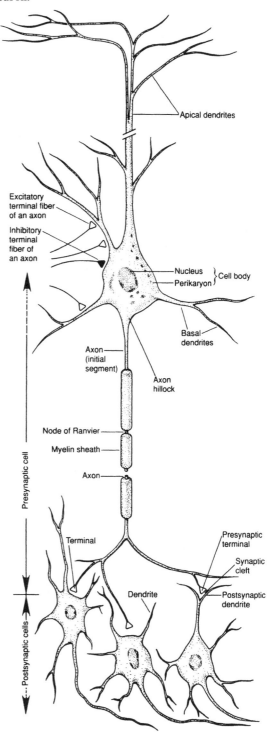

3. What is the basic function of the neuron?

Neurons come in many different shapes and configurations, but their basic function is to integrate activity impinging on the neuron and transmit this information from one place to another. Some neurons function primarily as processing elements in a network (e.g., the interneurons in the spinal cord gray matter), while others conduct information from one place to another along a long cylindrical cellular projection called the axon (e.g., corticomotorneurons projecting into the corticospinal tract).

4. How do neurons integrate and transmit information?

Via chemicals that are released at the **synapses**. These chemicals, called **neurotransmitters**, either excite the postsynaptic neuron by depolarizing its membrane and thus creating an excitatory postsynaptic potential, or inhibit the neuron by hyperpolarizing the membrane and thus producing an inhibitory postsynaptic potential. Any particular neuron is constantly bombarded through the synaptic inputs to its dendritic tree by both excitatory and inhibitory influences, which are integrated and then control the overall state of excitation of the neuron, determining when and how frequently it will become excited enough to generate an **action potential**. That action potential can then be conducted along the neuron's axon to other neurons via synaptic junctions. This continual, dynamic process of integration of inputs by the neuron is the basis of computation within the nervous system. All the "action" that takes place in the neuron occurs at its membrane and involves transient local changes in the electrical properties of the nerve cell membrane, or **neurolemma**.

5. Explain what is meant by resting membrane potential.

All cellular membranes have ATP-dependent ion-exchange pumps that are used to control the movement of sodium and potassium ions between the intracellular and extracellular spaces. The electrical voltage in the intracellular space of all cells, by virtue of the high intracellular concentration of nondiffusable anions together with the action of the ion-exchange pump, is relatively negative (by just under 100 mV) compared to the extracellular space. The membrane is thus said to be "**polarized**," with its inside surface being relatively negative at rest compared to its outside surface. This is an important fact since all excitable tissue phenomena in muscle and nerve cells assume a **resting membrane potential** that keeps the excitable cell quiescent in the presence of a lack of excitation. However, this is not really a "resting" condition since it is *actively* maintained.

6. What is an ectopic membrane potential?

Any problem with the membrane-based ion-exchange pump or the relative permeability of the membrane to any of the major ionic species can result in a major fluctuation of the resting membrane potential in nerve and muscle fibers. This fluctuation can lead to unconstrained depolarization of the membrane to the threshold level, resulting in spontaneous excitation and discharge of the membrane with the production of an aberrant, or **ectopic**, action potential. This is one of the main physiologic ways that excitable cells respond to pathologic conditions and is the basis for ectopic discharge in excitable tissues, producing such phenomena as muscle fiber fibrillation and motor unit fasciculation.

7. How does the voltage-dependent ion channel work in this system?

In neuronal and muscle membrane (the neurolemma and sarcolemma, respectively), **voltage-dependent ion channels**, primarily for sodium and potassium, pop open transiently when the intracellular voltage drifts positive (i.e., the membrane depolarizes). At the threshold voltage, an explosive electrochemical process is initiated in which **voltage-dependent sodium channels** open in rapidly increasing numbers, and the transmembrane voltage rises sharply as sodium ions rush into the cell from higher concentration in the extracellular space to lower concentration in the intracellular space, producing a further rise in intracellular voltage and further depolarization of the cell membrane. This regenerative explosion is the basis of the sharp upswing of the nerve action potential. The voltage eventually levels off as the sodium channels become less sensitive (i.e., less likely to open) to the increased voltage and as **voltage-dependent potassium channels** open allowing potassium to move out of the cell. The transmembrane voltage reverses, dropping toward the resting level. It actually overshoots the resting level, and the membrane becomes hyperpolarized for a short period called the **refractory period**, during which it is resistant to excitation.

8. Discuss the role of membrane refractoriness in conducting action potentials.

Postexcitatory refractoriness is a critical aspect of neural network dynamics that helps to constrain the excitatory phenomena in the nervous system. The duration of the refractory period determines how quickly a nerve can be repetitively excited and restricts the effective "bandwidth," or information-carrying capacity, of the neuron. This refractory mechanism produces an asymmetry of excitability around the area of depolarized membrane conducting the action potential. The membrane in front of the action potential remains excitable and ready to "fire up," while the membrane behind the action potential becomes transiently inexcitable and resistant to rebounding excitatory influence. This asymmetry prevents "backfiring" of the cell membrane and ensures that the action potential travels as a wave in one direction down the length of the fiber.

9. Where do calcium ions operate in the action potential?

A transient "spike" of membrane depolarization is conducted from the cell body of the neuron down the axon as a wave of excitation. When it reaches the distal end of the axon at the presynaptic terminal, the depolarization spike initiates the flow of calcium ions into the presynaptic terminal through voltage-dependent calcium channels concentrated in the membrane of the presynaptic terminal. This leads to release of neurotransmitter from the presynaptic terminal, leading to excitation or inhibition of the postsynaptic cell.

10. What are fibrillation and fasciculation?

In the mature neuromuscular system, a muscle fiber should normally generate an action potential and contract only when "it is told to" by a motor neuron. However, in muscle fibers with defective membranes that "leak" sodium ions from the extracellular to the intracellular space, spontaneous membrane depolarization leads to the spontaneous generation of a muscle fiber action potential and the autonomous contraction of the fiber. This autonomous contraction of a muscle fiber occurs in the presence of pathologic conditions that either remove the normal neural control over the muscle fiber or directly damage the muscle fiber membrane. This pathologic autonomous muscle fiber contraction is called a **fibrillation**, an invisible tiny twitch of an individual muscle fiber.

A similar type of electrical destabilization of the membrane of the motor neuron and motor axon leads to spontaneous generation of an ectopic nerve action potential, which is conducted through the terminal branching of the fiber to all muscle fibers innervated by the motor neuron. This results in a synchronous autonomous contraction of all the fibers in the motor unit, producing a significant, visible twitch of the muscle called a **fasciculation**. Both phenomena are physiologic results of the loss of normal constraint over the excitation of nerve and muscle fibers that can occur in various neuromuscular disorders.

11. What is a neural network? What does it do?

A neural network is a set of neurons that are interconnected in a specified pattern. Through the conduction of activity from one place to another within the network and through the convergence and divergence of activity in different parts of the network as it is dynamically active, patterns of activation emerge. A network may be considered to have a set of inputs impinging on input neurons, a set of outputs generated by output neurons, as well as a set of neurons that mediate activity back and forth between input and output neurons. The general structure of a neural network includes input neurons that convey afferent (i.e., in-flowing) information from the periphery and output neurons that convey efferent (i.e., out-flowing) information to the periphery. These two general flows of information can interact at multiple levels, allowing an efferent flow to modulate an afferent flow and an afferent flow to modulate an efferent flow. These interactions help control what moves along the pathway from the periphery to more central structures to eventually enable perception to occur, and what moves along the pathway from central structures to the periphery to generate movement.

12. Give an example of a neural network.

The interaction of afferent and efferent flows helps the nervous system to differentiate when apparent movement of an external object is due to actual object movement in the external world versus self-generated movement that makes it seem as if the object is moving (e.g., eye movement). These two situations are distinguished by a so-called efference copy signal that is sent from the efferent system to the afferent system to inform perceptual areas that the apparent movement is due to self-generated movement. This mechanism can sometimes fail, leading to illusory perceptions of object movement, as when a patient has nystagmus and feels that the external world is actually jumping around with each eye movement, a symptom referred to as oscillopsia. This illusion can be produced by pushing with one's finger on the lateral aspect of the globe of the eye.

13. Outline the parts and functions of the peripheral nervous system.

STRUCTURE	FUNCTION
Somatic	Controls voluntary movement
Afferent (sensory)	Transmits sensory information from periphery and surface (i.e., skin, muscles, joints) about the dynamic state of limbs, their articulation in space, and external environment
Efferent (motor)	Conducts voluntary motor control messages to skeletal muscle
Autonomic	Controls vegetative functions
Afferent	Receives sensory information about internal environment of body
Efferent	Sends control messages to smooth muscle of blood vessels, cardiac muscle, exocrine glands, and internal viscera
Parasympathetic	Maintains internal resources and internal homeostasis
Sympathetic	Involved in stress response and energy expenditure

14. What comprises the motivational subsystem of the CNS?

The CNS has three major interacting functional subsystems: the sensory, motor, and motivational subsystems. The hypothalamus and the nuclei of the limbic system, such as the hippocampus and amygdala, are important parts of the motivational subsystem. This subsystem interconnects sensory and motor subsystems by making decisions about actions based on the detection of sensory context from both the internal and external environments. For example, the motivational subsystem activates the motor system to reach for an apple when the sensed internal nutritional state indicates a need for nourishment. The motivational subsystem must work in close conjunction with both the autonomic and somatic peripheral nervous systems by taking in information from both systems and coordinating activity in both systems.

15. How are the sensory systems of the nervous system organized?

There are several major sensory systems in the brain: somatosensory, special visceral afferent (taste), vestibular, auditory, visual, and olfactory systems. The somatosensory system is divided into the lemniscal system subserving epicritic sensations of light touch and vibration sense and the spinothalamic system subserving the protocritic sensations of pain and temperature. All systems except for the olfactory system transmit information to specialized regions of the thalamus. The interaction between the thalamus and cortex is a mutually excitatory interaction, and each sensation (except for olfaction) has a specific thalamic nucleus that is reciprocally connected to a well-circumscribed cortical area that functions as a primary receiving zone for that particular sensation. Other nonspecific thalamic nuclei are more diffusely connected to the cerebral cortex. The olfactory system connects directly into the amygdala, a critical nucleus of the limbic (motivational) system, as well as to olfactory regions of the cerebral cortex. Unlike all other sensory systems, it does not connect through the thalamus to its cortical area.

16. How are the extrathalamic ascending neuromodulatory systems organized?

In addition to the sensory system projections to the cerebral cortex, a number of widely projecting systems connect to the cerebral cortex directly from nuclei in the reticular core of the brainstem and midbrain. These systems are characterized by the major neurotransmitter which each system utilizes to modulate cortical activity. These systems are extremely important in controlling the overall excitability and responsiveness (or tone), of different parts of the cerebral cortex and are especially important in regulating levels of consciousness and the sleep-wake cycle. They are also involved in the regulation of mood and emotional states. Disruption of these systems is associated with the loss of consciousness that occurs with the diffuse axonal injury to the subcortical white matter in cranial trauma. Many neurotransmitter-based psychoactive medications function by influencing the operation of one or more of these major systems.

Major Extrathalamic Neurotransmitter Systems

NEUROTRANSMITTER	MAJOR SOURCE NUCLEUS	TYPICAL MEDICATION(S)
Acetylcholine	Nucleus basalis of Meynert	Benzotropine mesylate (antagonist), donepezil (agonist)
Dopamine	Substantia nigra (pars compacta), ventral tegmental area	L-Dopa, bromocriptine (agonists); droperidol (antagonists)
Norepinephrine	Locus coeruleus	Methylphenidate, nortriptyline (agonists)
Serotonin	Raphe nuclei	Fluoxetine, sertraline, citalopram (agonists)

17. What other substances function as neurotransmitters in the brain?

Additional neurotransmitter systems in the brain include those utilizing epinephrine and histamine, amino acids (e.g., GABA, glutamate, glycine), neuropeptides, hypothalamic and hypophyseal peptide hormones, and opioids (endorphins and enkephalins).

18. What is a motor unit?

The motor unit is the *functional element of voluntary movement*. It consists of the anterior horn cell, motor axon, nerve terminals, neuromuscular junctions, and all the muscle fibers innervated by the anterior horn cell. The CNS activates the anterior horn cell, which in turn activates the muscle fibers in the motor unit to produce voluntary movement. Movement is controlled through motor unit recruitment and firing rate modulations.

19. How does the motor unit work?

The anterior horn cell controls a significant number of muscle fibers, ranging up to several thousand muscle fibers in a single motor unit. Each time the anterior horn cell fires an action potential, the end result is a **synchronous** twitch of all the muscle fibers in the motor unit. Tension is graded in muscle by recruiting additional motor units and by increasing the firing rate of the motor units in the available pool that have been activated. A motor unit cannot be normally fired at a tonic rate less than about 6/sec. The rate at which a motor unit starts firing when it is first recruited is called the **onset firing rate.** The rate at which a motor unit is firing when the next motor unit in sequence is recruited is called the **recruitment firing rate** or **recruitment frequency**.

The manner in which motor units in a muscle are recruited is generally very orderly and in a sequence from the population of smaller motor units innervated by motor neurons with smaller cell bodies, through to the population of larger motor units innervated by motor neurons with larger cell bodies. This process of recruitment from smaller to larger units is referred to as the **size principle**. The size principle has a number of important functional implications. The units recruited initially in a contraction are generally slow-twitch oxidative units, while those recruited at higher tension levels are generally fast-twitch glycolytic units, ensuring that sustained low-level concentrations are performed by fatigue-resistant muscle fibers. Furthermore, the amount of incremental force (ΔF) added to a muscle contraction at any point during a graded activation is approximately proportional to the current force (F) being produced by the muscle. Therefore, the ratio of ΔF to F is a constant during the development of tension in a graded contraction of the muscle.

20. What is muscular co-contraction and what does it accomplish?

High-force output motor units cannot be immediately accessed but can only be recruited after low-force output motor units have first been activated. To obtain the rapid deployment of a large amount of force, the muscle may need to be "preloaded" so that it is already operating up in the range in which the high-force output units are starting to be recruited. Agonist-antagonist muscle groups will sometimes oppose each other in a **co-contraction** in order to "bias" a muscle into its higher output range, which enables more immediate access to the large-amplitude, fast-fatigable motor units and facilitates rapid production of large bursts of muscular force.

Muscle co-contraction is also important for the stabilization of proximal joints during more distal movement and also for situations in which forces across a joint must be absorbed through muscle contraction. Co-contraction is also used to stabilize a limb in anticipation of a dynamic load whose exact direction of force cannot be predicted.

On the other hand, in many gross motor activities, gravity acts as a sustained force that serves as the primary propulsive force, which is then controlled by low-grade, sustained, eccentric muscle contractions. In this case, the muscles operate in their low range where the slow-oxidative, low-amplitude units predominate and co-contraction just adds an unnecessary and wasteful burden. In such instances, agonist-antagonist interaction is controlled with patterns of **reciprocal inhibition** that produce a "push-pull" alternating interaction between muscles to produce opposing forces. Mechanisms for controlling the interaction of agonist-antagonist pairs of muscles in either co-contraction or reciprocal inhibition relationships are programmed to a great extent at the spinal segmental level.

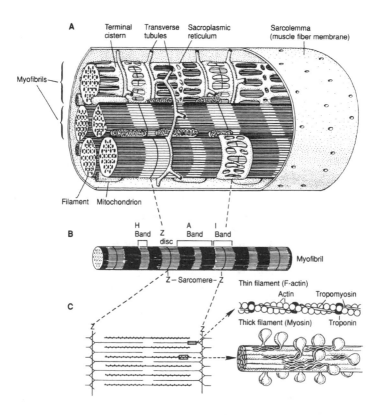

Muscle anatomy. (From Kandel ER, Schwartz JH, Jessell TM (eds): Principles of Neural Science, 3rd ed. New York, Elsevier, 1991; p 549, with permission.)

21. How does a muscle fiber contract?

A twitch of mechanical energy is produced through the transient shortening of a muscle fiber whenever an action potential travels along the sarcolemma (i.e., muscle fiber cell membrane).

The actual shortening of muscle is produced by the coordinated, relative movement of thin (**actin**) and thick (**myosin**) filaments within the myofibrils (see figure). Two factors are necessary for the contraction to develop: a supply of high-energy phosphate bonds for metabolic support of contraction (usually provided by ATP) and a supply of calcium ions. The movement is driven by cross-bridge molecules originating in the thick filaments and bridging across to the thin filaments. The binding of ATP to a cross-bridge causes it to release its contact with the actin-binding site on the thin filament. The ATP then splits, forming a high-energy state of the crossbridge which extends and binds itself to another binding site on the thin filament. The cross-bridge moves from a high-energy state to a low-energy state in the process of bending and shortening, thus moving the thin filament in toward the center of the thick filament and drawing the Z lines on the sarcomeres closer together. A new ATP molecule then must bind to the cross-bridge in order to facilitate its dissociation from the binding site on the thin filament. The dissociated cross-bridge is then cocked and ready to attach to another binding site on the thin filament. This cycle repeats itself over and over as long as there is ATP present to drive the process.

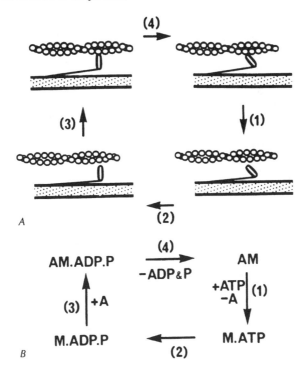

Steps in the contraction of a muscle fiber according to the sliding filament theory. Structural (A) and corresponding biochemical (B) changes. (From Engel AG, Franzini-Armstrong C (eds): Myology: Basic and Clinical, 2nd ed. New York, McGraw-Hill, 1994, p 162, with permission.)

22. What role does calcium play in muscle contraction?

The forming of a cross-bridge can only occur when there are receptor-binding sites available on the thin filament for the cross-bridge to attach. In the presence of calcium ions, there is a conformational change in the thin filament that exposes the binding sites. When calcium is not present in the myofibril, contraction cannot occur because the binding sites are retracted. Thus, control of the contractile process reduces to controlling the concentration of calcium ions in the myofibril. The spreading excitation of the muscle fiber causes a release of calcium into the myofibril through voltage-dependent calcium channels that open in the membranes of the sarcoplasmic reticulum as the wave of depolarization spreads down the fiber. Calcium ions flow into the myofibril and activate the contractile process. Calcium ions are then rapidly and efficiently pumped out of the myofibril and back into the sarcoplasmic reticulum as the muscle fiber relaxes.

This then is the basic process whereby the electrical phenomenon of transmitted membrane depolarization along the length of a muscle fiber is transformed into the mechanical phenomenon of muscle fiber shortening and muscle contraction.

23. Outline the sequence of events in muscular contraction.

Excitation-contraction coupling
1. Depolarization of sarcolemma with conduction of muscle fiber action potential
2. Internal fiber depolarization through transmission along T-tubule system
3. Release of Ca^{2+} from sarcoplasmic reticulum
4. Ca^{2+} diffuses into sarcomeres

Contraction
5. Ca^{2+} binds to troponin
6. Troponin–Ca^{2+} complex removes tropomyosin blockage of actin-binding sites
7. Myosin heads containing high-energy myosin–ADP–P_i complex attach to actin-binding sites and form cross-bridges between thick and thin filaments
8. Conformational energy-releasing changes occur in high-energy myosin heads that cause them to swivel, producing relative motion of the thick and thin filaments, releasing ADP and P_i and returning the myosin head to its low-energy state
9. A new ATP molecule binds to the myosin head, allowing the release of the head from the actin-binding site
10. ATP splits to ADP and P_i, producing a high-energy myosin–ADP–P_i complex
11. Return to Step 7 with repeating of cycle of steps 7–10 as long as actin-binding sites remain available for attachment

Relaxation
12. Ca^{2+} pumped back into sarcoplasmic reticulum
13. Ca^{2+} around thin filaments diffuses back toward the sarcoplasmic reticulum
14. Ca^{2+} released from troponin–Ca^{2+} complex
15. Troponin permits return of tropomyosin to blocking position
16. Myosin–actin cross-bridges break with addition of ATP to the myosin head, but new cross-bridges cannot form because the actin-binding sites are no longer available because of blocking action of tropomyosin

24. What is spasticity? Describe its neurophysiologic basis.

Spasticity is most often used to refer to abnormalities of movement in a limb in which there has been damage to centers that modulate the activity of the motor unit. A number of things go wrong with motor control and the process of voluntary activation of the motor units when centers above the level of the spinal segment are damaged. When motor control is dysfunctional, events can be viewed as **"negative"** phenomena, where activity that should normally be present is not or where normal activity patterns become abnormally attenuated, or **"positive"** phenomena, where activity patterns that are normally not present appear (e.g., pathologic reflex patterns) or where activity patterns that are normally present become abnormally exaggerated and distorted.

25. List the six major descending tracts from the brain.

The circuits in the spinal cord at the segmental level are controlled by descending tracts from the brain.

1. Corticospinal tract (including lateral and ventral tracts) projecting from the cerebral cortex
2. Vestibulospinal tract projecting from the vestibular nuclei in the pons
3. Medial reticulospinal tract projecting from the pontine reticular formation
4. Lateral reticulospinal tract projecting from the medullary reticular formation
5. Rubrospinal tract projecting from the red nucleus in the midbrain
6. Tectospinal tract projecting from the superior colliculus in the tectum of the midbrain

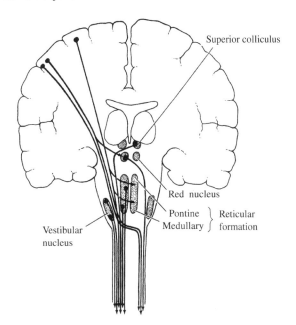

Descending fiber tracts from different parts of the brain to the spinal cord. (Figure reproduced from Nicholls JG, Martin AR, Wallace BG: From Neuron to Brain: A Cellular and Molecular Approach to the Function of the Nervous System, 3rd ed. Sunderland, MA, Sinauer Associates, Inc., 1992, p 534, with permission.)

26. How do each of the different descending tracts affect muscle tone?

Each of the descending pathways has a different influence on the background tone and dynamic activation of motor neuron pools and interneuronal circuits in the spinal cord.

The **vestibulospinal** and **reticulospinal** tracts are involved in the postural biasing of muscles and anticipatory postural adjustments that precede voluntary movements. The vestibulospinal and reticulospinal output neurons are generally excitatory to extensor motor neurons innervating extensor muscles in the arms and legs and are under inhibitory control from the cortical level. The loss of cortical inhibitory control over these pathways tends to facilitate extensor tone in the arms and legs, resulting in **decerebrate rigidity**.

The **rubrospinal** and **corticospinal** tracts both tend to balance the extensor drive by facilitating drive to flexor muscles. The rubrospinal tract in humans extends only into the cervical cord and thus can counteract extensor drive in the arms but not the legs. Thus, the **decorticate rigidity** in humans with large cerebral hemisphere lesions is primarily one of net facilitation of flexors in the arms and extensors in the legs. This is because loss of descending control from the cerebral cortex releases unopposed excitatory extensor drive from the vestibular and reticular formation areas to the lower limb extensor muscles, while flexor facilitation is released from the red nucleus to upper limb flexor muscles in projections in the rubrospinal tract.

27. What is the upper motor neuron syndrome?

When there is dysfunction of the descending inputs to the spinal cord, there is a degrading of the dynamic control of the motor neurons, and the patterns of activation of muscles in a limb that form the basis of normal limb function become disordered. This combination of findings—changes in response to passive sustained and dynamic stretch, disinhibition of antigravity postural subroutines, and disordering of voluntary patterns of muscle activation—depends on the exact way in which the descending pathways have been affected by the damage. This combination of changes can be thought of as a type of disordered motor control or as a syndrome, the **upper motor neuron syndrome** (UMNS), where the term "upper motor neuron" refers to any neuron in the central neuraxis which projects down to the spinal cord through one of the descending pathways.

The disorder of function associated with UMNS may be due to a wide variety of possible mechanisms, which could include altered response (usually exaggerated excitation) to passive stretch, an inability to generate voluntary activation of a muscle (i.e., decreased drive), or an inability to dynamically coordinate the activation of a set of different muscles in the limb. Additionally, over time in the paretic limb, there are changes in the fibrous architecture of the muscle that lead to changes in the passive viscoelastic properties of the muscle of an affected limb. Thus limitation of movement in chronic UMNS may be due to fixed contracture or may be exaggerated by a loss of distensibility of the fibrous matrix of the muscle.

28. What parts of the nervous system are involved in the control of voluntary movement?

The **motor cortex** is the cortical strip of the precentral gyrus. It is a somatotopically organized, electrically excitable region of the cerebral cortex that is involved in the execution of detailed aspects of voluntary fine movement, especially rapid, finely coordinated, "fractionated" movements of the fingers and toes.

Areas in the **parietal cortex** and **frontal cortex** (in the "premotor" cortex) are involved in translating the intent to act into more global aspects of the task, such as its timing, sequential linkage of different subtasks, trajectory through extrapersonal space, and coordination of the postural stabilization and distal limb control in movement.

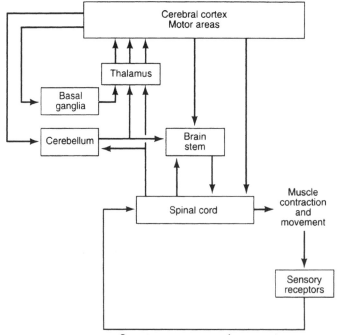

Levels of organization of the motor system. (From Kandel ER, Schwartz JH, Jessell TM (eds): Principles of Neural Science, 3rd ed. New York, Elsevier, 1991, p 539, with permission.)

The **cerebellum** receives two inputs and has one output. This input, from the cerebral cortex and from the spinal cord, keeps the cerebellum informed about what is going on in the limbs, particularly with muscle and tendon stretch information. The cerebellum generates output back to the cerebral cortex that can then influence the ongoing outflow of activity from the cortex. There is thus a circular loop involved in cerebellar circuitry, called a **re-entrant loop**, since the output re-enters the general part of the nervous system (the cerebral cortex) from which input originated.

The **basal ganglia** consist of the striatum (the caudate and putamen nuclei), the pallidal nuclei (the external and internal segments of the globus pallidus), and a set of nuclei in the mid-brain including the substantia nigra and subthalamic nucleus. The basal ganglia constitute a second, but differently connected, re-entrant loop with the cerebral cortex. Both the cerebellum and the basal ganglia reconnect to the cerebral cortex by way of distinct thalamic nuclei in the ventral region of the thalamus.

29. What is the role of the cerebellum in the control of voluntary movement?

The cerebellum is an important "meta-system" in voluntary motor control that enables *the refinement and fine-tuning of motor performance* through dynamic modulation of outflows from the motor cortex. This is done by correcting errors detected between the sampled outflow from the motor cortex, which conveys the details of the *intended* movement, and the sensory input from the periphery, which conveys the details of the *actual* movement.

The cerebellum can be viewed as being responsible for the discrete timing relationships within a pattern of muscle activations and may have some type of dynamic clocking function. The cerebellum rapidly performs precise adjustments of the dynamics of the sensorimotor linkage and muscle activation patterns to allow for progressively more rapid and accurate performance of a motor task as it is being practiced. As such, the cerebellum is an important site for *motor learning* and for the *development of procedural memories* (i.e., motor engrams). The automatization of motor skill performance frees up the cerebral cortex from the attentional load involved in taking care of all the details of execution.

30. What motor dysfunction is associated with cerebellar damage?

Deficient movement execution and coordination with the appearance of oscillations (ataxic tremor), inaccurate endpoint acquisition (**past-pointing**), and impairment of the timing of muscle activation in dynamic alternation and rhythmic movements (**dysdiadochokinesis**). There is a lack of precision in the timing of activation of bursts of EMG activity in agonist and antagonist muscle pairs, particularly for rapid "ballistic" movements which cannot be controlled with continuous feedback. A delay in the development of the braking effect of the antagonist burst that follows the acceleration produced by the initial agonist burst results in overshoot of the target, or past-pointing. This effect is exaggerated when movement speed increases, since the timing precision demands of the task become more severe. Errors are reduced by slowing down performance of the task and by focusing more attention on performance.

In the presence of cerebellar impairment, patients tend to try to simplify the problem of performing multijoint movements by focusing on the movement of one joint at a time in sequence, rather than attempting to move all joints simultaneously. The cerebellum adjusts stretch reflex gains to allow for appropriate dynamic load compensation necessary, for example, when an unexpected loading of the limb occurs. In the presence of cerebellar damage, load compensation responses are reduced or delayed, the gain of the stretch reflexes is reduced with resulting hypotonia, and the result is an underdamped limb that is prone to oscillation and overshoot.

31. What role does the basal ganglia play in voluntary movement?

Whereas the cerebellum is involved in the control and coordination of precise timing relationships between bursts of activity in different muscles firing within a pattern, the basal ganglia seem to be involved in the *more global control of the timing of the pattern as a whole*—i.e., its relative expansion or compression in time. This may be closely related to the clocking of internal ultradian rhythms. The striatum receive widespread input from all over the cerebral cortex, and the output of the globus pallidus goes to a limited area of the thalamus that interacts with a very limited region of the premotor and supplementary motor areas. The striatum appears to be subdivided into segregated modules, each of which receives inputs from different subregions of the cerebral cortex, suggesting a highly modularized system of re-entrant loops.

The basal ganglia may play a role in *selecting specific motor patterns* to be chosen from a vast repertoire of potential patterns based on current cortically processed sensory context. This probably occurs through a process of selective facilitation of a small subset of modular loops and massive inhibition of the remaining loops that allows only limited modules of the striatum to be allowed to inhibit regions of the globus pallidus, which then projects inhibitory output to the thalamus. Thus, the basal ganglia can be viewed as a selective filter of information flow converging on motor preparation regions of the cerebral cortex. They may therefore be involved in the process of selecting motor engrams to be activated in a certain context or setting up critical perceptuomotor linkages.

32. How does dopaminergic failure in the basal ganglia present clinically?

Dysfunction of the dopaminergic system within the basal ganglia results in problems with slowness of movement, impairment of initiation, and overall constriction of movement. Dopamine acts as a promotor and energizer of movement by playing a role in the selective facilitation of specific movements. It may also serve a role as a controlling influence on an internal sense of time. Thus, patients with dopaminergic insufficiency associated with parkinsonism have problems with estimating time intervals and accurately reproducing time intervals presented to them.

33. Explain the roles of different parts of the cerebral cortex in the planning and control of movement.

The cerebral cortex plays an important role in assuring that movements are integrated, coordinated, and contextually appropriate. Through emerging techniques, such as positron-emission tomography (PET) and functional MRI, that allow the activity of different parts of the brain to be imaged in the active human subject, we are able to learn more about the functional networks in the cerebral cortex that participate in conscious perception and volition.

One theory relates to how different parts of the cerebral cortex have evolved. The medial part of the cortex has evolved from the hippocampus, while the lateral part of the cortex has evolved from the primitive olfactory complex. This suggests that structures on the medial surface of the hemisphere, such as the **anterior cingulate cortex** and the **supplementary motor area**, are involved in the initiation and control of movements that are internally based, while the areas on the lateral surface of the brain, such as the **ventrolateral frontal lobe** and the **lateral parietal regions**, are involved in the detection and registration of external information and the integration of external cues into action control. In fact, the anterior cingulate cortex on the medial surface of the brain, just above the corpus callosum, appears to be part of an important **executive attention network** that is associated with conscious volition, while the lateral structures appear to be important elements of a perceptual orienting network and a **vigilance network** that focuses on external events. The cerebellum appears to be more closely associated with the lateral system, while the basal ganglia are most closely associated with the medial system. These different "premotor" systems, the medial and lateral, appear to relate to each other through reciprocal inhibition. Activation of the anterior circulate region and the executive attention network appears to be associated with the subjective experience of awareness or effort directed to performance—attention for action.

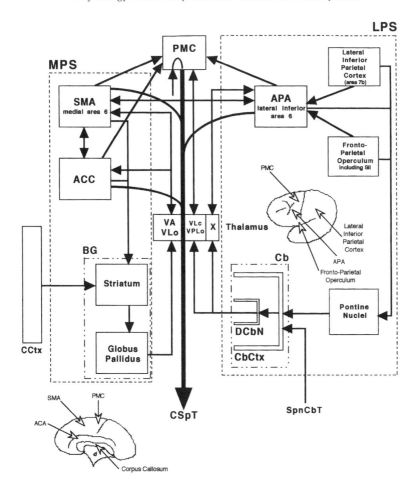

Structure and organization of the medial premotor system (MPS) on the medial surface of the hemisphere and the lateral premotor system (LPS) on the lateral surface of the hemisphere. In the MPS, the supplementary motor area (SMA) and the anterior cingulate cortex (ACC) project in topographically ordered fashion to the primary motor cortex (PMC). These areas are also in close relationship with the basal ganglia (BG). In the LPS, the arcuate premotor area (APA) on the lateral surface of the monkey brain projects similarly to PMC. The cerebellum (Cb) with the cerebellar cortex (CbCtx) and the deep cerebellar nuclei (DCbN) is part of the LPS and projects through the thalamus back to APA and PMC.The cerebellar cortex also receives direct afferents from the spinal cord by way of the spinocerebellar tract (SpnCbT). The BG receive input from broadly distributed regions of the cerebral cortex projecting to the striatum and project output back from the globus pallidus to the SMA and ACC via the VA and VLo nuclei of the thalamus. Outflow from the PMC, SMA, ACC, and APA projects to the spinal cord by way of the corticospinal tract (CSpT). Projections to the PMC influence the "gain" of sensorimotor "transcortical loops" that link sensory input to the PMC to the efferent projects from the PMC into the CSpT.

BIBLIOGRAPHY

1. Deecke L, Eccles JC, Mountcastle VB (eds): From Neuron to Action: An Appraisal of Fundamental and Clinical Research. New York, Springer-Verlag, 1990.
2. Dieber MP, Passingham RE, Colebatch JG, et al: Cortical areas and the selection of movement: A study with positron emission tomography. Exp Brain Res 84:393–402, 1991.
3. Dumitru D: Electrodiagnostic Medicine, 2nd ed. Philadelphia, Hanley & Belfus, 2002.

 4. Frackowiak RSJ, Weiller C, Chollet F: The functional anatomy of recovery from brain injury. In Chadwick DJ, Whelan J (eds): Exploring Brain Functional Anatomy with Positron Tomography (CIBA Foundation Symposium 163). New York, Wiley, 1991, pp 235–249.
 5. Glenn WB, Whyte J (eds): The Practical Management of Spasticity in Adults and Children. Philadelphia, Lea & Febiger, 1990.
 6. Goldberg G: From intent to action: Evolution and function of the premotor systems of the frontal lobe. In Perecman E (ed): The Frontal Lobes Revisited. New York, IRBN Press, 1987, pp 273–306.
 7. Goldberg G: Neurophysiologic models of recovery in stroke. Phys Med Rehabil Clin North Am 2:599–614, 1991.
 8. Goldberg G: Premotor systems, attention to action and behavioral choice. In Kien J, McCrohan CR, Winslow W (eds): Neurobiology of Motor Programme Selection. New York, Pergamon Press, 1992, pp 225–249.
 9. Jenkins WM, Merzenich MM, Ochs MT, et al: Functional reorganization of primary somatosensory cortex in adult owl monkeys after behaviorally controlled tactile stimulation. J Neurophysiol 63:82–104, 1990.
10. Kandel ER, Schwartz JH, Jessel TM (eds): Principles of Neural Science, 3rd ed. New York, Elsevier, 1991.
11. Latash ML: Control of Human Movement. Champaign, IL, Human Kinetics, 1993.
12. Pastor MA, Atreida J, Jahanshahi M, Obeso JA: Time estimation and reproduction is abnormal Parkinson's disease. Brain 115:211–225, 1992.
13. Patton HD, Fuchs AF, Hille B, et al (eds): Textbook of Physiology: Vol. 1. Excitable Cells and Neurophysiology, 21st ed. Philadelphia, W.B. Saunders, 1989.
14. Posner MI, Raichle ME: Images of Mind. New York, Scientific American Library, 1994.
15. Raichle ME, Fiez JA, Videen TO, et al: Practice-related changes in human brain functional anatomy during non-motor learning. Cerebral Cortex 4:8–26, 1994.

7. ANATOMY AND KINESIOLOGY OF THE MUSCULOSKELETAL SYSTEM

Carson D. Schneck, M.D., Ph.D.

PRINCIPLES OF KINESIOLOGY

1. How do agonist, antagonist, and synergistic muscles operate to accomplish joint motion?

1. An **agonist**, or prime mover, is any muscle that can cause a specific joint motion. For example, the biceps brachii contracts to cause elbow flexion.

2. An **antagonist** is any muscle that can produce a motion opposite to the specific agonist motion. For example, triceps brachii is an antagonist to elbow flexion. Antagonists are normally completely relaxed during contraction of an agonist (except during a rapid ballistic motion).

3. **Synergistic** muscles normally contract to remove unwanted actions of agonists or to stabilize other (usually more proximal) joints. For example, during elbow flexion by the biceps brachii, the forearm pronators contract to remove the undesirable supination that the biceps would produce.

2. What forces normally produce motion at joints?

Muscle contraction and gravity, with each serving as the prime mover for about 50% of all joint movements.

3. Name the three types of muscle contraction.

1. **Shortening, concentric, or isotonic** contraction occurs when the muscle's force exceeds the load. Hence, the muscle shortens to produce joint motion while maintaining constant tension.

2. **Isometric** or **static** contraction occurs when the muscle force equals the load. The muscle maintains the same length, and the joint does not move.

3. **Lengthening** or **eccentric** contraction occurs when muscle force is less than the load. This normally occurs when gravity is the prime mover. To control the effect of gravity, eccentric contraction occurs in the muscle(s) that opposes the direction that gravity is tending to move the joint.

4. Two muscles together often perform the same function. How can you eliminate one of the muscles to evaluate the other muscle in relative isolation?

Three muscle elimination procedures are used commonly:

1. Placing a muscle at a **mechanical disadvantage** by positioning the part so that the muscle to be eliminated will have no substantial vector component in the direction of the function to be tested.

2. Placing a muscle at a **physiologic** or **length disadvantage** by positioning the part so that the muscle is slackened or has much of its shortening capability used up by performing a function other than the one being tested.

3. If the muscle to be eliminated has several functions, it can be **reciprocally inhibited** from participating in the tested function by forcibly performing a function antagonistic to one of its other functions.

5. How is muscle strength graded?

Manual muscle strength assessment is accomplished by proceeding cephalad down in the order of innervation from the brachial plexus, through the lumbosacral plexus. If specific nerves are in question, examine muscles in the proximal-to-distal order in which they receive their motor branches. Resistance is best assessed using the "make and break" technique, in which the examiner overpowers a patient's fixed mid-muscle-length contraction.

In clinical practice, the following hierarchy of ordinal-ranked categories is used. For greater reproducibility, a continuous measure such as hand-held dynamometry is superior.

5 = Normal power against gravity and the usual amount of resistance
4 = Muscle contraction possible against gravity and less than the normal amount of resistance
3 = Muscle contraction possible only against gravity, not with resistance
2 = Joint movement possible only with gravity eliminated
1 = Flicker of contraction with no movement
0 = No contraction detectable

SPINE

6. Name the major ligaments of the spine.

Anterior longitudinal ligament
Posterior longitudinal ligament
Ligamenta flava
Interspinous and supraspinous ligaments

7. What are the parts of the intervertebral disc?

A peripheral, laminated, fibrocartilaginous **anulus fibrosus** and a central, gel-like **nucleus pulposus**. The anulus fibrosus contains the nucleus pulposus fluid between the adjacent vertebral bodies. The nucleus pulposus serves as a hydraulic load-dispersing mechanism, so that as the spine bends in any direction, the compressive loads borne by that side of the disc are redistributed over a larger surface area, thereby reducing the pressure.

8. Why do most intervertebral disc protrusions occur posterolaterally?

1. The disc is reinforced anterolaterally by the anterior longitudinal ligament and posteromedially by the posterior longitudinal ligament. Posterolaterally, there are no extrinsic supporting ligaments.

2. The nucleus pulposus is eccentrically located closer to the posterior aspect of the disc, causing the posterior anulus to have the smallest radial dimension and offer the least support.

3. The posterior anulus is thinnest in the superior-inferior dimension at cervical and lumbar levels, causing it to suffer the greatest strain.

4. Because flexion is the most predominant spine motion, the posterior anulus receives the most repetitive tensile stresses.

5. The posterolateral anulus is subject to the highest intralaminar shear stresses, causing intralaminar separation.

9. Describe the course of the spinal nerves in the spine.

At most levels, **dorsal** and **ventral roots** joint to form **spinal nerves** as they enter the intervertebral foramen. The **dorsal root ganglia** are located on the spinal nerve at this point. As spinal nerves exit the intervertebral foramen, they terminate by dividing into **dorsal** and **ventral rami**. Cervical spinal nerves exit above the vertebra of the same number. The C8 spinal nerve emerges between the C7 and T1 vertebrae, which causes all thoracic, lumbar, and sacral nerves to exit below the vertebrae of the same number. Because lower spinal nerves must descend to their intervertebral foramina from their higher point of origin from the spinal cord, they typically occupy the upper portion of their intervertebral foramen.

10. Why do herniated lumbar intervertebral discs commonly miss the nerve that exits at that level and instead affect the next lower spinal nerve roots?

Lumbar intervertebral foramina are large, and because the nerves occupy the upper part of the foramen and the disc is related to the lower part of the foramen, posterolateral disc herniations commonly miss the nerve in the foramen. Instead, they tend to affect the roots of the next lower spinal nerve, which occupy the most lateral part of the spinal canal before exiting from the next lower intervertebral foramen. For example, a herniated L4–5 disc will typically miss the L4 nerve and affect the L5 roots.

11. What are the uncovertebral or Luschka's joints?

The lower five cervical vertebrae contain uncinate processes that protrude cranially from the lateral margins of the superior surface of their bodies. Luschka's joints begin to develop in the second decade of life as degenerative clefts in the lateral part of the intervertebral disc just medial to the uncinate processes. Degeneration begins at this point because it is where the cervical discs are narrowest in their superior-inferior dimension and hence subject to greatest tensile stresses during motion. Hypertrophic degenerative changes can involve Luschka's joints or the posterior portion of the cervical disc, which is the next thinnest part of the disc. Hypertrophic bars developing in the posterior disc can encroach both nerve roots and spinal cord.

12. What are lateral recesses? What is their significance?

Lateral recesses are a normal narrowing of the anteroposterior (AP) dimension of the lateral portion of the spinal canal at the L4, L5, and S1 levels. They occur because the pedicles become shorter in their AP dimension at these levels. This brings the superior articular processes and facet joints close to the posterior aspect of the lateral part of the vertebral bodies. The pedicle forms the lateral wall of the recess.

As the L4–S1 nerve roots descend the spinal canal, they each course through a lateral recess before exiting their intervertebral foramen. When hypertrophic degenerative changes involve the superior articular process, it can reduce the distance between this process and the vertebral body to < 3 mm, producing **lateral stenosis** with the potential for nerve root encroachment. Hypertrophic changes involving the more medially situated inferior articular process will more likely produce a **central stenosis** of the spinal canal. Facet joints also form the posterior boundary of the intervertebral foramen, where hypertrophic changes can produce **foraminal stenosis**.

13. What anatomic and mechanical features of the lumbosacral junction predispose L5 to spondylolysis and spondylolisthesis?

The steep inclined plane of the sacral angle (commonly 50° from horizontal) predisposes the L5 vertebra to slide forward on S1 under a gravitational load. This slippage is resisted by the impaction of the inferior articular processes of L5 against the superior articular processes of the sacrum. These forces and their reactions concentrate substantial shearing stresses on the **pars interarticularis** of the L5 lamina. Hence, **spondylolysis** is most commonly a stress fracture. Whether a **spondylolisthesis** develops depends on the ability of the intervertebral disc, anterior longitudinal ligament, and iliolumbar ligaments to resist anterior displacement of the L5 vertebral body.

14. Are the deep back muscles contracted or relaxed in the upright position?

In the upright position, the spine is in relatively good equilibrium because the line of gravity falls through the points of inflection of each of the curves of the spine. As a result, activity in the major deep back muscles (erector spinae, semispinalis, multifidus, and rotators) is negligible, and the ligaments of the spine resist any applied moments.

15. Which muscles are responsible for producing the major spine motions?

Flexion—The **anterior abdominal muscles** initiate flexion, but as soon as the spine is out of equilibrium, gravity becomes the prime mover under the control of an eccentric contraction of the **deep back muscles**. A concentric contraction of the deep back muscles returns the spine to an upright position.

Extension—Spinal extension is initiated by the **deep back muscles**, with gravity becoming the prime mover as soon as the spine is out of equilibrium. The **anterior abdominal muscles** control gravity with an eccentric contraction and return the spine to an upright position with a concentric contraction.

Lateral bending—Lateral bending is initiated by the ipsilateral **deep back, abdominal, psoas major**, and **quadratus lumborum** muscles. Once started, gravity becomes the prime mover under the control of eccentric contraction of the same muscles on the contralateral side, which also contract concentrically to return the spine to the upright position.

Rotation—Rotation of the front of the trunk to one side is produced by the ipsilateral **erector spinae** and **internal abdominal oblique** muscles and the contralateral **deeper back** muscles and **external abdominal oblique**. Rotation of the face to one side is also produced by the ipsilateral **splenius**, contralateral **sternocleidomastoid**, and other **cervical rotators**.

16. What do dorsal rami of spinal nerves innervate?

Dorsal rami innervate the skin of the medial two-thirds of the back from the interauricular line to the coccyx (top of the head to the tip of the tail), deep muscles of the back, posterior ligaments of the spine, and the facet joint capsules.

UPPER LIMB

17. What structure provides the strongest support for the acromioclavicular joint?

The **coracoclavicular ligament**, which descends from the distal clavicle to the coracoid process. This ligament must be torn to produce the major stepdown of the acromion below the clavicle in grade 3 acromioclavicular joint injuries.

18. What structural features cause the shoulder (glenohumeral) joint to be a highly mobile but relatively unstable joint?

The relatively poor bony congruence between the glenoid and humeral head and a slack capsule.

19. What dynamic features help maintain shoulder joint contact through the full range of abduction?

The **rotator cuff muscles** stabilize the shoulder by varying their medially directed vector forces. In early abduction, the **deltoid** tends to sublux the humeral head superiorly. This is offset by increased tension in the superior capsule by the simultaneous contraction of the **supraspinatus** and by the slightly downward vector pull of the **subscapularis, infraspinatus**, and **teres minor** muscles. In the middle range of abduction, the **subscapularis** turns off to allow the **infraspinatus** and **teres major** to externally rotate the humerus and bring the greater tubercle posteriorly under the acromion (which is the highest part of the coracoacromial arch). This prevents its impingement against the arch.

20. How does medial and lateral winging of the scapula occur?

The medial border of the scapula is normally kept closely applied to the thoracic wall by the resultant vector forces of its medially and laterally tethering muscles, the **trapezius** and **serratus anterior**. If the serratus anterior is paralyzed, the medial border will wing away from the chest wall and be displaced medially by the unopposed retraction of the trapezius (medial winging). If the trapezius is paralyzed, the medial border will also wing but will be displaced laterally by the unopposed protraction of the serratus anterior (lateral winging).

21. What are the two major "crutch-walking" muscles of the shoulder?

The upward vector force of the crutches at the shoulder is primarily offset by the downward pull of the **pectoralis major** and **latissimus dorsi** muscles acting on the humerus.

22. Why is the elbow a relatively stable joint?

The trochlear notch of the ulna has a good grip on the humeral trochlea, and there are strong, relatively taut radial and ulnar collateral ligaments.

23. Where is the axis for pronation and supination of the forearm located?

Proximally, it passes through the center of the radial head; distally, it passes through the ulnar head. Hence, during pronation and supination, the radius scribes half a cone in space about the ulna.

24. How are major loads transferred from the radius at the wrist to the ulna at the elbow?

They are transferred across the **interosseous membrane**, whose fibers run primarily from the ulna upward to the radius. Hence, loads ascending the radius will tense this membrane and be transferred to the ulna.

WRIST AND HAND

25. Which carpal bones are most frequently injured?

The major weight-bearing carpal bones are most frequently injured: the **scaphoid** by a neck fracture and the **lunate** with a palmar dislocation. In one-third of scaphoid fractures, there is nonunion, because about one-third of scaphoids receive a blood supply only to their distal end. The lunate tends to dislocate palmarly during hyperextension injuries, because it is wedge-shaped with the apex of the wedge pointing dorsally.

26. Why doesn't carpal tunnel syndrome cause sensory abnormalities over the palm?

The palmar cutaneous branch of the median nerve passes superficial to the flexor retinaculum.

27. How can the flexor digitorum profundus be eliminated in order to test the flexor digitorum superficialis tendons in isolation?

To test the ability of the flexor digitorum superficialis to flex the proximal interphalangeal (PIP) joint of a finger, hold the rest of the fingers into forcible hyperextension by resistance over the distal phalanges. This is effective because the individual tendons of the profundus generally arise from a common tendon that attaches to its muscle mass, whereas each of the tendons of the superficialis has its own separate muscle belly. Hence, placing the other fingers into extension puts all of the profundus under stretch and eliminates it as a PIP joint flexor.

28. How can the extensor digitorum be eliminated to isolate and test the extensor indicis as the last muscle innervated by the radial nerve?

The extensor indicis is tested by metacarpophalangeal (MP) joint extension of the index finger with the other fingers held in flexion at their MP joints. This is effective because the tendons of the extensor digitorum are cross-linked over the dorsum of the hand by intertendinous connections. Therefore, if the rest of the tendons are pulled distally over their MP joints by forcible flexion, it tethers the tendon to the index finger distally and makes the extensor digitorum ineffective as an index finger MP joint extensor.

29. Why are the motions of the thumb at right angles to the similar motions of the fingers?

In the resting hand, the thumb is internally rotated 90° relative to the fingers. Hence, flexion and extension of the thumb occur in a plane parallel to the plane of the palm, and abduction and adduction of the thumb occur at right angles to the plane of the palm, with the thumb moving away from the palm in abduction and toward the palm in adduction. Opposition involves almost 90° of further internal rotation of the thumb at its carpometacarpal joint.

30. What is the normal digital balance mechanism of the fingers?

At the MP joint, there is one extensor, the extensor digitorum (though there is an additional extensor of the index and little fingers), balanced against four flexors: the interossei, lumbrical, and flexor digitorum profundus and superficialis. At the PIP joint, there are three extensors (interossei and the lumbrical and extensor digitorum) balanced against two flexors (flexor digitorum profundus and superficialis). At the distal interphalangeal (DIP) joint, there are three extensors—interossei and the lumbrical and extensor digitorum—balanced against one flexor, flexor digitorum profundus. The muscles contributing to the extensor balance form an extensor hood mechanism, which splits into lateral and central bands over the PIP joint, with the central band inserting into the base of the middle phalanx and the lateral bands inserting into the base of the distal phalanx. Over the PIP joint, all three bands are connected by the **triangular membrane**, which holds the lateral bands in their normal dorsal position. An **oblique retinacular ligament of Landsmeer** splits off the lateral bands to tether them ventrally to the proximal phalanx.

LOWER LIMB

31. What structural features make the hip a relatively stable joint?

1. Good congruence between the femoral head and the deeply concave acetabulum, which with its labrum forms more than half a sphere.

2. Strong capsular ligaments, two of which—the iliofemoral and ischiofemoral ligaments— are maximally taut in the extended upright position (the usual weight-bearing position).

32. What are the unique features of the hip joint capsule and its blood supply? What is their clinical significance?

The anterior hip joint capsule attaches to the **intertrochanteric line of the femur**, thereby completely enclosing the anterior femoral neck. The posterior capsule encloses the proximal two-thirds of the femoral neck. Therefore, the femoral head and most of the femoral neck are intracapsular. This has two clinically important effects. First, it requires that most of the blood supply to the femoral head (mostly from the **medial femoral circumflex artery**) must ascend the femoral neck. Hence, except for the small branch of the obturator artery that enters the head with the ligament of the femoral head (ligamentum teres), most of the blood supply to the femoral head is compromised by femoral neck fractures. Second, because the capsule attaches to the femoral neck so low, the upper femoral metaphysis is intracapsular. Because the metaphysis is the most vascular part of a long bone, hematogenously spread infection to the upper femoral metaphysis can easily produce a septic arthritis. In most other joints, the metaphyses are extracapsular.

33. Even though the long, obliquely situated femoral neck predisposes the hip to high shearing forces and fracture, are there any physiologic advantages to this unique design?

The long, obliquely situated femoral neck has the salutary effect of displacing the greater trochanter farther from the abduction-adduction axis of the femoral head, thereby lengthening the moment arm of the gluteus medius and minimus muscles. In standing on one leg, the gravitational vector acting on the adduction side of the hip joint is on a moment arm approximately three times as long as the gluteus medius and minimus moment arm. Therefore, these muscles have to produce a force approximately three times as great as the gravitational vector to offset the hip adduction tendency. If the femoral neck were any shorter or more vertically oriented, as in a valgus hip, the gluteus medius and minimus moment arm would be shortened, requiring these muscles to apply more force to offset the gravitational vector. The long moment arm of the normal femoral neck thereby reduces the loads across the hip and helps protect the hip from degenerative arthritis.

34. What is the best way to test the right gluteus medius and minimus muscles?

Ask the patient to stand on the right leg. If these muscles are weak or paralyzed, the left side of the pelvis will sag under the influence of the gravitational adduction vector (Trendelenburg sign).

35. At what point in the gait cycle is the gluteus maximus most active? Why?

At heel strike of the ipsilateral limb. This offsets the effect of the ground reaction vector, which acts anterior to the hip at this point and therefore tends to cause the trunk to flex on the thigh.

36. When is the iliopsoas most active during the gait cycle? Why?

At **toe-off**, the iliopsoas acts as a hip flexor to offset the ground reaction vector, which is then acting posterior to the hip to cause hip extension.

37. Why is the knee joint most stable in extension?

1. Because the anterior portion of the femoral condyle is less curved than the posterior condyle, the congruence and area of contact between the **femoral** and **tibial condyles** are greatest in extension. Hence, the pressures acting across the knee are lowest in extension.

2. The **tibial** and **fibular collateral ligaments** are maximally taut in extension.

3. The **anterior cruciate ligament** is completely tense only in extension.

38. Why are the gastrocnemius and soleus muscles the most active lower limb muscles in standing?

In quiet standing, the line of gravity falls slightly behind the hip joint, slightly anterior to the knee, and 2 inches anterior to the ankle joint axis. At the hip, the tendency of the line of gravity to hyperextend the hip is resisted by the tension in the iliofemoral (and ischiofemoral) ligaments. Therefore, hip flexor muscle activity is generally unnecessary. The line of gravity tends to hyperextend the knee, and tension in the posterior capsule probably helps resist this. However, the activity in the gastrocnemius muscle, which is primarily to stabilize the ankle, also helps prevent back-knee. At the ankle, the long moment arm of the line of gravity makes it a strong ankle dorsiflexor. The activity in the gastrocnemius and soleus muscles resists this ankle dorsiflexion tendency.

FOOT AND ANKLE

39. What is the most osteologically stable position of the ankle? Why?

Dorsiflexion. Both the talar trochlea and tibiofibular mortise have wedge-shaped articular surfaces that are wide anteriorly and narrow posteriorly. In dorsiflexion, the wide anterior part of the talar trochlea is wedged back into the narrow posterior part of the tibiofibular mortise.

40. At what joint does most of the pronation and supination of the foot occur?

The subtalar joint permits most of the pronation (eversion) and supination (inversion) of the foot, but the transverse tarsal and tarsometatarsal joints also contribute.

41. When are the ankle dorsiflexor muscles active during gait?

The ankle dorsiflexors are active isometrically during swing to prevent gravity from causing foot-drop and eccentrically from heel strike to flat foot (the loading response) to control the plantar flexion vector exerted on the calcaneus by the ground reaction.

42. Which nerve of the foot is homologous to the median nerve in the hand?

The medial plantar nerve. It generally supplies the plantar skin of the medial two-thirds of the foot and medial three and one-half digits, the intrinsic muscles of the great toe except for the adductor hallucis, the first lumbrical, and the flexor digitorum brevis (homologous to the flexor digitorum superficialis of the upper limb). The lateral plantar nerve is also homologous to the ulnar nerve.

BIBLIOGRAPHY

1. Bland JH, Boushey DR: Anatomy and physiology of the cervical spine. Semin Arthritis Rheum 20:1–20, 1990.
2. Cailliet R: Low Back Pain Syndrome. Philadelphia, F.A. Davis, 1995.
3. Hayashi K, Yabuki T: Origin of the uncus and of Luschka's joint in the cervical spine. J Bone Joint Surg 67A:788–791, 1985.
4. Inman VT, Saunders JB, Abbott LC: Observations on the function of the shoulder joint. J Bone Joint Surg 26A:1–30, 1944.
5. Johnson RM, Crelin ES, White AA, et al: Some newer observations on the functional anatomy of the lower cervical spine. Clin Orthop 111:192–200, 1975.
6. Schneck CD: Clinical anatomy of the cervical spine. In White AH, Schofferman JA (eds): Spine Care. St. Louis, Mosby, 1995, pp 1306–1334.
7. Schneck CD: Functional and clinical anatomy of the spine. Spine State Art Rev 9:1–37, 1995.
8. Turek SL: Orthopedics: Principles and Their Application. Philadelphia, J.B. Lippincott, 1984, pp 1123–1126.

II. Caring for People with Disabilities

8. COMMUNICATION STRATEGIES FOR REHABILITATION PROFESSIONALS: Disability Etiquette and Empowerment

Margaret G. Stineman, M.D., Susan M. Miller, M.D., Harlan Hahn, Ph.D., and Steven A. Stiens, M.D., M.S.

We reject the idea that institutions must be created to "care" for us and proclaim that these institutions have been used to "manage" us in ways that non-disabled people are not expected to accept. We reject the notion that we need "experts" to tell us how to live, especially experts from the able-bodied world. We are not diagnoses in need of a cure... We are human, with human dreams and ambitions.

—J. R. Woodward, *A Disabled Manifesto*

1. How and why is communication important?

The establishment of a patient-physician relationship requires interest and sensitivity. Effective listening and perceptive questioning lead to knowledge of the patient as a person. Each person has a unique experience and perspective of disablement. Understanding that perspective is essential for collaborative rehabilitation goal-setting. Maximum success is accomplished by designing a rehabilitation plan that leads to functional and social outcomes in a sequence that empowers the patient to be independent in accomplishing his or her broader life goals. Thus, regardless of disability, whenever possible, speak directly to the patient as a person rather than through any family or companion who is present. It is essential to hear and formulate an understanding of the patient as a person living with disablement. This evolving experience must be validated by the rehabilitation team.

2. What is the independent living movement?

The **independent living movement** was developed primarily by young people with disabilities wanting to be respected as equal members of society. Disability is experienced more as an environmental problem than a personal one. The most pervasive environmental barriers are the attitudinal. People with disabilities have been viewed as pathetic helpless victims deserving of charity or as less, useless to society. Pervasive attitudes of this nature led to the independent living movement which is exemplified by the *Disabled Manifesto* at the beginning of this chapter.

Like the civil rights and equal rights movements of the 1960s, the independent living movement in the 1970s has led to major changes in the way people with disabilities are viewed. For example, passage of the Americans with Disabilities Act (ADA) gives people with disabilities rights to pursue and participate in socially meaningful activities. It is essential at all times to recognize the individuality and humanity of the person over the disability. The dignity of persons with disability must be honored at all times. People with disabilities must be integrated into society as self-determining contributors.

3. Why do some people with disability object to being referred to as "patients"?

A number of individuals with disability do not like to be called "patients." They believe the word inherently implies too much passivity and subordination. Some also believe that the concept of being "a patient " permanently confines them to the "sick role." The sick role, as defined by Parsons, involves people's exemption from ordinary social obligations in exchange for the promise that they will follow medical directives without questions and devote themselves exclusively to the goal of "getting well." Most disabilities are, almost by definition, permanent and getting well, if it implies cure, is not always a realistic objective.

Yet there does not appear to be an obvious alternative choice to the word *patient*. The terms of *consumer* and *client* have been suggested as substitution but people who see clinicians are much more than consumers and clients of professional services and interventions. The controversy about the "patient" terminology within the disability community is a wake-up call to health professionals. It is not the word that is offensive, but rather the demeaning attitudes of some practitioners that have resulted from the medical mystique or traditional power structure.

4. What are some special issues with regard to communicating with people with life-long disabilities?

People who have life-long disabilities have the opportunity to integrate fundamental disablement experiences into their self-concept. They also have the benefit of an entire lifetime of sharpening their skills. Those who become involved in the independent living movement and its historic endeavor to extend and expand the definition of civil rights can gain a strong cultural self-identity as being a member of that community. Some people accept their disabilities as just one of the many traits that determine who they are.

Yet, they remain at a potential disadvantage by never having the exposure to any number of typical experiences that people without disabilities experience routinely. However, their unique experiences of life with disablement can result in creative perspectives that may escape the attention of others experiencing the world lived as able bodied. Most have difficulty living fully in a society designed for those with average capacity. Nevertheless, if disability is regarded as an experience rather than a source of pathology, it can provide a different perspective that can be enriching and innovative.

5. What are some special issues in communicating with the person who becomes disabled in later life?

People with disabilities are a minority that anyone is eligible to join at any time. Membership becomes more likely as people age. Loss of function and perceived loss of stature in society can be issues for those with new-onset disabilities in later life. Fortunately, people who become disabled later in life have the benefit of knowing how society works and have had the opportunity to develop their social skill sets as able-bodied people. Yet, they carry the burden of knowing what it is like to live without disability. The process of facing and living with the real and often extreme changes in their lives can be empowering, overwhelming, or depressing. The health professional through his or her communications with the individual has the opportunity to lead them toward empowerment and away from more self-destructive feelings.

6. Discuss the reactions and expectations that patients and doctors have for one another in the patient-doctor relationship.

Two terms from psychoanalysis are used in reflecting on emotions and meanings evoked in the encounters. **Transference** is the term for the patient's projection of feelings, thoughts, and wishes onto the physician or therapist. These are often unconscious and can be evoked by similarities between the practitioner and people in the patient's past or current life. **Countertransference** is the physician or therapist transference of emotional needs, expectations, and feelings about the patient. A thoughtful consideration of the perspectives that patients and practitioners may have is often helpful in guiding the therapeutic relationship toward the most successful patient outcome.

7. What about environmental accessibility for people using wheelchairs or other types of mobility aids?

Not only the ADA but also many state statutes compel physicians, businesses, and other institutions to obey the law by providing an accessible environment. Hence, office accessibility is a matter of compliance with the law. If the human-made environment is littered with obstacles and barriers that force people with disabilities to remain in their own domiciles, it cannot be truly said that rehabilitation has been fulfilled.

The task of measuring progress in removing or reducing such environmental barriers is a formidable one, and responsibility extends beyond the rehabilitation profession. The specific requirements for environmental modifications or accommodations for people using mobility aides have already been defined by ADA regulations. The ADA does not require accommodation of personal devices, individually prescribed devices, or services of a personal nature to patients. Adjustable-height examination tables, platform or sitting scales, and other accessible features would make the experience of seeking care as comfortable as for those without disabilities. Without these features, patients with disabilities are separated out and can receive less thorough evaluation and treatment.

8. How should I talk with a person with a new disability who needs to use a wheelchair or other type of visible equipment?

Some health professionals loath discussing need for a wheelchair with its symbolism of infirmity and loss. Loosing the ability to stand and walk is a deeply personal loss. Rehabilitation clinicians need to be familiar with the advantages and disadvantages of various types of wheelchairs, assistive technology, and durable equipment so that they can make the most appropriate recommendations given the individual's types of functional limitations, energy, living environment, and life requirements and goals. Furthermore, this permits a presentation of the wheelchair as an adaptive tool used to meet patient life goals. Never assume that a person once seated is comfortable, physically or psychologically. When a wheelchair is the wrong size, without adequate back supports, padding or appropriate seat angle sitting in it even briefly can be agonizing. Careful fitting is imperative. Choice of color and accessories that complement the person's wardrobe and personality makes the wheelchair a logical and aesthetic extention of the person. The appropriate wheelchair can open life to new possibilities, give tremendous relief, and provide a wonderfully liberating feeling to a person whose life had become restricted.

9. How can I communicate effectively with a person using a wheelchair?

Remember, people who use wheelchairs live below the eye level of average-sized standing adults. Even positioned in the full view of others, those with disabilities are commonly ignored. Communication is facilitated by being at the person's eye level. Sitting down goes a long way in establishing contact. People without disabilities need to be conscious of their gait speed while accompanying a person using crutches or a manual wheelchair.

10. If you believe a person with physical disabilities may need help getting into your office, undressing, or getting onto your examination table, how should you approach this need?

Apologize for limitations in accessibility. Ask the individual if they would like some help. Put them in charge; empower them and enable them. Respect the person's answers. People with physical disabilities are sometimes touched by well-meaning strangers without warning. Unless the circumstance clearly warrants quick action to avoid injury, do not provide physical assistance unexpectedly to a person who you think needs help who is already walking or standing. Grabbing an arm suddenly could cause the person to lose balance and fall. Never assume that a person needs help just because he or she has some visible physical disabilities.

11. What are some common pitfalls in examining and caring for people who use wheelchairs?

People with disabilities do not always consult health professionals for reasons related to their disabilities. Real problems arise when the attention of the physician is diverted by the presence of the disability. In some cases, physicians may mistakenly attempt to treat the disability rather than the presenting signs or symptoms for which patients are seeking medical attention. As a result, there is a danger that the signs and symptoms of routine health problems can be ignored or neglected. Moreover, physicians are trained to make quick observations. Disabilities can lead to physiological changes that may confound the interpretation of studies or affect outcomes. Disabilities can also affect persons' abilities to communicate. Thus, a lot can be missed with quick observation. It is important not to make assumptions about function, personality, or character based only on physical appearances.

Doing an examination while a patient remains in a wheelchair can lead to a suboptimal pulmonary, abdominal, musculoskeletal, and neurologic assessment compared to a person who is disrobed and on an examining table. Determining the degree to which the person is able to stand, walk, and move around on the examination table is an essential part of the examination. Of course, if the patient has serious mobility difficulties take appropriate safety precautions. Ask the individual who is using a wheelchair if he or she is able to stand and transfer onto the examination table. Determine how much assistance is needed. It is essential to plan transfers carefully. Too often, a diverse collection of inexperienced people are rounded up at the spur of the moment to move patients. It is essential for the rehabilitation professional to receive training in how to transfer patients safely from wheelchair to an examining table or x-ray apparatus. Never move a wheelchair or other walking aid out of the person's reach.

12. What is the "lump syndrome"?

In hospitals, medical equipment, food or laundry carts, and people sitting in wheelchairs or lying on litters are all hauled about and left sitting in corridors for future transport. Never begin pushing patients in wheelchairs or on litters without greeting them and saying where you are taking him or her. Pushing a wheelchair without permission takes away the power of self-direction and may even cause the person to fall forward if the movement is unexpected. Never leave a person sitting somewhere without an explanation. State why you are placing the person. Thoughtful gestures may take little time and go a long way. For example, "I am going to leave you here in the waiting room until transportation comes for you" or "Would you like a magazine to read?" Remember, some people who use wheelchairs are stuck where you leave them. Effective and thoughtful communication is the only way to avoid the lump syndrome.

13. Why must I consider specialized adaptive techniques and equipment in order to achieve a better understanding when communicating with people who live with sensory disabilities?

In order to make a specific diagnosis and provide patient-centered care, it is necessary to glean a rudimentary appreciation of the patient's illness experience and life goals. It is the health care provider's responsibility to make certain that effective communication is established and maintained with all those individuals who are seeking services, receiving services, or responsible for an individual seeking services. So, for example, if the physician's patient is a hearing child, a deaf parent may need an auxiliary aid or service in order to provide or receive information about the child's condition. It is the obligation of the physician's office to provide these aids or services.

According to Title III of the ADA, public accommodations must provide "appropriate auxiliary aids and services where necessary to ensure effective communication with individuals with disabilities." Such aids and services include means by which educational or informational content, normally presented verbally, can be communicated to those with hearing impairments. Similarly, such materials usually delivered by visual methods (i.e., written information) must be otherwise furnished to those with visual impairments.

14. What kind of aids and services are required to be furnished?

Communication accommodations must be offered to those who need them, unless these aids and services represent either an undue burden for "the health care provider" or would "fundamentally alter" the nature of the services being offered. For those with hearing impairments, a few examples of typical aids and services include qualified interpreters, video text displays, exchange of written notes, and telecommunication devices for the deaf. For those with visual impairments, braille and large-print material may be appropriate as well as qualified readers and audio recordings.

The ADA allows the health care provider to choose from a myriad of communication options available, as long as the end result ensures "effective communication" for all patients and families. The expense of accommodation is to be treated as part of the overhead cost of doing business. However, it is expected that health care providers will confer with the individuals who have disabilities and consider their self-appraisals of communication needs before any specific aid or service is obtained for use.

15. How should the office staff and interdisciplinary team provide mobility assistance to a person with visual impairments?

Any staff member in your office who has contact with a visually impaired person should introduce him or herself, because that individual may not be able to recognize faces. Furthermore, all staff members should speak in a normal voice when addressing a visually impaired individual. As with any person who has a disability, staff should always *ask first* if and what kind of assistance is needed. If necessary then, basic sighted guide techniques can be used to assist those with visual impairments through your waiting and exam rooms.

If mobility help is needed, the following techniques can be followed:

1. Inform the visually impaired individual that you will touch his or her hand with the back of your own hand and then ask him/her to take hold of your arm just above the elbow. The individual may take your arm either from its internal or external aspect. You should walk to the side of and approximately half a step in front of the person you are helping (his or her shoulder should be behind yours).

2. If more support is needed, bend your elbow 90° and ask the individual you are helping to grasp onto your forearm. When walking in this manner, the individual should not be behind you, but instead at your side.

3. If you are walking through a room full of people or through a narrow space, move your guide arm to the center of your back, thus directing the visually impaired individual behind you. Ask the person you are guiding to extend the arm by which you are being held to its full length— this prevents you from getting stepped on. If the person you are guiding is too unsteady for this type of positioning, have him or her stand behind you and place one hand on your waist, if necessary changing the arm used to grasp your own.

4. When going through a doorway, position yourself so that the individual whom you are assisting is standing to your side, closest to the door hinges. Ask that person to hold the door open while you advance through it; then guide him/her through. If the individual does not have the strength to hold open the door, hold it open yourself and either guide the person ahead of you or go through the door together if it is sufficiently wide.

5. To help seat a visually impaired person in a chair, guide the individual to it and describe its position. As he or she is facing the chair, place one of the person's hands on its back or armrest and ask him or her to feel the seat with the other hand. Then have the individual turn around and sit down.

16. How should you assist a visually impaired person who uses a mobility aid?

Ask if and how the individual would like to be guided. Many persons prefer a description of the area and wish to find their own way. Others may want to follow the sound of a guiding voice or a voice giving explicit directions (e.g., "turn right here"). If hands-on assistance is requested and the individual uses a cane, walk on the opposite side from this device. If using a walker, the person you are assisting may need only for you to place one of your hands on one of theirs and walk along side. If asked to push a wheelchair, do so—but those who independently use a wheelchair may ask you to guide them by placing your hand on one of their shoulders. Always remember to adjust your pace to that of the equipment user.

17. Are there any other tips to help a visually impaired person be more comfortable in my waiting or exam rooms?

Once you have escorted the individual to his or her final destination, describe the environment and what may be going on in the room. Let the person know if you are leaving and how he or she may access further aid as needed.

18. How can I place a visually impaired individual at ease during an examination?

When entering the room, introduce yourself verbally before touching your patient. Talk to the person directly and use a normal tone of voice. Verbally describe the actions you wish the individual to perform or that you are about to do (being very specific). Name all body parts being examined and all equipment being used. Allow your patient to examine any appropriate pieces of equipment with his/her tactile senses.

19. How can I make it easier for those with visual impairments to complete necessary paperwork as well as to provide them with appropriate written material?

For those with partial sight, high-contrast text makes for more readable material. Light letters (white or light yellow) on a black background may be more easily read than dark letters on a light background, but there are ways of making the latter (the more traditional scheme of printing) legible to those with visual impairments.

Office documents such as brochures and forms are most easily read when they are printed in black and white. Placing a piece of yellow acetate filter over the print or using yellow clip-on filters over the patient's eyeglasses tends to make the print look blacker. For information that is written on-site at the office, use a black bold-tip pen or type the information in capital, double-spaced letters.

Other means of making written materials more legible include using nonglossy paper which can reduce glare. Type should be large (at least 16 to 18 points). Decorative, cursive, italic, and condensed fonts should not be used; Roman and sans serif typefaces may be more readable. Spacing between lines should be at least 25–30% of the point size; spacing between letters should be wide with mono-spaced fonts being chosen preferentially over proportionally spaced fonts. Because many optical devices that make it easier to read for those who are partially sighted work best on flat surfaces, extra-wide margins are useful when preparing written materials as is spiral binding. Clinicians and staff members should not raise their voices when speaking to a vision-impaired patient.

20. How can I make my waiting or exam rooms more accessible and comfortable for those with impaired vision?

Appropriate illumination can be key to the visual abilities of those with partial sight. A flexible-armed or necked lamp can be helpful as it can be positioned for each individual task (e.g., reading, completion of forms) to avoid glare. Modifying a light from a window that is producing a glare is also helpful. Adequate color contrast between furniture and carpeting may help those with visual impairment avoid mobility related accidents. At least a few large-print publications should be provided. In addition, ample space between pieces of furniture should be provided in waiting rooms and examination areas for patients with low vision and wheelchairs.

21. How can my office staff and I communicate more effectively with a person who is hearing impaired?

First, you must capture the attention of the person you wish to speak with. A light tap on the shoulder, or a wave (if the individual has vision) is suggested, before you identify yourself. As you speak, make certain that you face the person squarely and that the light is in front of you, on your face, so that you can be clearly seen. If the person is sitting, sit near them. Keep objects, including your hands, away from your mouth. Mustaches and beards should be well trimmed.

Do not shout; instead talk as naturally as possible. Eliminate background noise as much as possible. Speak clearly, but do not talk in slow motion or overemphasize your words. If a sentence is misunderstood, do not repeat it—rephrase it. If you change topics, inform your listener; and if appropriate, write down vital pieces of information or ask the individual with the hearing loss to repeat what you have said to make certain you have been understood. Remember that a minority of hearing-impaired persons can read lips proficiently. Never have the expectation that spoken messages will be understood. An interpreter or individual who knows sign language may be required. Always have written materials available to describe treatments for common rehabilitation problems.

22. How can I help my patients who wear hearing aids be more comfortable in clinical setting?

It is important to remember that hearing aids do not restore normal hearing—they are merely devices that amplify all sounds, including noise. The hearing-impaired individual must discriminate speech from extraneous sound. To help this process, all background noise should be eliminated. If you have television, music, or radios in your office lobby, or simply a great deal of conversation, staff should move to a quieter area to speak with the patient.

Some individuals who have severe hearing loss wear cochlear implants. It is important to remember that an MRI scan may impart significant damage to the cochlear implant. Unless absolutely critical to the patient's care, other means of obtaining necessary imaging information should be applied. Prior to using diathermy, electroconvulsive shock, ionizing radiation, and electrosurgical instruments, specialists in the field of cochlear implants should be consulted.

23. If a person who is hearing impaired can lip-read, do I need to provide an interpreter?

People with hearing impairments rarely rely on lip-reading alone to exchange important information. When communicating or receiving medical information, you need to consider the use of an interpreter. However, all interpreters are not equally skilled. Interpreters (and those they serve) may speak one of a few different languages. Some interpreters speak **American Sign Language (ASL)**, a form of communication that has grammar and syntax different from the English language. On the other hand, some individuals use **Signed English**, a language that has the same word order as does English. There are also **oral interpreters**, who can articulate words in a specialized manner for those with hearing loss, as well as **cued speech interpreters**, who furnish visual cues to aid lip-reading.

Because there are so many different kinds of communications transmitted and received by those with hearing impairments, it is important to remember the following facts:

1. Written notes back and forth between the health care provider and patient may not be sufficient. Many who are hearing-impaired consider ASL to be their first language. Because this method of communication also has a grammar and syntax different from English, the writing of notes between a person who does and does not understand ASL may not be effective.

2. All individuals with hearing impairments do not necessarily read lips, even if they speak clearly. Particularly in the medical setting, terminology is complex, yet exacting. Lip-reading may not present an effective means of communication between health care provider and patient.

3. It may not be appropriate for family or friends to provide interpreter services. Besides the issues concerning confidentiality of patient information, a family member or friend may not be able to handle the complexity of technical processing nor the emotionality of medical issues necessary to provide effective communication to the patient.

Therefore, when considering those services needed by an individual with a hearing loss, the health care provider is required by the ADA to consult with that person and consider that individual's own self-appraisal of communication needs, including whether or not an interpreter is necessary.

24. Are there other "indirect" methods by which communication can be improved for a person with hearing impairment?

Architectural changes can be made to improve communication. Flashing alarm systems should be considered mandatory. The installation of appropriate sound buffers in selected areas of the office can be extremely helpful to persons with hearing loss or brain injury.

25. Is it possible to sensitize health care professionals to the needs of those with disabilities?

Surprisingly, health care professionals often have negative attitudes towards those with disabilities. Unfortunately, evidence also exist that some physicians with poor attitudes provide a lower level of care to these patients and thus can negatively affect the achievement of medical and rehabilitation goals as well as the success or failure of community reintegration.

Graduate and undergraduate programs in disability studies are emerging in many universities. Much of the impetus for the study of this subject emerged from a "minority-group model" of disability which identifies social and attitudinal discrimination as a problem for people with disabilities that rivals or even eclipses the difficulties produced by their impairments. The best way for clinicians to become familiar with the problems faced by people with disabilities (as well as other oppressed and disadvantaged segments of the population) entails the study of their history, their culture, and the major discriminatory barriers they face. Disability studies is an important component of the curriculum for rehabilitation professionals.

The attitude of medical students about people with disabilities may require some favorable influence. Curricula developed to help students understand the societal, economic as well as medical impact of impairments, limitations in activity (disability) and participation restrictions (handicap) should be presented in the first 2 years. Through disability studies, role playing and exposure to faculty and patients with disabilities a more realistic perspective can develop. Outpatient contact visits with appropriate patients in their community settings further illustrates options for patient adaptations. Then clinical exposure to patients with disabilities undergoing comprehensive rehabilitation can be better understood in the medical context. Exposure to very successful self-actualized people with disabilities helps students set goals with their patients that are not too limiting.

26. How can the health professional help patients feel more comfortable talking about their disabilities?

Patients have been socialized to communicate with their doctors by describing symptoms rather than disabilities. Paradoxically, disabilities or fear of disabilities at times can be viewed as most problematic by the patient. They may fear that professionals see disability as a weakness or they may be afraid of being placed in a nursing home. They may not want to bother the physician or believe that such issues fall outside the usual interest of doctors. Others may avoid health professionals altogether because of unfavorable experiences with the medical profession encountered in childhood or in the immediate aftermath of a disabling accident. Still others may prefer to be seen as strong and self-sufficient, thus choosing to remain silent. The rehabilitation professional can help the patient feel more comfortable about talking about disabilities by being aware of the following.

1. **Recognize the possible biasing effects of medical training.** Pathology-focused training tends to see cure as success and chronic disease and progressive disability as failure. The rehabilitation physician overcomes this bias by assessing the social implications of disability and by making the social, environmental, and functional review of systems an essential component of the medical history and physical examination. The taking of a functional review of systems provides patients with excellent opportunities to openly discuss concerns about their disabilities. It should include ADLs, IADLs, mobility and environmental barriers, and facilitators.

2. **Recognize masked concerns.** Sometimes patients raise issues explicitly—noting difficulty getting out of the house for social occasions or excessive fatigue. Digging deeper, the professional might find that the patient fears falling (because of weakness) or is limited in ambulatory endurance by severe arthritis. Questions that evoke discussions of disability experience shift focus toward life activities and personal goals. Adaptive mobility equipment such as an ambulation aid or a wheelchair might offer a solution. Patient attitudes regarding the use of such devices might be elicited by the question: have you thought of any equipment that might help you meet these challenges away from home? For another example, if a patient was complaining about incontinence, follow-up questioning might acknowledge that it is very difficult to live with. Then ask the patient what has worked and not worked for him or her and why.

3. **Recognize the facilitating role.** The rehabilitation physician should maximize effectiveness by recognizing his or her role as the facilitator of a team of experts. Shortened appointment times, particularly with physicians, force the discussion of acute concerns over long-term ones, creating a vicious cycle that inhibits the discussion of chronic issues that could have a more lasting influence on the quality of the patient's life. Through focus on patient's short and long term goals, the rehabilitation physician is uniquely positioned to help patients improve the quality of their lives. Maintaining a complete problem list and knowing the patient's life passions and aspirations all contribute to a more wholistic approach, even in a short problem focused visit. The realities of physician practice today may leave insufficient time to personally take all problems through to their optimal resolution, making timely referral to other rehabilitation providers essential. Referrals should be made in ways that aid those providers in understanding the patients' viewpoint. An important role is talking with the patient about the outcomes of that referral at the next visit.

27. Why should the physician be concerned about the living arrangements for their patient with disabilities?

Many people with mobility restrictions become virtually "incarcerated" in their own bedrooms because their homes are not accessible. Some are needlessly placed in nursing homes before even exploring the option of creating a first-floor set-up or moving to a ground-floor apartment. Living in an institution or isolated bedroom may deprive the individual of social interactions, undermining health. The physician may assist the patient in recognizing the limitations of their living arrangements and help in seeking the least restrictive living environment.

28. Some people with disabilities use animals (often dogs) to guide them or help with certain tasks. How should the health professional relate to these animals?

Service animals are working and should never be distracted. Never touch or feed the service animal unless invited to do so.

29. What is disability etiquette?

Etiquette refers to being polite and courteous to all people including those with disabilities. Beyond this, disability etiquette puts the humanity of the person first and any disabilities second. The golden rule is: "Do unto the person with disabilities as you would have others do unto you with understanding, sensitivity, and respect for dignity and autonomy." Any disability etiquette principle must be rejected that implies dominance and subordination that is incompatible with the principle of equality. That person has all the same needs for respect, dignity, appreciation, and autonomy as anyone.

When selecting types of medical care, treatment options, and rehabilitation goals, recognize that a person with disabilities, as anyone, should remain master of his or her own life. As physical dependency on others for basic needs increases, it becomes easier to overlook even basic human rights. Social institutions (such as medical institutions) should operate in ways that maximize opportunities for patient and family togetherness, self-direction, and freedom while minimizing the restrictiveness of the environment. Good etiquette respects the rights for personal freedom and avoids judgment. Principles of good communication with people who have disabilities hold to the same principles as communication with anyone.

30. What is appropriate terminology for communication with or about people with disabilities?

The language we use and the images we promote through that language mirror attitudes we have toward particular groups of people. There is power in naming. When communicating with or about people with disabilities, most (but not all people with disabilities) argue that it is essential to use **person-first language** and to avoid focusing on the disability before recognizing the whole person. Saying a person with a disability or who uses a wheelchair recontextualizes the relationship rather than defining the person with these characteristics. Also, avoid using "normal" as the opposite of disabled. "Normal" implies that people with disabilities are not normal. Use "nondisabled" or "persons without disabilities." Disability concepts and language used to describe it are evolving. Some people with disabilities proclaim that disability is "the most important" part of their life and that they are "proud to be disabled." In many medical settings, the focus is on aspects of the disability for treatment. Special effort must be taken to avoid allowing those characteristics to eclipse the person that is the patient.

Person-first Terminology

POOR TERMS	BETTER TERMS	EXPLANATION
Cerebral-palsied	Has cerebral palsy	Use person-first, nonemotional language that describes the condition.
Cripple	Has a disability	
Invalid	Has paralysis *or* is paralyzed	
Lame	Person with spinal curvature	
Paralytic	Is deaf	
Hunchback		
Deaf and dumb		*Table continued on following page*

Person-first Terminology (Continued)

POOR TERMS	BETTER TERMS	EXPLANATION
Wheelchair bound Wheelchair confined Home bound Home confined	Uses a wheelchair Is limited by barrieres outside the home	Wheelchairs are liberating to people who have severe walking impairments. People are not tied to the device. Homes should be places of refuge and hopefully comfort.
Physically challenged	Has a limitation in activity	"Physically challenged" implies that people are made stronger by having to overcome barriers. People should not be subjected to unnecesary barriers. Communities (and physicians) should be committed to identifying and removing them. The terms *disabled* and *handicapped* are still accepted by many but are being replaced by more neutral terms. Avoid "tragic" but "brave" and "courageous" stereotypes. Emphasize abilities, but do not describe successful people with disabilities as "superhuman."
Afflicted Victim	Simply state that the person has a particular condition	Avoid terms that imply serious misfortune and emotional disability.

31. What is "the shock response"? How can the health professional guard against this normal response to unusual pathology?

The shock response occurs when the professional is distracted by the most visible or unusual aspects of the patient's physical presentation. This can eclipse recognition of symptoms, signs, and other patient attributes that could potentially contribute to the best outcome. In rehabilitation, this may lead to an aberrant focus on the most visible aspects of disability rather than those features of disablement that are most life-limiting for the patient. We must remember that our interactions and reactions to patients are potent influences on their body images and self-perceptions.

The best ways to avoid the shock response is to listen to the patient, look at all aspects of the presentation, seek guidance when needed, and always start with addressing the same fundamentals as in any patient. Another way to guard against the shock response is to bring any hostile or negative feelings toward the disability to the surface. Many nondisabled persons, especially health professionals, may resist the suggestion that they might harbor adverse or hostile emotions. By confronting and analyzing such feelings directly, rehabilitation professionals might be able to prevent them from emerging inadvertently in their interactions with patients.

32. What are "turn-offs" and invalidating statements? How can they be avoided?

Invalidating statements arise from partial truths, where the physician judges (prejudges) the patient through the misuse of general medical information. With invalidating statements, nonspecific medical knowledge is used in ways that are insensitive or distorted or that fail to address the full circumstances of the patient's life. The "turn-off" occurs after the physician has alienated or embarrassed the patient in a way that he or she no longer wants to communicate about an important issue or need.

One of the most common forms the invalidating statements relates to some physician's belief and verbal or non-verbal implications that wheelchair use is always a sign of patient incapacity and physician failure and needs to be put off for as long as possible. The partial truth is that by giving in to an appliance, the person will become weakened. It is clearly important for a person with some remaining walking ability to maintain it. Part-time use of a wheelchair or other ambulatory aide (depending on life demands) may enhance function, increase opportunities for participation, and prolong productivity. In many cases, powered mobility is liberating. The rehabilitation physician emphasizes function over form.

An additional source of invalidating statements and turn offs may emerge from the behavior of physicians' imposing their authority during the aftermath of a disabling incident in a way that indicates that they are taking complete control of the patient's life. Such perceptions may be reinforced by prolonged periods of hospitalization or institutionalization. Some disabled patients feel like "guinea pigs." To minimize these feelings, clinicians need to be especially mindful to return choice and autonomy to patients as soon as they are able to make decisions for themselves.

It is also essential to avoid excessively dire predictions. Ed Roberts, founder of the disability movement, often told the story that when he was diagnosed with polio, he was told that he would "never be anything more than a vegetable." He would frequently add, "So I want you to know that today I feel like a turnip."

Invalidation also occurs when the physician has a faulty perception of how a disease is influencing a person's abilities or makes a broad generalization and then expresses it in a way that causes the patient to have nagging and inappropriate self-doubts. Invalidation is a conversation stopper. One example is attributing a legitimately cheerful mood to the "inappropriate euphoria of MS."

Avoid invalidation by using medical knowledge to affirm the patient. This requires creativity, the ability to listen, and the ability to see beyond medical aspects to the humanity of the person. It is essential to use medical knowledge to empower and not to tear down the patient. Avoid conflicts with the patient that pit "medical knowledge" against the patient's "knowledge of him- or herself." Again, see the person as separate from the processes of his or her diseases and disabilities. Disability is not the same as being sick and incapacitated.

33. What are some issues in the medical mainstream that are resisted, even feared, by some people with disabilities?

Physicians and other health professionals need to be aware that some people with disabilities have values which cause them to refuse efforts to eliminate functional impairments. Individuals with hearing impairments, for example, may resist cochlear implants because they regard such interventions as a threat to the preservation of their deaf culture. Hence, physicians must refrain from becoming too aggressive in promoting treatments that seem logical scientifically and functionally but are not desired by the patient.

People with disabilities resent and fear concepts such as **disability-adjusted life years**, which suggest that each year of life with a disability is of less value than a year without a disability. In multiple studies clinicians consistently underestimate the quality of life that their patients report. For similar reasons, many people with disabilities are concerned about policies of assisted suicide, fearing that those policies pose a disproportionate threat to people with disabilities.

34. What is empowerment medicine?

Empowerment medicine is person-first medicine. The empowerment process seeks to enhance patients' potential for interaction with the environment by maximally restoring personal function through medical and rehabilitation practices, by expanding access to the environment through assistive technology, and by removing physical, attitudinal, societal, and legal barriers. The restoration of personal function and environmental enhancement should occur simultaneously and in harmony. While emphasis on pathology and its treatment remains essential to the medical management of acute injury and illness, such an approach is too narrow for chronic disabilities.

Admittedly, health professionals are not adequately trained in medical and professional schools in environmental issues. Yet, there is no reason why education about environmental concerns can not occur during primary training or continue after graduation. When clinicians ask patients with disabilities routinely about barriers in their own homes and neighborhoods, descriptive evidence of these barriers becomes available for presentation to local policy-makers and even publication. Such information must be brought forth by professionals on behalf of people with disabilities in efforts to yield positive change at the community level.

Clinical and environmental concerns necessarily go hand in hand in the field of rehabilitation. To pursue one of these objectives without the other can only yield outcomes that are intrinsically incomplete. To practice empowerment medicine, the rehabilitation professional first must have a solid foundation in evidence-based practices. Next the clinician needs familiarity with a basic disability studies bibliography and to remain current with prominent disability issues as reported in magazines such as *Mouth, New Mobility,* and *Ragged Edge.* Knowledge of disability studies will enhance clinical skills, forge a deeper connection with patients, and make it possible for health professions to recommend readings to people with disabilities that can provide valuable sources of meaning and purpose to their lives.

ACKNOWLEDGMENT

The authors wish to thank Ms. Nicholle N. M. de Leon for her contributions to this manuscript.

BIBLIOGRAPHY

1. Batavia IA: Independent living centers, medical rehabilitation and managed care for people with disabilities. Arch Phys Med Rehabil 80:1357–1360, 1999.
2. Cohen J: Disability Etiquette. Jackson Heights, NY, Eastern Paralyzed Veterans Association, 1998.
3. DeJong G: Health care reform and disability: Affirming our commitment to community. Arch Phys Med Rehabil 74:1017–1024, 1993.
4. Glick PB: Communication Access: Everyone's Right: A Handbook for Meeting Planners, Conference Site Managers and People Who are Deaf or Hard of Hearing. Jackson Heights, NY, Eastern Paralyzed Veterans Association, 1998.
5. Grabois EW, Nosek MA, Rossi CD: Accessibility of primary care physicians' offices for people with disabilities: An analysis of compliance with the Americans with Disabilities Act. Arch Fam Med 8:44–51, 1999.
6. Hahn H: An agenda for citizens with disabilities: Pursuing identity and empowerment. J Voc Rehabil 9:31–37, 1977.
7. Iezzoni LI: When walking fails. JAMA 276:1609–1613, 1996.
8. Iezzoni LI: What should I say? Communication around disability. Ann Intern Med 129:661-665, 1998.
9. Messiah College: Disability-related language [on-line]. Grantham, PA, Messiah College, 1999. Available: http://www.messiah.edu/disability/terms.htm.
10. Murray CJ: Quantifying the burden of disease: the technical basis for disability-adjust life years. Bull World Health Org 72:429–445, 1994.
11. Nagler M (ed): Perspectives on Disability, 2nd ed. Palo Alto, CA, Health Markets Research, 1993.
12. National Center for Law and Deafness: ADA Questions and Answers for Health Care Providers. Washington, DC, Gallaudet University [800 Florida Avenue, NE, Washington, DC 20002-3695].
13. Nosek MA: Women with disabilities and the delivery of empowerment medicine. Arch Phys Med Rehabil 78:S1–S2, 1997.
14. Parsons T: The sick role and the role of the physician reconsidered. Milbank Mem Fund Q Health Soc 53:257–258, 1975.
15. Stiens SA: Personhood, disablement, and mobility technology: Personal control of development. In Gray DB, Quantrano LA, Liberman M (eds): Designing and Using Assistive Technology: The Human Perspective. Towson, MD, Paul Brookes, 1998, pp 29–49.
16. Stineman MG: Medical humanism and empowerment medicine. Disabil Stud Q 20:11–16, 2000.
17. Stineman MG: The spheres of self-fulfilment: A multidimensional approach to the assessment of assistive technology outcomes. In Gray DB, Quatrano LA, Lieberman ML (eds): Designing and Using Assistive Technology. The Human Perspective. Baltimore, Paul H. Brookes Publishing Co., 1998, pp 54–74.
18. Stineman MG: Defining the population, treatments, and outcomes of interest: Reconciling the rules of biology with meaningfulness. Am J Rehabil Med 80:147–159, 2001.
19. Tate DG, Rasmussen L, Maynard F: Hospital to community: A collaborative medical rehabilitation and independent living program. J Applied Rehabil Counseling 23:18–21, 1992.
20. United Nations ESCAP: Asian Pacific Decade of Disabled Persons, 1993–2002. Using the Correct Terminology 1999 [on-line]. Available: http://www.unescap.org/decade/terminology.htm.
21. U.S. Access Board: ADA Accessibility Guidelines for Buildings and Facilities (ADAAG), as amended through January 1998. Available on-line at http://www.access-board.gov.
22. Woodward JR: A Disabled Manifesto. Available on line at http://www.empowermentzone.com/manifest.txt.
23. World Health Organization: International Classification of Functioning, Disability and Health. Final Draft, Full version. (ICIDH-2). Geneva, WHO, 2001.
24. World Health Organization: International Classification of Impairments, Disabilities, and Handicaps.
25. Young MA, Morgan SB: Strategies for fostering communication between physician and patients with siabilities. Wis Med J 96:36–37, 1997.

9. REHABILITATION OF PATIENTS WITH SEVERE VISUAL IMPAIRMENTS OR BLINDNESS

Stanley F. Wainapel, M.D., M.P.H.

1. Is vision rehabilitation relevant to physiatric practice?

Vision loss is one of the most common causes of functional disability among adults, and its impact on mobility, activities of daily living (ADLs), or both is often profound. Moreover, severe vision impairment is likely to be a frequent concomitant of the conditions traditionally treated by physiatrists—i.e., stroke, amputation, hip fractures—and has been seen in 7% of patients admitted to an inpatient rehab unit. Maximizing visual perception is one component of a plan to maximize adaptive compensational outcome. Finally, in an environment where primary care is a favored model of medical management, it would be wise for physiatrists to have basic knowledge of the treatment of this highly prevalent sensory impairment.

2. What are common causes of visual impairment?

Among the elderly (those at highest risk for such problems), four conditions dominate all other etiologies of vision impairment:

Common Causes of Visual Impairment Among the Elderly

	AGE		
	< 65 YR (%)	65–75 YR (%)	75+ YR (%)
Senile cataracts	2.6	9.6	33.7
Glaucoma	0.7	1.7	2.9
Diabetic retinopathy	1.1	1.7	3.0
Macular degeneration	0.6	4.1	15.4

Adapted from Morse A, Friedman D: Vision rehabilitation and aging. J Vis Impair Blind 80:803–804, 1986.

Among young and middle-aged adults, **diabetic retinopathy** is the most frequent cause of vision loss, with diseases such as retinitis pigmentosa also beginning to assume greater importance. In children, congenital disorders (**cataract**) and disorders related to prematurity or neurologic disease (retinopathy of prematurity, cortical vision loss following anoxia or CNS infection) are among the more frequent etiologies.

3. How are visual impairments described and classified?

Visual impairment is usually described as **central** (visual acuity) or **peripheral** (visual field) deficits. Central deficits are either discrete (e.g., scotomas) or diffuse (e.g., lens opacity). Peripheral deficits are described as concentric (loss of peripheral vision resulting in "tunnel vision," as in retinitis pigmentosa or glaucoma) or central (retention of peripheral fields only, as in age-related macular degeneration). Visual impairment can also be classified in terms of its severity—i.e., legal blindness or low vision.

Legal blindness was defined by the Social Security Act of 1935 as:

1. Visual acuity of 20/200 or less in the better eye despite use of corrective lenses, or
2. Visual field of $\leq 20°$ in the better eye.

This arbitrary definition includes many people with some residual vision (only 15% of those who are legally blind are actually totally blind by virtue of having no light perception), and it unfortunately excludes many people with significant vision problems. These latter individuals are described as having **low vision**, which is usually defined as corrected visual acuity of less than

20/70 but better than 20/200, or visual field exceeding 20°. Those who are legally blind have greater access to state-funded vision rehabilitation services.

4. Does visual impairment affect physical function?

It most certainly does, which is a major reason for physiatrists to know about it. Several studies in the geriatric population have demonstrated that isolated visual impairment in older people produces significant deficits in basic ADLs as well as instrumental ADLs. Additional effects of visual impairment are social isolation and low employment rates.

It should also be noted that vision is one of the three major components of sensory feedback to maintain normal upright stance (proprioception and vestibular function are the other two), and its loss can be associated with increased risk of falling in the elderly, with a consequent rise in the risk of hip fractures.

5. How can visually impaired patients gain access to vision rehabilitation services?

An ophthalmologic evaluation documenting the presence of "legal blindness" requires the submission of a form certifying the presence of this degree of visual impairment. The form goes to a state commission for the blind (this may vary from state to state), which then coordinates vision rehabilitation services to which such individuals are entitled. These may include social or vocational services, mobility and ADL training, low-vision equipment and other technology, and referral to the talking books library services. People with low vision may not be entitled to all these services, but they often can receive some of them through local facilities specializing in vision rehabilitation services.

6. What are the basic components of vision rehabilitation?

Vision rehabilitation techniques can be broadly grouped into two types, vision enhancement and vision substitution. These can be seen as analogous to orthotics and prosthetics, respectively. **Vision enhancement** uses devices or techniques that maximize the utility of any remaining visual function, whereas **vision substitution** uses technology or techniques that do not require any vision at all.

7. What are some vision enhancement techniques?

Vision enhancement techniques can be remembered with the mnemonic **IMAGE**:

I = **I**llumination
M = **M**agnification
A = **A**ltered contrast
G = **G**lare reduction
E = **E**xpanders of visual field

8. Classify the common vision substitution techniques into related groups.

• **Mobility**—cane, guide dog, sonic devices
• **Tactile**—Braille books/devices, raised markings
• **Recorded**—talking books, radio reading services
• **Synthetic speech**—computers with verbal output, talking watches/calculators, etc.
• **Computer-generated vision systems**
• **Special ADL techniques**—cooking techniques, money identification

9. Name some low-vision aids.

Vision enhancement
Magnifiers (hand-held, stand-alone, illuminated)
Telescopic lenses (monocular or binocular)
Closed-circuit television (CCTV), video magnifiers
Computer software providing magnification
Prisms for visual-field expansion
Nonoptical aids
Appropriate lighting (illumination)
Visors, tinted eye glasses (reduce glare)

Heightened color contrast (bold print pens, paper with extra-thick lines, white-on-black reversal images for slides)

10. What kinds of mobility aids are used by blind or visually impaired patients?

Special mobility devices include the long **white cane**, **laser cane**, **ultrasonic devices**, and the **guide dog**. The guide dog is usually reserved for those with near-total blindness and is more likely to be used by younger adults. Finally, a friend or willing helper can offer his or her arm and walk alongside the person with a visual impairment (sighted guide technique).

11. How can computer technology contribute to the rehabilitation of visually impaired people?

On a basic level, simple "talking" devices, such as the talking watch, talking calculator, and talking glucometer (for blind diabetics), are obviously helpful ADL aids. At a more elaborate level, computers with synthetic speech output in combination with optical character recognition scanners, braille output, or voice-activated operation can open a world of informational and professional opportunities for people unable to read the computer screen or ordinary output from a printer.

12. What about some simple self-care devices that are low-tech?

Inexpensive ADL devices include the "talking" technology mentioned previously, raised-dot labeling of dials on kitchen equipment, high-contrast color surfaces in work areas, simple labeling systems for clothing (such as the use of variously shaped labels for each color), and the folding of dollar bills in particular ways to identify each denomination. The assessment of self-care needs of visually impaired persons and training in such strategies is customarily done by rehabilitation teachers, but in recent years occupational therapists have sometimes provided such services in selected settings.

13. What are the expected functional outcomes in patients with combined visual and neuromusculoskeletal disabilities (e.g., blind amputee)?

They are surprisingly good, particularly when vision loss preceded the more familiar physiatric diagnosis. In a study of 12 blind amputees, 75% became functional prosthetic users, and blind stroke patients have had similar results in inpatient settings.

14. Who pays for vision rehabilitation services?

Usually these services are covered through a state Commission for the Blind rather than by standard third-party payers such as Medicare and Medicaid. This funding (or lack of funding) is a reflection of the separate nature of the vision and medical rehab systems as they currently operate. A recent trend is the use of occupational or physical therapists as providers of vision rehab services. Under these circumstances, such services have been reimbursed by Medicare or Medicaid.

15. Where can patients get more information on vision impairment and rehabilitation?

American Council of the Blind
1155 15th Street, NW, Suite 720
Washington, DC 20005
202-467-5081
800-424-8666

American Foundation for the Blind
11 Penn Plaza, Suite 300
New York, NY 10001
800-232-5463
212-502-7600

National Federation of the Blind
1800 Johnson Street
Baltimore, MD 21230
410-659-9314

Jewish Guild for the Blind
15 West 65th Street
New York, NY 10023
212-769-6200

The Lighthouse
111 East 59th Street
New York, NY 10022
212-821-9200
800-334-5497 (Information/referral)
800-829-0500 (Mail order products)

National Library Service for the Blind and Physically Handicapped
1291 Taylor Street, NW
Washington, DC 20542
800-424-8567

Council of Citizens with Low Vision International
5707 Brockton Drive, #302
Indianapolis, IN 46220
800-733-2258
317-254-1155

Resources for Rehabilitation
33 Bedford Street, Suite 19A
Lexington, MA 02173
617-862-6455

BIBLIOGRAPHY

1. Altner PE, Rusin JJ, De Boer A: Rehabilitation of blind patients with lower extremity amputations. Arch Phys Med Rehabil 61:82–85, 1980.
2. Branch LG, Horowitz A, Carr C: The implications for everyday life of incident self-reported visual decline among people over age 65 living in the community. Gerontologist 29:359–365, 1989.
3. Carabellese C, Apollonio I, Rozzini R, et al: Sensory impairment and quality of life in a community elderly population. J Am Geriatr Soc 41:401–407, 1993.
4. DiStefano AF, Aston SJ: Rehabilitation of the blind and visually impaired elderly. In Brody SL, Ruff DL (eds): Aging and Rehabilitation Advances in the State of the Art. New York, Springer Publishing, 1986.
5. Faye EE: Clinical Low Vision. Boston, Little, Brown, 1984.
6. Felson DT, Anderson JJ, Hannah MT, et al: Impaired vision and hip fracture: The Framingham Eye Study. J Am Geriatr Soc 37:495–500, 1989.
7. Greenblatt SL: Providing services for people with vision loss. Lexington, MA, Resources for Rehabilitation, 1989.
8. Wainapel SF: Rehabilitation of the blind stroke patient. Arch Phys Med Rehabil 65:487–489, 1984.
9. Wainapel SF: Visual impairments. In Felsenthal G, Garrison SH, Steinberg FU (eds): Rehabilitation of the Aging and Elderly Patient. Baltimore, Williams & Wilkins, 1993, pp 327–337.
10. Wainapel SF, Kwon YS, Fazzari PJ: Severe visual impairment on a rehabilitation unit: Incidence and implications. Arch Phys Med Rehabil 65:487–489, 1984.
11. Wainapel SF, Bernbaum M: Rehabilitation of the patient with visual impairment. In DeLisa JA, Gans BM (eds): Rehablitation Medicine: Principles and Practice, 3rd ed. Philadelphia, W.B. Saunders, 1998, pp 1733–1748

10. REHABILITATION STRATEGIES IN THE HEARING IMPAIRED

J. Michael Anderson, M.D., Denise W. Thrope, M.S., CCC-A, and Linda J. Anderson, O.T.R.

The best and most beautiful things cannot be seen or even touched...they must be felt with the heart.

—Hellen Keller

1. When is hearing loss a rehabilitation problem?

Difficulty hearing impairs many functional activities, including communication, education, the exchange of ideas, carrying out of orders, and the pure pleasure of listening and responding. A person begins to be socially incapacitated when hearing loss in both ears reaches 40 dB in the speech frequencies (500–3000 Hz). Only when the hearing loss is total or near-total (> 85-90 dB below normal) do we apply the term *deafness*. Hearing loss implies a partial loss of function; only the profoundly damaged ear is unable to respond to amplified sound. When a physician learns that a patient's hearing cannot be corrected medically or surgically, suitable rehabilitation must be advised.

2. What can rehabilitation personnel do for hearing problems?

Evaluation for medical or surgical approaches to underlying problems should first be undertaken to identify correctable hearing problems. Hearing aids and augmentative hearing devices can be provided by an audiologist and are often used in conjunction with aural rehabilitation techniques. Other professionals who may help treat hearing impairment include educators of the deaf, speech therapists, and occupational therapists.

3. What are the signs and symptoms of hearing problems? How often do they occur?

Although people with hearing impairment may report their difficulty in hearing, often they may noy be aware of their problem. Others may first note a person's poor response to auditory stimuli. In the elderly patient, hearing loss may "masquerade" as dementia. The patient who is unable to hear speech or who has poor speech discrimination may not be able to respond to verbal or other aural stimuli and appear confused or demented. Other symptoms, such as tinnitus, sometimes may be the initial presentation of an underlying hearing problem.

4. How many people does hearing impairment affect?

Hearing problems that require some form of assistance affect over 20 million people in the United States, and a minimum of 12 million persons have a hearing loss great enough to handicap them. Over 2 million Americans are either totally deaf or lack sufficient hearing to understand speech.

5. What are the four types of hearing problems?

1. **Conductive hearing loss** occurs in patients with external or middle-ear disorders, such as otitis media, otosclerosis, and perforated eardrum. These patients have a normal inner ear and are hard of hearing because of a defect in the mechanism by which sound is transmitted to the inner ear. These persons can hear perfectly if the sound is amplified sufficiently and so are usually able to use hearing aids.

2. **Sensorineural hearing loss** is due to processes within the inner ear, cochlea, eighth cranial (cochlear) nerve, or brain and is associated with infection, trauma, toxic substance, degenerative disease, or congenital abnormality.

3. **Combined hearing loss** with both conductive and sensorineural components

4. **Central auditory loss** occurs when the brain's hearing center is not properly functioning. Sound of sufficient loudness may reach the center, but understanding is impaired, especially in a noisy environment. Such disorders are the most difficult to diagnose and treat and can be caused by various conditions, including tumors or head injury.

6. How are hearing problems clinically assessed on a rehabilitation service?

Easily administered hearing tests include use of whispered and spoken voice, watch tick, tuning forks, or similar devices. Audiometry screening with a portable pure-tone audiometry device (to test speech frequencies of 250–3000 Hz) can be done by trained personnel (i.e., audiologist, speech therapist, nurse, occupational therapist, or physician).

The 128-cycle tuning fork, commonly used to test vibration sensation, should not be used, as patients often have difficulty differentiating between feeling the vibrations and hearing them. The most useful tuning forks for testing hearing are those with frequencies of 256, 512, or 1024 Hz. The tuning fork should be stroked between the thumb and index finger, gently tapped on the knuckle, or carefully activated with a rubber reflex hammer. Striking the fork too hard produces overtones as well as too intense a sound.

7. What are compensatory strategies and how are they used?

When a patient has a significant hearing problem, it impairs communication with every team member. The rehab team and hospital staff can "ignore" the hearing problem to minimize inconvenience or use compensatory strategies. **Compensatory strategies** include hand signs, gestures, written communication, speaking clearly and distinctly at a normal to slow speed in a well-lit environment (so the listener can observe facial expressions), and use of assistive listening devices (such as battery-powered voice amplifiers). A quiet area with a minimum of background noise is recommended. The family should be instructed in these techniques and may be better able to interpret communicative gestures and nonverbal cues than will the rehabilitation staff.

8. How reliable is a hearing test in an aphasic or neurologically impaired patient?

Very often, an individual can be tested reliably even when neurologically impaired. The ability to detect tones does not require the higher centers of the brain. If the individual can be trained to respond to tones, a valid hearing test can be obtained. If such training cannot be completed, often speech threshold can be obtained with a little creativity, whether it be following instructions such as clapping hands or finishing the words to a familiar song. In a nonresponsive patient, physiologic tests can be utilized, such as brainstem evoked audiometry.

9. What are the parts of an audiology evaluation?

Air conduction threshold testing obtains pure-tone thresholds at octaves from 250–8,000 Hz, as well as using speech stimuli in both ears under headphones. **A speech reception threshold** is obtained by presenting two-syllable words, called "spondee words" spoken down to a level where 50% of the words can be heard and repeated. **Speech recognition testing** is completed by presenting monosyllabic words at comfort levels. Generally, a list of 50 monosyllabic words is presented, and the percent correct is obtained for a speech recognition score. In **bone conduction threshold** testing, the bone oscillator is placed on the mastoid, and again pure-tone thresholds are obtained, from 250–4000 Hz, to determine whether the hearing loss is conductive, sensorineural, or mixed. **Impedance audiometry** may also be performed to assess middle ear function and to check the acoustic reflex. An audiologist who specializes in identifying, assessing, and providing nonmedical or surgical interventions, holds a masters degree, and is certified by the American Speech-Language-Hearing Association (ASHA) performs the evaluation.

10. Describe the treatment options for various hearing problems.

Treatment interventions for sensorineural and conductive loss may include hearing aids, assistive listening devices, and aural rehabilitation. For the profoundly deaf, **cochlear implants** are available. The cochlear implant is surgically implanted to stimulate the auditory nerve and provides awareness of sound, although not sound as a "normal" hearing person knows it. Some conductive losses can be helped through medical intervention, depending on the cause of the hearing loss. A **hearing aid** generally does not help a purely central hearing loss, as the problem is not one of decreased volume. **Aural rehabilitation**, using speech-language pathology or audiology services, can be useful as a focusing technique. An **assistive listening device** can also be useful to improve the signal-to-noise ratio and to focus on the auditory information during therapy sessions.

11. How does a hearing aid work?

A hearing aid is a small electronic instrument that makes sound louder and thus easier to detect and understand. It does not correct a hearing loss, overcome reduced discrimination, or even provide normal hearing the way eyeglasses can provide normal vision, but it can make a tremendous improvement in quality of life. A hearing aid consists of a **microphone** to pick up the signal, an **amplifier** to make the sound louder, and a **receiver**, which is a mini-loudspeaker to deliver the sound. It relies on a battery for power.

12. Describe the different types of hearing aids.

A number of different styles and types of hearing aids exist. The different styles vary in size from a **completely-in-the-canal** (CIC) hearing aid, which can barely be seen from the outside; to the **full-concha in-the-ear** (ITE) hearing aid, probably the most prevalent; to a **behind-the-ear** hearing aid, which fits over the ear and relies on an attached ear mold to direct the sound into the ear. An **in-the-canal** style is also very popular. It is not quite as invisible as a CIC, but smaller than an ITE.

Body-type hearing aids also exist but are rarely used, in which the user wears a small box that serves as the hearing aid on the body with a cord or cords that snap into the ear molds. **Bone conduction aids** often look like headbands and are used by individuals who cannot place the ear mold or hearing aid in the ear, possibly because of constant drainage or a malformation. They are also rather uncommon. A **contralateral routing of the signal** (CROS) hearing aid is appropriate for the user with one unaidable ear and one ear with normal or near normal hearing. The poorer ear side picks up the signal and routes it either through a hard wire or FM waves to the better ear. This provides auditory information to be picked up from a nonhearing ear. When the better ear requires amplification, a biCROS aid is utilized, meaning the better ear side is aided and wired to pick up from the poorer ear.

13. What types of technologies are available in hearing aids?

Conventional hearing aids using analog technology have been on the market for many years. They are available in all sizes and use a manual volume control to regulate the intensity of the signal. **Programmable hearing instruments** were introduced in the 1990s. They use a computer to program the response and provide greater precision and flexibility than conventional instruments. These hearing aids are considered nonlinear, meaning loud stimuli receive less amplification than soft. Often more than one response can be programmed as memory for different listening environments. These devices are sufficiently automatic to not require a manual volume control, but are analog instruments. **Digital hearing aids** are said to provide the most natural sound using digital signal processing. Also programmed by computer, they are extremely flexible, nonlinear, and can offer noise suppression and feedback management. They are completely automatic and have the least amount of distortion of the technologies on the market.

14. Where does one obtain hearing aids?

Hearing aids may be obtained through an audiologist or a hearing aid dispenser. An **audiologist** is the professional with a minimum of a masters degree trained in evaluating and managing hearing loss. This individual works with other professionals, including physicians and speech language pathologists, to help determine the best course of treatment for a person with hearing loss, including hearing aids and aural rehabilitation. An audiologist is usually certified by a professional organization. A **hearing aid dispenser** is trained in the sales of hearing instruments and may require licensing, depending on the state in which he or she practices.

The sale of hearing aids through the internet has become a concern in some states. Prior to obtaining amplification, an audiological evaluation should be completed and the condition of the ears should be evaluated. An earmold impression should be taken by someone experienced in doing so. Once evaluated, a hearing aid user should have a professional able to fine tune hearing aids and make adjustments when necessary. This is usually a process that takes a few to several visits. Some internet companies will refer to a local dispenser to do the actual fit, but the buyer must remain cautious in knowing whether follow-up services will be covered for the warranty period of the device or whether each visit will require additional charges. The internet cost advantage may not exist in these situations.

15. What is an assistive listening device?

An assistive listening device is any equipment or system that helps the hearing-impaired individual communicate more effectively, often in conjunction with or in place of a conventional hearing aid. These devices may be for personal use or part of a large room system. A **personal system** may use a hard wire from a speaker's microphone to the listener's headset or hearing aid or use FM radio waves or infrared light to transmit the sound information. The signal must be picked up by some type of receiver, which may be the telephone switch built into the hearing aid. **Room systems** usually rely on FM, infrared, or an audio loop system (which creates an electric current in a length of wire looped around the room). The signal can be picked up by a receiver obtained from the facility or through use of the telephone switch on the hearing aid, if it has one. Assistive listening devices, especially the personal type, are helpful to those who have difficulty in noisy situations, because only the message sent over the device is amplified and the background noise is not made louder.

More familiar assistive listening devices include **closed captioning** for television and **telephone amplifiers**, both of which can be purchased inexpensively. Other devices recommended for the severely or profoundly hearing impaired person include alerting devices such as a light connected to the telephone, doorbell, or fire alarms.

16. What is aural rehabilitation?

Aural rehabilitation is a process that addresses the effect of impaired hearing on the individual and attempts to provide strategies for coping with the communication deficit as well as psychosocial aspects of hearing loss. The most obvious form of aural rehabilitation is the fitting of a hearing aid and follow-up to teach the user realistic expectations and proper use of the device. Auditory training attempts to teach the hearing-impaired person to use residual hearing to its maximum. One goal is to relearn the sounds of both speech and the environment. Lessons in speech reading (lip-reading) are another aspect of aural rehabilitation. Counseling the hearing-impaired individual, along with his or her family, to understand the degree that a communication deficit can impact upon life is also a part of aural rehabilitation. Thus, aural rehabilitation may involve a number of rehab professionals.

17. How can you tell which type of hearing aid is best for an individual patient?

The degree of hearing loss is important. A severe to profound hearing loss cannot be effectively corrected with a tiny, mini-canal hearing aid. The person's lifestyle, tolerance, and ability to manipulate the hearing aid are all important. Someone whose cognition is impaired may be a candidate for an assistive listening device, not a hearing aid, which requires some manipulation. It should be understood that the individual is being fit, not the hearing loss.

18. Why may some people dislike hearing aids? What barriers exist to use of the aids?

1. The primary reason people reject hearing aids is because they think it makes them seem old or disabled.

2. Hearing aids are not usually covered by insurance, and Medicare does not reimburse for the devices. Prices range from $500 to over $3000 for digital instruments.

3. Some patients report difficulty in manipulating the tiny controls and in inserting the aids into the ear canal.

4. Hearing aids, as mentioned previously, do not provide normal hearing or amplify just what the user desires to hear. Expectations of hearing improvement with use of a hearing aid must be realistic.

19. What factors impact the satisfaction of hearing aid use in older persons with hearing loss?

Relatively few older adults with hearing loss currently use hearing aids. Improved screening and intervention programs to identify older adults who would benefit from amplification are needed to improve hearing-related quality of life for this large segment of the population.

Hearing impairment in older adults is a chronic condition with high prevalence that shows negative correlations with communication, social integration, well-being, and cognition. It s suggested that elderly persons with pure-tone averages at 30 dB hearing loss are in need of hearing aids. First-time hearing aid candidates in a nursing home situation were less successful to become users if they were not concerned about their hearing difficulties and reported themselves as not wanting or needing a hearing aid. An attitude that use of a hearing aid will be stigmatizing was not predictive of hearing aid use, but did correlate with increaed complaints of dificulty in handling the aid. Studies show candidates for amplification tend to expect more benefit than they will achieve from hearing aid use, particularly when listening to speech in noise or without visual cues.

Generally hearing aid benefits cannot be reliably predicted based on perceived need or expectation. Extroverted patients report more hearing aid benefits in all speech-comunication situations. Other personality variables explain a relatively small amount of variance in satisficaton of hearing aid use. Older persons with mild to moderate hearing loss showed positive effects on self-perceived hearing handicap after receiving hearing aids.

20. When should I refer my patient for an ENT evaluation?

A patient complaining of a unilateral hearing loss, tinnitus, ear pain or drainage, and vertigo or dizziness not associated with other known factors should be referred. Any patient complaining of a hearing problem can be referred to rule out an underlying medical process. A patient with significant cerumen impaction may be an appropriate referral.

21. What types of hearing problems occur in children?

All types of hearing problems occur in children. Conductive hearing loss caused by otitis media is the single type seen more in children than in adults.

22. At what age can training begin in hearing-impaired children?

With the advent of infant hearing screening programs in the past several years, significant hearing loss is being identified in infancy and often treated by 3 months of age with amplification. The important speech development period is, therefore, not lost. When amplification is not adequate, cochlear implants may be an option. In all cases, aural habilitation is imperative to provide proper stimulation and auditory training.

23. How can hearing be assessed clinically in neonates and young children?

Infant screening programs utilize physiological techniques such as brainstem evoked responose audiometry (BAER) and otoacoustic emission testing (OAE) often within 1–2 days of birth prior to leaving the hospital. Generally, if the screening is not passed initially, it is repeated. With a second abnormal result, the infant should be referred for an otologic consult to rule out a medical problem, such as middle ear pathology. The child will also be seen for a complete audiological evaluation with more extensive physiological testing. Behavioral testing can be attempted in children as young as 6 months of age. It must be performed in a sound-treated room. The presence of a unilateral hearing loss is difficult to establish.

Conditioning techniques are helpful in testing small children. This is done by presenting auditory stimulation through loud speakers and associating the sound with a light or toy. A child of 2–3 years of age can frequently be taught "play audiometry." For example, the child is instructed to throw a block into a box when hearing a tone. Speech is also an effective tool to use with a hard-to-test child. This child may localize to his or her own name, wave "bye-bye," or identify body parts even at very-low-intensity speech levels. Although a child's response to spoken voice is not a complete frequency response, at least some hearing within the speech range can be implied from these responses.

24. How are physiologic hearing tests done?

The best known of the physiologic techniques is brainstem auditory evoked response (BAER), also known as auditory brainstem response (ABR) and brainstem evoked response audiometry (BSER). BAER involves placing electrodes on the child and presenting a stimulus, picked from the computerized system. A specific waveform response is recorded from the brainstem if the stimulus is heard. When the intensity of the stimulus is decreased, the response should show a decrease in amplitude and an increase in latency. A click stimulus or tone pips are utilized to assess higher frequencies. The test requires the infant to be quiet and preferably asleep.

25. What is otoacoustic emission testing?

An otoacoustic emission (OAE) test refers to a quick, noninvasive screening procedure that can identify a properly functioning cochlea if the sound can reach the inner ear. The otoacoustic emission refers to an "echo" from the hair cells of a normally functioning cochlea, which is reflected back through the middle ear where it is picked up by a microphone connected to a microcomputer. This procedure is used in a number of newborn screening programs to detect hearing loss of > 35 dB.

26. How old should a child be before using a hearing aid or other device?

With accurate physiologic testing now available, infants can be fitted with hearing aids as soon as the hearing loss is verified. A child of 3–4 months of age can wear a hearing aid with the hopes that speech and language development can begin. A hearing loss of a moderate to severe degree or worse warrants intervention.

27. Can a hearing-aid induced progressive hearing loss occur in the pediatric population?

Hearing aids are needed for treatment of profound sensorineural hearing loss in infancy and early childhood in order to obtain auditory and speech development. Concerns exist that the use of powerful hearing aids in this population could cause a progressive loss of hearing. Recent studies have shown no correlation between the duration of the hearing aid usage and the maximum output level of the hearing aid on progressive hearing loss in infancy and early childhood. It is currently recommended that all children with profound sensorineural hearing loss receive hearing aids.

28. What factors impact the accetance of hearing aid use in children?

The majority of children (58.6%) with persistent hearing impairment who were fitted for a hearing aid had excellent or good acceptance of the device as determined by wearing time. Wearing acceptance was reduced with children having unilateral hearing impairments. Stigma of an aid was reported as minimal under the age of 7. Hearing aid acceptance did not correlate with the severity of the hearing disorder

29. Besides hearing aids or other devices, what interventions are needed to ensure their safety and allow communication and education for infants or young children with hearing problems?

Early parental intervention and safety. Basic issues are addressed, such as being careful when opening doors which the child may not hear, replacing auditory fire alarms with intense visual alarms with flashing lights, and obtaining deaf signs to warn neighborhood motorists.

Enrichment of visual and tactile sensory environment. Normal toys can be purchased to provide a variety of visual, tactile, and auditory stimulation. Hammers, drums, rattles, and other "musical" toys can encourage participation in an experience of rhythm, vibration, and auditory stimulation for musical enjoyment. Use of talking books, audio tapes, and spoken language are to be encouraged. Toys using sound frequencies that are within the child's unimpaired range should be encouraged.

Basic sign language. Parents should learn basic sign and use it with the child from the time the hearing loss is detected.

Protection of the child's remaining hearing. Use of ear plugs for swimming or bathing may be advised. Seeking early medical care for suspected ear infections or "allergies" will help prevent further damage. Physicians should be told of the child's hearing loss before prescription medications are given, so as to avoid inadvertent ototoxic injury associated with medications.

30. What resources are available for hearing-impaired children and their parents?

As soon as a child or infant is identified with a hearing loss, the best referral is to an audiologist or a school for the deaf. If neither of these is available, the child's school system, local United Way agencies, and social workers may offer further advice. Very often, a school system will have a child-find or parent-infant program that can be helpful. Parental support groups may educate the parents in the various school options available within a community and about their rights and responsibilities. Parental support groups are also important for preventing child abuse, which occurs more commonly to the handicapped child. The American Speech-Language-Hearing Association (ASHA) and Self-Help for Hard of Hearing People, Inc. (SHHH) provides information, offer support groups, and serve as advocates on issues of concern for the hearing-impaired.

BIBLIOGRAPHY

1. Bille M, Jensen AM, Kjaerbol E, et al: Clinical study of a digital versus an analogue hearing aid. Scand Audiol 28:127–135, 1999.
2. Brooks DN, Hallam RS: Attitudes to hearing difficulty and hearing aids and the outcome of audiological rehabilitation. Br J Audiol 32:217–226, 1998.
3. Garstecki DC, Erler SF: Hearing loss, control, and demographic factors influencing hearing aid use among older adults. J Speech Lang Hear Res 41:527–537, 1998.

4. Hoekstra CC, Snik AF, van den Bornse S, van den Broek P: Auditory training in severely and profoundly hearing impaired toddlers: The development of audtory skills and verbal communication. Int J Pediatr Otorhinolaryngol 47:201–204, 1999.
5. Klein AJ, Weber PC: Hearing aids. Med Clin North Am 83:139–151, 1999.
6. Leake FS, Thompson JW, Simms E, et al: Acauisition of hearing aids and assistive listening devices among the pediatric hearing-impaired population. Int J Pediatr Otorhinolaryngol 52:247–251, 2000.
7. Popelka MM, Cruickshanks KJ, Wiley TL, et al: Low prevalence of hearing aid use among older adults with hearing loss: The Epidemiology of Hearing Loss Study. J Am Geriatr Soc 46:1075–1078, 1998.
8. Schum DJ: Perceived hearing aid benefit in relation to perceived needs. J Am Acad Audiol 10:40–45, 1999.
9. Yoshinaga-Itano C: Benefits of early intervention for children with hearing loss. Otolaryngol Clin North Am 32:1089 1102, 1999.

11. SEXUAL SATISFACTION DESPITE DISABLEMENT

Steven A. Stiens, M.D, M.S., Ruth K. Westheimer, Ed.D., and Mark A. Young, M.D.

1. What is sexuality?

Sexuality is the expression of a person's femaleness or maleness through personality, body, dress, and behavior; it is the personification of biologic gender, gender identity, and sexual orientation. It develops through physiologic cues from the body, experiences of self, maturation, socialization, societal reflection of the person, and intimate relationships. Sexuality, therefore, requires an evolving self-understanding, an ongoing opportunity for communication of self-perception, and responses from those around us. The context of sexual rehabilitation is the affirmation of the person's sexuality and enablement of sexual self-expression. The anticipation of patients' sexuality as a facet of their role in relationships is but one example of the power of therapeutic expectation.

2. What is sexual literacy?

Sexual literacy is the working knowledge of anatomy, physiology, and recent research pertaining to human sexuality theory and practice. The "sexually literate" health professional must be comfortable with his or her own sexuality, able to suspend judgment, and express genuine willingness to pursue understanding and solutions with the patient and partner.

3. What are the subcomponents of personal sexual expression?

- **Sexual identity**—phenotypic sex with objective expression and function of secondary sexual characteristics, anatomy, and physiology
- **Gender identity**—the person's subjective sense of self as man or woman
- **Orientation**—the focus of desire for sexual relationship, sexual orientation is a fluid continuum ranging from exclusively heterosexual to with many homosexual
- **Intention**—degree of aggression inherent in sexual fantasy and behavior
- **Sexual desire**—interest in a variety of activity, frequency

4. How does disability affect body image and sexual self-concept?

Body image is the mind's picture of our own bodies, the perception we have of ourselves. It is closely associated with the awareness of our body (the afferent sensory barrage and central processing, "the experienced homunculus"). The expression and practice of sexuality are affected by self-esteem, body image, and interpersonal attachment. It is continually evaluated by the self. Despite adaptation to self, individuals often confront a society with a stigma and risk devaluation by others. Rehabilitation specialists must strive to help patients become fully self-aware, construct a body image, accept it, like it, and share it.

5. Isn't it important to have a relationship first?

Personal relationships begin with our attitudes about ourselves. Beyond self-perception is self-acceptance, self-esteem, and self-worth as a potential partner for another. The rehabilitation team must successfully reflect patients' unique personal attributes, reinforcing the value of their companionship to others. People who project self-respect and satisfaction are most fully capable of attracting partners, graciously accepting others' attention and sensitively meeting their needs. People who recognize their capabilities are most able to contribute them to a mutually complementary relationship. Consequently, rehabilitation must teach patients the necessity for risking the rejection of others in social interactions and recognition of their unique assets and capabilities.

6. What communication must there be with the patient's partner?

For patients who have a sexual partner, intervention is most effective if the partner is included in any communication between the rehabilitation professional and the patient on matters of sexual functioning. This is particularly true after a myocardial infarction, when the partner may be fearful about engaging in sexual activity that might produce another "attack" and perhaps even cause the patient's death.

Sexual issues must be integrated into the entire rehabilitation plan; partners in life need full inclusion in the rehab process. If possible, it is desirable to maintain a separation between roles of caretaker and sexual partner. This can be achieved with proactive planning for attendant care.

7. What are the physiologic changes associated with the four stages of the human sexual response as outlined by Masters and Johnson?

Excitement stage I: muscle tension, sympathetic activity, nipple erection
    Female: clitoris swelling, vaginal lubrication
    Male: penile erection, testes rise
Plateau stage II: heightened excitement, pulse 100–160 bpm, sex flush
    Female: clitoris withdrawals, vaginal vasocongestion
    Male: testes enlarge, Cowper's secretion
Orgasm stage III (seconds to minutes): rhythmic muscle contractions
    Female: uterus, vagina, and anus contract
    Male: ejaculation, bladder neck closes
Relaxation stage IV (minutes to hours): return to baseline, refractory period

8. Describe the physiology of the sexual response in women.

The uterus and ovaries receive only sympathetic innervation from the hypogastric nerve. Clitoral swelling and vaginal secretion are parasympathetically driven. At orgasm, the pelvic floor (pudendal nerve) contracts rhythmically.

9. How do neurologic injuries affect female sexual function?

Menstruation may not occur for 3 or more months after central nervous system (CNS) trauma. Vaginal lubrication occurs with reflex stimulation as long as the conus and autonomic connections remain intact. After complete spinal cord injury at level T6 and above, psychogenic subjective arousal does not produce vaginal lubrication; manual clitoral stimulation produces reflex lubrication and increased vaginal pulse amplitude.

Fertility generally is not significantly affected by spinal cord injury. Pregnancy may be complicated by urinary tract infection, decubitus ulcers, constipation, and mobility limitations. Labor is initiated and driven hormonally. The delivery can be vaginal but should be anticipated and monitored, with autonomic dysreflexia prevention with anesthesia and preparedness for forceps use or cesarean section.

10. How do erections occur?

Male erection is initiated by arterial vasodilatation and venous outlet constriction, which result in engorgement of the sinusoids. Autonomic penile innervation is via the pelvic plexus lateral to the rectum, which carries the parasympathetic **nervi erigentes** (S2,3,4) and sympathetic

hypogastric nerve (T12, L1) fibers to the penis. Somatic sensation and pelvic floor motor control are via the pudendal (S2,3,4) mixed nerve. Psychogenic (imaginative) erections are mediated by the lumbar sympathetics (T10–L2). Reflexogenic (contact) erection is primarily cholinergic (parasympathetic, S2,3,4), and the ejaculation detumescence process is primarily sympathetic, but a complex interplay of autonomic systems and other neurotransmitters also have roles in the process.

11. Describe the physiology of the sexual response in men.

Psychogenic stimuli can produce erection and emission containing spermatozoa through sympathetic facilitation. **Emission** is the sympathetically (T10–L2 emission center) controlled process of deposition of seminal fluid in the posterior urethra. **Ejaculation** is the forceful delivery of the semen out of the urethra by the pudendal-innervated bulbocavernous and ischiocavernosus muscle contractions. Ejaculation is typically ineffective after complete spinal cord injury (SCI) and can result in retrograde ejaculation (semen into the bladder). Ejaculation can be facilitated with a vibrator stimulus (2.5 mm amplitude, 100 Hz frequency) under the glans at the frenulum or inhibited by the squeeze technique (firm grasp of glans). **Orgasm** is the cortical experience of extreme pleasure followed by a feeling of well-being and satisfaction.

12. How do neurologic injuries affect the process of erection?

Past reviews have reported an overall 54–87% incidence of erection after SCI (60–90% upper motor neuron reflex, 10–30% lower motor neuron psychogenic or reflex). A recent study using physiologic recordings defined erections as an increase in penile circumference of 3–6 mm and demonstrated 100% reflexogenic erection in upper SCI and in 80–90% of patients with lower motor neuron lesions. The capacity for tumescence with partial innervation is encouraging, but penile rigidity facilitates successful **intromission**, vaginal insertion of penis (not to be confused with "intermission").

13. What are the rehabilitation options for producing erections after neurologic injuries?

Without erection, satisfying intromission can be accomplished with the **stuffing technique** (pushing the flaccid penis into the vagina and stimulating the woman with friction and sustained pressure at the introitus). Erection can be produced noninvasively with **vacuum tumescence constriction therapy** and expansion of the penis; cavernosal engorgement can be maintained with a custom circular rubber-tension ring at the base of the penis.

Pharmacologic adjuncts have included **yohimbine** (not used in SCI) and **testosterone** (increases libido, minimal improvement of erections [use only if serum levels are low]). Intracorporal injections with **papaverine** (a nonspecific smooth muscle relaxant) or **prostaglandin E₁** produce erections if dosed properly, with initial trials in the clinic. Injection is into the lateral aspect of the base of the penile shaft to avoid neurovascular structures. These agents act by causing relaxation of smooth muscle and vasodilatation. Venous outflow is decreased through relaxation of corporal smooth muscle that occludes draining venues. Oral **sildenafil** (Viagra) works best if patients have at least partial reflexogenic erections. It is a potent selective inhibitor of eGMP—specific for PDE-5, which maintains higher concentrations of eGMP and nitric oxide to sustain reflexogenically stimulated erections. Dosing of 50–100 mg orally enhances erections for up to 4 hours. Sildenafil is contraindicated in patients who uses organic nitrates such as nitropaste for control of autonomic dysreflexia. Prevention and management of side effects such as priapism (cavernosal needle aspiration reduces pressure and removes medication) and corporal fibrosis with repeated injections require physician supervision and a 24-hour emergency plan.

Penile implants may be noninflatable (rigid or semirigid, not currently used in SCI) or inflatable and facilitate retention of condoms for urinary management. Rigid or malleable penile implants are not recommended for SCI or neurologic disorders because they can cause tissue erosion at insensate areas.

14. Does spinal cord injury affect male fertility?

Deficits in spermatogenesis documented by testicular biopsy have included tubular atrophy, spermatogenic arrest, and interstitial fibrosis. Seminal parameters show decreased sperm counts and motility as well as abnormal morphology. Repeated ejaculation reduces stasis and can improve sperm quality.

15. How can sexual history-taking and intervention be made less of an ENIGMA?

The ENIGMA model is a series of steps that makes the process more conceivable.

Engage the patient in conversation by establishing mutual rapport by finding common ground and recognizing them as a person.

Normalize sexuality and sexual activity by embedding them in a structure for addressing the patients care such as the problem list which becomes an agenda for interaction.

Inform and educate the patient and their partner.

Guide them by mirroring their style of interaction about togetherness by validating their success and suggesting alternative for next steps. Use their lingo!

Maximize achievement by prescribing and providing adjuncts such as educational materials, equipment, therapy and experiences.

Assess and reassess by checking in on the issue as one in the spectrum of problems addressed on regular visit.

16. What is the PLISSIT model of sex therapy?

P =   Permission to be sexual
LI =   Limited Information
SS =   Specific Suggestions
IT =   Intensive Therapy

This model presents a spectrum of interventional areas that can be addressed in part by each member of the interdisciplinary team.

17. Explain the components of the PLISSIT approach.

Permission—Sensitive questions regarding sexual function in history-taking are therapeutic affirmations of the patient's sexuality and role in the lives of others. Recognition and sensitive discussion of potentially embarrassing situations—bathing, bowel and bladder care—provide permission for the patient to discuss their emotional reactions and fears and to begin communications about adaptive solutions. Teaching patients the management techniques for angina, bronchospasm, autonomic dysreflexia, and prevention of incontinence prepares them for their own problem-solving in sexual exploration.

Limited information—All rehabilitation programs should include lectures and discussion that educate the patient about the basic physiology and pathophysiology of the sexual response cycle and reproduction. One-to-one explanation of the unique effects of a patient's disease or injury should complement this review. This primary education should be the designated responsibility of one rehabilitation team member, with appropriate referral to another team member as needed for elaboration.

Specific suggestions—Ideally, all team members contribute to successful sexual adjustment and function. For example, the training of the patient by the primary nurse for skin examination for sores can lead to reflections on body image. A suggestion might be an assignment for the patient or couple to experiment with visual body exploration and survey patient sensation. Such a couple can later be assigned sensate focus exercises and then advance to a search for new erogenous zones. Physical therapy education for a spouse on transfers and mat mobility might easily be adapted by couples for use in sexual positioning.

Intensive therapy—The presence of impairments that contribute to role performance deficits demands formal attention and the response of a rehabilitation team member. On most teams, this is the psychologist.

18. How are sexual problems elicited?

Being in a medical environment may help a patient achieve openness and honesty about sexual issues. Evaluations of sexual function start with the social history and move from the review of symptoms out through the physical examination to goal setting. This framework for questioning will make sexual questions "matter of fact" when you arrive at the urogenital system. Descriptions of sexual function will lead to opportunities to discuss situations and partners.

The mirror is the most important tool for the physical exam. The mirror allows the physician to visualize areas of the body with the patient and partners. An examination that includes the aid of a spouse for positioning lends itself to review of the patient's sensory, motor, and autonomic impairments. Potential for lubrication, reflexogenic erections, and positioning for intercourse can be sensitively addressed in such sessions.

19. Is there sex after stroke?

Sensory impairment, as opposed to mobility deficits, has been associated with decreased libido, decreased intercourse frequency, and erectile and perceptual disturbance. The basal hypothalamus has been suggested as a center for sexual desire although cortical involvement can lead to disinhibition, hyposexuality, or hypersexuality (Klüver-Bucy syndrome). Issues related to aphasia, distortion of body image, and frontal limbic damage affect interest and performance. Women often experience difficulty with lubrication and require adjunctive creams to prevent dyspareunia.

20. Do people still want sex after going through a severe disability adjustment?

Depression, attitude, and self-perception all affect arousal. Use of explicit materials, memories, or conversations in person or by phone are often effective in reawakening desire. Self-exploration and stimulation reacquaint one with the recipe for satisfaction. Such self-knowledge provides a guide for pleasuring with partners.

21. When should a sex therapist be consulted?

Good sexual functioning depends not only on the physical health of the patients but also on their libido. Although the physical limitations caused by a disease or old age may require only some trial and error, the detrimental effects on the libido may be an issue that cannot be handled without guidance, particularly as the patient's sex partner may also be in need of assistance. Sex therapy need not be long-term, but even a few visits to a sex therapist should be recommended whenever issues involving difficulties of arousal are suspected by the primary physician.

22. Is there sex after a heart attack?

Yes! Myocardial infarction or heart disease in general need not preclude resumption of sexual activity. Contrary to popular myth, sexual activity is not associated with the risk of sudden death in coronary patients. In fact, Ueno found that > 1% of sudden deaths in Japan happened during sex. The metabolic cost of sex in middle-aged married men is no more than 5 METs. Metabolic cost of intercourse in a familiar position is lower than that in an unfamiliar position. Rest before intercourse, postpone for 3 hours after meals and alcohol, and take nitrates as needed before intercourse to prevent chest pain. For people resuming sexual activity after heart disease, foreplay may be a metabolically favorable "warm-up" (training) activity. Initial explorations can include masturbation to give the patient full control of the process. Thereafter, successive approximation of the previous routine can follow.

23. How important is it for the physician to give permission for sexual activity?

Change, especially a negative one occurring from an accident, disease, or aging, is often accompanied by fear. Patients frequently worry that they may aggravate their condition through sexual activity. This anxiety can affect sexual function as much as pathophysiology. Hearing the physician give permission to engage in sexual activity is a therapeutic step toward healthy sexual activity.

24. What experiences do women with new neurologic impairments report as they adapt sexually?

The process of sexual readjustment after paralysis varies and may include three stages.

1. **Cognitive genital dissociation**—Sexual ennui is accompanied by dysphoria and pessimism about desirability. There may be fear of rejection or abandonment. Therapeutic support

includes exploration of the role sexuality played before injury and validates the patient's current experience as common but not necessarily persistent.

2. **Sexual disenfranchisement**—Sexuality becomes less of a priority although activity may occur out of curiosity. Experiences may produce sexual dissonance and disappointment in lack of sensation of the pleasure that was.

3. **Sexual rediscovery**—Sexual readjustment continues and includes exploration and discovery of alternative approaches to arousal and orgasm.

25. Can the location of erogenous zones really change after injury to the CNS?

Recent primate and human data demonstrate central sensory reorganization in response to injuries to the spinal cord or peripheral nerve. People with SCI have reported areas in the zone of partial sensory preservation that are sexually exciting with stimulation. These areas can lead to the experience of orgasm with associated tachycardia and flushing above the lesion.

26. What is there to be afraid of?

Overcoming attitudinal and cultural taboos of intervention transcends barriers. Practices that bring together mutually sensate erogenous zones can become particularly satisfying parts of couples' repertoires: possibilities for **cunnilingus** (oral and lingual vulva stimulation) and **fellatio** (oral and lingual penile stimulation) should be explored. Unfortunately, a major barrier to sexual fulfillment after disability is our fears. This starts with fears of poor acceptance by a partner. Issues related to involuntary loss of urinary or bowel control are particularly ominous. Planning for sexual encounters reduces anxiety and makes them more conceivable.

27. How can humor help with sex after disability?

Humor puts people at ease. Disability often reduces physical control of situations. Humor offers a response to surprises and produces a playful atmosphere for persons to explore and bring pleasure to one another.

BIBLIOGRAPHY

1. Annon J: The PLISSIT model: A proposed conceptual scheme for the behavioral treatment for sexual problems. J Sex Educ Ther 2:1, 1976.
2. Donahue J, Gebbard P: The Kinsey Institute/Indiana University Report on Sexuality and Spinal Cord Injury. Sex Disabil 13:7–85, 1995.
3. Gilbert DML: Sexuality issues in persons with disabilities. In Braddom RL (ed): Physical Medicine and Rehabilitation, 2nd ed. Philadelphia, W.B. Saunders, 2000, pp 616–644.
4. Kreuter M, Sullivan M, Siostee A: Sexual adjustment after spinal cord injury: Comparison of partner experiences in pre- and post-injury relationships. Paraplegia 32:759–770, 1994.
5. Lemon MA: Sexual counseling and spinal cord injury. Sex Disabil 11:73–97, 1993.
6. Monga M, Bernie J, Rajasekarran M: Male infertility and erectile dysfunction in spinal cord injury: A review. Arch Phys Med Rehabil 80:1331–1338, 1999.
7. Sipski ML, Alexander CJ: Sexual Function in People with Disability and Chronic Illness: A Health Professional's Guide. Gaithersburg, MD, Aspen Publication, 1997.
8. Sipski ML: Sexual function in women with neurologic disorders. Phys Med Rehabil Clin North Am 12:79–90, 2001.
9. Tepper M: Providing Comprehensive Sexual Health Care in Spinal Cord Injury Rehabilitation: Continuing Education and Training for Health Care Professionals. Huntington, CT, Sexual Health Network, 1997.
10. Westheimer RK: Sex. In Ruskin SA (ed): Current Therapy in Physiatry: Physical Medicine and Rehabilitation. Philadelphia, W.B. Saunders, 1984, pp 530–535.
11. Westheimer RK: Sex for Dummies, 2nd ed. Foster City, CA, IDG Books, 2000.

12. ENVIRONMENTAL ADAPTATIONS

Shoshana Shamberg, OTR/L, M.S., Steven A. Stiens, M.D., M.S.,
and Aaron Shamberg, OTR/L, M.S.

Rehabilitation is often like surgery from the skin...out.
—Steven A. Stiens

1. Describe the relationship between the physical environment and personhood?

Essentially, behavior is carried out against or through the medium of the physical environment. The human maturation process requires physical interaction with the environment to develop functional mobility and facilitate physical adaptation. The variety of physical capabilities acquired in this interaction defines our freedom to move about and modify the environment to our personal specifications. These experiences of "mastery" are internalized as self-discovery and development. Our mastery becomes a behavioral pattern that is successful and is acted out in our relationship to the world that surrounds us. It is uniquely human to adapt to the environment and to adapt the environment to our specifications. Rehabilitation can be considered as a process of acquisition of disability-appropriate behaviors and extinction of maladaptive disability-inappropriate behaviors. The adaptive habits needs to be cued, supported, and enabled by the adapted habitat.

2. How does a new injury or illness affect this relationship?

Immediately after a catastrophic illness or injury, the experience of the lived body is radically distorted. The **body image** is altered due to new deficits in perception, sensation, motor performance, and loss of body parts. Environmental perception may be altered due to sensory deficit or neglect. This situation is compounded by the **depersonalization** of hospitalization; the person is separated from the familiar immediate environment of their clothes and personal objects (keys, watch, jewelry) and is confined to a bed, horizontal. Communication as a means to share personal identity and to alter the physical environment frequently dominates the interaction. Patients may be labeled as "problems" due to repeated requests for assistance.

This situation of **person in a new body in the environment** can be compared to that of an infant in a crib who is testing the environment. This testing and modifying the environment through verbal and physical interaction are crucial for beginning the problem-solving process and eliminating potential barriers to independence. The patient carries memories, impressions, and attitudes about their new physical state in this reality. Early "experiments" of environment interaction in the new state confirm or refute such impressions and color the person's future expectations. The ongoing process of adaptation is an **operant process** that is facilitated by multiple repetitions, spontaneous activities, and a variety of perceptual and physical interactions.

3. The environment is a big place. How can it be subdivided in order to focus on the parts of the environment that are most pertinent for my patient?

Many of the limitations persons experience can be attributed to the environment. As such these areas are substrate for rehabilitation intervention. These environments can be thought of as similar to the hierarchy of systems that make up the biopsychosocial model.

1. Rehabilitation treatment within the **immediate environment** includes specialized dressings, orthotics, prosthetics, adaptive clothing and mobility devices. These aspects can be addressed in the clinic or hospital.

2. The **intermediate environment** is adapted and arranged to maximize function and safety based on activity of daily living (ADL) needs and activities unique to those using the space.

3. The **community environment** is where the home, jobsite, and social support are located. It includes the structures, people, and institutions located within the sphere of the person's domain.

4. In the last decade, the **built environment** has become more accessible. Many structural changes have been implemented in accordance with the American with Disabilities Act (ADA) and fair housing legislation.

5. Finally the **natural environment** presents access challenges that can be overcome with adaptive landscaping and terrain-specific mobility aids.

4. What is the role of the rehabilitation team in this process?

The rehabilitation professionals should facilitate the patient's articulation of feelings and memories of satisfaction with past physical "prowess" and experiences with the physical world in the new relationship. Adaptation of the patient's immediate and intermediate environment catalyzes the success of their efforts and enables the person to interact successfully with the physical environment despite disability. The patient is set up for independent trials of self-feeding, dressing, and use and manipulation of environmental controls (bed, call light, TV, phone). Achievements in therapy need to be reinforced with equipment at the bedside and updated orders specifying assistance required.

The goal is for the patient to rediscover a healthy interaction with the environment, which the patient can generalize to the achievement of his or her personal goals for the future. This may require the demonstration of "solutions" offered through technology or environmental design early in the rehabilitation process.

5. What assessment techniques can be used by the interdisciplinary team to target environmental barriers and formulate solutions to maximize functional independence?

The full capabilities of the patient are difficult to predict early in the rehabilitation process. Initial emphasis must be placed on the team's knowledge of the patient's activity before the injury. Such knowledge can be elicited through **retrospective sociobehavioral mapping** (review a typical 1-week period for patient location, activity, and companionship).

The chronology of the rehabilitation process can be understood as a continuum that starts with the design of the person's immediate environment (braces, wheelchair, etc.) and progresses to the intermediate environment (their home). The community and natural environments are emphasized during the latter phases of the process.

Assessment of the home environment can include floor plans, photographic/video depictions, or home visits. The progression to home must include experimentation and interaction with the environment after physically entering it (therapeutic leave of absence, pass, predischarge home visits, community outings). In essence, the goal is to progressively design an environment that enhances personhood (the objectives are safety and independence) and reflects the characteristics and goals of the patient in concert with others living in the home.

6. Describe two transitional environments in current use as part of community rehabilitation units today.

1. **Independent living trial apartment** is an environment designed to simulate a patient's home, where he or she may reside for a brief period before actual discharge. The patient's family or other social support may choose to visit or live in this simulated home environment to receive comprehensive training and to practice assistive care. Problem-solving and generalization of skills attained during the inpatient rehabilitation process allow adaptation to the traditional home environment and identification of new foci for rehabilitation intervention.

2. **Simulated community environments** provide safe challenges to the patient, while he or she works on refining maximum functional skills. For example, functional skills must be combined in real-world challenges requiring memory and problem-solving as well as mobility.

7. How are the intermediate (residential) environmental needs of a person assessed and met before discharge home?

The rehabilitation team and patient collaborate to determine present and to anticipate evolving patient capabilities and demands imposed by the change in environment. These solutions for the removal of barriers in the home include environmental modifications, assistive devices, and ADL training in the home environment.

A building contractor or designer knowledgeable in accessibility issues, in consultation with the patient and interdisciplinary team, can then determine the structural feasibility of the suggestions, the cost of each recommended modification, and equipment and installation costs. To determine which modifications will be implemented initially and in the future, the patient must prioritize them in terms of immediate requirements to maximize safety, independence, and use of the environment for daily activities, as well as in terms of financial constraints.

Before discharge, the modifications should be phased in to ensure safe and direct access to at least one exterior entrance, a bathroom, and the bedroom. If the patient is able to move and function in the environment, renovations can be phased in until full access is achieved to the areas used by the patient.

8. How can you ensure optimal return to the community for the patient?

To answer this question, consider the following case example: Forest is a 39-year-old landscape contractor and a father of three. Iris, Forest's wife, is a landscape architect. Two years after the couple had purchased their dream home, a 75-year-old farmhouse, Forest fell out of the children's treehouse and sustained a T4-level spinal cord injury. During rehabilitation, he and his team of medical professionals worked together to plan his discharge to the home and community. Forest made good progress in rehabilitation and achieved independence in basic ADLs, wheelchair skills including wheelies, and cooking and driving. The family goal was for Forest to return home to the farmhouse. Comparing the very different outcomes of the following two postdischarge scenarios illustrates the best way to achieve desired rehabilitation goals.

Scenario 1. Approximately 2 weeks prior to Forest's planned discharge, Iris provided photographs of their farmhouse to his rehabilitation team of a social worker, an occupational therapist, a physical therapist, a rehab nurse, and a physician.

Suggestions included a ramped entrance; bedside commode for toileting, since the bathroom on the second floor is located at the end of a long hallway opposite the master bedroom; sponge bathing until modifications could be made; plans for an eventual stairglide or wheelchair stairlift to connect the first and second floors, where the bedrooms are located; and an accessible sink in the kitchen, created by removing the doors underneath. Adaptive equipment was provided with training for Forest and Iris at discharge. Home care, occupational therapy (OT), physical therapy (PT), and adaptive driver training were recommended. A home visit by his rehabilitation therapist to conduct an environmental assessment had to wait to be covered by home care therapy.

Forest's friends built him a makeshift ramp, but it was too steep for him to navigate himself, and two people had to wheel the chair up to the door. A single hospital bed was set up in the dining room with a curtain as a doorway. A commode was set up by the bed for toileting. A portable shower unit was set up in the dining room for bathing. Forest had no privacy, was exposed to a great deal of noise, and was on display for all visitors from the neighborhood who often came by to say hello by peering in the bay window. He did like being the center of attention for his kids; they could watch him do things and get a better understanding of his disability and how he adapts. At night, he watched TV with Iris, but there was no room in his bed for them to sleep together and little space for them to position themselves for reestablishing intimacy. He was "in the hospital at home." This was not the empowering independence that he had imagined. Home care OT and PT maximized his ability to perform ADLs and increased his muscle strength within his very limited intermediate environment, though it was certainly not the lifestyle he had imagined while awaiting discharge home.

Scenario 2. At admission, the physician requested that a floor pan of their house and a few photographs be submitted to the occupational therapist. Five weeks before discharge, a home visit was made and recorded on videotape. Four weeks prior to Forest's discharge, a referral was made to an occupational therapist/architect with expertise in disability assessment, adaptive design, accessible construction, and assistive technology. This accessibility consultant provided a variety of funding resources to assist in the cost of modifications. The accessibility consultant attended a team meeting within 2 days of the initial referral and watched videotapes of the home environment, both exterior and interior. The goals and concerns were expressed by the patient, his wife and rehabilitation team members. The accessibility consultant visited their home and conducted a thorough environmental assessment of each area of Forest's intermediate environment.

This evaluation targeted environmental barriers and problems in each area of the home, specifically parking, driveway, walkways, entrances, type of lighting, door hardware, hallways, floor surfaces, space planning in each room, type of furniture, kitchen/bathroom layout and use of appliances and fixtures, stairs, bedrooms, basement, safety, utilities, security, environmental controls, adaptive equipment, home and lawn maintenance, and leisure space. A week of family activity was reviewed in order to design modifications that would allow Forest to participate more fully. Where environmental demands exceeded Forest's functional abilities, a list of barriers and problems was generated and organized by area. Recommendations to remedy these problems generated a list of solutions that included specialized equipment, rearranging the environment, and structural alteration of the environment. These recommendations were formulated to include adaptability, the possibility of Forest's changing status, and the need to create an environment in which both Forest and Iris could raise a family.

Forest and Iris prioritized these recommendations. The reconstruction plan included two accessible parking spaces. A gradually sloped ramp with side rails was installed that led to a widened door with an automatic opener. Forest's home office space was rearranged to provide an unobstructed route. Forest's top desk drawer was removed, providing adequate access for his wheelchair. An intercom system allowed him to communicate with children upstairs and downstairs as well as with landscape employees that would visit or work in the home.

The family bathroom was enlarged by taking some space from the hallway and modified with by widening the doorway and installing levered door handles and faucet controls, an accessible height sink with an open bottom, an automatic hand dryer and soap dispenser, paper towel dispenser, a high rise toilet with a flusher extension and grab bars, and accessible height light switches.

Upon Forest's return to his home on a weekend pass, he was comfortable, self-reliant, and able to immediately integrate his rehabilitation skills into his day-to-day life. After discharge, the home care therapists were able to carry over the progress and skills achieved in the rehabilitation center, resulting in a lot less frustration from unnecessary environmental barriers and inadequate or inappropriate equipment.

Conclusion. Successful rehabilitation requires specification of the immediate and the intermediate needs and the community environment. Early identification of needs facilitates discharge and optimizes patient adaptation. A discharge from rehabilitation should be an admission into the community.

9. After the patient is relocated to home, what other assessments are needed to help change the immediate environment to meet personal needs?

Once the patient is home and using the environment, further biosocial and functional assessment by an occupational or physical therapist or an accessibility consultant may be necessary to continue to maximize functional independence in self-care. *Role changes* may result from disabilities that prevent the patient from returning to a previous job or to duties in the home. Transitions to this new status can be less stressful if adequate preparation is accomplished through **family scenario mapping** (verbal review of family activities to define tasks by interest and aptitude). In addition, transition can be facilitated by practice with therapy as needed in such areas as bathroom and kitchen activities, housekeeping, gardening, home maintenance, childcare, and marital relations.

10. What areas of the home are considered in a functional home assessment?

An occupational therapist follows the sequence of movements the patient would take through the home. The therapist considers such environmental elements as:

Parking	Location of telephones
Exterior walkways and driveway	Interior stairs and handrails

Steps
Exterior lighting
Lawn maintenance
Security
Entrances and doorways
Interior hallways
Living/dining room layout and furniture
Floor surfaces
Switches and environmental controls
   (e.g., heating, lighting, air conditioning)
Interior lighting

Accessing anduse of bathroom (especially
   toilet and tub/shower)
Kitchen layout and appliances
Storage (including closets and dressers)
Laundry facilities
Basement access
Location of breaker/fuse boxes
Need for environemental control units (ECUs)
Need for personal emergency response system
Locations and use of fire extinguisher and
   smoke alarms

11. How is accessibility defined in the community environment?

Government legislation has established accessibility guidelines at the federal, state, and local levels. These regulate the type, location, design, and layout of public and, in some cases, private spaces. Most building design is based on the use of space by an average person and may not meet the needs of individuals with disabilities, tall or short stature, or any other physical or cognitive characteristics that do not fall into society's norm. The **Access Board**, a federal agency responsible for developing these guidelines, has organized numerous task forces, comprised of disability advocates and national experts in the design and construction industry, to develop accessibility guidelines that address construction of all types of environments. The goal is eventually to develop a single set of design and construction guidelines that can be adopted by any state to comply with all previous federal legislation dealing with accessibility of environments for children as well as adults with a variety of abilities and disabilities. Due to separation of church and state, religious organizations are exempt from complying with federal accessibility guidelines unless they house a service open to the general community.

12. What rights does a tenant with a disability have?

The **Fair Housing Act of 1988** mandates accessibility compliance and civil rights protection in private housing. Persons with disabilities are provided equal access to housing and a mechanism for filing complaints if their civil rights are violated. According to this law, the resident cannot be denied the opportunity to modify the rented home to meet individual needs for accessibility. However, the cost of the modification is the responsibility of the renter. The landlord may require that the work be done by a professional approved by him, and an escrow account may be established in which the tenant must place funds for returning the residence to its original state. Modifications that may be easily used by other tenants and do not change the nature of the residence (e.g., widening doorways, levered handles, grab bar solid blocking) would not be required to be remodified. A physician's order stating that these modifications are a medical necessity would enable the tenant to deduct the cost as a medical expense on his or her income taxes. **Section 504** of the **Rehabilitation Act of 1973** mandates that public housing and housing subsidized with federal funds be accessible and adaptable to meet the needs of tenants with disabilities.

13. What exterior elements should be considered when making an apartment accessible?

Parking spaces should be level and located near an accessible entrance. Each space should be at least 96 in wide and have an adjacent access aisle at least 60 in wide. Two accessible parking spaces may share a common access aisle. One **no-step entrance** may be created by grading the entrance to the ground level, by constructing a porch lift or stair glide, or by constructing a ramp. The **ideal grade** on an exterior uncovered ramp is 1:20 (20 inches of ramp length for every inch of height)—the maximum grade should not exceed 1:12; if an entrance is 2 ft from ground level, the ideal ramp length is 40 ft. A level **platform** at the top of the ramp should provide adequate turning radius for a wheelchair to maneuver and turn, and a 24-in area on the latch side of the door to allow approach.

All door thresholds should be 1/2 in high or less, removed, or beveled. All **doorways** should be 36 inches wide with at least a 32-in clearance when the door is open. An alternative to widening existing doorways is to install **swing clear hinges**, which allow the door to open clear of the doorframe, thereby increasing the door clearance by approximately 2 inches. Door-closing pressure should be 5 lbs or less. **Automatic door openers** and **keyless locks** create easy access for any resident of the apartment building with limited upper body strength and hand function. **Levered door handles** or doorknob adapters may make it easier to use door hardware.

14. What elements should be considered in making interior spaces and hallways accessible?

Motion sensitive, photosensitive, or automatically timed lighting along walkways and entrances provide security and visual cueing for safety and direction. Walkways and hallways should be 48 in wide. Elevator controls must be located at an accessible height from a wheelchair and should have tactile and auditory indicators for each floor. Outlets and switches should be located approximately 18 in from the floor.

The turn radius in each room of the apartment should allow enough space for a wheelchair to turn and maneuver, usually a minimum of 60 in in diameter. In tight spaces, such as in a kitchen and bathroom, open areas underneath countertops and sinks and open shower stalls can be utilized for this turning area.

15. Discuss environmental adaptations needed in bathrooms.

Multilevel or adjustable sink heights and counter tops provide accessibility from standing and seated positions. Plumbing should be installed toward the back wall with hot water pipes insulated and water temperature set to prevent burns. **Single-levered faucet handles** are universal. Automatic faucets, hand dryers, wall-mounted electric toothbrushes, and soap/shampoo dispensers may be installed for a person with limited hand function and upper body strength. **Toilet height** of 17–19 in allows horizontal transfers from the wheelchair and limits the degree that an adult must bend when getting up and down. However, for a child or short adult this may be too high.

An adequate **grab bar system** provides support throughout the tub and toilet areas and must be located at the height that promotes safe movement and good body mechanics. A **hand-held showerhead** on an adjustable-height track can be used for bathing from a seated and standing position. **Tub lifts**, which lower a person into a tub, can be controlled by hydraulic, battery, or manual mechanisms. A rubberized mat and tub strips provide a nonslip surface. An angled mirror and a side-mounted medicine cabinet can be used from a standing or seated position.

Adequate lighting is of the nonglare type, preferably with sconces and multiple bulbs or adjustable intensity. A **ground fault intercept (GFI) outlet** prevents electrocution from the use of electrical appliances near a sink or other source of water. **Contrasting the color of surfaces**, especially background and foreground, enables people with visual or cognitive impairments to see and define surfaces.

16. Discuss environmental adaptations for kitchens.

Cabinets should allow enough toe space for wheelchair clearance. A U-shaped or L-shaped kitchen design provides efficiency of movement and work. Use a side-by-side refrigerator with adjustable shelves and drawers. A stove installed in an accessible countertop or one with adjustable height should have staggered burners and side- or front-mounted controls to prevent accidental burns when reaching. An angled mirror installed on the back wall allows a seated person to view the contents of pots. A side-swing wall oven is advisable. A pull-out shelf or cutting board installed beneath the oven or near the stove and sink areas provides a stable surface for transferring hot items from the oven as well as a working surface usable from a seated position.

All appliances and sinks should have counter space on both sides so those heavy items can be slid from one place to another without excessive lifting. The sink should have a maximum depth of 6 inches. A **long, retractable water hose** on the sink makes cleanup and filling pots on the burners easy if installed nearby. **Task lighting** over work areas affords extra lighting. **Lazy**

Susan's in the cabinets and the refrigerator allow access to items toward the back of shelves, and **easy-glide, pull-out shelving** creates accessible storage in cabinets while decreasing the need for reaching and bending.

A **fire extinguisher** located at an accessible height and location is very important. A message board or tape recorder can be used for notes and directions on the use of small appliances. Large knobs or buttons on the stove, dishwasher, and microwave controls are helpful, but existing ones often can be adapted. A strip outlet with a single on/off switch for small appliances can be installed toward the front of a lower cabinet under the countertop work surface.

17. What adaptations may be considered in the living room?

Seating should be firm and high enough for smooth transfers and movement from sitting to standing. Sturdy armrests with a good grasping surface provide stability for good body mechanics. An electric-powered, lounge lift chair or a spring-loaded seat lifter can also promote safety and increase independence. Tight, short-loop **carpeting**, preferably glued to the floor or with a dense, firm, thin pad, allows easier and safer movement. **Environmental control units (ECUs)** enable regulation of thermostats, lighting, stereos, and television from a single location or portable control unit. Intercoms to entrances and other rooms and remote door openers decrease the need to move quickly.

18. What is visitability? Why is this movement important?

Visitability is a design concept for residential households that promotes the creation of communities in which people of all abilities and disabilities, especially mobility impairments, can get into the door and use at least one bathroom when visiting neighbors. Key features of visitability include at least one no-step entrance, at least 32-in clearances on all doorways with ½-inch or less thresholds, and a bathroom door and interior space that is large enough for wheelchair access, especially to the toilet and sink areas. This concept provides a bridge from the intermediate to the surrounding community environment and fosters social interdependence (neighbor role) and relationships that can offer natural supports for persons with disabilities. This concept is being promoted by **Concrete Change**, an organization based in Atlanta and created by Eleanor Smith, a wheelchair user.

19. Give some examples of accessible features for visually impaired persons.

1. **Increased lighting with reduced glare.** Situate lighting to reduce shadows; use shades, sconces, or recessed lighting to diffuse direct lighting.

2. **Contrasting solid color of surfaces.** Defines objects and spaces, especially background and foreground (e.g., contrasting the color between the floor and wall and/or door, toilet seat and floor).

3. **Raised letters** or **voice output** on controls and signage. Use of large print with high contrast.

4. **Varying textures** provide cues for direction, dangerous situations, and boundaries (e.g., different floor textures, simple patterns).

5. **Illuminated switches** for appliances, lights, etc.

6. **Nonskid, matte-finish floor surfaces** decrease glare and perceptual distortions.

20. Give some examples of accessible features for hearing-impaired persons.

1. Use of **TDDs** for telephone communication, fax machine, and telephone relay systems.

2. Handy access to **paper and writing implement** for communication.

3. **Vibrating devices** such as alarms on clocks, smoke alarms, telephone, doorbell, and baby monitor.

4. **Smoke alarms** and other signals (e.g., doorbells, telephone) with visual-alerting devices. Access to oral and sign language interpreters when needed.

5. **Amplification devices** to eliminate background noises and increase volume of desired noise.

6. **Furniture arrangement** so that seating is facing and adequate lighting so that the person can use visual cues when speaking.

21. A single woman with mild dementia had to be discharged home. Suggest possible environmental solutions for challenges she may face.

1. Provide environmental cues to address safety, memory, and communication deficits.

2. Personal emergency response system with medication management. Training in the use of the devices and monitor ability to learn.

3. Automatic medication management system that is set up weekly by a home care nurse.

4. Burglar alarm and posted fire escape plan that has been learned, practiced, and monitored regularly.

5. Smoke alarms that are hot-wired with battery back-up.

6. Emergency lighting in case of power failure.

7. Daily call to monitor ability to care for herself.

8. Meals on wheels and use of microwave with electric hot-water pot.

9. Electric range or microwave oven. Avoid use of a gas stove. Automatic turn-off controls to address memory deficits.

10. Post instructions on the step-by-step use of all appliances and their safety issues.

11. Preprogram telephone numbers used most for one-button speed calling.

12. Use of a tape recorder to record daily instructions or for message taking.

13. Provide opportunities for the patient to access as many community resources as needed to maintain her independence, health, and safety and promote socialization—e.g., support groups, religious associations, social service agencies, transportation.

22. Which is the most dangerous room in the house?

The bathroom. Bathroom accidents are one of the leading causes of death and disability in the older population. Shower and tub falls rank as the third leading cause of accidental death in the 50-plus age group. More than half of all accidents could be prevented with some sort of environmental modification.

23. What does the phrase "aging in place" mean?

According to a 1990 study by the American Association of Retired Persons, 86% of seniors (65 years and older) want to "age in place," i.e., remain in their present homes as long as possible. In 1986, the figure was 78%. This shows an increasing desire for older adults to do whatever is possible to make their homes fit their changing needs as they age or become disabled.

One in 10 elderly move against their wishes due to the environmental limitations of their present homes. Most of these people are homeowners who have occupied the home for 20+ years, and 86% of these homes are mortgage-free. Many spouses or family members provide partial or full-time caregiving when needed, rather than choosing a nursing home or specialized senior housing. Environmental modifications, adaptability of the environment, specialized equipment, services, and ADL training can assist in providing seniors and people with disabilities with this goal, maximizing quality of life, autonomy, and health.

BIBLIOGRAPHY

1. Freiden L, Cole JA: Independence: The ultimate goal of rehabilitation for spinal cord-injured persons. Am J Occup Ther 39:734–739, 1985.
2. Grandjean E: Fitting the Task to Man: An Ergonomic Approach. London, Taylor & Francis, 1986, pp 263–357.
3. Kornblau B, Shamberg S, Klein R: Americans with Disabilities Act position paper: Occupational therapy and the ADA. Am J Occup Ther 54:622–625, 2000.
4. Pedretti LW: Occupational Therapy:Practical Skills for Physical Dysfunction. St. Louis, Mosby, 1985, pp 436–461.
5. Shamberg S: The accessibility consultant: A new role for occupational therapist under the ADA. Occup Ther Pract 4(4):14–23, 1993.

6. Shamberg A, Shamberg S: Re-entry begins at home: Maximizing independence through environmental modifications. Natl Head Inj Found TBI Challenge 2:4–8, 1994.
7. Stiens DW, Stiens SA: Environmental modifications and role functions: Redesign of a house for a family with a paraplegic father. J Am Parapleg Soc 16:278–279, 1994.
8. Stiens SA: Personhood disablement and mobility technology: Personal control of development. In Gray DB, Quatrano LA, Liberman M (eds): Designing and Using Assistive Technology: The Human Perspective. Towson, MD, Paul Brookes, 1998, pp 29-49.
9. Wylde M, Baron-Robbins A, Clark S: Building for a Lifetime:The Design and Construction of Fully Accessible Homes. Newtown, CT, Taunton, 1994.

RESOURCES

Access Board Checklists: UFAS and ADAAG, www.access-board.gov *or* 202-272-5434.

American Association of Retired Persons, Fulfillment, K St. NW, Washington, DC 20049.

Abilities OT Services, Inc—comprehensive functional and environmental assessments, accessibility consultations, and educational programming. 1-410-358-7269; www.blackboard.com/courses/ADTS2000.

Abledata—database of free information, listing over 17,000 adaptive devices. 1-800-346-2742.

Access Board-ATBCB—technical assistance and resource manuals on accessibility guidelines and compliance issues. ADA resources. 1-202-272-5434 (voice), 1-202-272-5449 (TTD), 1-800-872-2253.

American Occupational Therapy Association (AOTA)—information for employers and consumers concerning ADA and accessibility and the OT ADA Consultant Network. 1-800-SAY-AOTA (members), 1-800-755-8550 (consumers and employers).

A Comprehensive Approach to Retrofitting a Home for a Lifetime—National Home Builders Research Center, 400 Prince George's Blvd., Upper Marlboro, MD 20772-8731; www.nahbrc.org.

A Consumer's Guide to Home Adaptations—Adaptive Environments Center 374 Congress Street, Ste 301 Boston, MA 02210 617-695-1225

CEAC (Certificate in Environmental Access for Consultants & Contractors)—PRIME (Professional Resources In Management Education, Inc.), 1820 S.W. 100th Avenue, Miramar, FL 33025; 954/436-6300; 954/436-0161 (fax); http://www.accessrehab.com

Center for Universal Design—one of the major national resource and educational centers for environmental design for people with disabilities and universal access. They carry extensive publications and conduct trainings nationwide. http://www.design.ncsu.edu/cud.

Department of Housing and Urban Development (HUD)—1-800-795-7915.

Design School of North Carolina State University—Box 8613, Raleigh, NC 27695-8613; 800-647-6777.

Equal Employee Opportunity Commission and Department of Justice (1991), Americans with Disabilities Act Handbook, JS Government Printing Office.

Hensen J: *Building a Ramp* (1988)—Arkansas Department of Human Services, Division of Rehabilitation Services, Donaghey Plaza West, Slot 3440, P.O. Box 1437, Little Rock, AR 72203-1437; (501) 682-8650.

Institute for Technology Development, Advanced Living Systems Division—research and information on accessible design and products. 1-601-634-0158.

National Association of Home Builders, Research Center—publications on senior housing and accessible products. 1-301-249-0305, 1-800-368-5242.

National Easter Seal Society—videos, publications, resource information, and sensitivity training on a variety of disability issues. 1-312-726-6200, 1-312-726-4258 (TDD).

National Organization on Disability (NOD)—publications and newsletter concerning ADA, disability rights, and accessibility; also specializing in accessibility for places of worship. 1-202-732-1139, 1-202-732-5316 (TDD).

National Resource Center on Supportive Housing & Home Modification—University of Southern California/Andrus Gerontology Center, 3715 McClintock Avenue, Los Angeles, CA 90089-0191; 213/740-1364; 213/740-7069 (fax); http://www.homemods.org.

Paralyzed Veterans Administration (PVA), Access Information Bulletin—discusses issues in accessible design, construction, and retrofitting. 1-800-424-8200.

Trace Research and Development Center, University of Wisconsin—database of products and organizations on computer access for persons with disabilities. 1-608-262-6966.

Volunteers for Medical Engineering (VME)—future home resource center for assistive technology and adaptive design. 1-410-666-0086, 1-410-666-9023 (fax).

13. LEGISLATIVE ISSUES IN THE FIELD OF PHYSICAL MEDICINE AND REHABILITATION

Leighton Chan, M.D., M.P.H., Mary Richardson, Ph.D., M.H.A., and Richard Verville, J.D.

1. How has legislative action addressed the needs of persons with disabilities?

Currently, over 54 million people in the U.S. have a disability. At least 20% of the population have one or more disabilities. The federal government has continually attempted to protect the rights of these citizens and provide opportunities for them to live the fullest of lives in freedom. Legislation has addressed rights to education, public access, income, health care, housing, vocations training, and employment for about 15% of the U.S. population. These laws have a potent and pervasive affect on patient outcomes by specifying many aspects of the social and physical environment in which they live.

2. How has the federal government attempted to protect the civil rights of persons with disabilities?

Attempts were made to include individuals with disabilities in the Civil Rights Act of 1964. However, these efforts failed, and it was not until the Rehabilitation Act of 1973 that the federal government began to address the issue of discrimination against those with disabilities. More recently, the Americans with Disabilities Act (ADA) has further expanded the rights of persons with disabilities.

3. What is the Americans with Disabilities Act?

The ADA was signed into law by President George Bush in 1990. Most people are aware that the ADA requires the removal of architectural barriers in some facilities; however, the ADA is much more that just a set of building codes and regulations. The ADA takes aim at discrimination and articulates goals for equal opportunity, full participation, independent living, and economic self-sufficiency. It documents that people with disabilities, as a group, occupy an inferior status in our society and are severely disadvantaged socially, vocationally, economically, and educationally. It calls for a "clear and comprehensive national mandate for the elimination of discrimination against individuals with disabilities" and provides enforceable standards for doing so.

Specifically, the ADA is designed to prevent discrimination against those with disabilities in several settings: employment, public services, public accommodations, and telecommunications and transportation. These rights had been partially protected by The Rehabilitation Act of 1973, which prohibited discrimination in programs receiving federal assistance. The ADA extends these rights to cover entities not receiving such funds. This means that private concerns, such as businesses and restaurants, must abide by the ADA.

Like much federal legislation, the ADA's language is specific in some places and vague in others. Therefore, it has been up to the judicial system to sort out some of the operational details of the ADA through a series of ongoing legal actions. Thus, many of the ADA's implementation issues are not yet resolved. In addition, state and local laws may duplicate or contradict ADA guidelines. Complete, up to date information on specific regulations in your area can be obtained by contacting your regional DBTAC (Disability and Business Technical Assistance Center) [1-800-949-4232 U/TTY].

4. How does the ADA define disability?

The ADA defines **disability** as "(A) a physical or mental impairment that substantially limits one or more of the major life activities of such individual, (B) a record of such an impairment,

(C) being regarded as having such an impairment." Thus, those with physical disabilities *or* mental disabilities are covered under the act. The drug and alcohol provisions of the ADA protect those who are recovering alcoholics and former drug abusers. The ADA will not protect an alcoholic who is unable to perform their job due to alcoholism, nor will it protect current drug abusers.

5. What are the employment provisions of the ADA?

The ADA defines an **employer** as anyone engaged in an industry effecting commerce who has 15 or more employees. The ADA prohibits discrimination by the employer against any *qualified individual* with a disability in regard to hiring, promotions, discharge, compensation, training, or other privileges of employment. Qualified individuals are those who "with or without *reasonable accommodation,* can perform the *essential functions* of the employment position that such person holds or desires." Reasonable accommodations must be made by the employer unless it poses *undue hardship* on the operation of the business.

The ADA specifically prohibits an employer from using screening methods and selection criteria that do not pertain to the requirements of the job and/or are meant to deny opportunity to the candidate because of his or her disability. Furthermore, the employer must clearly articulate the skill demands of the position and the performance expectations. If a person can meet those demands and expectations with reasonable accommodation by the employer, then he or she must be considered equally with other candidates, regardless of disability.

The **Equal Employment Opportunities Commission** (EEOC) is in charge of issuing regulations concerning employment and the ADA, and many of these rules are published in the Code of Federal Regulations. In general, however, the Commission has opted for a case-by-case approach to resolving important issues, such as defining what constitutes reasonable accommodation, undue hardship, and the essential functions of employment. Fortunately, many of these definitions were resolved during the legal challenges to section 504 of the Rehabilitation Act of 1973, which contained similar wording. EEOC has published guidances on reasonable accommodations.

6. What are the public service provisions of the ADA?

Title II of the ADA states that "no qualified individual with a disability shall be excluded from participation in or be denied the benefits of the services, programs, or activities of a public entity or subjected to discrimination by such entity." Public entities are defined as state and local governments and the National Railroad Passenger Corporation.

The title goes on to describe specific requirements for public transportation. In general, all public rail systems must have accessible cars. Retrofitting existing public buses is not required, but all new vehicles purchased or leased must be accessible, and good-faith efforts must be made to acquire accessible used vehicles.

7. What are the public accommodation provisions of the ADA?

Title III of the ADA specifies that "no individual shall be discriminated against on the basis of disability in the full and equal enjoyment of the goods, services, facilities, privileges, or accommodations of any place of public accommodation by any person who owns, leases (or leases to), or operates a place of public accommodation." The title lists places of public accommodation to include hotels, restaurants, professional offices, museums, etc. Religious organizations are exempted from this portion of the ADA.

Title III of the ADA requires that preexisting places of public accommodation remove architectural barriers only if this is readily achievable—i.e., "if this is easily accomplished and able to be carried out without difficulty or expense". Among the basic changes that may be needed for compliance are:
   a. Making curb cuts
   b. Installing ramps
   c. Widening doorways
   d. Assuring an accessible path from parking lot to areas of service provision
   e. Removing high-pile carpeting to allow wheelchair accessibility

f. Installing paper cup dispensers at water fountains

g. Installing accessible toilets

8. What are the telecommunications provisions of the ADA?

Title IV of the ADA encourages the Federal Communications Commission to make telecommunications facilities available for hearing-impaired and speech-impaired individuals. It requires development of relay services for TTY users and that all federally funded public service announcements on television include closed captioning (subtitles). Title IV also requires the telecommunications industry to create the infrastructure necessary to utilize closed captioning.

9. What is the role of the physiatrist in regard to the ADA?

A good physiatrist must know the **rights** afforded to persons with disabilities by the ADA and make sure the patient andrehabilitation team are well versed in them so these goals can be achieved. In regard to the **employment provisions** of the ADA, a physiatrist may be called upon by an employer to state the work limitations of a particular patient and specify any job modifications that might be necessary. Therefore, a physiatrist must be aware of what questions to ask an employer and have a good grasp of assistive technology that might help a patient perform specific job-related tasks.

10. How do individuals with disabilities acquire medical insurance?

For those who do not have private insurance, the most common way is through Medicare and Medicaid. Persons who are injured while working may have their medical bills covered through Workers' Compensation.

11. What is Medicare?

Medicare was created under the Social Security Act of 1956. It is a federally run program that provides health care coverage to those who have paid a Medicare payroll tax during their working years. In addition, family members of those who qualify may also be covered. In 1999, Medicare provided health care coverage for 39.5 million people.

In general, Medicare benefits begin when one retires and applies for Social Security benefits, but no earlier than age 65. An eligible individual can apply for benefits earlier in life if they are disabled or have renal disease and require dialysis.

12. How is Medicare organized?

Medicare coverage is divided into two parts. **Part A** covers the cost of inpatient hospitalization and home health services, as well as stays in skilled nursing facilities and hospices. **Part B** is a voluntary program requiring additional payments by the beneficiary, and it covers the services of physicians, outpatient clinic visits, and many ancillary services such as x-rays, lab tests, and durable medical equipment. Many private insurance companies offer Medicare supplemental coverage for those items not covered in Part A or B.

13. How does Medicare pay for inpatient rehabilitation?

Medicare's payment system for inpatient rehabilitation is currently transitioning from a **fee-for-service** system defined by the Tax Equity and Fiscal Responsibility Act of 1982 (TEFRA) to a new **prospective payment system**.

Critics of the old TEFRA payment system point to the rapid increase in rehabilitation facilities as a sign of over-utilization. Indeed, from 1985 to 1991 the number of rehabilitation facilities in the U.S. grew from 335 to 816. In addition, over that same time period, the percentage of Medicare patients in these institutions grew from 50% to 70%, suggesting that the increase was largely fueled by individuals with Medicare coverage.

In the Balanced Budget Act of 1997, Congress mandated that the Centers for Medicare and Medicaid Services (formerly the Health Care Financing Administration), the federal body charged with administering Medicare, implement a new prospective payment system for inpatient rehabilitation.

While the system is still under development, it will likely be based on a **per episode** system, not unlike the Diagnostic-Related Groups system that determines payment for acute care hospitalization. Patients will be placed in certain groups based on characteristics such age, diagnoses, and functional status. Rehabilitation facilities will be given a fixed amount of money for each patient based on the category they fall into, no matter how long the patient stays. Additional payments may also be given to facilities based on their location, the income status of their patients, and for "outliers" (patients whose extended stay might be particularly expensive). The current plan is for this new prospective payment system to start in 2001 and be in full effect several years later.

14. What is Medicaid?

Authorized under Title XIX of the Social Security Act, Medicaid provides health insurance to low income patients as well as to some disabled and medically needy individuals. The Medicaid program is funded jointly by federal and state dollars. The federal government issues broad guidelines to the states, and they administer the programs. Regulations concerning eligibility, coverage, and reimbursement vary from state to state. In 1999, Medicaid provided medical assistance to about 36 million people.

15. How does a person qualify for Medicaid?

In general, Medicaid is a means-tested program. That is, if a qualified individual has an income and resources below a certain level, then they are eligible for coverage. However, not all poor individuals qualify. For instance, healthy adults without children cannot be covered by Medicaid regardless of their income and resources. Individuals who might qualify include pregnant women, families with children, as well as the aged, blind, medically needy, institutionalized, and disabled. Often these individuals have to "spend down" their resources until they qualify.

To qualify for Medicaid on the basis of disability, an individual needs to be receiving Social Security Insurance (SSI) payments for that disability. The SSI program requires that an individual must be "unable to engage in any substantial gainful activity by reason of a medically determined physical or mental impairment expected to result in death or that has lasted or can be expected to last for a continuous period of at least 12 months." In addition, recipients may also have to pass a means test.

16. What is covered under Medicaid?

Medical coverage varies widely from state to state. In general, Medicaid requires that states cover the cost of hospital stays, physician care, and nursing homes. Several states, such as Oregon, have Medicaid waivers to design their own package of benefits. Coverage of many items, such as prescription drugs and dental care, is optional and states are not required to include them in their Medicaid package.

17. How can individuals with disabilities receive income assistance?

Poverty is a commonly associated with disability. With costly medical bills and poor earning potential, many people with disabilities are economically disadvantaged and can come to rely on public assistance. There are two major federal programs to provide income assistance to individuals with disabilities: Social Security Insurance (SSI) and Social Security Disability Insurance (SSDI).

SSI is linked to the Medicaid system and provides financial assistance to low income individuals who are aged, blind, or disabled. To qualify on the basis of disability, a person must be "unable to engage in any substantial gainful activity by reason of a medically determined physical or mental impairment expected to result in death or that has lasted or can be expected to last for a continuous period of at least 12 months." (Note: SSI determination for children is different and based on a categorical definition of disability.) In 1999, an estimated 6.5 million individuals received SSI payments, including 20% who were older Americans, 79% who were disabled and 1% who were blind.

SSDI is similar to SSI but it is linked to the Medicare system. Therefore, to get SSDI benefits, one has to have worked and paid into the Social Security system. Applicants for SSDI must meet a definition of disability similar to that for SSI. Physicians assess when a person cannot work or is ready to return to work. Eligibility is reevaluated approximately every 3 years. In 1999, 6.5 million former workers received SSDI payments.

18. What has the federal government done to encourage vocational rehabilitation for persons with disabilities?

Federal involvement in vocational rehabilitation for people with disabilities was greatly expanded by the Rehabilitation Act of 1973. Title I of the Act provided federal grants to state vocational rehabilitation agencies and outlined guidelines under which these agencies operate.

In general, to be eligible for vocational rehabilitation, a person must have a physical or mental impairment that results in a substantial impediment to employment. Since vocational rehabilitation is not an entitlement program, states are not mandated to provide services to all those who qualify. In fact, states are required to prioritize services to those with the most severe disabilities, including amputees and individuals with paraplegia, quadriplegia, stroke, and other neurological disorders. Title I requires that each person receiving vocational rehabilitation have an individualized plan for employment (IPE) that outlines goals and the specific services required. This IPE is written collaboratively with the program participant.

Title I of the Rehabilitation Act of 1973 authorizes a wide range of services for vocational rehabilitation. These include "evaluation, counseling, guidance, referral, and placement." The title also establishes the Rehabilitation Services Administration to oversee the programs and the National Institute on Disability and Rehabilitation Research to fund research efforts.

Physiatrists should know the specific vocational resources available in their area so they can help their patients reenter the work force if this is desired. While physiatrists are not involved directly in writing the IPE, they can be very helpful in detailing specific limitations, defining a prognosis, and most importantly, clarifying functional strengths and potential.

19. What has the federal government done to educate children with disabilities?

Federally mandated education for children with disabilities began in the mid-1970s, when several studies revealed that only a few states attempted to educate more than half their disabled children. In 1975, Congress passed the Education for All Handicapped Children Act. This Act was later incorporated into Individuals with Disabilities Education Act (IDEA), and together, they have served to define state obligations in regard to education of the children with disabilities.

20. Who is covered under IDEA?

By law, any state that accepts federal funds under IDEA, must have a "zero reject" policy and provide assistance to all who qualify. In general, all children aged 3 to 21 years are eligible for educational assistance under IDEA if they meet specific eligibility criteria. A child must have 1 of 13 specific conditions listed in the Act or they can come under the category of "other health impairment." In addition, this health condition must "adversely affect educational performance" and require special education.

21. What type of education is the state required to provide?

Under IDEA, all qualified children must be provided with a free appropriate public education, including special education and related services in the least restrictive setting. The Act "further mandates that 'to the maximum extent appropriate, children with disabilities...are educated with children who are not disabled." States are obligated to provide the necessary assistive technology and other personnel to achieve these goals.

The intent of IDEA is to promote the "mainstreaming" of children with disabilities into regular classrooms with the rest of their peers. It is felt this improves the education of both disabled *and* nondisabled students. Clearly, however, "mainstreaming" is not appropriate for all children with disabilities, and for some individuals, a more controlled setting may represent the "least restrictive environment." The educational goals for children with disabilities, including the educational setting, are set out in an Individual Education Plan (IEP) produced by the school district for each student. Educational goals vary depending on the student's capabilities. The goals may be similar to students without disabilities or they may be focused on achieving "self-help skills."

22. What is the physiatrist's role in the education of children with disabilities?

While the physiatrist is not directly involved in creating the IEP, they can be very helpful in (1) identifying children who might be candidates for educational assistance; (2) providing written guidance to the school concerning the educational impact of the disability; and (3) outlining a child's health maintenance activities, such medication prescription, urinary catheterization, and g-tube feedings, as well as writing therapy orders.

23. What has the federal government done to promote assistive technology?

The Technology Related Assistance for Individuals with Disabilities Act (Tech Act) was signed into law in 1988 in response to the growing awareness of the role of technology in the field of rehabilitation. The Act defines assistive technology as a combination of both devices and services. The term assistive technology device is defined as "any item, piece of equipment, or product system whether acquired commercially off the shelf, modified, or customized that is used to increase, maintain, or improve the functional capabilities of individuals with disabilities." Assistive technology services means "any service that directly assists an individual with a disability in the selection, acquisition, or use of an assistive technology device." These definitions were later amended into the Individuals with Disabilities Education Act in 1990. In addition to providing definitions, the Tech Act also provides funding to the states for research efforts, demonstration projects, educational programs, as well as direct provision of assistive technology to patients.

BIBLIOGRAPHY

1. Brandt EN, Pope A: Enabling America. Washington, DC, National Academy Press, 1994, p S-2.
2. Public Law. Americans with Disabilities Act of 1990, pp 101–336.
3. Federal Regulations Vol. 56, no. 45, March 7, 1991, pp 9623–9626.
4. Federal Regulations Vol. 56, no. 144, Appendix A to Part 36.
5. US Department of Health and Human Services: 1999 Rockville, MD, Health Care Finance Administration Statistics: Health Care Financing Administration, 2000, HCFA publ mo. 03421.
6. Prospective Payment Assessment Commission, Interim Report on Payment Reform for PPS-Excluded Facilities. Congressional Report C-92-05, Oct. 1, 1992, p 21.
7. Chan L, Koepsell T, Deyo RA, et al: The effect of Medicare's payment system on patient length of stay, charges, and payments in rehabilitation hospitals. N Engl J Med 337:978–985, 1997.
8. Chan L, Ciol M: The effect of Medicare's payment system on discharges to skilled nursing facilities from rehabilitation hospitals. Arch Phys Med Rehabil 81:715–719, 2000.
9. Medicare Cost Reports Data for PPS-Excluded Facilities, 1985–91.
10. Balanced Budget Act of 1997. Public Law 105-33. Subtitle E, Chapter 2, sections 4401–4421.
11. Carter GM, Relles DA, Wynn BA, et al: Interim Report in an Inpatient Rehabilitation Facility Prospective Payment System. No. DRU-2309-HCFA. Santa Monica, CA, Rand Corp., 2000, pp 1–235.
12. Price R: Medicaid: Eligibility for the Aged, Disabled, and Blind. CRS Report for Congress, 94-297 EPW, April 4, 1994, p 39.
13. Pope A., Tarlov A: Disability in America. National Academy Press, 1991, p 47.
14. Richardson M: The impact of the Americans with Disabilities Act on employment opportunity for people with disabilities. Annu Rev Public Health 15:96, 1994.
15. Fast Facts and Figures about Social Security. Social Security Administration, Office of Research, Evaluation and Statistics. Aug 2000.
16. Rothstein L: Disabilities and the Law. New York, McGraw-Hill, 1992, p 55.
17. Melvin D: The desegregation of children with disabilities. DePaul Law Rev 44:603, 1995.
18. Julnes R., Brown S: Assistive technology and special education programs: Legal mandates and practice implications. Law Educ Desk Notes 3(4):54, 1993.
19. Perlman L, Kirk F: Key disability and rehabilitation legislation. J Appll Rehabil Counsel 22(3):25, 1991.

RESOURCES

Disability Business Technical Assistance Center (DBTAC)
1-800-949-4232 U/TTY
www.ADATA.org

Job Accommodation Network (JAN)
1-800-ADA-Work U/TTY
www.50.pcepd.gov/pcepd/JAN.htm

Tech Act Projects
www.resna.org/tap/person/p_direct.htm

III. Rehabilitation Evaluation

14. THE PHYSIATRIC CONSULTATION: Interdisciplinary Intervention and Functional Restoration

Steven A. Stiens, M.D., M.S.

1. What is a physiatric consultation?

In the old days, a consultation was one physician asking another to come to the bedside and evaluate the patient together. In these times, the deliberation between physicians may be separated by space and time. A **consultation** is the process of giving expert medical advice to the physician directing the care of the patient. The relationship between the patient and the consulting physician develops through the steps of suspension of judgment, examination, reporting, and treatment. The physiatric consultant becomes a part of the treatment effort directed by the attending physician and cooperates by making recommendations or conducting the rehabilitation of the patient as delegated by the attending. A physiatric consult includes not only a medical evaluation with treatment recommendations but also a functional assessment that includes rehabilitation recommendations and interventions to minimize impairments, disabilities, and handicaps.

2. Why are PM&R consultations requested?

Inpatient hospital care and outpatient practice are the two most common settings for consultation. Typically, almost all patients who come to physiatric practice are presented through these conduits. Inpatient consultation usually includes a request for transfer of a patient to inpatient rehabilitation. These requests are notoriously late and may not seek any therapeutic advice whatsoever. Less frequently, physiatrists are consulted for concurrent rehabilitation of an inpatient who is receiving acute treatment or surgery. These patients often can be treated with acute rehabilitation then followed up with home care or outpatient therapy. The call for outpatient consultations includes persistent musculoskeletal complaints, new disability with need for disability determination, assuming care of persons with disabilities, pain management, electrodiagnosis, and disability determination. Studies have demonstrated that rehabilitation needs often go unrecognized, that medical student rotations in PM&R increase recognition and referral for disabilities, and that proximity of PM&R services increases utilization.

3. What is the medical continuum?

The medical continuum is a construct for viewing medical intervention in three phases. **Preventive medicine** (public health) focuses on interruption of disease processes, hygiene, immunizations, screening for early disease indicators, and safety. **Acute treatment** (medicine and surgery) is called for if prevention fails. **Rehabilitation**, in theory, occurs after treatment.

4. Should rehabilitation be limited to this late stage of medical care?

Although Rusk referred to rehabilitation as the "third phase of medical care," the interdisciplinary team can intervene throughout the medical continuum. Early intervention with rehabilitation during or before acute treatment can shorten the overall time required for rehabilitation and prevent morbidity and mortality, especially in stroke, cardiac, spinal cord, and amputation rehabilitation. For example, contemporary rehabilitative intervention for a patient who requires a limb prosthesis includes a collaborative effort among vascular surgery, orthopedic surgery, and the interdisciplinary rehabilitation team to prompt appropriate medical attention as soon as infection, ischemia, or other processes threaten a limb. In this consultative model, the physiatrist contributes throughout the medical continuum. If a wound is discovered, the rehabilitation team can advise on dressings, protective footwear, bracing, assistive devices for ambulation, and foot care for the opposite limb. Should preventive efforts fail, the physiatrist and prosthetist can contribute during the acute phase of the medical continuum by planning for level of amputation and applying rigid dressings with pylons immediately after surgery, as indicated for early weight bearing and ambulation. Thereafter, the rehabilitation team will define and fit the definitive prosthesis and continue prevention with systemic interventions to interrupt pathophysiology and treatment for risk factors and risk behaviors. Preventive measures to protect the opposite limb include diabetes management, prevention of platelet adhesion, foot care training, and foot protection with custom footwear with Plastizote inserts and a large toe box. Inclusion of the physiatrist in this early intervention produces the best results for the patient.

5. What skills and knowledge are necessary for the savvy consulting physiatrist?

First and foremost physiatrists are patient-centered function doctors. Therefore, the physiatrist should be knowledgeable about the potential personal experiences of patients with new impairments and disabilities. The primary benefit of the physiatric visit is that rehabilitation can help the patient maximize his or her abilities for the most promising future. The physiatrist must know people, personalities, and coping styles and be able to estimate patient's tolerance for treatment and equipment (**gadget tolerance**). The consultant should know the hospital very well: diets, supplies stocked, therapies, other ancillary support, and pass policies. Finally, it is good to know the "territory" of the community that your patients come from and return to. Knowledge of the surrounding community, landscape, housing designs, and access to places of business helps the physiatrist prepare the patient for the fullest participation upon discharge.

6. What are the objectives of a comprehensive physiatric consultation?

1. Confirm the diagnosis and relate it to functional performance.
2. Quantify functional level. Establish a baseline.
3. Develop a rehabilitation problem list.
4. Provide a functional prognosis.
5. Answer the question of the initial consultation and then inform the team of the proposal for comprehensive rehabilitation interventions.
6. Formulate short, intermediate, and long-term rehabilitation plans.
7. Translate the plans and interventions for the originators of the physiatric consultation and for the patient and family.
8. With the approval of the attending physician, explain the intervention plan to the patient and family (interdisciplinary family conference), emphasizing their participation in the process.
9. Orchestrate the consultations and direct interventions through the interdisciplinary process to achieve goals on schedule.

7. When you go into the room to take the patient's history, how many experts will be present?

At least two: the **patient** and (hopefully) the **physiatrist**. Every experience of an injury or disease is unique because the course of injury and recovery always varies and the person impacted by the bodily changes has a unique development, life experience, and goals. The patient is an expert on his or her illness experience (a subjective sense of not being well) and the impact of disablement (sum total of impairment, disability, and handicap impact). Other "experts" in the room may include family, close friends, attendants, and roommates. Each has his or her own picture of the challenges the patient faces and may have a vision of what recovery is or adaptation should be. These expectations need to be elicited and addressed in the design of a cohesive rehabilitation plan that the patient and the interdisciplinary team accept. In acute inpatient cases, it is often necessary to do ward-based patient, family, and team goal-setting meetings to explain the rehabilitation process and decide on the facility for future postacute rehabilitation.

8. How do you elicit information on actual and specific help the patient gets at home from family, friends, and attendants?

After paralysis, patients often depend on others to accomplish basic activities of daily living (ADLs). In a society that values independence, the facts of practical adaptations are not always casually volunteered by the patient. The establishment of an **atmosphere of acceptance** permits honest expression of functional solutions and requests for improvement in the system that is in place. Keep the patient in charge of his or her life activity. Ask: "Whom do you direct in assisting you with transfers [dressing, bathing, meal preparation, etc.]?" The role of the clinician is to frame the interaction as a learning activity. Each patient is embedded in a physical, social, and economic matrix that includes a variety of current and potential solutions. It is the work of the physiatrist to plan and orchestrate the solution and understand the perceived options in the context of the patient's life. Then a series of person-centered goals can be derived, and a plan can be developed to sequence the achievements that maximize the patient's independence soonest and allow continuance of the plan outside the hospital. Once goals are identified, the team aggressively works on small improvements that will meet the patient's health needs and life goals. Indeed, each situation is a psychosocial and economic equation in itself. The challenge is to understand the patient's specific self-care methods and compliment these processes to precipitate a refinement.

9. What options are there for sequencing the history with the patient?

The first step is introduction and explanation of the services provided by rehabilitation medicine. This is accomplished through introductions and explanation to the patient that his physician consulted with you to work with the patient to review his medical and functional needs and design a rehabilitation plan. Thereafter, rapport is established with the patient by doing a general review of his lifestyle and supports within the home. One sequence option is to record the history chronologically, starting by asking the patient: "When were you last perfectly well?" Proceeding from the assessment or baseline function from history also provides options for adapted improvements in performance that meet the patient's needs. The various aspects of disablement as experienced by the patient can be elicited by asking what bothers her or limits her most. Another option is to focus on the patient's function before the injury or illness and then review the changes afterward in a format that is guided by the problem list. The history can provide some patient education as the problems are carefully explained to the patient and connected to the primary pathophysiology. When carrying out the review of symptoms, be sure to elicit comments about function as well as symptoms.

10. How can the examination be an education for the patient and provide therapy that could contribute to recovery?

Many patients with pain, paralysis, and anesthesia are not fully aware of their capabilities and learn much from a guided examination. In addition, spouses, attendants, and nurses caring for the patient may have questions about methods for improving the patient's care. Sensory testing allows for a discussion of the receptive fields of various peripheral nerves and dermatomes. In the patient with myelopathy, sacral sparing can be explained and used as an incentive to be attentive to and attempt to regain control of bowel, bladder, and sexual function. Range of motion (ROM) testing allows for instruction in self-stretching and ROM with assistance. Strength testing permits instruction in proprioceptive neuromuscular facilitation techniques. Functional motor and coordination testing can lead to demonstration of exercises prescribed for the patient. At the conclusion of a visit, the patient can be set up for independent exercise as is practical.

11. What kind of format best communicates the course and results of the consultation?

The objective of the database is to record the questions to be answered, problems uncovered, functional deficits, adaptive capabilities, recommended interventions, and anticipated future needs. The following information should be recorded:

Section 1. Introduction. Record referring physician and reason for referral.

Section 2. Current Treatment

A. **Identifying statement.** For example: The patient is a [age]-year-old, [occupation, life activity] with [diagnosis or injury], since [date of injury].

B. **Current history and management.** Record details of injury or disease severity. Record active treatment.

C. **Medication, treatment, and exercise.**

Section 3. Past History. Record past medical history, family medical history, social history, review of systems.

Section 4. Current Function

A. **Mobility**—bed, transfers, and ambulation.

B. **ADLs**—hygiene, bathing, eating, urine/bowel management, dressing.

C. **Leisure function**—activities for enjoyment.

D. **Vocational function**—include volunteer work and work in home, parenting.

E. **Equipment** and home **architecture**.

Section 5. Examination. Focus on areas of rehabilitation intervention and assessment of severity of injury or diagnosis. Identify any risks or cause for precaution for therapies. Results of the **functional neuromuscular examination** should be included to assess mobility, ADLs, cognition, and mental status.

Section 6. Problem List. This should include primary diagnosis, date of onset, secondary diagnoses with onset and severity, impairments, disabilities, and handicaps. Follow each problem with a brief assessment description.

Section 7. Recommendations. List these in the same order as problem list. Include short- and long-term goals. Describe an immediate plan (acute rehab), an intermediate plan (transfer to comprehensive inpatient unit), and a future plan (e.g., discharge home, community reintegration).

12. Whose consult is it anyway?

Whose life is it anyway?…The patient's, of course. In practicing patient-centered medicine we must receive confirmation of the patient's interest and willingness to participate in the evaluation process and treatment. Sensitivity and perceptiveness are required as the patient's needs are elicited and the current plan of care is reviewed. The physiatric assessment and treatment recommendation should be communicated to the attending physician or directly responsible resident first for discussion and concurrence. Immediately thereafter, a report should be made to the patient for his or her concurrence with the plan. This minimizes misunderstanding, promotes consistency in information transmitted to the patient, and maximizes cooperation.

13. How is the problem list organized in consultation report notes?

As the chart is reviewed, a problem list is derived that includes **diagnoses, impairments, disabilities,** and **handicaps**, arranged in that order. Specifics of hospital course need not be recorded. The diagnoses themselves, duration of time under treatment, and recent severity measure are most useful in each problem. Each problem should be a short phrase that describes the unique situation of that patient. **Potential problem domains** are primary injury or diagnosis, other diagnoses, spine stability, neurogenic bowel, neurogenic bladder, pressure ulcers, mobility, ADLs, communication, psychological adaptation, social role function, architectural accessibility, community reintegration, and discharge management.

14. How would you carry out a consultation on a 55-year-old married white man with a new left-middle cerebral artery stroke?

On approach to the ward, identify the patient's nurse for a review of his current condition and particular needs. A review of his chart should yield the date of the cerebrovascular accident (CVA), risk factors, complications, and medical stability. Separate the information into a problem-oriented format that includes location, size, and etiology of the stroke, and list the risk factors for CVA as problems as well. Document other associated diagnoses and severity of involvement. For example, a description of diabetes mellitus might read, "IDDM for 10 years with Hb AIC of 8." Separate the problems that can be listed for risks of various complications such as risk for deep venous thrombosis (DVT), edema, and skin breakdown. Then list the disabilities, mobility, ADLs, communication ability, cognitive perception, leisure activities, community reintegration, and spirituality. The assessment should focus on the list of major sensory and mobility limitations, which can be summarized under one problem of mobility. Functional limitations in self-care be summarized in the list of problem ADL limitations. Thereafter, problems at the handicap level can be listed: psychological adaptation (depression), social role function (e.g., husband, neighbor), and architectural access (ramp to door, bathroom access). Recommendations, interventions, and prioritization of short-term goals should be mobilized as soon as possible, making sure to include the family in training, and the patient should be transferred to the least restrictive setting for continued rehabilitation.

15. What is a physiatric prescription?

A *prescription* is a written formula for the preparation and administration of a therapeutic remedy. The physiatrist leads the interdisciplinary rehabilitation team by prescribing specific interventions to meet short- and long-term goals of various patient problem domains. Prescriptions for treatment come in the form of orders for nursing care and consultative referrals to allied health professionals and other members of the rehabilitation team. The physician as team leader must balance specific requests for interactions with the objective or outcomes that may be achieved through a variety of means. Therefore, therapeutic prescriptions are often an amalgamation of objectives, specific requests for treatment, and requests for evaluation and problem-solving to achieve outcomes.

16. How do you write a prescription for treatment that integrates other members of the interdisciplinary team into the rehabilitation process?

The basic components of the physiatric prescription are:
• Identification of discipline consulted (e.g., physical, recreational, occupational therapy)
• Major and significant secondary diagnoses
• Pertinent impairments, disabilities, and handicaps that may be a focus of therapy
• Precautions: cardiac, weight bearing, pulmonary (O_2 sat monitoring)
• Short- and long-term goals and objectives of therapy. Include a copy of physiatric consult as needed
• Specific therapeutic prescription including: areas to be treated, modality, intensity, duration, frequency, as needed
• Frequency of visits and over what period of time
• Date of reevaluation, request for a summary report detailing response to therapy

17. What is a clinical pathway?

A clinical pathway or a **clinical care map** is a uniform procedure for intervention by a variety of medical disciplines in patients within a given diagnostic group. The development of a clinical pathway requires a sufficient number of cases seen per year to justify pathway design. Management of past cases is reviewed by all disciplines that care for patients with the diagnosis. The sequence schedule and details of interventions are designed and agreed upon. A form for the chart is drawn up that has the interventions and disciplines listed. The pathway is typically triggered by one order done by the attending physician. Other referrals and orders are made automatically through the clinical pathway. As a result, time is saved and the quality of care is enhanced.

18. How can the PM&R consultation service be used as a mechanism for teaching?

A PM&R consultation service can fulfill many teaching missions. Bringing rehabilitation to other floors of the hospital clinics or to patients' homes showcases rehabilitation in process and functional outcomes. Bringing medical students and premedical students on PM&R consultation rounds introduces them to patients with a wide spectrum of diagnoses and a variety of impairments, disabilities, and handicaps that are treated in various settings throughout the hospital. The consult service offers an opportunity to provide a broad overview of various medical problems and solutions with rehabilitation.

ACKNOWLEDGMENT

The author thanks Walter Stolov, M.D., for his PM&R consult format, used for decades at the University of Washington.

BIBLIOGRAPHY

1. Fredrickson M, Cannon NL: The role of the rehabilitation physician in the postacute continuum. Arch Phys Med Rehabil 76:SC5–SC9, 1995.
2. Grabois M, Bloodworth D, Bodenheimer C: Consultation and prescription writing. In Grabois M, Garrison SJ, Hart KA, Lehmkuhl LD (eds): Physical Medicine and Rehabilitation: The Complete Approach. Malden, MA, Blackwell, 2000, pp 375–393.
3. Marin EL, Colandner AS: Therapeutic prescription. In O'Young B, Young MA, Stiens SA (eds): PM&R Secrets. Philadelphia, Hanley & Belfus, 1997, pp 509–512.
4. Stiens SA, Berkin DI: A clinical rehabilitation course for college undergraduates provides an introduction to biopsychosocial interventions that minimize disablement. Am J Phys Med Rehabil 76:462–470, 1998.
5. Zimmermann KZ, Brown RD: Rehabilitation technology prescription: Determinations of failure and elements of success in advances in rehabilitation technology. Phys Med Rehabil State Art Rev 11:1–12, 1997.

15. NEUROLOGIC EVALUATION OF THE REHABILITATION PATIENT

Rajiv R. Ratan, M.D., Ph.D., and Adriana Conforto, M.D.

1. Summarize the major parts of the neurologic examination.
Mental status
Cranial nerves
Motor function—tone, power, adventitial movements, reflexes
Sensory function—pain, temperature, vibration, proprioception, stereognosis, two-point discrimination
Cerebellar function
Gait

2. What should bedside cognitive or mental status testing include?
Standard mental status testing is extensive, making it difficult for physicians to remember. To encourage use of the examination, the mnemonic *COMO ESTAS*, the Spanish phrase for "how are you?", can be used to denote the components of the examination:

   C = Cognitive functions; i.e., calculation, concentration, insight, judgment
   O = Overview; i.e., appearance, attitude, level of consciousness, movements
   M = Memory; i.e., recent and remote
   O = Orientation; i.e., to person, place, and time

   E = Emotion; i.e., affect and mood
   S = Speech; i.e., fluency, form, comprehension
   T = Thought; i.e., process, content, perceptual disturbances
   A = Attention; i.e., abstract thinking, recall, intelligence
   S = Something else that the practitioner has forgotten that might be important for the patient—The level of wakefulness and attention should be evaluated and taken as a guideline to interpret performance on other tasks. If arousal is significantly compromised, testing of memory, language, and other cognitive functions may not be valid.

3. What are often the earliest unequivocal symptoms of metabolic or toxic encephalopathy?

Metabolic encephalopathies are among the most common causes of changes in mental status. Etiologies include recreational or prescribed drug intoxication, electrolyte imbalance, hypoxia, and liver disease. **Attention** and **cognition** are the most sensitive indicators of metabolic encephalopathy but are difficult to evaluate if the examiner does not know the premorbid personality or intellect. Under such circumstances, defects in **orientation** and **grasp of test situation** are the most sensitive indicators of brain dysfunction.

Specific questions to be asked include: What time is it? What day is it? How long does it take to reach home from the grocery store [or other well-defined place familiar to the patient]? Disorientation to person and place but not time is rarely observed in structural disease and can be a sign of nonorganic illness or hysteria.

4. Define dementia. What is required for its diagnosis?

Dementia is a clinical state characterized by a significant loss of function in multiple cognitive domains, to the point of interfering with activities of daily living (ADLs). Dementia does not necessarily indicate any specific etiology. Thus, its diagnosis is not synonymous with a progressive course, and it does not imply irreversibility.

The diagnosis requires serial examinations over time that document a decline in intellectual function or a single evaluation of cognitive function with evidence of a higher level of intellectual function in the past. Delirium, psychiatric problems, and focal central nervous system (CNS) abnormalities such as stroke must be excluded. An altered level of consciousness is incompatible with an initial diagnosis of dementia. Once dementia is clinically suspected, a work-up must be done to ascertain its etiology.

5. How can aphasia be distinguished from dysarthria?

Aphasia is a disorder of language; dysarthria is a disorder of articulation. In dysarthria, naming, fluency, repetition, and comprehension are normal. Additionally, the patient can read and write with no errors.

6. What should a bedside evaluation for aphasia include? What abnormalities are seen in the major syndromes of aphasia?

1. **Anomia**—A cardinal feature of many aphasic syndromes. Naming of common objects, such as a pen or watch, is a good initial test of aphasia.

2. **Fluent or nonfluent**—Fluency refers to normal speech rhythm and output. Circumlocutions, use of empty word and incorrect words (e.g., "coon" for car), and syntactical errors can be associated with fluent speech. In nonfluent aphasias, speech is constipated and generated only with a great deal of effort. Nonfluent aphasias are generally associated with cerebral damage anterior to the Rolandic fissure (motor cortex), while fluent aphasias are believed to be posterior to this anatomic structure (sensory cortex).

3. **Comprehension**—Ask the patient to point to the door, window, or electric light. Ask two- to three-step commands, such as "Take your right hand, touch your nose, stick out your tongue." Hearing loss, motor paralysis, or apraxia should be excluded as reasons for not following commands. Comprehension can also be tested by yes/no questions or by commands that require only a pointing response.

4. **Repetition**—Ask the patient to say: "No ifs, ands, or buts" or "Around the rugged rock, the ragged rascal ran."

7. Name some types of aphasias.

Broca's—abnormal naming, nonfluent, normal comprehension, abnormal repetition
Wernicke's—abnormal naming, fluent, abnormal comprehension, abnormal repetition
Global—abnormal naming, nonfluent, abnormal comprehension, abnormal repetition
Conduction—abnormal or normal naming, fluent, normal comprehension, abnormal repetition
Anomic—abnormal naming, fluent, normal comprehension, normal repetition

8. Does the severity of aphasia correlate with the efficiency of communication?

While the severity of aphasia correlates significantly with communication difficulty, other factors need to be considered in maximizing communication skills of the aphasic patient. Information about impairment and training in compensation should be given to the spouse and family as well as the patient. Evaluation of the aphasic patients should include a neuropsychological assessment to differentiate aphasia from apraxia, visuoconstructive difficulties, and neglect.

9. Define unilateral neglect.

Unilateral neglect is a lack of orienting responses to stimuli presented unilaterally. Neglect cannot be diagnosed unless the primary sensory or motor modalities required to sense or orient the particular stimulus are intact. Neglect can be unimodal (i.e., visual neglect) or multimodal (i.e., performing complex tasks, such as dressing, where the patient fails to cover the neglected side). Hemineglect is most commonly associated with right hemisphere strokes but can be seen with strokes or with tumors affecting either hemisphere. Neglect is prognostic of poor functional recovery.

10. After excluding visual field defects and disorders of eye movements, how does one evaluate neglect at the bedside?

1. **Line bisection**—Have the patient mark the center of five horizontal lines, each presented separately on a sheet of paper.

2. **Line cancellation**—Present the patient with a single sheet of paper on which 20 lines in varying orientations are drawn on each half of the page.

3. **Letter cancellation**—Instruct the patient to mark all the A's on a sheet of paper. There should be 8 A's on the sheet, 4 on each side, with 70 distractor letters (e.g., D, L, F, R).

4. **Clock construction**—Have the patient place numbers as they would appear on a clockface with an outline circle on a piece of paper.

With the above tests, performance on the left side can be compared with performance on the right side.

CRANIAL NERVE EVALUATION

11. How should one evaluate the integrity of the patient's visual fields?

Stand about 3 feet in front of the patient, and ask him or her to view your nose. Hold your hands to either side of your face, midway between your eyes and the patient's. Briefly present one or two fingers from each hand, and ask the patient to indicate the number of fingers on each hand. Give the patient one or two trials to make sure that the nature of the trial is understood. The hands should be moved so that all four quadrants of the visual field are tested. These tests will enable detection of a field defect or neglect.

During testing encourage the patient to maintain fixation of your nose. If the patient is uncooperative, bedside confrontation of the visual fields can provide diagnostic information. In the uncooperative, dysphasic, or lethargic patient, visual threat may cause an asymmetric blink response if there is field deficit or neglect.

12. What do defects in the separate visual fields indicate?

Deficits confined to one eye are usually caused by disease of the globe, retina, or optic nerve. Deficits in both eyes (binocular) can be nasal (the half of the visual field of each eye toward the nose) or temporal (the half of the visual field of each eye toward the temple). Bitemporal deficits imply impairment of fibers crossing the optic chiasm (e.g., from pituitary tumor) or homonymous (i.e., the same field of vision for both eyes), indicating disease of the optic tract radiation, or cortex. Temporal lobe (inferior) lesions usually result in superior homonymous field defects, whereas parietal lobe (superior) lesions usually produce lower homonymous field defects.

13. How do you distinguish a field defect due to malingering or hysteria from an organic field defect?

In nonorganic field loss, the most frequently encountered defect remains the same size regardless of distance from the eye and is often described as tunnel vision. In organic field loss, the size of the intact field increases as the distance from the eye increases.

14. What is the first question to ask a patient who complains of diplopia (double vision)?

"Does the diplopia go away when you cover one eye?" Monocular diplopia (double vision that persists with only one eye viewing) is usually due to a problem with the lens or cornea. Binocular diplopia (double vision that disappears with only one eye viewing) is usually due to a paralysis of extraocular muscles.

15. How does one evaluate the seventh cranial nerve?

Paying particular attention to the nasolabial folds and palpebral fissures, look for facial asymmetry at rest and during spontaneous facial movements. Then systematically test the frontalis muscle ("raise your eyebrows"), orbicularis oculi ("Close your eyelids and don't let me open them"), buccinator ("Blow out your cheeks"), elevators of the lips ("Show me your teeth, smile"), orbicularis oris ("Purse your lips and don't let me open them").

Upper motor lesions generally cause lower facial weakness, with slight assymmetry of the palpebral fissures and little or no weakness of the orbicularis oculi or frontalis muscles. Lower motor neuron lesions result in weakness of the upper and lower parts of the face and can involve taste (chorda tympani) and tearing (greater superior petrosal nerve).

16. Define the different types of dysphagia.

Dysphagia can be due to **mechanical factors** or **neurologic dysfunction**. Each of these types of dysphagia can be **oropharyngeal** or **esophageal**.

17. Name some common neurologic causes of oropharyngeal dysphagia.

Stroke	Demyelinating disease	Myasthenia gravis
Brainstem tumor	(multiple sclerosis)	Myopthies
Motor neuron disease	Syringobulbia	Parkinson's disease

MOTOR FUNCTION

18. Define spasticity and rigidity.

Spasticity is the increased resistance appreciated by the examiner when he or she moves a joint briskly. The hypertonicity is sometimes called *clasp-knife spasticity* because, like a pocket knife blade, the initial resistance fades away as the joint is flexed. Spasticity usually involves some specific groups of muscles more than others. For instance, after a brain lesion, a patient may become hemiplegic and have a greater increase in flexor muscles in the upper extremity and extensor muscles of the lower extremity.

Rigidity is defined as increased resistance appreciated by the examiner throughout the range of joint movement. It is like bending a lead pipe and thus is referred to as *lead pipe rigidity*. The *cogwheel sign* corresponds to an intermittent but regular resistance to passive motion. The resistance affects flexor and extensor muscles in the involved limb equally.

19. Name some diseases commonly associated with spasticity.

Diseases that involve damage to the corticospinal tracts (upper motor neurons), such as stroke, brain tumors, multiple sclerosis, traumatic brain and spinal cord injury, cerebral palsy, and cervical spondylosis.

20. What diseases are commonly associated with rigidity?

Diseases that involve damage or dysfunction of the extrapyramidal system (basal ganglia) such as idiopathic Parkinson's disease or drug-induced parkinsonism (e.g., metoclopramide, haloperidol, reserpine).

21. What historical features suggest proximal muscle weakness?
Legs
  Inability to get up from a chair or toilet without using one's hands
  Inability to get out of a car
Arms
  Inability to comb's one hair or brush one's teeth
  Inability to carry grocery bags or young children

22. What are the clinical features of myopathy?
Nearly asymmetric proximal muscle weakness without muscle wasting, with normal sensory examination, and with intact or slightly decreased reflexes.

23. List some of the common causes of myopathy in the rehabilitation setting.

Steroids	Duchenne's muscular dystrophy
Alcohol	Polymyositis
Zidovudine (AZT)	AIDS
Hypothyroidism	Mitochondrial diseases

24. What is the critical clinical difference between myopathies and disorders of the neuromuscular junction (e.g., myasthenia gravis)?
While the distribution of weakness is similar in these disorders, neuromuscular diseases are characterized by **fatigability**. They worsen with use and recover with rest.

25. What historical features suggest distal weakness?
Arms—inability to button, open jars, or hold onto things
Legs—frequent tripping or unusual wear on the toes of the shoes

26. What are the clinical features of peripheral neuropathies?
Distal weakness which may be asymmetric or symmetric, with atrophy, possible fasciculations, sensory loss, and absent reflexes.

27. How can peripheral neuropathies be distinguished from spinal cord lesions?
Spinal cord lesions usually cause weakness that is distal more than proximal. They are characterized by a sensory level below which there is a decrease in sensation, distal symmetric weakness, hyperreflexia, and bowel and bladder problems. Peripheral neuropathies can have a glove-and-stocking sensory loss, dermatomal sensory loss, or sensory loss in the distribution of a single nerve. They are characterized by loss of reflexes rather than hyperreflexia. Finally, some types of neuropathies involve the bladder or bowel. However, peripheral neuropathies cause bladder disorders of emptying, whereas spinal cord lesions usually cause bladder disorders of storage.

28. What pattern of weakness is commonly seen after hemispheric stroke?
Hemispheric stroke involving the internal capsule (subcortical) or cortical motor strip results in hemiparesis of the contralateral limb. The pattern of weakness is typically extensors greater than flexors in both the upper and lower extremity. In subcortical strokes, the face, arm, and leg are usually affected equally, whereas in cortical strokes, the face, arm and leg are usually affected unequally.

29. Describe one grading system for reflexes.
  0 = Absent reflex
  1 = Hypoactive reflex, or normal reflex that can only be elicited with reinforcement
  2 = Normal reflex
  3 = Hyperactive reflex. A clear indicator is elicitation of other reflex responses when testing one reflex. For example, if testing the biceps, and the brachioradialis and finger flexor reflexes are also elicited; this suggests hyperreflexia.
  4 = Clonus

30. What can you do if you get no response when eliciting a reflex?

Make sure to strike the blow crisply on the muscle, vary compression of the tendon with your finger, or try reinforcement. Reinforcement can be done by having the patient perform a strong voluntary contraction of a muscle you are not testing. For example, have the patient bite down to facilitate elicitation of the biceps reflex.

31. How is clonus at the ankle elicited?

Quick dorsiflexion of the foot followed by continuous light pressure against the ball of the foot. The continuous light pressure opposes the reflex plantar flexion elicited by quick dorsiflexion.

32. What does the presence of clonus indicate?

Hyperreflexia due to an upper-motor-neuron lesion. Nonsustained clonus can also be elicited in patients who are anxious.

33. What happens to the abdominal and cremasteric reflexes in a cervical spinal cord lesion?

They are usually absent. When testing this reflex, remember that the abdomen should be relaxed. The abdominal reflex response is difficult to obtain if the muscles are too tense.

34. What is the Babinski sign?

The Babinski sign is dorsiflexion of the great toe in response to a plantar stimulus. It indicates an interruption of upper-motor-neuron tracts to the lumbosacral reflex centers as seen in diseases such as spinal cord injury, stroke, and multiple sclerosis.

SENSORY EXAMINATION

35. Define the primary and secondary sensory modalities.

Primary sensory modalities include pain sensation, temperature sensation, light touch, proprioception, and vibration sense. Primary sensory loss can be due to a lesion in the periphery, spinal cord, brainstem, or thalamus. Stereognosia (form sense, as in identifying a nickel or penny placed in the hand) and topognosia (ability to localize skin stimuli) are **secondary sensory** or cortical sensory modalities.

36. What is the proper way to test pain sensation?

With a clean safety pin. The advantage of a safety pin is that it has a blunt end and a sharp end, thus allowing the reliability of the patient to be tested. The pin should be disposed of after the examination.

37. What is the proper way to test position sense?

Position sense should be tested in the hands or feet. The distal end of the third or fourth digit or toe should be used, as these have the least cortical innervation and are thus the most sensitive to a loss in position sense. The digit should be grasped laterally and moved up or down or maintained in the neutral position. It is helpful to perform the test a few times with the patient's eyes open to be sure communication is established. With the eyes closed, the patient should make no mistakes on five trials. If abnormalities are found in one digit or two, other digits or toes should be tested.

38. What frequency tuning fork should be used for vibration testing?

256 cps.

39. How is the Romberg test performed? What does a positive Romberg sign signify?

The Romberg test examines the integrity of the dorsal columns. It is not a test of cerebellar function. The proper procedure for the Romberg test is to ask the patient to stand with his or her heels together. With the patient's eyes open, note whether he or she sways. Then have the patient close his or her eyes. If the swaying is dramatically worse and the patient almost falls, the

Romberg is considered "positive," and a dorsal column or proprioceptive defect is suggested. Patients normally sway slightly with the eyes closed, but never fall. Patients with cerebellar disease usually sway more with the eyes open as well as closed. In the Romberg test, the visual information for balance is being removed (by having the patient close his/her eyes), thus placing the responsibility for balance solely on the proprioceptive system.

40. Name the anatomic landmarks that mark different dermatomes.

C2—angle of the jaw	T10—umbilicus
C6—thumb	L4—knee cap
C7—middle finger (third digit)	L5—big toe
C8—little finger (fifth digit)	S1—lateral foot
T4—nipple	S4,5—perianal area

CEREBELLAR TESTING

41. What are the clinical features of cerebellar disease?
The main features of cerebellar dysfunction can be remembered by the mnemonic **HANDS Tremor**:

H = **H**ypotonia
A = **A**synergy (lack of coordination)
N = **N**ystagmus (ocular oscillation)
D = **D**ysarthria (speech abnormalities)
S = **S**tation and gait (ataxia)

Tremor = coarse intention tremor

42. How can cerebellar ataxia be distinguished from a sensory ataxia?

Cerebellar ataxia	Sensory ataxia
Nystagmus	Loss of vibration and position sense
Hypotonia	Hypotonia
Coarse intention tremor	Loss of reflexes
Dysarthria	Ataxia worse with eyes closed (positive Romberg sign)

43. What is the best way to describe someone with cerebellar dysfunction?
They look drunk.

44. What is the typical stance of someone with cerebellar dysfunction?
A broad-based gait.

45. How can gait coordination be tested?
Have the patient tandem walk. Ask him or her to step along a straight line, placing the heel of one foot directly in front of the toe of the other foot.

46. How can coordination of the arms be tested?
Have the patient perform a finger-to-chin test. The patient is instructed to touch the examiner's finger, then touch his or her own chin. This sequence is repeated several times with the examiner altering the position of his or her finger with each trial. The chin is used instead of the nose because many patients with cerebellar dysfunction have such poor coordination that they are in danger of poking their own eye. If the patient undershoots or overshoots the examiner's fingers, the test is considered indicative of cerebellar dysfunction.

47. What is the heel-to-shin test?
This is another test of leg ataxia. With the patient lying down or sitting, he or she is instructed to place the heel of one leg on the opposing knee and to run the heel down to the shin.

48. Name some common causes of cerebellar dysfunction seen in the rehab setting.

Strokes, multiple sclerosis, and anticonvulsants (phenytoin, phenobarbital, carbamazepine)

BIBLIOGRAPHY

1. Astrachan JM: Como estas, a mnemonic for the mental status examination [letter]. N Engl J Med 324:636, 1991.
2. Butter C, Kirsch N: Combined and separate effects of eye patching and visual stimulation on unilateral neglect following stroke. Arch Phys Med Rehabil 73:1133–1139, 1992.
3. Caplan L: The Effective Clinical Neurologist. Oxford, Blackwell, 1990.
4. DeMeyer W: Technique of the Neurologic Examination: A Programmed Text, 3rd ed. New York, McGraw Hill, 1980.
5. Johnson RT, Griffin J: Current Therapy in Neurological Diseases, 4th ed. Philadelphia, B.C. Decker, 1994.
6. Sundet K: Assessment of aphasia in relation to communication and cognitive impairments among stroke patients. Scand J Rehabil Med Suppl 26:60–69, 1992.
7. Kirschner HS: Speech and language disorders. In Samuels MA, Feske S (eds): Office Practice of Neurology. New York, Churchill Livingstone, 1996.
8. Wintraub S: Examining mental state. In Samuels MA, Feske S: Office Practice of Neurology. New York, Churchill Livingstone, 1996.

16. MANUAL MUSCLE TESTING AND RANGE OF MOTION MEASUREMENT

John J. Nicholas, M.D., and Ian B. Maitin, M.D.

MANUAL MUSCLE TESTING

1. Why perform manual muscle testing (MMT)?

Results help define impairment and develop a program to improve function.

2. In MMT, how are muscles graded?

0/5 = No motion at all
1/5 = Trace motion observed
2/5 = Poor strength; full range of motion (FROM) when not against gravity only
3/5 = Fair strength; FROM against gravity, but not against additional resistance
4/5 = Good strength; FROM against gravity and moderate resistance
5/5 = Normal strength; FROM against gravity and normal resistance

3. What does MMT test?

The one-repetition maximal contraction of the muscle.

4. How is muscle endurance tested?

It is tested by counting the seconds that muscle contraction is maintained or by counting repetitions against a given weight.

5. What factors may limit the results of MMT?

Lack of full effort. The patient should try his or her hardest. The examiner can determine this by observing or feeling other muscle groups contracting. A person cannot maximally contract one muscle without contracting many others.

Inappropriate positioning. The patient must be stable while being tested. The examiner should place hands on both sides of the joint of the muscle being tested so that the patient does not lose balance. If the patient feels off balance, he or she will not be able to perform maximal contraction.

Abnormal muscle tone. Spasticity, for example, may give a false result.

6. Does deconditioning cause focal muscle weakness?
No. Deconditioning leads to decreased endurance in all muscles.

7. What can cause focal muscle weakness?
Focal neuropathies, nerve entrapment, mononeuritis, injuries, trauma, or myopathies.

8. Is MMT mostly concentric or eccentric muscle contractions?
Mostly concentric.

9. What does a hand-held dynamometer measure?
It measures force in pounds or kilograms of the contracting muscle.

RANGE OF MOTION EXERCISES

10. Define active range of motion (AROM) and passive range of motion (PROM).
AROM is the ROM through which the patient can move the joint. PROM is the ROM through which the examiner can move the joint.

11. When is PROM less than AROM?
Never. PROM must be greater than or equal to AROM.

12. Can fluid in the knee limit ROM?
Yes. Small amounts of fluid in the knee (bulge sign) probably limit flexion and extension of the joint.

13. What joints do the ROM of shoulder abduction measure?
Glenohumeral and scapulothoracic.

14. In shoulder abduction ROM, how does the glenohumeral joint move as the scapulothoracic joint moves?
There is approximately 2° of glenohumeral joint motion for every degree of scapulothoracic joint motion.

15. What is the instantaneous axis of rotation (IAR) of a joint?
The IAR of the joint is the center about which both members of the joint move. IAR varies throughout the ROM of a joint, and, thus, it is difficult to maintain the axis of the goniometer always on the axis of the joint.

16. Does the straight-leg-raising test measure full ROM of hip flexion?
No, the knee must be flexed to measure the full extent of hip flexion.

17. Approximately how much variation occurs with repeated ROM examinations of the same joint by the same examiner?
10%.

18. Early inflammatory arthritis of the hip usual limits what ROM?
Internal rotation.

19. What does the Shober test measure?
Loss of mobility of the spine. The posterior spinous processes don't spread apart, and flexion occurs because of hip motion.

20. What does the Spurling test detect?

Cervical spine radiculopathy demonstrated by simultaneous cervical lateral flexion and cervical spine extension.

21. What does the Thomas test evaluate?

The presence of a hip flexion contracture. It is measured when the patient is lying flat on a firm surface, and the hip opposite the side measured is flexed to the chest as much as possible.

22. Are there other forms of ROM besides PROM and AROM?
- Active-assisted ROM (AAROM)—patient is assisted by the therapist
- Self ROM (SROM)—e.g., a hemiparetic patient uses one arm to assist the other.

BIBLIOGRAPHY

1. American Medical Association: Guides to the Evaluation of Permanent Impairment, 4th ed. Chicago, AMA, 1993.
2. Anderson H, Jakobsen J: A comparative study of isokinetic dynamometry and manual muscle testing of ankle dorsal and plantar flexors and knee extensors and flexors. Eur Neurol 37:239–242, 1997.
3. Bickley LS: Bates Guide to Physical Examination and History Taking, 7th ed. Philadelphia, Lippincott Williams & Wilkins, 1999.
4. Hoppenfeld S: Physical Examination of the Spine and Extremities. New York, Prentice-Hall, 1976.
5. Kendall FP, McCreary EK, Provance PG: Muscles Testing and Function, 4th ed. Baltimore, Williams & Wilkins, 1993.
6. McPeak LA: Physiatric history and examination. In Braddom RL (ed): Physical Medicine and Rehabilitation, 2nd ed. Philadelphia, W.B. Saunders, 2001.
7. Mulroy SJ, Lassen KD, Chambers SH, Perry J: The ability of male and female clinicians to effectively test knee extension strength using manual muscle testing. J Orthop Sports Phys Ther 26:192–199, 1997.

17. ANALYSIS OF GAIT AND KINESIOLOGY

D. Casey Kerrigan, M.D., Susan Ehrenthal, M.D., and Richard Mazzaferro, D.O.

1. Why is gait more costly in energy terms than wheelchair ambulation?

The body's center of mass must rise and fall with each step during gait, while in wheelchair ambulation, the center of mass does not rise and fall. There is much work associated with this rise and fall. To estimate the work done in walking a certain distance, multiply the vertical displacement of the center of mass by the body weight and the number of steps.

2. What is a gait cycle?

A **gait cycle** can be considered the functional unit of gait. It is also referred to as a stride. **Stride length** is the distance between sequential corresponding points of contact by the same foot. **Step length** is the distance between sequential corresponding points of contact by opposite feet. Each stride or gait cycle comprises two steps.

3. What is cadence?

The number of steps per unit time. The average adult cadence is 90–120 steps/minute, with an energy cost of approximately 100 cal/mile.

4. What is a normal adult step length and step width?

Normal step length: about 38 cm

Normal base (or the distance between the center of the heels): 6–10 cm

5. Describe the terminology of gait analysis.

The classic terminology of gait, such as heel strike, heel-off, and toe-off, is dated since these terms are often not applicable in certain disabilities. Current terminology divides gait into three functional tasks: **weight acceptance, single limb support,** and **limb advancement**. These first two terms comprise the stance period, while the latter comprises the swing period. Stance can be further subdivided into the following phases: **initial contact, loading response, midstance, terminal stance,** and **preswing**. Swing consists of three phases: **initial swing, mid-swing,** and **terminal swing**.

6. How much of a typical walking cycle is spent in the stance phase? How much in the swing phase?

At normal walking speed, approximately 60% of a gait cycle is spent in stance and 40% in swing. The relative amount of time in stance decreases as the speed of walking increases.

7. What is the difference between walking and running?

Double support usually comprises 20% of a normal walking gait cycle. The relative amount of time spent in double support decreases as the speed of walking increases. Walking becomes running when there is no longer a period of double support.

8. What is the significance of the determinants of gait?

These factors are utilized in normal human gait to minimize the movement of the center of mass as predicted by the simple compass model of gait described by Saunders, Inman, and Eberhart. The center of mass usually travels along a sinusoidal up-and-down and side-to-side formal path with each step. If instead of having a mobile pelvis, knees, and ankles, we had inflexible lower limbs, we would walk much like a compass. With such a compass gait, the center of mass goes up and down much more, resulting in a much more inefficient gait. These determinants are mechanisms or events we utilize to reduce and smooth out the path of the center of gravity.

9. What are the determinants of gait?

The determinants of gait reduce the center of mass displacement. They include the following: **heel rise, pelvic rotation, pelvic tilt, knee flexion, foot motion, knee motion,** and **pelvic lateral displacement**. Recently, it has been shown that pelvic rotation, pelvic tilt, and knee flexion play less significant roles in reducing the center of mass displacement than was once thought. Heel rise, not previously thought to be a main determinant of gait, has recently been shown to be the major contributor to reducing center of mass displacement.

10. How do the determinants of gait work?

The first four determinants of gait primarily deal with raising the center of gravity's would-be lowest point at double support or lowering its would-be highest point at midstance. The fifth and sixth effectively smooth out the sinusoidal curve. The seventh determinant has to do with reducing the center of mass' (COM's) horizontal displacement.

1. **Heel rise:** During normal walking, heel rise from foot flat has a considerable role in raising the height of the COM when it is at its lowest, reducing its overall displacement by approximately 6–8 mm.

2. **Pelvic rotation:** With 4° of pelvic rotation in either direction during double support, the limbs are essentially lengthened. This effectively raises the COM's would-be lowest point by approximately 20–25 mm.

3. **Pelvic tilt:** Occurs at midstance. The pelvis normally dips 4° on the swing side and carries the COM along with it. This lowers the COM's would-be highest point by approximately 2–3 mm.

4. **Knee flexion:** Occurs at midstance. Also effectively lowers the COM's would-be highest point by 2 mm.

5 & 6. Foot and knee motion: The ankle pivots on the posterior heel at initial contact. The pivot point progresses to the forefoot by terminal stance. The knee and foot motions act to smooth the motion into a sinusoidal curve.

7. Lateral displacement of the pelvis: The hip joints are separated in the horizontal plane by the pelvic width. Valgus alignment at the knees combined with hip adduction places the feet closer together. This allows less excursion of the center of gravity in the horizontal plane.

11. Where is the normal center of mass? How much does it move during ambulation?

It is approximately 5 cm anterior to the second sacral vertebra. The average total displacement of the center of gravity is about 5 cm in the vertical axis and 5 cm in the horizontal axis for an average adult male step. Were it not for the determinants of gait, the displacement would be about 10 cm. The actual displacement of the center of gravity varies depending on a person's height and step length, but it is always approximately one-half of what it would be if it were not for the determinants of gait.

12. When is the center of gravity at its highest and lowest points in walking? In running?

In walking, it is highest in midstance during single limb support and lowest at initial contact during the double support. Interestingly, in running, it is at its highest point in the "flight" phase and at its lowest point in midstance of single limb support.

13. What is considered a comfortable walking speed?

A comfortable walking speed is one in which the energy cost per unit distance is at a minimum (i.e., comfort equates with efficiency). This is about 80 m/min or 3 mph, with an energy cost of 4.3 kcal/min. Abnormal biomechanics result in an increased energy cost, which is usually compensated for by a slower walking speed.

14. Does a plastic or metal ankle-foot orthosis (AFO) reduce the energy cost of hemiparetic ambulation?

Both types of braces can significantly increase walking speed and reduce energy expenditure. An AFO reduces energy cost by simulating pushoff and raising the center of gravity in terminal (most important). Also, foot-drop is prevented in the swing phase. In hemiplegic subjects, energy expenditure per unit distance is 74% above normal using an AFO but 88% without one. There is no significant difference in energy expenditure between the types of AFOs. Interestingly, it was easier to negotiate stairs when an AFO was used.

15. How do different assistive devices affect energy expenditure?

In healthy subjects, the use of either a cane or crutches with a partial weight-bearing gait requires approximately 18–36% more energy per unit distance. Non-weight-bearing gaits using forearm crutches requires 41–61% more energy per unit distance. There are no differences in energy expenditure when comparing the use of axillary or forearm crutches with one another.

16. What is the difference between kinematics and kinetics?

Kinematics is the study of the motions of joint and limb segments. **Kinetics** is the study of forces or torques that cause joint and limb motion.

17. When is a gait laboratory analysis indicated?

It is particularly useful in cases of upper motor neuron pathology. In many cases, the static evaluation of strength and tone may be deceptive. For instance, spasticity evident on static examination may not be apparent during ambulation. Gait analysis provides a respectable quantifiable measure of the requirement and result of a therapeutic intervention. It can be useful to assist in selecting the correct orthosis, therapy program, or surgical procedure. It may suggest a different treatment plan for a patient whose performance has plateaued.

18. What is antalgic gait?

In an ambulator with lower-extremity pain, gait is modified to reduce weight-bearing on the involved side. The uninvolved limb is rapidly advanced to shorten stance on the affected side.

Gait is often slow and steps are short to limit the weight-bearing period. Initial contact is avoided to decrease jarring.

19. What is steppage gait?

It is a compensatory gait using excessive hip and knee flexion to assist a "functionally long" lower leg and foot to clear the ground. For instance, it may be seen with an equinus (plantarflexion) deformity, gastrocsoleus spasticity, or weak dorsiflexors.

20. Which gait can be detected *before* the patient enters the room?

The foot-slap of a patient with a partial foot-drop can be heard as the foot rapidly moves from initial contact to loading response. Moderately weak (grade 4 or 3) dorsiflexors are the cause. During the period from initial contact to loading response, they must eccentrically contract to slow the forward fall of the body. If dorsiflexors are very weak (grade 2 or worse), a steppage gait is used as there is not enough strength to lift the forefoot off the ground; this gait is silent.

21. What are the possible causes of equinus in swing?

Excessive plantar flexion in swing may be caused by:
1. Heel cord contracture
2. Spasticity of the soleus, gastrocnemius, or posterior tibialis muscles
3. Weak dorsiflexors

22. What are possible causes of genu recurvatum during the stance period of gait?

1. Plantar flexion contracture (causing a knee extension moment through the closed kinetic chain)
2. Quadriceps weakness
3. Plantar flexor spasticity
4. Quadriceps spasticity

23. What is Trendelenburg gait?

A Trendelenburg gait is characterized by lateral trunk-bending toward the supporting limb during the stance phase. The trunk will bend toward the affected side to keep the center of gravity directly above the hip joint. This maneuver eliminates the need for hip abductors and decreases the forces across the hip joint. A useful intervention is the introduction of a cane to be used contralaterally during the stance period of the affected side.

24. What are the two causes of a Trendelenburg gait?

The most common cause is **hip pain**, usually from osteoarthritis. Lateral trunk-bending serves to reduce the forces across the hip joint. The second cause is **weak hip abductors**. If hip abductors are weak bilaterally, the trunk will sway side to side, causing a "waddling" gait.

25. What is the gait pattern in a person with weak hip extensors?

The person walks with an **extensor lurch**. The trunk is hyperextended at the hip to prevent rapid forward fall at initial contact (jack-knifing).

26. When does an infant acquire the ability to walk supported? To walk unsupported? To run?

An infant generally walks with support by 1 year, walks unsupported by 15 months, and runs by approximately 18 months. By 3 years old, a mature gait pattern is established.

27. How does a toddler's gait differ from that of an adult?

Toddlers walk with:
1. A wider base of support
2. A reduced stride length with a higher cadence
3. No heel strike

4. Little knee flexion during standing
5. Absence of reciprocal arm swing
6. External rotation of the entire leg during the swing phase

28. In the erect body position, where is the line of gravity relative to the hip, knee, and ankle joints?
The line of gravity passes behind the hip and in front of the knee and ankle. This allows the hip to be supported by the iliofemoral ligament and the knee to be supported by the posterior popliteal capsule with no muscular effort. Ankle stability is maintained by continuous contraction of the gastrocsoleus.

29. When walking with a heavy load, what features of the gait cycle are altered?
The step length is decreased. The period of double support is prolonged.

30. During which activity is leg length discrepancy most apparent?
Running.

31. At how many degrees does a knee flexion contracture significantly interfere with gait?
At 30°, all phases of the gait cycle will be abnormal. Contractures of this severity or greater essentially produce a leg-length discrepancy.

32. Do high-heeled shoes increase the risk for osteoarthitis of the knees?
It appears so. Gait analysis of women wearing high-heeled shoes showed findings consistent with increased force across the patellofemoral joint and a greater compressive force on the medial compartment of the knee (23% greater) during walking in high heels versus barefeet. Thus, since osteoarthritis of the knee is twice as common in women as it is in men and usually occurs bilaterally, it appears likely that high heels can predispose to osteoarthritis of the knees.

33. What are the major lower-extremity joint parameter differences in the elderly versus young adults?
There are many differences in lower-extremity joint parameters in the elderly when compared to young adults. However, the only difference that persists when elderly subjects walk at an increased speed consistent with younger subjects is decreased peak hip extension. Peak hip extension has also been found to be further reduced in elderly patients with a history of falls when compared to elderly patients who have no history of falls.

34. What are the major kinetic and kinematic differences between elderly fallers and non-fallers?
Elderly fallers have been found to have all of the following differences versus their non-falling counterparts:
1 Decreased hip extension
2. Increased hip flexion
3. Decreased knee flexion moment in preswing
4. Decreased knee power absorption in preswing

BIBLIOGRAPHY

1. Berger N, Edelstein J: Lower limb prosthetics [dissertation]. New York, New York University Post Graduate Medical School, 1990.
2. Fisher S, Gullickson G Jr: Energy cost of ambulation in health and disability. Arch Phys Med Rehabil 59:124–133, 1978.
3. Gard SA, Childress DS: The effect of pelvic list on the vertical displacement of the trunk during normal walking. Gait Posture 5:233–238, 1997.
4. Gard SA, Childress DS: The influence of stance-phase knee flexion on the vertical displacement of the trunk during normal walking. Arch Phys Med Rehabil 80:26–32, 1999.

5. Gonzalez E, Corcoran PJ: Energy expenditure during ambulation. In Downey JA (ed): Physiological Basis of Rehabilitation Medicine, 2nd ed. Boston, Butterworth-Heinemann, 1994.
6. Harris GF, Wertsch JJ: Procedures for gait analysis. Arch Phys Med Rehabil 75:216–225, 1994.
7. Hoppenfeld S: Physical Examination of the Spine and Extremities. Norwalk, CT, Appleton-Century-Crofts, 1976.
8. Kerrigan DC, Della Croce U, Marciello M, Riley PO. A refined view of the determinants of gait: Significance of heel rise. Arch Phys Med Rehabil 81:1077–1080, 2000.
9. Kerrigan DC, Lee LW, Collins JJ, et al: Reduced hip extension during walking in healthy elderly and fallers versus young adults. Arch Phys Med Rehabil 82:26–30, 2001.
10. Kerrigan DC, Lee LW, Nieto TJ, et al: Kinetic alterations independent of walking speed in elderly fallers. Arch Phys Med Rehabil 81:730–735, 2000.
11. Kerrigan DC, Riley PO, Lelas JL, Della Croce U: Quantification of pelvic rotation as a determinant of gait. Arch Phys Med Rehabil 82:217–220, 2001.
12. Kerrigan DC, Todd MK, Della Croce U, et al: Biomechanical gait alterations independent of speed in the healthy elderly: evidence for specific limiting impairments. Arch Phys Med Rehabil 79:317–322, 1998.
13. Kerrigan DC, Todd MK, Riley PO: Knee osteoarthritis and high-heeled shoes. Lancet 351:1399–1401, 1998.
14. Lehmkuhl LD, Smith LK (eds): Brunnstrom's Clinical Kinesiology, 4th ed. Philadelphia, F.A. Davis, 1987.
15. Perry J: Gait Analysis: Normal and Pathological Function. Thorofare, NJ, Slack, 1992.
16. Rose J, Gamble JG (eds): Human Walking, 2nd ed. Baltimore, Williams & Wilkins, 1993.
17. Saunders JBCM, Inman VT, Eberhardt HD: The major determinants in normal and pathological gait. J Bone Joint Surg 35A:543–548, 1953.

18. EVALUATION OF THE GERIATRIC PATIENT

Susan J. Garrison, M.D., and Gerald Felsenthal, M.D.

1. Describe the characteristics of the geriatric population.

The difference in physiologic age compared to chronological age can be amazing. People tend to become exaggerations of their adult selves as they age. Research shows that people who live through their middle years (ages 45–65) without major illness will live to be a part of the geriatric population. Medicare benefits begin at age 65.

2. How do the basic principles of rehabilitative management differ for the geriatric patient?

The basic rehabilitation principles are the same for all adults. Those specific to the geriatric population include physiologic changes, multiple impairments, and a focus on small improvements.

3. What neurologic changes are found in the elderly? How are these significant?

Neurologic Changes and Their Significance in the Elderly

SYSTEM	FINDINGS	SIGNIFICANCE
Visual	Diminished ROM on convergence and upward gaze Small, irregular pupils Diminished reaction to light and near reflex	Combination of restricted vertical gaze and cervical motion can make it difficult to see information posted on walls, such as exit signs
Motor	Decreased muscle strength, legs > arms, proximal > distal Atrophy of interossei Short-stepped or broad-based gait with diminished associated movements	Hip extensors may no longer be strong enough to lift the body from sitting to standing; arm strength used to push up

Table continued on following page

Neurologic Changes and Their Significance in the Elderly (Continued)

SYSTEM	FINDINGS	SIGNIFICANCE

Sensory	Diminished vibratory, legs > arms
	Mildly increased threshold for pain,
	  temperature, and light touch
	Possible change in proprioception
		Poor sensory input from feet indicates risk
		  for falls
		At risk for injury from topical heat modali-
		  ties

Reflexes	Absent or diminished ankle jerks
	Reduction in knee, biceps, and triceps reflexes
	Babinski's sign may not be present when
	  it normally would occur
		Radiculopathies may be overlooked or
		  misdiagnosed

Adapted from Ham RJ: Assessment. In Ham RJ, Sloane PD (eds): Primary Care Geriatrics: A Case-Based Approach. St. Louis, Mosby, 1992, p 87.

4. What changes in biologic functions occur in response to aging, as compared to inactivity and exercise?

Changes in Biologic Functions in Response to Aging, Inactivity, and Exercise

FUNCTION	AGING	INACTIVITY	EXERCISE
VO_2max	Decreased	Decreased	Increased
Cardiac output	Decreased	Decreased	Increased, not for older
Systolic blood pressure	Increased	—	Decreased
Orthostatic tolerance	Decreased	Decreased	Increased
Body water	Decreased	Decreased	—
Red blood cell mass	Decreased	Decreased	—
Thrombosis	Increased	Increased	Decreased
Serum lipids	Increased	Increased	Decreased
High density lipoprotein	Increased over age 80 yr	—	Increased
Lean body mass	Decreased	Decreased	—
Muscle strength	Decreased	Decreased	Increased
Calcium	Decreased	Decreased	—
Glucose tolerance	Decreased	Decreased	Increased
EEG dominant frequency	Decreased	Decreased	Increased

Adapted from Felsenthal G, Garrison SJ, Steinberg FU: Rehabilitation of the Aging and Elderly Patient. Baltimore, Williams & Wilkins, 1994, p 512.

5. How does functional impairment affect this population?

As one ages, comorbidities accumulate and result in functional impairment and difficulty with simple tasks. This is particularly true for women, who may live 7–12 years longer than their same-aged spouse.

6. Which geriatric patients are candidates for rehabilitation, and where should this care be delivered?

Candidates should be physically well enough to participate in therapy sessions. If an acute care inpatient cannot tolerate a rigorous program of 3 hours of therapy per day, they should be considered for admission to a skilled nursing facility (SNF = Slower, Not Faster) or long-term acute care. Other options include a subacute care facility, nursing home, home healthcare, and outpatient services.

7. How should "motivation" be utilized in addressing this population?

"Lack of motivation" is not a reason to exclude a person from therapies. The person is motivated to do something; it may simply be to stay in bed. Many older patients are against "exercise" after a life of physical labor. They may also succumb to their own ageism. Make certain that the patient is not medically/surgically ill, depressed, or nutritionally impaired.

8. What is the concept of functional presentation of disease?

While a young adult may quickly become febrile in response to an acute infection, the elderly patient may become confused or begin falling rather than demonstrating a temperature elevation. Stopping eating or drinking, urinary incontinence, acute confusion, weight loss, falling, dizziness, dementia, and failure to thrive are functional presentations of disease.

9. Why is cognition important in this group?

Most rehabilitation is based on learning compensatory skills for lost functional abilities. Standard rehabilitative techniques do not benefit severely demented patients. Also, medications a patient may be taking can affect cognitive performance.

10. Does diagnosis of vascular dementia prevent participation in rehabilitation?

Patients with vascular dementia are often excluded because of their inability to learn new material and retain information. Today, earlier diagnoses and more effective treatments can modify the usual progression of vascular dementia. Medications such as SSRIs can improve responses and performance. A multidisciplinary approach may involve psychiatrists, risk-management personnel, adult protective services, legal counsel, and neuropsychologists. Discharge requires 24-hour supervision for safety.

11. What is polypharmacy? How can this problem be addressed?

Polypharmacy, the use of multiple medications, often results in compliance problems. Patients become confused about dosage and scheduling and may forget to take medications, causing potential adverse drug effects. Attempt to limit the total number of medications. Additionally, medications may represent a significant out-of-pocket expense.

Seven Steps for Writing Safer Medication Prescriptions for the Elderly

PHYSICIAN BEHAVIOR	PURPOSE
1. Start at ½ of the lowest recommended dose and increase slowly to obtain the desired effect: "start low and go slow."	The desired response in the elderly occurs at a lower dosage than that required in the younger population.
2. Use a simple dosing regimen, with the fewest medications possible; encourage lifestyle modifications rather than drugs.	Noncompliance and the incidence of adverse drug reactions decrease as the total number of doses and medications decline.
3. Whenever adding a new medication or changing the dosing of a current one, make certain that the instructions are understood.	Detailed information can assist in preventing problems. Write explicit instructions for the patient or significant other.
4. Be aware of medication costs.	Patients are unlikely to be compliant with numerous expensive medications. Also, they may continue to take a previously prescribed medication because they have already paid for it.
5. Periodically review patient medications, including over-the-counter drugs. Eliminate those not being used; keep the total number low.	This assists in preventing the possibility of drug-drug interactions, potentially reduces costs, and may prevent the accidental ingestion of medication.

Table continued on following page

Seven Steps for Writing Safer Medication Prescriptions for the Elderly (Continued)

PHYSICIAN BEHAVIOR	PURPOSE
6. Create a written prescription list for the patient to keep with him/her at all times.	This record is helpful to other physicians and pharmacists who may then review the list for possible drug problems. It is invaluable for the geriatric traveler and for ER visits.
7. Instruct home health nurses or aides to communicate directly with the physician about any medication problems.	The sooner a problem is noticed, the sooner action can be taken to correct the situation.

Adapted from Stein BE: Avoiding drug reactions: Seven steps to writing safe prescriptions. Geriatrics 49:28–36, 1994.

12. Why is nutrition important?

Nutrition is important for maintaining good health and quick healing. The description "malnourished" can signify obesity or cachexia. Obesity causes immobility and poor endurance. The underweight are at risk for skin breakdown, poor exercise tolerance, and peripheral edema due to low serum albumin levels.

13. Why is the maintenance of routine physical activity important?

"Use it or lose it." Muscle groups must be exercised in order to stay strong.

14. What are typical reasons for falls in the elderly?

Typical reasons for falls include syncope, visual problems, peripheral vascular disease, poor balance, inappropriate footwear, inappropriate use of gait devices, and use of sedative hypnotics. Falls are a serious threat to functional ability and can result in major life changes.

15. What housing options are available for the elderly who can no longer live independently?

Living arrangements are related to the patient's financial status and functional abilities and deficits. Alternatives to living independently include a nursing home, assisted living, homecare, or living with relatives.

16. How should you communicate with the elderly patient?

Talk directly to the patient whenever possible. Make certain that the individual's wants, needs, and goals are expressed directly to you.

17. Are there specific equipment needs in the elderly?

Many elderly patients resist using gait devices or use inappropriate ones. They may also request scooters or other electric mobility when standard wheelchairs are best. Remember that less is more. Too many adaptive devices may overwhelm people. Other concerns include environmental modifications such as entrance ramps and grab bars in bathrooms. Also, equipment is expensive, even when partially reimbursed by third-party payors, and must be maintained.

18. Why is a hip fracture of such concern in a geriatric patient?

Poor balance following hip fracture is significantly associated with increased hospitalizations and nursing home placement. The mortality rate in the year following hip fracture is 14–36%, and 25–75% experience prolonged functional impairment.

19. What treatment is best for osteoarthritis? When is surgery indicated?

The drug of choice is acetaminophen. Other options include NSAIDs, topicals (salicylate/capsaicin), or tricyclic antidepressants. Therapeutic modalities such as heat, cold, TENS, and exercise may be helpful in pain management. Intra-articular joint injections of glucocorticoids should be limited to four. At that time, total joint replacement should be considered. Indications for total knee replacement include varus angulation of greater than 10°, ligamentous instability and valgus deformity, severe knee pain unrelieved by medications, and back pain. Total hip replacement is indicated when nonsurgical strategies have failed to provide functional improvement and pain relief.

20. What are the rehabilitative goals of total knee replacement in this population?

Ability to ambulate household distances of approximately 100 ft using a rolling walker and achieve assisted ROM of the affected knee approaching full extension and greater than 90° of flexion.

21. What is significant about undergoing total hip replacement secondary to osteoarthritis?

Postoperative rehabilitation involves teaching the patient independence in bed mobility, sitting to standing, and dressing, while following hip precautions. Joint protection and nutrition should also be stressed.

22. Explain the rehabilitative issues concerning osteoporotic vertebral fractures.

Rehabilitation problems include acute pain upon movement and immobility, which may progress to severe deconditioning and loss of function. These patients cannot tolerate trunk movement due to protective paravertebral muscular spasm. A typical rehabilitation program includes bed rest in a position of comfort. Sitting should be limited to 10 minutes at a time for 7 to 10 days, with time added as pain allows. Localized paravertebral muscular spasm is treated with local heat such as hot packs and ultrasound, in addition to oral muscle relaxants and TENS.

23. What are the risk factors for stroke in this population?

The primary risk factor for stroke is age; the second is previous stroke. Use the Functional Independence Measure (FIM) to predict the need and projected outcome of stroke rehabilitation. Dynamic sitting balance is a good indication of the ability to participate in an intensive stroke rehabilitation program.

24. What is the goal of stroke rehabilitation? How can patients maximize their learning efforts?

The goal is to teach compensatory skills to substitute for lost functional abilities. Cognitive strengths and weaknesses should be identified, and the strengths are emphasized.

25. Can the geriatric stroke patient regain the ability to walk?

All unilateral-hemispheric nonoperative stroke patients eventually regain some ability to ambulate, if they do not sustain a second stroke or die of some other cause first.

26. Why is preservation of the knee joint important in amputation?

Amputation is usually a result of dysvascular problems, such as ischemia or diabetic or hypertensive neuropathy or a combination of the two. In the past, a gangrenous leg often required transfemoral amputation. However, due to revascularization techniques, transtibial amputation is now the most common level. Preservation of the knee joint is extremely important due to the high energy cost of ambulation after transfemoral amputation, compared to transtibial amputation.

27. What factors may hinder lower limb prosthetic restoration in the geriatric amputee?

Limiting factors include inability to learn, neurologic deficits; poor endurance, hip or knee contractures of either leg, upper limb strength, skin integrity of the residual limb, and emotional effects.

28. Describe the specific prosthetic modifications that may be helpful for the geriatric lower-limb amputee.

Various suspension methods, safety-type joints, and energy-storing feet may assist in providing more stability during ambulation. A cosmetic lower limb may be emotionally beneficial.

29. What is the risk of contralateral limb loss in the geriatric amputee?

Approximately 15% to 20% experience contralateral limb loss within 2 years. After 4 years, it increases to 40%. The remaining limb should be protected with meticulous foot care, use of an appropriate shoe, and maintenance of joint AROM and muscular strength.

30. Why is pain control significant in the geriatric population?

Pain must be controlled in order to maximize functional abilities.

BIBLIOGRAPHY

1. American Geriatrics Society: The management of chronic pain in older patients: AGS Panel on Chronic Pain in Older Persons. J Am Geriatr Soc 46:635–651, 1998.
2. Braddom RL (ed): Physical Medicine and Rehabilitation. Philadelphia, W.B. Saunders, 1996.
3. Egbert AM: Postoperative pain management in the frail elderly. Clin Geriatr Med 12:583–599, 1996.
4. Felsenthal G, Garrison SJ, Steinberg FU (eds): Rehabilitation of the Aging and Elderly Patient. Baltimore, Williams & Wilkins, 1994.
5. Garrison SJ, Lindeman J (eds):Vascular dementia: Implications for stroke rehabilitation. Top Stroke Rehabil 7(3), 2000.
6. Grabois M, Garrison SJ, Hart KA, Lehmkuhl LD (eds): Physical Medicine and Rehabilitation: The Complete Approach. Malden, MA, Blackwell Science, 2000.

19. IMPAIRMENT EVALUATION AND DISABILITY RATING

Richard T. Katz, M.D., and Robert D. Rondinelli, M.D., Ph.D.

1. How do impairment, disability, and handicap differ?

Impairment is an abnormality of structure, appearance, and/or function at the end-organ level. **Disability** is the inability to perform an activity because of an abnormality of the person as a whole. For example, when a nurse can no longer bend over on a frequent basis, which most job analyses require for a ward nurse, she can no longer work full duty and must be placed temporarily or permanently on light duty. **Handicap** is an environmentally defined abnormality reflecting societal bias experienced by the individual trying to fulfill a role.

While these definitions provide a useful construct, they unfortunately are not how these terms are used in the real world. Insurance companies use *disabled* to imply that the person can no longer perform the "substantial and material duties of an occupation." For the Social Security Administration, a person must be disabled for all "substantial gainful activity" in order to receive benefits. Finally, there are important modifiers to the concept of disability. A patient may be on temporary or permanent disability (i.e., no improvement after > 6 months of treatment), or the disability may be total (100% of the whole person) or partial.

2. How do Worker's Compensation and Social Security define disabilty?

Worker's Compensation is a federally mandated social program adopted state by state in the United States. The critical language of Workers' Compensation statutes is that employees must suffer "accidental . . . personal injury . . . arising out of and in the scope of employment." Another key concept in the Worker's Compensation statutes is that of no-fault or tort immunity; in exchange for the employer caring for the injured worker, the worker (theoretically) offers the employer tort immunity from legal suit in response to being injured. Workers usually receive 50% to 70% of preinjury wages as an incentive to return to work.

The physician has four key responsibilities when determining disability under Worker's Compensation statutes: (1) Is there a causal relationship between the injury and the impairment?

(2) Has the patient completed the healing period? (3) Is there a permanent impairment? and (4) What are the work capacity and restrictions (can the worker return to the same job, similar job with modifications, similar job with a different employer, with a different employer, on the job training with same employer, or job retraining?)?

Social Security is the second major system providing a social safety net for persons with disability. For a worker to become eligible for Social Security disability benefits, he or she must have a medical condition that will result in death, last longer than 12 months, preclude any gainful employment, or result in a loss of the ability to earn > $500 per month.

3. How is the functional capacity evaluation used to determine if a patient with low back pain can return to work?

The physician can determine when and to what job the patient may return, based solely on his or her clinical judgment, or he or she may rely on a *functional capacity evaluation* (FCE). An FCE is simply a quantified physical ability test in which various parameters are measured over time—i.e., how long and how much a patient can perform in a given day. Although there is an intuitive attractiveness to FCEs, there are some significant questions: Are these tests valid and reproducible (possibly)? Does patient motivation compromise the value of the test? The key question with FCE is, "Does physical testing predict successful return to work?"

4. What considerations does the Americans with Disabilities Act (ADA) mandate with regard to disability and return to work?

The ADA defines disability as a "physical or mental impairment that substantially limits one or more of the major life activities of the individual, or a record of such an impairment, or being regarded as having such an impairment." The ADA is intended to protect persons who can perform the essential functions of a job with *reasonable accommodation*. An employer may not inquire about a potential employee's impairment or medical history when he or she applies for a job. When the potential employee is offered a job, a medical examination may be performed, and the position may be withdrawn if the medical officer, based on receiving more information about the worker's abilities, impairments, and past medical history, feels that the particular position offered would be a direct threat to the health of the worker or those around him. However, the ADA asks the employer to consider whether some type of machine or coworker could help to perform certain activities which would let the employee complete the essential functions of the job. That is, could the employer make a reasonable accommodation?

5. How is permanent disability determined?

The method depends on the jurisdiction. In a Workers' Compensation case, the first task is to find out the laws in that state. These can be obtained by contacting a human resources department of any large employer, contacting a litigation attorney who handles Workers' Compensation, or looking in textbooks. There are certain periods of time in which the worker must notify the employer of the injury, and a certain period after which compensation begins (waiting period). States also vary in whether the physician care is employer- or employee-directed. For example, in Illinois, workers may select a practitioner of their choice (e.g., physician, surgeon, osteopath, chiropractor), but in Missouri the insurance underwriter selects the physician or other practitioner to whom that patient must go for care if costs are to be assumed by the insurer.

In many jurisdictions, the physician will be asked to provide a disability rating, and the best available document for doing that is the *AMA Guides to the Evaluation of Permanent Impairment*. The AMA Guides is not based on demographic or epidemiological data but is developed by a panel of informed experts who have formed a relative consensus. One basic principle of the *AMA Guides* is that it rates *permanent* partial disability. A suitable period of time must elapse before the disorder is considered to be permanent. Secondly, the concept of *regional* versus *whole person* impairment is incorporated in the *Guides*. Impairments of the hand or foot (regional impairment) must be converted to whole person impairments utilizing certain tables, whereas spine impairments are all considered impairments of the whole person.

It is estimated that 40 million Americans are protected by **long-term disability**, largely through their workplace. There are no uniform criteria for determining when a person becomes disabled with low back pain according to a long-term disability insurer. Typically, the insurer will ask the treating physician for information about lifting, bending, stooping, and other tasks, which the physician may feel awkward about answering unless an FCE has been performed. An important feature of long-term disability policies is whether there is *own occupation* versus *any occupation* coverage. *Own occupation* coverage provides the insured with disability benefits (typically in the range of 60% of normal salary) if the patient is not able to perform the essential elements of a particular job. *Any occupation* coverage means that, within limits, the employee would be reimbursed only if he or she could no longer perform meaningful work in any related occupation. Again, the criteria vary according to the insurer.

6. How does the independent medical examination (IME) differ from the usual history and physical?

When a physician sees a patient for an IME, certain features of the interaction differ from a traditional patient evaluation. First, and most importantly, the physician is not assuming care of the patient. This must be clearly stated orally to the patient as well as documented in the report. The evaluation is for IME purposes, and there is to be no ongoing physician-patient relationship.

The expert role in an IME has eight steps: (1) give a diagnosis and severity of the condition, (2) determine causality, (3) determine if necessary tests have been performed, (4) suggest any additional tests that are required to complete the work-up, (5) determine whether maximal medical improvement has been reached, (6) determine an impairment rating, (7) determine apportionment, and (8) determine what restrictions are needed.

IMEs are often obtained for the purpose of Worker's Compensation or for the solicitation of expert testimony in a tort liability case. One of the components of tort liability is to determine if there was a proximate or direct cause (i.e., the accident caused the impairment to the patient). The concept of causality or proximate or direct cause often places the examiner in an ethical dilemma. When there is loss of limb due to an accident, the physician feels quite comfortable in stating, for example, that a nail gun pierced the popliteal artery causing below-knee amputation to occur. However, it is more difficult to state that a particular job-related injury clearly caused lower back pain. Nevertheless the physician will generally be asked: "Within a reasonable degree of medical certainty, can you state that A caused B?" The real question the attorney is asking is, "Is it more likely than not (> 50% probability) that A caused B?" If you can say yes, you are satisfying the legal requirement that it is "probably true," and this is the level of certainty that the attorney is requesting—it is not the standard of "beyond a reasonable doubt" that holds in criminal cases. If you answer that A *possibly* caused B, the real meaning is that it is less than likely (≤ 50% probability) that A caused B and would suggest evidence against causality.

Maximal medical improvement refers to the point when it is judged that the patient's condition is either resolved or plateaued. Generally, 6 months might be a reasonable period before certain spinal disorders might be considered permanent, although they certainly may resolve earlier. Patients who undergo complex surgeries may not reach maximal medical improvement for several years.

Impairment rating and apportionment are additionally precarious. Physicians may be asked, "is the patient's back condition worthy of a 20% whole person impairment?" But if the patient had prior back injuries, how much of that 20% do you apportion to each injury?

Finally, physicians may be asked to provide restrictions for a patient in terms of lifting, carrying, stooping, and other activities. Restricting patients in the workplace without at least attempting an FCE is no better than speculation. If a patient participates in an FCE but you feel that the results do no reflect his or her best effort, one can still offer more liberal restrictions and comment on the level (or lack) of motivation of the patient participating in the FCE.

BIBLIOGRAPHY

1. American Medical Association: Guides to the Evaluation of Permanent Impairment, 5th ed. Chicago, American Medical Association, 2000.
2. Rondinelli RD, Katz RT: Impairment Rating and Disability Evaluation. Philadelphia, W.B. Saunders, 1999.
3. Rondinelli RD, Katz RT (eds): Disability Evaluation. Physical Medicine and Rehabilitation Clinics of North America, vol. 12, no. 3, 2001.

IV. *Electrodiagnostic Fundamentals*

20. GENERAL PRINCIPLES OF ELECTRODIAGNOSIS

Mooyeon Oh-Park, M.D., and Dennis D.J. Kim, M.D.

1. What is the role of electrodiagnosis in the evaluation of a patient?

Electrodiagnosis can only be an extension of the history and physical examination. It assists to narrow the differential diagnosis and at times confirm the diagnosis. To perform the electrodiagnosis efficiently, one should have a clear reason for each and every step in the study.

2. What are the limitations of the nerve conduction and EMG studies?

1. The nerve conduction studies selectively examine only the large myelinated fibers and do not define diseases of the smaller nerve fibers. Nerve conduction velocity does not correlate with **functional deficit**.

2. Motor conduction study is currently not available for most proximal or most distal segment of the nerves.

3. Sensory nerve conduction studies (SNCS) only evaluate the post-ganglionic lesions and not the preganglionic lesions. SCNS does not correlate with pain. SNCS is not useful for evaluating conduction block due to the great degree of temporal dispersion and excessive cancellation.

4. Needle EMG evaluates mainly the small motor units and cannot be used to differentiate the large motor units recruited later. The needle electrode only detects signals several millimeters away from the tip of the needle. Needle EMG provides only pathophysiologic information and not the etiology.

3. How are the electrodiagnostic parameters affected by the frequency of the filters?

The changes of compound muscle action potential (CMAP) parameters are similar to those for sensory nerve action potentials (SNAPs). CMAP is more profoundly affected than SNAP by elevating the low-frequency filter since the CMAP contains mostly low frequencies. On the other hand, CMAP is not significantly affected by lowering the high-frequency filter.

PARAMETERS OF SNAP	ELEVATED LOW-FREQUENCY FILTER	LOWERED HIGH-FREQUENCY FILTER
Onset latency	No change	Increased
Peak latency	Decreased	Increased
Amplitude	Decreased	Decreased

Fibrillation and initial sharp component of positive sharp waves can be affected by lowering the high-frequency filter since these are potentials with predominantly high frequencies.

4. What are the commonly observed spontaneous discharges?

After insertion of an EMG needle into normal muscle at rest, no electrical activity is seen unless the needle is near an endplate zone. Spontaneous activity refers to electrical activities recorded in resting muscle after movement of the recording electrode has ceased.

5. Name the commonly observed spontaneous activities and their characteristic sounds.

Fibrillation potential—Clicking noises, like raindrops on the roof or static

Positive sharp waves—Pop, pop, pop, regular 2–20 Hz

Endplate spikes—Irregular clicks

Fasciculation potentials—Spontaneous isolated loud snaps

Complex repetitive discharges—Motor boat or dive bomber that misfires occasionally, stops abruptly

Myokymic discharges—Marching soldiers

Neuromyotonic discharges—High-pitch whining sound of a race car

6. What are the EMG characteristics of a fibrillation potential?

Fibrillation potential is defined as a spontaneous action potential recorded from a single muscle fiber by a needle electrode located outside the endplate zone. The precise mechanism for generation of fibrillation potentials is not known, although the prevalent hypothesis is "denervation hypersensitivity." When a muscle fiber loses innervation, there is increased production of acetylcholine receptors and other membrane proteins, which are widely distributed on the muscle cell membrane. Subsequently, increased sensitivity of muscle membrane may be responsible for fibrillation potentials. Fibrillations are also found in myopathies, neuromuscular transmission disorders, periodic paralysis, and occasionally in healthy individuals.

Fibrillation potentials are usually regular. The amplitude of the fibrillation may not exceed 100 µV after 1 year of denervation. Endplate spike can be confused with fibrillation potential if recorded outside the endplate zone. Repeated observation is necessary to identify the rhythmic nature of fibrillation potentials.

7. What are positive sharp waves (PSWs) and their EMG characteristics?

PSWs are usually seen together with or followed by fibrillations. A PSW is a spontaneous depolarization of a single muscle fiber recorded close to the tip of the needle electrode. This waveform is believed to represent a similar clinical significance as the fibrillation potential. PSWs can be seen in the foot intrinsic, gastrocnemius, and paraspinal muscles of normal individuals, probably due to large endplate zone in these muscles. When the recording electrode is near the tendon area, upcoming propagation of motor unit action potentials may look like PSWs.

8. Describe the EMG characteristics of endplate spikes.

Endplate spike is a single muscle action potential originating from the endplate zone, triggered by the needle electrode. It usually has an initial negative muscle fiber action potential, although it can be initially positive if recorded just outside the endplate zone. EPSs are irregular in rhythm and unlike fibrillation; they are not recorded away from the endplate zone. **Endplate noises** are nonpropagating potentials recorded from the endplate zone representing spontaneous release of acetylcholine vesicles during the resting state. These potentials are not recorded in denervated muscles.

9. What are complex repetitive discharges?

Complex repetitive discharges are continuous trains of polyphasic or serrated action potentials that may begin spontaneously or after needle movement. They have a uniform frequency, shape, and amplitude, with abrupt onset or change in configuration. They probably originate from ephaptic activation of groups of adjacent muscle fibers and are seen in both neuropathic and myopathic disorders. The term complex repetitive discharges is preferred to "bizarre high-frequency discharges" or "pseudomyotonic discharges."

10. What are fasciculation potentials?

Fasciculation potential results from the spontaneous discharge of a portion of or entire muscle fibers belonging to a **motor unit**. Fasciculations are often visible in the superficial muscles but may not be visible in the deep muscles. Their sources can stem anywhere from the brain or spinal cord to the terminal motor branches.

Many studies indicate that most fasciculations originate distally. Fasciculations can be seen in normal individuals and therefore cannot be considered pathologic by themselves. EMG cannot differentiate between benign and malignant forms of fasciculations.

11. What are the EMG characteristics of myokymic discharges? Neuromyotonic discharges?

Myokymic discharges are spontaneous bursts of a group of motor unit potentials probably resulting from ephaptic transmission between the motor units.

Neuromyotonic discharges are bursts of motor unit action potentials which originate in motor axons, fire at high rates (150–300 Hz) for a few seconds, and often start and stop abruptly. These discharges can be seen in many conditions including neuropathies, tetany, spinal muscular atrophy, and Isaac syndrome.

12. Define a motor unit and describe the EMG characteristics of motor unit action potential (MUAP).

The **motor unit** consists of the motor neuron, the axon and its branches, and all the muscle fibers (10–1500 fibers) innervated by that motor neuron. A motor unit territory is 5–10 mm in diameter. Normally, each muscle fiber produces an action potential duration of about 1–3 ms. It is often difficult to differentiate the small motor unit with short duration (i.e., facial muscles) from "myopathic motor unit potentials" or fibrillation potentials.

The most important parameters of MUAP are duration, firing rate, variability, and amplitude in decreasing order. The **duration** is the most reliable and informative parameter (6–15 ms). The duration of MUAP becomes longer with monopolar needle recording, lower temperature, larger motor unit size, advanced age, and neuropathy. **Firing rate** and **variability** can provide additional clues for differentiating neuropathy, neuromuscular transmission disorders, and myopathy. MUAP **amplitude** is determined by fiber density (the number of muscle fibers in the same motor unit in close proximity to the recording electrode) and not by the total number of muscle fibers in that motor unit (size), since only several fibers close to the needle determine the amplitude.

13. What are "myopathic" MUAPs?

MUAPs with short duration and small amplitude are often called myopathic MUAPs. These MUAPs can be seen in conditions involving decreased number of contributing muscle fiber action potentials (i.e., neuromuscular transmission diseases, regeneration of nerve fibers after injury, neuropathies affecting the terminal branches of the nerve fiber, myopathies). Instead of describing a condition as "myopathic MUAP," it is recommended that the parameters of the observed MUAP be described.

14. Explain the size principle in motor unit (MU) recruitment. What is the recruitment rate and ratio?

The primary mechanism for increasing muscle force is the additional activation of more MUs (**spatial recruitment**) rather than an increased firing rate of MUs (**temporal recruitment**). MUs are recruited in size order from small to large, which require greater facilitation for depolarization than smaller MUs (**size principle**). The recruitment is a function of CNS, not a function of peripheral nerve.

Recruitment rate is defined as the firing rate of the first MU when the second is recruited (usually 10–12 Hz, < 15 Hz in normal individual). Single MU firing rate can be up to 50 Hz in pathologic conditions. **Recruitment ratio** is calculated by the highest firing rate of MU among all on the screen, divided by the number of MUs recruited. Recruitment ratio is normally < 5.

In the early phase of proximal nerve or root lesions (i.e., early discogenic radiculopathy), the only electrodiagnostic clue is poor recruitment with high firing rate of MUs. Early recruitment signifies that too many MUAPs are recruited in proportion to the level of muscle force upon initiating contraction. This can be observed in myopathies, neuromuscular transmission disorders, or even end-stage neuropathy in which the force contributed by each MU is decreased due to the loss of the muscle fibers.

15. What information can be obtained with a nerve conduction study (NCS)?

An NCS induces and detects the waves of depolarization along the nerve axons and muscle depolarization. The types of nerves tested are either sensory, motor, or mixed. Nerve conduction velocity (NCV) represents the velocity of the fastest fibers depending on **axon diameter, quality/thickness of the myelin sheath, internodal distance**, and **temperature**. NCV is decreased in demyelinating disease with relatively preserved amplitude unless significant conduction block coexists. NCV may remain normal with reduced amplitude in diseases with axonal degeneration, until the nerve trunk loses most of the fast fibers.

16. What is the mixed nerve study (MNS) and when is it useful?

MNS is technically the same as sensory NCS utilizing an **orthodromic sensory** and **antidromic motor** to avoid volume conduction from compound muscle action potentials. Median and ulnar MNS across the wrist is useful for diagnosis of carpal tunnel syndrome. Medial and lateral plantar MNS across the ankle is useful for diagnosing tarsal tunnel syndrome since sensory nerve action potential (SNAP) is difficult to obtain.

The EMG machine should be set for the sensory conduction study mode because it is recording nerve potentials only. The initial deflexion of the compound mixed nerve potential probably represents the large myelinated sensory fibers.

17. How does temperature affect electrodiagnostic measurements?

Nerve conduction velocities: Cooling results in a longer time for the action potential to propagate and a net slowing of conduction.

SNAP and CMAP amplitude: When cool, the duration of an action potential gets longer and the amplitude gets larger. In addition, when the duration of the action potential becomes longer, there will be less phase cancellation, resulting in a higher amplitude of SNAP or CMAP. The degree of these effects may vary depending on whether cooling is local (a few Ranvier nodes) or general (major neural segment).

Conduction block: With low temperature, slow opening and even slower closing of ion channels lead to prolonged ion channel opening time and increased influx of Na^+, resulting in prolonged action potential duration. This extra duration may be just long enough to excite or skip a short demyelinated segment. Therefore, conduction block can be overcome by cooling. In local cooling of the recording area, the amplitude and duration of compound nerve action potentials increase due to the increased duration of individual nerve action potentials. The regional cooling of the nerve segment may result in opposite effects.

Neuromuscular transmission: Neuromuscular transmission improves with cooling because of complex mechanisms which include increased number of acetylcholine vesicles released, enhanced sensitivity of the postsynaptic endplate, and decreased hydrolysis of acetylcholine.

Spontaneous and voluntary EMG potentials: Cooling leads to desynchronization, which results in an increase in the duration of the MUAP and increased polyphasicity. The amplitude of the MUAP may or may not increase depending on the pattern of cooling. Fibrillations and positive waves decrease in frequency with cooling; fasciculations may increase.

Myotonia: In myotonic dystrophy, cold causes an increase in myotonia on EMG. In congenital myotonia and myotonia congenita, cold causes no significant changes. In paramyotonia congenita, there seems to be two different responses to cold. In patients with hypokalemic and hyperkalemic periodical paralysis, exposure to cold can precipitate weakness and/or myotonia.

18. What characteristics of nerve pathologies should be defined during an electrophysiologic study?
   • Sporadic, diffuse, or localized
   • Motor, sensory, or both
   • Axonal or demyelinating, or both
   • Old, new, or progressive
   • Neuromuscular junction or muscle

19. What are the clinical features suggesting axonal or demyelinating lesions?

NATURE OF THE LESION	AXONAL	DEMYELINATING
Onset	Subacute/slow	Acute/subacute
Weakness pattern	Distal, rarely proximal	Distal and proximal
Reflex	Relatively preserved	Loss of reflex common
Sensory symptoms	Burning or painful sensation	Numbness or tingling
Ataxia of gait	Less common	More common

20. How does the F-wave differ from the H-reflex?

F-wave is a late motor potential recorded with supramaximal stimulation as a result of back-firing of 3–5% of the motor neuron pool. The rule of thumb is that F-wave latency is about < 30 msec in upper extremity (side-to-side difference < 2 msec), < 50 msec in lower extremity (side-to-side difference of < 4 msec). **Hoffman (H) reflexes** are the electrical equivalent of the muscle stretch reflex. F-wave and H-reflex are most useful for suspected proximal-segment pathologies when the other electrodiagnostic parameters are normal, especially in the early stage of disease.

	F-WAVE (NOT A REFLEX)	H-REFLEX
Afferent arc	Alpha motor neuron	I-A fiber
Efferent arc	Alpha motor neuron	Alpha motor neuron
Stimulation intensity	Supramaximal	Submaximal
Stimulation duration	Same as motor conduction study	Long duration (> 500 msec for I-A fibers)
Muscles recorded	All muscles	Soleus, flexor carpi radialis, quadriceps
Consistency	Variable latency and configuration	Consistent latency and configuration
Amplitude	3–5% of M-response	Can be higher than M-response
Side-to-side difference	< 3 msec in upper extremity < 4 msec in lower extremity	< 2 msec in soleus

21. What is the "blink response" and what is its significance?

The blink response is an electrical analog of the corneal reflex. The afferent loop is the supraorbital branch of the trigeminal nerve, and the efferent loop is the facial nerve. **R1** is ipsilateral only, probably disynaptic or oligosynaptic. **R2** is polysynaptic and bilaterally corresponding to the clinical corneal reflex. This is used to evaluate cerebellopontine angle tumors, demyelinating diseases (Guillain-Barré syndrome, multiple sclerosis) and facial nerve palsy. Blink reflexes can be observed in facial muscles other than orbicularis oculi in cases of synkinesis from aberrant reinnervation or ephaptic transmission.

22. What is the Martin-Gruber anastomosis?

The Martin-Gruber anastomosis involves the motor axons destined for the ulnar nerve, joined up with the median nerve in the brachial plexus, returned to the ulnar nerve in the forearm and then supplying various hand muscles. The anastomosing axons innervate the first dorsal interosseous, hypothenar, and thenar muscles.

23. What are the clinical and electrodiagnostic clues for Martin-Gruber anastomosis? How is the diagnosis confirmed?

Clues:
- No thenar muscle weakness or atrophy despite severely abnormal median sensory studies
- Initial positive deflection of median CMAP on elbow stimulation

- Higher amplitude of median CMAP on elbow stimulation than those on wrist stimulation
- Spuriously fast median NCV across the forearm as compared to norm or ulnar NCV
- Ulnar motor conduction study shows unusually low amplitude at elbow stimulation as compared to wrist stimulation mimicking conduction block

This anastomosis can be confirmed by recording from the first dorsal interosseous or other ulnar intrinsic muscles while stimulating the median nerve at the elbow. Recordable CMAP at elbow stimulation with no CMAP on wrist stimulation suggests crossing nerve fibers. Volume conduction should be avoided with wrist stimulation.

24. Describe the types of nerve injury according to the Seddon and Sunderland classifications.

SEDDON	SUNDERLAND*	PATHOLOGIC BASIS
Neuropraxia	Type 1	Local myelin injury, axonal continuity, no wallerian degeneration
Axonotmesis	Type 2	Disruption of axonal continuity with wallerian degeneration; endoneurium, perineurium, and epineurium intact
	Type 3	Loss of axonal continuity and endoneurial tube; perineurium and epineurium preserved
	Type 4	Loss of axonal continuity, endoneurium, and perineurium; epineurium preserved
Neurotmesis	Type 5	Severance of entire nerve

* Sunderland classification is not practical for electrodiagnosis.

Neuropraxia: Refers to the failure of impulse conduction across the affected nerve segment and normal conduction above and below the affected segment. The electrophysiological and clinical signficance is its reversibility.

Axonotmesis: Refers to a nerve injury involving only the axons and not the enveloping endoneurium and the supporting connective tissue structures, perineurium, and epineurium.

Neurotmesis: Complete disruption of the nerve and all of its supporting connective tissue structures. Clinical significance is poor prognosis, and surgical repair likely for functional recovery.

25. What is the purpose of electrodiagnosis soon after nerve injury (first 72 hours)?

The most important step at the early stage is to differentiate **axonotmesis** from **neurotmesis**. Axonotmesis is confirmed by the presence of CMAP or SNAP across the injured segment and voluntary motor unit(s) in the paralyzed muscles, while neurotmesis is supported by their absence. It is important to be aware that denervation potentials seen within a few days after a surgical procedure may represent a presurgical nerve lesion rather than damage from the surgical procedure.

For axonotmesis caused by blunt contusion, traction, or compression (not sharp objects), it is usually treated nonsurgically since good endoneural alignment is likely. The axonotmetic electrodiagnostic findings in sharp cutting injury should be interpreted differently because they represent a "neurotmetic lesion" for those "particular fascicle(s)" involved. Early surgical repair may be justified.

26. Can electrodiagnosis help in assessing the prognosis in Bell's palsy?

Conventional conduction study can only examine the segment distal to the compromised section of the facial nerve, and the latency value is not helpful in prognostication. The examiner should perform side-to-side comparison of amplitude/area of the CMAPs after completion of the wallerian degeneration. If CMAP amplitude remains **> 10%** of the unaffected side, there is a 90% of chance of satisfactory recovery. Some authors advocate the **30% CMAP amplitude** criteria for excellent functional recovery within a 2-month period. Good voluntary motor unit recruitment and return of R1 component of the blink reflex has some value. The needle EMG examination is the only objective way to document reinnervation.

27. What is the meaning of preganglionic lesion?

In most cases of radiculopathy, the pathology is proximal to dorsal root ganglion. Since the postganglionic sensory fibers continue to be supplied by axoplasmic flow from the dorsal root ganglion, the routine sensory conduction studies show no abnormalities. This is the reason why the routine nerve conduction study and EMG may fail to detect root pathology if the patient's complaint is "pain" without muscle weakness or atrophy.

It is possible, however, for the dorsal root ganglion to be situated slightly more proximal in the foramina affected by direct compression or indirectly by vascular insult and edema formation. The dorsal root ganglion can also be damaged in diseases such as diabetes mellitus and herpes zoster (ganglionopathy). In these conditions, SNAP may be abnormal, but abnormal SNAP occurs rarely in discogenic radiculopathy.

28. How can I differentiate between C8–T1 radiculopathy and ulnar neuropathy at the elbow?

1. Positive Spurling test, clinical sensory involvement of the ring finger without splitting and the medial arm and forearm, entirely normal ulnar SNAP, and concurrent involvement of the thenar and extensor indicis proprius muscles favor C8–T1 root pathology.

2. Sensory splitting of the ring finger, involvement of dorsal ulnar sensation with intact medial forearm sensation, low-amplitude or absent ulnar SNAP, and atrophy of the ulnar intrinsic muscles without concurrent median thenar atrophy favor ulnar neuropathy at the elbow.

3. However, this over-simplified picture can be complicated by **thoracic outlet syndrome** (thenar atrophy with ulnar sensory involvement), low trunk of the brachial plexus lesion, and **ulnar neuropathy at the palm**.

29. List five common reasons for a fluctuating baseline during electrodiagnostic studies.

- Poor contact between ground electrode and patient
- Broken recording electrode wire (G1 or G2)
- Cathode/anode reversal and anodal block: placing stimulating cathode near the recording electrode and stimulating anode away from the nerve trunk minimize anodal block. Excessive stimulus duration and intensity
- Crossing of stimulation wire leads with the other leads and cables
- Recording electrodes contacting parts of body other than recording electrodes

30. List five common pitfalls in reporting electrodiagnostic results.

1. Vague terminology and the inclusion of too many findings and differential diagnoses can often confuse the referring physicians. The pertinent normal or abnormal findings are not grouped together.

2. Diagnosis is outlined in a random order without explanation instead of presenting possible diagnoses from the most likely to least likely.

3. Absence of explaining the limitations of electrodiagnosis to the referring physician.

4. Semiquantitative grading of the lesion by "mild to severe" (radiculopathy, carpal tunnel syndrome) or "one plus to four plus" (fibrillation, positive sharp waves) should be done cautiously because the grading is rather subjective.

5. The lesion should be described in terms of neuromuscular localization rather than musculoskeletal localization. For example, a radial nerve lesion should be described as "distal to innervation of the triceps, proximal to innervation of brachioradialis" instead of "lesion in spiral groove" since the specific fascicular lesion at proximal site can mimic the lesion at distal location.

BIBLIOGRAPHY

1. Denys EH: AAEM minimonograph #14: The influence of temperature in clinical neurophysiology. Muscle Nerve 14:795–811, 1991.
2. Dumitru D, King JC: Nerve conduction study pitfalls. [AAEM Workshop Handout]. Sep 1994.

3. Dumitru D, Walsh NE, Porter LD: Electrophysiologic evaluation of the facial nerve in Bell's palsy: A review. Am J Phys Med Rehabil 67:137–144, 1988.
4. Dumitru D: Electrodiagnostic Medicine, 2nd ed. Philadelphia, Hanley & Belfus, 2002.
5. Gatens PF, Saeed MA: Electromyographic findings in the intrinsic muscles of normal feet. Arch Phys Med Rehabil 63:317–318, 1982.
6. Gutmann L: AAEM Minimonograph #2: Important anomalous innervations of the extremities. Muscle Nerve 16:339–347, 1993.
7. Henneman E, Somjen G, Carpenter DO: Functional significance of cell size in spinal motor neurons. J Neurophysiol 28:560–589, 1965.
8. Johnson EW: Why and how to request an electrodiagnostic examination and what to expect in return. Phys Med Rehabil Clin North Am 1:149–158, 1990.
9. Stolov WC: Instrumentation and measurement in electrodiagnosis: AAEM minimonograph #16. Muscle Nerve 18:799–811, 1995.

21. RADICULOPATHIES

Timothy R. Dillingham, M.D.

1. What are radiculopathies?

Cervical and lumbosacral radiculopathies are conditions resulting from pathologic processes affecting the spinal nerve root. Commonly, the cause is a herniated nucleus pulposus that anatomically compresses a nerve root within the spinal canal. Another common etiology is spinal stenosis resulting from a combination of degenerative spondylosis, ligament hypertrophy, and spondylolisthesis. Inflammatory radiculitis is another pathophysiologic process that can cause radiculopathy. It is important to remember that other more ominous processes, such as malignancy and infection, can present with the same symptoms and signs of radiculopathy as the more common causes.

2. What are the nondiscogenic radiculopathies?

- Tumors: meningiomas, neurofibromas, lipomas (cauda equina and conus medularis)
- Leptomeningeal metastasis (leukemias, lymphoproliferative diseases)
- Abscess, hemorrhage, cysts
- Infection: herpes zoster, tuberculosis, Lyme disease, syphilis, HIV infection
- Arachnoiditis: myelogram, surgery, anesthetics, steroid injections
- Sarcoidosis, Guillain-Barré syndrome, diabetes

3. Which anatomic structures are involved in radiculopathies?

In the lumbar spine, the attachment and shape of the posterior longitudinal ligament predisposes to herniation of the nucleus pulposus in a posterolateral direction where it is the weakest. The dorsal and ventral lumbar roots exit the spinal cord at about the T11–L1 bony level and travel in the lumbar canal as a group of nerve roots in the dural sac. This is termed the "horse's tail," or cauda equina. Radicular lesions from T11 to the sacrum can involve one or more roots due to this anatomic relationship.

In contrast to the lumbar spine, in the cervical spinal cord the location of an exiting nerve root is closer to its origin. This makes it easier to determine if an anatomic finding is causing a cervical radiculopathy.

4. What do patients complain of when they have a radiculopathy?

Generally pain that radiates from the neck or back into the limb. Numbness, weakness, and paresthesias are common complaints as well. Lumbosacral radicular pain is often increased with bending, sitting, or Valsalva manuevers such as coughing. Cervical radicular pain may be aggravated by neck extension, which causes narrowing of the intervertebral foramen.

5. What conditions can mimic cervical radiculopathy?

The symptoms of cervical radiculopathy are nondescript and not specific for radiculopathy. Many other neurologic and musculoskeletal conditions can produce pain, weakness, and sensory symptoms. In addition to the standard peripheral neurologic examination, one of the most helpful maneuvers is to ask the patient where it hurts, then carefully palpate that area. If pain is reproduced by this palpation, then the examiner should have a heightened suspicion for a musculoskeletal disorder. Common musculoskeletal disorders that produce symptoms similar to those produced by a cervical radiculopathy are shown in the table.

Common entrapment neuropathies also can present with symptoms similar to those of radiculopathy (see Chapter 23). Plexopathies such as idiopathic brachial neuritis can pose diagnostic dilemmas for the electrodiagnostician as well.

Musculoskeletal Conditions that Commonly Mimic Cervical Radiculopathy

CONDITION	CLINICAL SYMPTOMS/SIGNS
Fibromyalgia syndrome	Pain all over, female predominance, often sleep problems, tender to palpation in multiple areas
Regional myofascial pain syndrome	Trigger point reproducing localized or radiating pain
Polymyalgia rheumatica	Age > 50 yr; pain and stiffness in neck, shoulders, and hips; high ESR
Sternoclavicular joint arthropathy	Pain in anterior chest, pain with shoulder movement, pain on direct palpation
Acromioclavicular joint arthropathy	Pain in anterior chest, pain with shoulder movement, pain on direct palpation, pain with crossed adduction of shoulder
Shoulder bursitis, impingement syndrome, bicipital tendinitis	Pain with palpation, positive impingement signs, pain in C5 distribution
Lateral epicondylitis, "tennis elbow"	Pain in lateral forearm, pain with palpation and resisted wrist extension
deQuervain's tenosynovitis	Lateral wrist and forearm pain, tender at abductor pollicis longus or extensor pollicis brevis tendons, positive Finkelstein test
Trigger finger, stenosing tenosynovitis of finger flexor tendons	Intermittent pain and locking of digit in flexion

ESR, erythrocyte sedimentation rate.

6. What conditions may mimic lumbosacral radiculopathy?

Common Musculoskeletal Disorders Mimicking Lumbosacral Radiculopathy

CONDITION	CLINICAL SYMPTOMS/SIGNS
Fibromyalgia, myofascial pain syndrome, polymyalgia rheumatica	See Question 5
Hip arthritis	Pain in groin and anterior thigh, pain with weight-bearing, positive Patrick's test
Trochanteric bursitis	Lateral hip pain, pain with palpation over lateral and posterior hip
Iliotibial band syndrome	Pain along outer thigh, pain with palpation, tight iliotibial band (positive Ober test)
Knee arthritis	Pain with weight-bearing
Patellofemoral pain	Anterior knee pain, worse with prolonged sitting, positive patellar compression test
Pes anserinus bursitis	Medial proximal tibia pain, tender to palpation

Table continued on following page

Common Musculoskeletal Disorders Mimicking Lumbosacral Radiculopathy (Continued)

CONDITION	CLINICAL SYMPTOMS/SIGNS
Hamstring tendinitis, chronic strain	Posterior knee and thigh pain, can mimic positive straight-leg raise, common in runners
Baker's cyst	Posterior knee pain and swelling
Plantar fasciitis	Pain in sole of foot, worse with weight-bearing activities, tender to palpation
Gastrocnemius-soleus tendinitis, chronic strain	Calf pain, worse with sports activities, usually limited ROM compared to asymptomatic limb

Neuralgic amyotrophy (due to nerve ischemia) from diabetes is a condition that is often very difficult to distinguish from lumbosacral radiculopathy. It often presents with thigh pain and on EMG appears more like proximal lumbosacral plexus mononeuropathies with frequent involvement of the femoral nerve. Mononeuropathies such as peroneal, tibial, and femoral, pose diagnostic challenges as well. Electrodiagnostic testing is useful to identify these entities.

7. What physical findings are helpful in identifying a radiculopathy?

A focused neuromuscular examination that assesses strength, reflexes, and sensation in the affected limb and the contralateral limb is important. Patients with radiculopathy may demonstrate subtle weakness, a reduced reflex, or sensory loss. The sensory loss is either nondescript or in a dermatomal distribution. For many persons, the examination is normal. A positive straight-leg-raise test may be noted in the absence of motor, sensory, or reflex changes.

Special tests such as those mentioned in questions 5 and 6 that indicate common musculoskeletal disorders are easy to perform and may identify a nonneurologic cause of the patient's symptoms. The clinician must remember that CNS disorders such as stroke or spinal myelopathy may result in sensory loss and weakness similar to that found in radiculopathy; however, reflexes are usually increased in these CNS conditions.

8. Which diagnostic tools are useful in evaluating patients with suspected cervical or lumbosacral radiculopathy?

To assess these patients, plain x-rays, MRI, and electrodiagnostic tests are available and provide the primary means of evaluation. Other tests, such as an erythrocyte sedimentation rate, can screen for a bone or disc infection or polymyalgia rheumatica. Electrodiagnostic testing consists primarily of electromyography (EMG) and nerve conduction studies. Electrodiagnostic testing provides an assessment as to whether motor axonal damage is occurring and can help determine when an imaging finding is of clinical relevance.

Plain x-rays assess bony alignment. Lateral flexion and extension views should be obtained when plain x-rays are ordered, as these dynamic views assess for spondylolisthesis or spinal instability.

9. How often are MRI findings false-positive?

The false-positive rates for MRI of the lumbar spine are high, with 27% of normals showing a disc protrusion. For the cervical spine, the false-positive rate is much lower, with 19% of subjects demonstrating an abnormality but only 10% showing a herniated or bulging disc. Radiculopathies can occur without structural findings on MRI and, likewise, without EMG findings. The sensitivity of MRI for identifying pathologic conditions of the spine is very high, but the trade-off is the correspondingly high rate of false-positive findings.

10. Can MRI screen for spinal malignancy?

Yes, it is an excellent diagnostic test for bony invasion by primary and metastatic tumors, extradural tumors, and intradural tumors. Gadolinium enhancement must be used if a tumor is suspected, as without enhancement, intramedullary tumors and other malignancies may be missed.

11. Can MRI adequately assess for spinal stenosis?

Yes, it can readily identify patients with spinal stenosis in both the lumbar and cervical regions. Sometimes, a myelogram with computed tomography is helpful to better delineate bony anatomy. However, the ever-increasing quality of MRI imaging of the spine provides ample evidence of spinal stenosis when present.

12. Is MRI as helpful in detecting spinal infections?

Again, the answer is yes. MRI with and without gadolinium enhancement is a great screening test for epidural abscesses, disciitis, and osteomyelitis. MRI is a key diagnostic tool that rules out the most serious of spinal pathologies.

13. Can a radiculopathy at a specific root level be diagnosed simply on the basis of positive paraspinal findings?

No. The diagnosis of radiculopathy can be made, but the root level cannot be specified unless EMG abnormalities are found in two or more muscles innervated by a single root and by different peripheral nerves, yet muscles innervated by adjacent nerve roots are normal. The paraspinal muscles are innervated by multiple nerve roots and not by one nerve root alone.

14. Are nerve conduction studies (NCSs) helpful in assessing for radiculopathy?

NCSs are not helpful in identifying radiculopathy. Sensory NCS findings should be normal as the dorsal root ganglion is situated in the intervertebral foramen, and for this reason, intraspinal problems (radiculopathies) do not affect the sensory NCSs in the limbs. Motor NCSs are usually normal unless marked axonal loss is present, in which case the amplitudes may be reduced.

Late responses, such as F-waves and H-reflexes, are not much help in identifying a radiculopathy, although they are excellent screening tests for polyneuropathy. H-reflexes evaluate the S1 reflex and demonstrate about a 50% sensitivity for S1 root involvement and can distinguish S1 from L5 radiculopathies. Typically, the side-to-side H-reflex latency differences are examined when considering whether an S1 radiculopathy is present. The upper limit of normal is considered to be approximately 1.8 msec.

15. How sensitive is EMG for diagnosing radiculopathy?

It is rather unimpressive. Various studies place the sensitivity of needle EMG for lumbosacral radiculopathies somewhere between 50% and 80%, depending upon the diagnostic gold standard used—clinical standards, imaging standards, or intraoperative confirmation. For cervical radiculopathies, the sensitivity is roughly 60–70%.

The value of EMG resides in its ability to define, localize, and grade the severity of a radiculopathy with high specificity. This makes EMG a complementary test to MRI. When MRI suggests an anatomic explanation for a patient's symptoms, such as a herniated nucleus pulposus with nerve root impingement, the EMG can provide evidence as to whether there is axonal damage from this lesion. EMG and NCS can exclude other disorders such as polyneuropathy.

16. Why is the EMG normal for many people with radiculopathies?

The needle EMG assesses only the motor axons. For this reason, a radiculopathy that involves only the sensory nerve roots and causes radicular pain and numbness will demonstrate a normal EMG. Radiculopathies that cause motor neuropraxia at the nerve root level will not show spontaneous activity (fibrillations and positive sharp waves) on EMG. Radiculopathies that result in chronic, slow axonal loss that is balanced with reinnervation may not show spontaneous activity, but rather may show more subtle findings such as polyphasic motor units or large motor units firing in a reduced recruitment pattern.

17. How many muscles must be studied in order to confidently identify a radiculopathy by EMG?

The electrodiagnostician is compelled to perform a study sufficient to confidently identify or exclude radiculopathies that can be delineated by EMG. Studies that include a large number of muscles, however, are uncomfortable to the patient. For this reason, delineating an optimal EMG screening exam that allows the examiner to identify a radiculopathy (when one can be electrodiagnostically confirmed) yet minimizes the number of muscles studied is of great clinical interest. *For optimal identification while minimizing harm, study six in the leg and six in the arm.*

Six lower limb muscles, including paraspinal muscles, consistently identify over 98% of electrodiagnostically confirmable lumbosacral radiculopathies. Studying additional muscles leads to marginal increases in identification. A suggested lower-limb EMG screen with optimal identification includes the vastus medialis, anterior tibialis, posterior tibialis, short head of biceps femoris, medial gastrocnemius, and lumbar paraspinal muscles.

Six upper limb muscles, including paraspinal muscles, also consistently identify over 98% of electrodiagnostically confirmable cervical radiculopathies. For upper-limb EMG evaluation, a suggested screen includes deltoid, triceps, pronator teres, abductor pollicis brevis, extensor digitorum communis, and cervical paraspinal muscles. For both lumbosacral and cervical symptoms, when paraspinal muscles are not reliable to study, then **eight** distal muscles are necessary to achieve optimal identification.

18. If a person has a herniated disc pressing on a lumbosacral spinal nerve as the cause of symptoms should he or she be immediately referred for discectomy?

No. The indications for an urgent referral to a spine surgeon include a cauda equina syndrome with bowel or bladder dysfunction, progressive weakness, or relentless pain that cannot be controlled by other means. Fortunately, these are rare circumstances, and for over 90% of persons with an acute herniated disc, conservative treatments are effective. These conservative management strategies include medications (anti-inflammatories and opiate pain medications), brief periods of rest, intraspinal corticosteroid injections, and gradual introduction of a lumbar stabilization exercise program. Surgery for herniated lumbar discs may be slightly more effective at pain control at 1 year, but the longer term outcomes are no different for surgical and nonsurgical management.

19. For persons with a herniated cervical disc and radiculopathy, what is the best treatment?

Surgery is indicated if there are signs and symptoms of a myelopathy in addition to a radiculopathy. These include gait disturbance, absent vibration perception in the legs, upgoing toes to plantar stimulation, or leg weakness. Otherwise, conservative treatments are effective.

20. What are the long-term outcomes for persons with a herniated lumbosacral disc who are managed conservatively?

They are quite good. It has become apparent over the last two decades that the natural history of both lumbosacral radiculopathy, with or without structural findings on MRI, is very favorable. A classic investigation by Henrik Weber, a randomized prospective study of surgery versus conservative care for herniated nucleus pulposus, demonstrated that surgery was somewhat more effective at pain control during the first year. Beyond 1 year, however, conservative treatment had equal results compared to the surgically managed group. Of particular note was the fact that even for persons with motor weakness, a good outcome with conservative treatment was the norm, and surgery did not improve motor return. Other investigators in cohort outcome studies have demonstrated that the majority of persons suffering lumbosacral radiculopathy can resolve their symptoms. In fact, on follow-up MRI studies, lumbosacral disc herniations and disc fragments resolve in 76% of patients.

21. What are the long-term outcomes for persons with a herniated cervical disc who are managed conservatively?

The outcomes for persons with cervical radiculopathy without myelopathy who are managed nonoperatively are quite good. Saal, Saal, and Yurth demonstrated that persons with cervical disc herniations have a favorable clinical course. Their cohort of patients were managed with pain management strategies incorporating medications, rehabilitation with cervical traction and exercises, and epidural or selective nerve root injections if medications failed to control pain. In this series, the majority (24 of 26) of patients with herniated cervical discs achieved successful outcomes without surgery.

BIBLIOGRAPHY

1. Boden SD, McCowin PR, Davis DO, et al: Abnormal magnetic resonance scans of the cervical spine in asymptomatic subjects. J Bone Joint Surg 72A:1178–1184, 1990.
2. Bush K, Cowan N, Katz DE, Gishen P: The natural history of sciatica associated with disc pathology: A prospective study with clinical and independent radiological follow-up. Spine 1:1205–1212, 1992.
3. Dillingham TR, Lauder TD, Andary M, et al: Identifying lumbosacral radiculopathies: An optimal electromyographic screen. Am J Phys Med Rehabil 79:496–503, 2000.
4. Dillingham TR: Electrodiagnosis of radiculopathies: How many and which muscles to study. AAEM Lecture presented at AAEM Annual Scientific Meeting, 1999, Vancouver, BC.
5. Dumitru D (ed): Electrodiagnostic Medicine, 2nd ed. Philadelphia, Hanley & Belfus, 2002.
6. Honet JC, Puri K: Cervical radiculitis: Treatment and results in 82 patients. Arch Phys Med Rehabil 57:12–16, 1976.
7. Jensen MC, Brant-Zawadzki MN, Obuchowski N, et al: Magnetic resonance imaging of the lumbar spine in people without back pain. N Engl J Med 331:69–73, 1994.
8. Knutsson B: Comparative value of electromyographic, myelographic and clinical-neurological examinations in diagnosis of lumbar root compression syndrome. Acta Orthop Scand (Suppl 49), 1961.
9. Kuruoglu R, Oh SJ, Thompson B: Clinical and electromyographic correlations of lumbosacral radiculopathy. Muscle Nerve 17:250–251, 1994.
10. Lauder T, Dillingham TR, Huston C, et al: Lumbosacral radiculopathy screen: Optimizing the number of muscles studied. Am J Phys Med Rehabil 73:394–402, 1994.
11. Lauder TD, Dillingham TR: The cervical radiculopathy screen: Optimizing the number of muscles studied. Muscle Nerve 19:662–665, 1996.
12. Lauder TD, Dillingham TR, Andary M, et al: Effect of history and exam in predicting electrodiagnostic outcome among patients with suspected lumbosacral radiculopathy. Am J Phys Med Rehabil 79:60–68, 2000.
13. Nardin RA, Patel MR, Gudas TF, et al: Electromyography and magnetic resonance imaging in the evaluation of radiculopathy. Muscle Nerve 22:151–155, 1999.
14. Olmarker K, Rydevik B: Pathophysiology of sciatica. Orthop Clin North Am 22:223–234, 1991.
15. Partanen J, Partanen K, Oikarinen H, et al: Preoperative electroneuromyography and myelography in cervical root compression. Electromyogr Clin Neurophysiol 31:21–26, 1991.
16. Robinson LR: Electromyography, magnetic resonance imaging, and radiculopathy: It's time to focus on specificity. Muscle Nerve 22:149–150, 1999.
17. Saal JS, Saal JA, Yurth EF: Nonoperative management of herniated cervical intervertebral disc with radiculopathy. Spine 21:1877–1883, 1996.
18. Saal JA, Saal JS, Herzog RJ:The natural history of lumbar intervertebral disc extrusions treated non-operatively. Spine 15:683–686, 1990.
19. Sampath P, Bendebba M, Davis JD, Ducker T: Outcome in patients with cervical radiculopathy: Prospective, multicenter study with independent clinical review. Spine 24:591–597, 1999.
20. Weber H: Lumbar disc herniation; a controlled, prospective study with ten years of observation. Spine 8:131–140, 1983.
21. Wilbourn AJ, Aminoff MJ: AAEM Minimonograph 32: Electrodiagnosis of radiculopathies. Muscle Nerve 21:1612–1631, 1998.

22. CARPAL TUNNEL SYNDROME AND/OR MEDIAN NEUROPATHY AT THE WRIST

Janet C. Limke, M.D., Steven A. Stiens, M.D., M.S., and Larry Robinson, M.D.

1. What is the carpal tunnel?

The carpal tunnel is the small, oblong pathway in the wrist through which the median nerve and nine tendons pass (four tendons each from the flexor digitorum superficialis and profundus muscles and one from the flexor pollicis longus). On the volar side, it is bounded by the taut transverse carpal ligament, or flexor retinaculum, and on the dorsal side by the carpal bones.

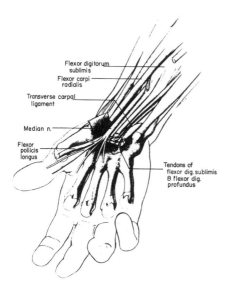

Carpal tunnel. (From Liveson JA, Spielholz NI: Peripheral Neurology: Case Studies in Electrodiagnosis. Philadelphia, F.A. Davis, 1991, p 20; with permission.)

2. How does carpal tunnel syndrome (CTS) present?

CTS is the most common focal nerve entrapment syndrome. The presentation includes major specific symptoms of pain and paresthesias (tingling, burning, and numbness) in the median nerve distribution. In advanced cases, weakness of the median-innervated hand musculature is present. Minor, nonspecific symptoms include wrist pain, clumsiness, tightness, and complaints of dropping things easily. Pain commonly involves the hand or wrist but may also be felt proximally in the forearm, elbow, or shoulder. Symptoms are often brought on by overuse of the hand, especially forceful gripping or repetitive hand/wrist motion. Nocturnal symptoms are frequently reported and are associated with the characteristic **"flick" sign** (shaking the hand to relieve nocturnal paresthesias)

3. How is the diagnosis of CTS made?

Median nerve impingement, which produces the spectrum of pathophysiologic changes known as CTS, can be discerned with nerve conduction studies (NCS), MRI, or open surgical exploration. The clinical evaluation includes a systematic history, eliciting of signs with provocative maneuvers, as well as confirmatory physiologic and anatomic tests.

Some clinicians rely solely on clinical history and physical exam and recommend surgery after conservative measures have failed. However, because many conditions can be confused with CTS, treating solely on the basis of physical signs and symptoms can be problematic. Whereas some investigators define CTS as a clinical diagnosis, others define it with combined clinical and electrodiagnostic changes (median neuropathy at the wrist) supportive of CTS. It may be argued that more stringent criteria, i.e., nerve conduction abnormalities, should be present before surgery is considered.

4. List the differential diagnosis of CTS.

Neurologic: cervical radiculopathy (C6,7,8); brachial plexus lesions, including thoracic outlet syndrome; ulnar, radial, or proximal median nerve lesions or generalized polyneuropathies; syringomyelia or other central sensory and motor phenomena

Musculoskeletal: tenosynovitis including deQuervain's (inflammation of synovial tendon sheaths), osteoarthritis of the metacarpal-trapezial joint (thumb carpometacarpal arthritis), Kienböck's disease (avascular lunate necrosis), scaphoidal-trapezial arthritis, and digital neuritis

Vascular: Raynaud's phenomenon, radial artery thrombosis

5. What is the difference between CTS and median neuropathy at the wrist?

CTS is a *clinical* diagnosis that may or may not be associated with electrodiagnostic findings, whereas median nerve entrapment is an *electrophysiologic* diagnosis. In the absence of clinical findings, an electrodiagnostic finding of median neuropathy at the wrist is referred to not as CTS but as median neuropathy at the wrist.

6. Are tests that attempt to objectify sensory impairment useful in screening for CTS?

Yes, but none are substitutes for NCS, currently the only truly objective measurement of nerve impairment. Tests of sensibility (sensory perception) can be divided into two general categories: threshold tests and innervation density tests.

The **thermal threshold test** quantifies dysfunction in the small myelinated and unmyelinated axons, whereas NCS tests large myelinated fibers. When compared to NCS as the gold standard, thermal threshold measurements are sensitive but not specific in early CTS.

Like NCS, **vibrometry** evaluates larger myelinated fibers. However, in an excellent study, vibrometry was not sensitive in picking up early CTS in an industrial population. According to the researchers, axonal injury must be present, as in more severe CTS, before abnormalities will be detected.

Another threshold test, the **Semmes-Weinstein monofilament test**, assesses touch perception of the thinnest detected filament applied to the digit. In general, the threshold tests are more sensitive than innervation density tests, such as the **Weber two-point discrimination**. Normal two-point discrimination is 5 mm or less. All of the sensibility tests have been used in documenting recovery of CTS, particularly after surgery.

7. Explain the important components of the electrodiagnostic consultation in suspected CTS.

The electrodiagnostic medical consultation evaluates nerve and muscle function as an extension of the clinical neuromuscular physical examination. The role of the electrodiagnostic consultant in management of CTS varies with referral requests. At the least, the consultative record should render an interpreted review of the patient's history (obesity, family history of CTS, diabetes, thyroid disease, employment and other risk factors), symptoms (acroparesthesias, weakness duration, distribution and symptoms, exacerbating/relieving facts), physical findings (weight, temperature, sudomotor changes, atrophy, edema, reflexes, strength, sensation, evocative maneuvers), and electrodiagnostic data. Neuromuscular or systemic conditions that could masquerade as CTS or predispose the patient to CTS should be uncovered, studied, and reported (e.g., diabetes).

8. How is the Phalen wrist flexion test carried out?

Dr. George S. Phalen, former Chief of Hand Surgery at the Cleveland Clinic and a founding member of the American Society for Surgery of the Hand, recommended that the patient place his or her flexed elbows on a table and allow the wrists to fall freely into maximum flexion (no forced flexion by patient or examiner). The median nerve is compressed between the proximal edge of the transverse carpal ligament and the flexor tendons. This position is expected to elicit numbness and tingling in a median distribution in 75% of persons with CTS symptoms and median neuropathy after 1 to 2 minutes and in > 25% of normals after 10 minutes.

9. Are any other tests used to elicit CTS?

The examination should include a bilateral directed evaluation of the cervical, shoulder, forearm, wrist, and hand regions. Provocative tests complement the examination by demonstrating a relationship between symptoms and mechanical manipulation of the median nerve. All are plagued with false-negative and false-positive results.

1. **Tinel's sign**—Percussion over the nerve produces tingling sensations in the distribution of a regenerating injured nerve. Light percussion with a reflex hammer along the nerve while the wrist is extended increases sensitivity, but false-positives have been reported to range from 6% to 45%.

2. **Tethered median nerve stress test**—The index finger is hyperextended and dorsal pressure is applied at the volar distal finger pad with the wrist extended and supinated to pull or stretch the nerve. A positive test produces median dysesthesias or forearm pain.

3. **Carpal compression test**—150 mmHg pressure is applied over the volar wrist at the median nerve for 30 seconds. The test is positive if median dysesthesia is reported.

4. **Reverse Phalen test**—The wrists are extended to 90° in a praying-hands position for 60 seconds. Paresthesias in the median distribution indicate a positive result.

10. If median neuropathy of the wrist is suspected, what is the current standard electrodiagnostic approach?

A combined committee of the American Association of Electrodiagnostic Medicine, in collaboration with the American Academy of Neurology and American Academy of Physical Medicine and Rehabilitation, published a practice parameter for electrodiagnostic studies in CTS. After a thorough review of the literature, recommendations include:

1. Sensory NCS of the median nerve across the wrist, and if the latency is abnormal, comparison to another sensory study in the symptomatic limb.

2. If the initial median sensory NCS across the wrist has a conduction distance > 8 cm and the results are normal, additional studies as follows:

- Median sensory NCS across the wrist over a short (7–8 cm) conduction distance or
- Comparison of median sensory NCS across the wrist with radial or ulnar sensory conduction across the wrist in the same limb.

The practice parameter also recommends motor NCS of the median nerve with comparison to one other motor nerve in the symptomatic limb and an option for EMG study of the limb.

More recent studies have shown it is more sensitive and reliable to perform three latency comparisons of the median nerve (median with ulnar across the palm, median with ulnar to the ring finger, and median with radial to the thumb) rather than a single test, and add the three latency differences. This combined sensory index is normally < 1.0 msec in asymptomatic individuals.

11. How do imaging studies contribute to the clinical data?

Plain x-rays of the wrist may be useful if one suspects arthritic disorders that may lead to degenerative spurs or calcified lesions in the carpal tunnel. MRI reveals anatomic as well as chemical changes of the nerve and surrounding tissues. Morphologic changes suggesting median nerve impingement include enlargement with edema, flattening, narrowing, and loss of normal fat in the carpal tunnel. Postsurgical changes may include hematomas, abscesses, and excess scar formation. MRI may reveal peripheral nerve lesions involving axonotmesis as early as 4 days after the onset of symptoms or injury by picking up an altered signal from denervated muscle. Neurapraxic injuries (conduction block without axon loss) result in normal signal from median innervated muscles. Despite these capabilities, the sensitivity and specificity of MRI are not well established, and MRI is not part of a routine workup for CTS.

12. What patient factors are associated with false-positive results in CTS?

In a recent study of over 900 industrial workers, new normative data were defined that support using a higher median-to-ulnar latency difference than in the general population. Similarly, patients with concomitant diabetes require more significant latency differences in order to distinguish peripheral neuropathy alone from a superimposed median neuropathy at the wrist.

- *Cold temperature* of the hand will slow conduction, prolong distal latencies, and increase the amplitude of a response.
- *Increasing age* is correlated with slower conduction times and smaller amplitude responses. Median digital amplitudes recorded antidromically fall slightly more than 2 μV per decade.
- *Height*, and therefore *axon length*, is directly correlated with latency and inversely related to amplitude; hence, taller people have longer latencies.

• *Finger circumference* is inversely related to the amplitude, as the intervening soft tissue causes attenuation of the recorded response on the skin surface.

• *Gender* does not appear to play as much of a role when the above factors are considered.

13. Which technical problems can result in inaccurate results?

Proper technique is essential to ensure the accuracy of NCS. The extremity should be warmed to ≥ 32°C when looking at absolute latencies, however, latency differences between two nerves in the same limb are not significantly affected by cold. A submaximal stimulus intensity may lead to an erroneously small amplitude response and possibly a longer latency since the fastest fibers may not be depolarized. Exact distances should be measured and rechecked if abnormal values are noted. Consistent amplifier gain, sweep speeds, and filter settings should be utilized that are appropriate for the given study and allow for comparison to reference values. Techniques to minimize stimulus artifact interference and overcome electrode and skin resistance should be adhered to.

Sensory studies with less than 4-cm electrode separation between active and reference electrodes may result in a smaller amplitude and shorter peak latency, since both electrodes will detect the nerve action potential at nearly the same time and therefore the difference between the two potentials is not maximized. For motor studies, the recording electrode must be centered over the main muscle belly or motor point and the reference over the tendon or adjacent joint. If the recording electrode is not properly placed, a positive deflection will be recorded before the negative deflection and may confuse the latency measurement. Activation of the nearby ulnar nerve will produce a similar initial positive deflection.

14. Describe anomalous innervations affecting the NCS and interpretation in CTS.

The **Martin-Gruber anastomosis**, typically a median-to-ulnar connection in the forearm motor fibers via the median or anterior interosseous nerve, occurs in 15% of individuals and affects both median and ulnar recordings. In an individual without median neuropathy at the wrist, this variation will result in a larger CMAP amplitude when stimulating the median nerve at the elbow than at the wrist. In median neuropathy, the anastomosis causes an initial positive deflection when stimulating over the elbow, despite proper centering of the recording electrode over the belly of the thenar muscles. The same deflection is not noted on distal wrist stimulation. The early positive deflection represents volume conduction from the stimulation of the anomalous ulnar axons that are conducting the impulse quicker since they do not pass through the carpal tunnel.

15. How do various innervations of hand muscles affect EMG interpretation of median neuropathy?

Many variations exist in the innervation of the thenar muscles. Approximately one-third of patients have all median-innervated thenar muscles: flexor pollicis brevis, abductor pollicis brevis, and opponens pollicis. Another third show median innervation to opponens pollicis and abductor pollicis brevis and ulnar innervation to the entire flexor pollicis brevis, while 15% show dual innervation of flexor pollicis brevis. Up to 2% of hands show an all-ulnar-innervated pattern. This knowledge of anatomy calls for caution in interpreting EMG abnormalities in thenar muscles, since ulnar lesions may account for changes in some patients.

16. What does the needle EMG exam contribute to the diagnosis of CTS?

1. It provides evidence of motor axon injury and/or reinnervation of the thenar muscles. Thus, along with NCS abnormalities consistent with a median nerve process at the wrist, it confirms axon loss in severe CTS and may help to determine chronicity.

2. It is useful in assessing separate or concomitant pathology, such as proximal median neuropathy, cervical or thoracic radiculopathy, plexopathy, or polyneuropathy. Proximal lesions along any part of the origins of the median nerve from the cervical spine and distal, in addition to median neuropathy at the wrist, are sometimes called a "double-crush" syndrome, though scientific evidence for the existence of this phenomenon is minimal. The distribution of abnormalities will lead the skilled electromyographer to the correct diagnosis or diagnoses.

17. What other lower motor neuron problems may present with similar symptoms?

The sensory dermatomal distribution of the hand is C6–8 going lateral to medial (or radial to ulnar side of the hand), while motor innervation to thenar muscles is C8–T1. A *cervical radiculopathy* will typically show abnormalities in the muscles innervated by the corresponding nerve root *without* sensory conduction changes since the dorsal root ganglion is typically spared. A *plexopathy* may present with a variety of patterns affecting the median nerve, since it arises from all three trunks of the brachial plexus. Tracing the changes back through the plexus will usually reveal the point or points of plexus involvement. A *polyneuropathy* results in multiple NCS findings in more than one limb.

18. What other common sites of median nerve compression should be considered in the evaluation of CTS?

1. At the supracondylar *ligament of Struthers* (an anomalous ligament) or *lacertus fibrosis* (bicipital aponeurosis) before it enters the pronator canal in the distal upper arm

2. Between the two heads of the *pronator teres* or under the edge of the *flexor sublimis* (sublimis arch), which spares the innervation to pronator teres and flexor carpi radialis

3. At the *anterior interosseous branch*, a pure motor branch of the median nerve in the forearm to flexor digitorum profundus I and II, flexor pollicis longus, and pronator quadratus

Proximal motor stimulation, transcarpal assessment, and careful EMG of proximal as well as distal median-innervated muscles help demonstrate these other entrapments.

19. Describe a practical severity rating scale for CTS and median neuropathy (MN) for use when reporting electrodiagnostic findings.

There are different ways to report severity. Many electromyographers do not report severity since there is usually a poor correlation between symptoms and latencies. One logical system that incorporates both latency and amplitude changes follows:

- **Mild MN:** Median sensory nerve conduction slowing without motor nerve conduction slowing *and/or* loss of median sensory amplitude of < 50% of the reference value.
- **Moderate MN:** Median sensory and motor slowing *and/or* loss of median sensory amplitude of > 50% of the reference value.
- **Severe MN:** Absence of median sensory potential along with median motor slowing, *or* median motor slowing along with reduction of median motor amplitude, *or* median NCS abnormalities along with evidence of axonal injury on EMG of the thenar muscles.

20. Discuss the nonoperative treatment of CTS.

Once CTS has been confirmed, basic laboratory tests for thyroid or renal disorders and diabetes should be obtained. Any underlying disorders should be treated.

Nonoperative therapy may include hand splinting in neutral wrist position, passive stretching of the transverse carpal ligament, ROM exercises, medications such as diuretics and NSAIDs, ergonomic modifications, and steroid injections in the wrist. Modest doses of pyridoxine (vitamin B_6) have been advocated, although no well-designed study has demonstrated its efficacy.

21. List five identified factors that predict failure of nonoperative treatment.

Less than 10% of persons with 3 of the 5 following risk factors improve with medical management alone:

- Age > 50 years (12–23% of patients are < 40 years of age)
- Symptom duration > 10 months (CTS is most commonly an insidious process that may develop over months or years)
- Constant paresthesias (constant symptoms suggest more significant nerve pathology)
- Stenosing flexor tenosynovitis (chronic synovial inflammation of the flexor tendons translates into higher pressures in the carpal tunnel)
- Positive Phalen test in < 30 sec

22. What are the ergonomic risk factors for CTS?

High force, high repetition, vibration, awkward posture, and temperature extremes have all been implicated as ergonomic risk factors for occupational hand and wrist disorders, including CTS. Obesity is also an independent risk factor.

23. What surgical treatments are possible for CTS?

Overall, the success rate for surgical treatment of CTS approaches 90%. Persons who have longer duration of symptoms or more severe nerve lesions have a worse prognosis, as do those with underlying polyneuropathies.

The most traditional technique for CTS release is an **open procedure** using a 4–5-cm, curved, longitudinal incision with good exposure of the transverse carpal ligament to minimize nerve injury. Occasionally, the palmar branch of the medial nerve and rarely the motor branch to the thenar muscles are transligamentous. When these variations are present, the branches are identified and dissected free from the ligament.

Endoscopic techniques have been described for release of the transverse carpal ligament. A recent analysis of published series indicates comparable rates of nerve injury complications between open and closed techniques. However, case reports indicate a small risk of unacceptable complications with endoscopic release, such as transection of the median nerve. In a separate review of outcomes, endoscopic release was associated with higher levels of physical functioning and fewer days to return to work when compared to open release. Further longer-term studies are needed to evaluate not only the complications but also the long-term efficacy of the endoscopic approach.

24. What are the possible complications of surgery?

Surgical complications occur in about 2% of cases. These include excessive scar formation (particularly with longitudinal incision proximal to the palmar flexor crease), infection, nerve injuries (including the motor branch or palmar cutaneous branch of the median nerve or the digital sensory nerves), pain (at the scar or reflex sympathetic dystrophy), and bowing of the tendons of the wrist with loss of grip strength.

25. Discuss follow-up after CTS surgery. How quickly does nerve function recover and NCS abnormalities resolve?

After surgery using the traditional surgical procedure, the wrist is splinted in extension for 1–3 weeks, and the fingers are gently exercised. A patient having an open surgery may be excused from work for 1–6 weeks (most would return to light duty much earlier) depending on the demands of the job, and those having the endoscopic technique may return to work in 1–3 weeks. Pain and paresthesias usually improve in the first several weeks, while numbness and weakness may require 6 to 9 months for optimal recovery. Patients with preoperative thenar muscle denervation are less likely to have resolution of paresthesias after surgery. With a median follow-up of 5.5 years, 86% of patients with surgical decompression showed at least partial improvement of NCS. Pain is the most significantly improved symptom. Poorer outcome has been observed in patients who have strenuous work activities. Nonoperative approaches also show a poor outcome in the heavy labor population, suggesting a need for ergonomic or vocational adjustments if CTS is to be relieved. Following surgery, NCS abnormalities typically improve, although complete normalization often does not occur; thus persistence of postoperative nerve conduction abnormalities does not necessarily imply an unsuccessful surgery.

BIBLIOGRAPHY

1. American Association of Electrodiagnostic Medicine, American Academy of Neurology, and American Academy of Physical Medicine and Rehabilitation: Practice parameter for electrodiagnostic studies in carpal tunnel syndrome: Summary statement. Muscle Nerve 16:1390–1391, 1993.
2. Andary MT, Werner RA: Using electrodiagnosis in clinical decision making: Carpal tunnel syndrome. AAEM Course, 1997.

3. Boeckstyns ME, Sorensen AI, Does endoscopic have a higher rate of complication than open carpal tunnel release? An analysis of published series. J Hand Surg [Br] 24:9–15, 1999.

4. Franzblau A, et al: Workplace surveillance for carpal tunnel syndrome: A comparison of methods. J Occup Rehabil 3:1–14, 1993.

5. Feuerstein M, Burrell LM, Miller VI, et al: Clincal management of carpal tunnel syndrome: A 12-year review of outcomes. Am J Ind Med 35:232–245, 1999.

6. Jarvik JG, Kliot M, Maravilla KR: MR nerve imaging of the hand and wrist. Hand Clin 16:13–24, 2000.

7. Katz RT: Carpal tunnel syndrome: A practical review. Am Fam Physician 49:1371–1378, 1994.

8. Kaplan SJ, Gickel SZ, Eaton RG: Predictive factors in the non-surgical treatment of carpal tunnel syndrome. J Hand Surg 15B:107, 1990.

9. Johnson EW, Kraft GH (eds): Carpal Tunnel Syndrome. Physical Medicine and Rehabilitation Clinics of North America, vol. 8, no. 3. 1997.

10. Robinson LR, Micklesen P, Wang L. Strategies for analyzing nerve conduction data: Superiority of a summary index over single tests. Muscle Nerve 21:1166–1171, 1998.

11. Stetson DS, Albers JW, Silverstein BA, Wolfe RA: Effects of age, sex and anthropometric factors on nerve conduction measures. Muscle Nerve 15:1095–1104, 1992.

12. Werner RA, Albers JW: Relation between needle electromyography and nerve conduction studies in patients with carpal tunnel syndrome. Arch Phys Med Rehabil 76:246–249, 1995.

23. ENTRAPMENT NEUROPATHY

Jaywant J. P. Patil, MBBS, FRCPC

1. How are nerve injuries classified?

Seddon has classified three categories of nerve injury, based on the severity of the injury:

1. **Neurapraxia:** There is loss of physiologic conductivity, and the axon is unable to propagate an action potential across the site of injury.

2. **Axonotmesis:** There is loss of anatomic continuity of the axon due to *irreversible damage*, with immediate conduction block across the site of the injury. Initially, the distal segment continues to remain excitable, making it difficult to distinguish between axonotmesis and neurapraxia on the basis of distal nerve excitability. *Wallerian degeneration* proceeds distal to the injury within a few days after the injury.

3. **Neurotmesis:** In addition to irreversible axonal damage, the supportive structures are damaged, including the *perineurium* that covers axon bundles and the *epineurium* that covers the nerve trunk.

2. List the common sites of nerve entrapment in the upper and lower limbs.

	SITE OF ENTRAPMENT	EXAMPLE
Upper Limbs		
Median nerve	Wrist	Carpal tunnel syndrome
	Forearm	Anterior interosseous syndrome
Ulnar nerve	Elbow	Tardy ulnar nerve palsy
	Wrist	Guyon's canal syndrome
Lower Limbs		
Peroneal nerve	Knee or fibular head	Cross leg syndrome
Lateral femoral	Medial to anterior	Meralgia paresthetica
Cutaneous nerve of thigh (ASIS)	Superior iliac spine	
Tibial nerve	Under laciniate ligament	Tarsal tunnel syndrome

3. Which electrodiagnostic test demonstrates physiologic changes due to mixed nerve entrapment?

Sensory conduction studies are more sensitive in detecting mixed nerve entrapment. For example, the distal sensory latency of entrapped median nerves is twice as likely to be prolonged compared with median distal motor latencies. The sensory fibers, which are the fastest conducting (1A alpha) nerve fibers, are first to be affected. The conduction velocity increases with axonal diameter and density of myelination. Nerve compression results in demyelination along the segment of nerve, resulting in increased internodal distances at multiple levels, which in turn slows down saltatory conduction (where waves of depolarization jump from one node to the next). Techniques that compare latencies between short nerve segments are more sensitive to effects of focal compression than latencies measured over a longer segment (where there is a dilution of the abnormality).

4. What is Saturday night palsy? Honeymoon palsy?

Saturday night palsy is one of the "sleep palsies" that result from focal compression due to limb position. It occurs secondary to compression of the radial nerve at the brachium as it pierces the lateral intermuscular septum in the upper part of the arm and then continues to travel into the anterior compartment of the arm distally. Compression often occurs in patients who, in an alcoholic stupor, fall asleep with the arm resting against a firm edge of a chair or couch.

Honeymoon palsy is another "sleep palsy," in which the compression of the radial nerve occurs more distally in the arm. It results from the bed partner's head resting in the crook of the patient's arm.

Most of these lesions are no more severe than axonotmesis. Prognosis for recovery within a couple of months is fairly good.

5. Describe the anatomy of Guyon's canal and the entrapment of the ulnar nerve there.

In 1886, Phillip Guyon, a French physician, originally described the Guyon's canal at the wrist. Guyon's canal is bordered medially by the *pisiform bone* and laterally by the *hook of the hamate*. This canal is covered on its volar aspect by the volar carpal ligament. The *ulnar nerve*, along with the *ulnar artery*, passes through this canal (see figure on following page).

While in the canal, the ulnar nerve divides into a superficial and a deep branch. The *superficial branch* gives a twig to the palmaris brevis and continues as a sensory branch to the ring and little fingers, as well as supplying sensation to the area of the hypothenar eminence. The *deep branch* along with the ulnar artery winds around the hook of the hamate and runs between the adductor digiti quinti and the flexor digiti quinti brevis and eventually supplies the dorsal and palmar interossei, the third and fourth lumbricals, the adductor pollicis, the first dorsal interosseous, and the deep head of the flexor pollicis brevis.

Compression of the ulnar nerve in Guyon's canal can occur secondary to a ganglion cyst, occupational trauma, local trauma, and less commonly, fracture, contracture scars, and ulnar artery pathology.

6. Describe the various clinical presentations of compressive ulnar neuropathy at the wrist.

There are three distinct compression syndromes:

1. Compression of the **superficial and deep branches** within Guyon's canal, resulting in weakness of the ulnar intrinsic muscles and loss of sensation over the little finger and ulnar half of the ring finger.

2. Compression of the **ulnar nerve** occurring after it exits Guyon's canal, resulting in weakness of the ulnar-innervated intrinsic muscles with sensory sparing.

3. Compression of the **superficial branch of the ulnar nerve** in Guyon's canal, resulting in sensory deficit over the ulnar-volar aspect of the palm and the volar aspect of the little and ring fingers.

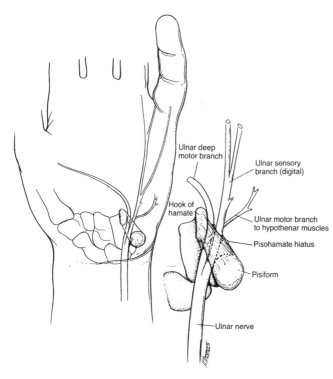

Ulnar deep
motor branch

Ulnar sensory
branch (digital)

Hook of
hamate

Ulnar motor branch
to hypothenar muscles

Pisohamate hiatus

Pisiform

Ulnar nerve

Guyon's canal. (From Liveson JA, Spielholz NI: Peripheral Neurology. Philadelphia, F. A. Davis, 1991, with permission.)

7. What is the differential diagnosis of numbness of the little and ring fingers?

C8 and/or T1 root lesion: Examination may reveal hypoesthesia (decreased touch sensation) or hypoalgesia (decreased pain perception) along the ulnar aspect of the forearm. There also may be evidence of Horner's syndrome (myosis and anhydrosis of the involved side of the face) due to interruption of the preganglionic sympathetic fibers that exit with the T1 (C8) root on their way to the paravertebral sympathetic ganglia. In this situation, the patient is literally in trouble "up to their eyeballs."

Neurogenic thoracic outlet syndrome: This is often associated with vascular thoracic outlet syndrome. Vascular impingement is suggested by the Adson's test, which reproduces the symptoms and obliterates the radial pulse. This maneuver reduces the space in the triangle between the scalenus anticus, scalenus medius, and the dome of the pleura. Classically, neurogenic thoracic outlet syndrome is associated with numbness in the little finger and more thenar than hypothenar atrophy.

Ulnar nerve palsy at the elbow: This is associated not only with numbness in the little and ring fingers but also decreased sensation on the dorsum of the hand along the distribution of the ulnar dorsal cutaneous branch.

Ulnar nerve entrapment at the wrist: This results in sparing of sensation supplied by the dorsal cutaneous branch of the ulnar nerve on the dorsum of the hand.

8. List the three potential sites of entrapment of the neurovascular bundle in thoracic outlet syndrome.

Thoracic outlet syndrome commonly presents with discomfort in the shoulder/arm area that is often precipitated by elevation of the hand during work. This syndrome may present due to entrapment of the neurovascular bundle at the following sites:

Scalenus anticus syndrome—entrapment between the anterior and posterior scalenes and the first rib

Costoclavicular syndrome—entrapment between clavicle and first rib

Pectoralis minor syndrome—entrapment between the pectoralis minor, rib cage, and coracoid process

9. What is "double-crush syndrome"? Give an example.

The double-crush nerve entrapment syndrome was described in 1973 by Upton and McComas. In this syndrome, the sensory nerves or motor nerves of a particular root can be compressed proximally as well as distally. This commonly occurs in patients with a C6 or C7 radiculopathy who also have evidence of entrapment of the median nerve at the wrist. One must assess which of the two compressions is giving the patient more symptoms and treat it appropriately.

10. What clues from the patient's history help the clinician to differentiate between carpal tunnel syndrome and cervical radiculopathy?

The patient with cervical radiculopathy often complains of pain in the neck, anterior chest, shoulder area, and interscapular region on sneezing or Valsalva-associated pain. The symptoms of carpal tunnel syndrome are localized to the upper extremity and appear to be worse at night. In cervical radiculopathy, the patient is more likely to complain of numbness which starts proximally and moves distally. The electrodiagnostic examination should always explore the possibility of both lesions.

11. What are the clinical and electrodiagnostic features of anterior interosseous nerve entrapment?

Typically, the patient complains about vague aching pain of the forearm, which starts suddenly or gradually. The patient may be unaware of weakness, but physical examination reveals weakness in the muscles supplied by the anterior interosseous nerve (i.e., the flexor pollicis longus, flexor digitorum profundus [lateral head], and pronator quadratus). These muscles work together to make the "okay sign" with the hand. There is no sensory deficit. The anterior interosseous nerve can be entrapped at the forearm by a fibrous band. Patients with sudden onset of this condition often give a history of prolonged focal compression or prolonged periods of repetitive pronation and supination.

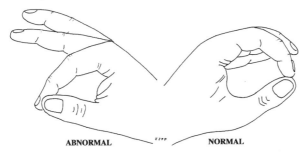

ABNORMAL   **NORMAL**

The okay sign.

12. How can one differentiate between a radial nerve palsy and a C7 radiculopathy?

Generally, the nerve conduction studies of the radial nerve are not affected significantly in C7 radiculopathy. In C7 radiculopathy, acute or chronic neurogenic alteration would be observed in the flexor carpi radialis, which is a median-innervated C7–8 muscle. Both conditions can coexist as a result of the "double-crush syndrome." Paraspinous muscle EMGs of the segment at the C7–8 vertebral level may show membrane instability, confirming a C7 radiculopathy.

13. Differentiate between C5–6 radiculopathy and a lesion of the suprascapular nerve.

After suprascapular nerve impingement, the supraspinatus and infraspinatus muscles may show atrophy and weakness on clinical exam as well as membrane instability and/or chronic neurogenic alterations on EMG study. The deltoid, rhomboid, and biceps muscles would be normal.

14. How can you differentiate between lesions of the brachial plexus involving the posterior cord and those of the radial nerve?

In radial nerve palsy, the deltoid muscle (axillary nerve) is spared. In posterior cord lesion of the brachial plexus, if the lesion is at or above the takeoff of the axillary nerve, the deltoid muscle will show abnormalities.

15. How does one differentiate between C5–6 radiculopathy and long thoracic nerve palsy?

Long thoracic nerve (C5,6,7) palsy results in weakness of the serratus anterior muscle, which presents with scapular winging. In C5 radiculopathy, one may observe weakness of the deltoid muscle and, to a lesser degree, biceps muscle. In C6 radiculopathy, the weakness would be greater in the biceps and lesser in the deltoid muscle. With either isolated C5 or C6 radiculopathy, there is no significant winging of the scapula observed.

16. Describe the clinical features of meralgia paresthetica. How is it treated?

Meralgia paresthetica occurs secondary to compression of the lateral femoral cutaneous nerve of the thigh (purely sensory), which passes beneath or through the inguinal ligament approximately one fingerbreadth medial to the anterior superior iliac spine (ASIS). Often, this condition is associated with pregnancy or obesity, when a relatively large protuberant "belly" hangs over the ASIS. It can also be precipitated by the use of tight belts, corsets, and underwear. There may be tenderness, a positive Tinel's sign, or a positive compression test just medial to the ASIS. The patient usually complains of paresthesias and pain on the anterolateral aspect of the thigh where one can demonstrate evidence of sensory disturbance.

Treatment includes eliminating the causative factor, be it weight reduction, decreasing abdominal flabbiness, or increasing abdominal muscle tone. For symptomatic relief, a temporary block with a local anesthetic and a small amount of steroid around the lateral femoral cutaneous nerve can be helpful in reducing painful dysesthesias. Surgical release of the nerve might be considered if other methods of treatment fail.

17. What clinically distinguishes meralgia paresthetica and lumbosacral radiculopathy?

In **meralgia paresthetica**, the patient presents with a purely sensory syndrome on the lateral aspect of the thigh, further confirmed clinically by a positive Tinel's sign over the entrapment site which lies just medial to the ASIS.

In **lumbosacral radiculopathy** involving the L2, 3, or 4 root, the sensory symptoms and disturbances are not just limited to the lateral aspect of the thigh but also involve the anterior aspect (femoral nerve). One may also find that the phasic stretch reflex (tendon tap reflex) in the iliopsoas (L1,2) or quadriceps (L3,4) may be decreased or absent. The sensory disturbance in the case of an L4 radiculopathy may extend below the level of the knee. The patient also may have symptoms of back pain, often radiating to the anterior aspect of the thigh, and a positive femoral nerve stretch test (with the patient prone, the hip is extended with the knee flexed, resulting in discomfort on the anterior aspect of the thigh). In addition to the clinical examination of the back, electrodiagnostic studies and appropriate imaging studies may confirm the diagnosis.

18. What are the common sites of entrapment in the sciatic nerve and the tibial nerve?

Though the sciatic nerve can be injured as a result of neoplasm, pelvic fractures, pelvic infection, gravid uterus, penetrating injuries, surgical trauma, or intramuscular injection, entrapment of the nerve is uncommon. The sciatic nerve can be entrapped especially by the piriformis muscle (piriformis syndrome). In this situation the gluteus medius, gluteus minimus, and tensor fasciae latae muscles are generally not affected. The sciatic nerve can also be compressed between the greater trochanter and the ischial tuberosity or between the hamstring muscle and adductor magnus. A large cystic swelling, such as a Baker's cyst, in the popliteal fossa can compress the sciatic nerve after it bifurcates into the tibial and peroneal nerves. Tibial nerve can be entrapped at the ankle in the tarsal tunnel.

19. Where does entrapment of the tibial nerve commonly occur?

The tibial nerve travels into the posterior compartment of the calf and is protected from trauma until it reaches the medial ankle. Entrapment of the tibial nerve occurs under the flexor retinaculum or just posterior to the medial malleolus. This is popularly known as **tarsal tunnel syndrome** and can occur as a result of tenosynovitis, venous stasis, edema, trauma, pronated foot (pes planovalgus), arthritis of the subtalar joint, or ganglia arising around the area of the medial aspect of the ankle. Lesions distal to the flexor retinaculum can either compress the medial or lateral plantar branches of the tibial nerve.

20. Describe the clinical presentation of tarsal tunnel syndrome.

- Presents in middle age
- Painful dysesthesias of the soles and toes, associated with sensory deficit on the plantar aspect of the foot and toes and with weakness in the intrinsic muscles of the feet
- Pain occurs at rest, while the patient is sitting or in bed
- Positive Tinel's sign (paresthesias in the nerve distribution with percussion over the nerve at the entrapment site) posterior to the medial malleolus
- Latencies of medial and/or lateral plantar branches may be prolonged
- Possible membrane instability of the abductor hallucis and/or abductor digiti quinti

21. How can you differentiate between scapular winging secondary to long thoracic nerve injury as opposed to spinal accessory nerve injury?

In **long thoracic nerve** injury or neuropathy, the serratus anterior weakness allows the vertebral border of the scapula to drift closer to the midline and the inferior angle to rotate medially. The winging increases with protraction of the scapula when the patient forcefully pushes forward with his or her arm against resistance; however, attempts at abduction of the shoulder decrease the winging.

Injury to the **spinal accessory nerve**, which supplies the trapezius muscle, is associated with a lesser degree of winging at rest, with the inferior angle of the scapula becoming more prominent. The inferior angle of the scapula is rotated medially as in serratus anterior weakness, but the scapula drifts away softly from the midline. The shoulder in this condition droops down due to atrophy of the superior part of the trapezius muscle. Attempts at shoulder abduction tend to increase winging initially, but as the shoulder approaches 90°, the winging diminishes.

22. How can one clinically differentiate between peroneal nerve palsy and L5 radiculopathy?

In **peroneal nerve palsy**, one may find weakness of the dorsiflexors and the evertors of the foot. Unlike in **L5 radiculopathy**, generally there should also be weakness of significance detected in the inverters of the foot as a result of weakness in the posterior tibial muscle.

23. How are L3 radiculopathy and femoral neuropathy differentiated?

In **L3 radiculopathy**, one detects abnormalities in the hip adductors (supplied by the obturator nerve L2,3,4 roots) as well as in the quadriceps muscle. In **femoral neuropathy** these abnormalities are confined to the quadriceps muscle.

24. What is Morton's neuroma?

Entrapment of the interdigital nerve between either the third and fourth or second and third metatarsal heads. The symptoms include shooting pain and burning of the second, third, or fourth toes. There is a cramping sensation at the metatarsal heads that is relieved with massage. Examination reveals tenderness of the sole and affected web spaces. Dorsal tenderness of the metatarsophalangeal joints may be indicative of extensor tendinitis or synovitis. Conservative treatment of Morton's neuroma includes a pad just proximal to the metatarsal heads and/or an injection of bupivicaine and corticosteroid.

25. Outline the approach to treatment of entrapment neuropathies.
Prevention
- Avoid sustained or intermittent extreme pressure or tethering at the entrapment sites.
- Avoid vitamin deficiencies, especially with B_{12}, folic acid.
- Monitor and optimally control diabetes. (Diabetics are more vulnerable to developing not only polyneuropathy or peripheral neuropathy but also entrapment neuropathies.)

Treatment
Nonoperative
- Splint the limb in a neutral position that maximizes space for the entrapped nerve.
- Maintain good blood flow to the limb and reduce swelling and edema in order to prevent further compression.
- Modify activity, and avoid positions that can be a source of nerve trauma.
- Reduce inflammation and consider the use of ice, NSAIDs, and corticosteroid injections in structures around the nerves that may be inflamed.

Operative
- If, despite nonoperative treatment, there is evidence of continuing axonal degeneration in the entrapped nerve, consider referral for surgical decompression.

BIBLIOGRAPHY

1. Liveson JA, Spielholz NI: Peripheral Neurology: Case Studies in Electrodiagnosis. Philadelphia, F.A. Davis, 1991.
2. Upton ARM, McComas AJ: The double crush in nerve-entrapment syndromes. Lancet 2:359, 1973.

24. PERIPHERAL NEUROPATHY

Peter D. Donofrio, M.D. and Yadollah Harati, M.D.

This world is but a canvas to our imagination.—Henry David Thoreau

1. How common is diabetes and diabetic neuropathy?
Diabetes affects approximately 7% of the U.S. population. Four percent are cognizant of the diagnosis, whereas approximately 3% are not aware that they have diabetes. The prevalence of neuropathy in this group depends on the way in which neuropathy is defined, i.e., by symptoms, abnormalities on neurologic examination, electrophysiology, nerve pathology, or a combination. In a large study of 4400 patients followed for 25 years, Pirart reported the prevalence of polyneuropathy to be 8% in diabetics at the time of diagnosis. After 20 years, approximately 40% of diabetics had neuropathy, and this percentage rose to 50% at 25 years. Neuropathy occurs in approximately the same frequency in both type I and type II diabetics.

2. What are the different types of diabetic neuropathy?
Several classifications have been proposed for diabetic neuropathy, some based on the major clinical presentation (weakness, ataxia, or pain), others based on symmetry, focality, anatomy, or pathology. The classification created by Dyck and colleagues divides diabetic neuropathy by symmetry, anatomy, and distribution of symptoms and signs.

Classification of Diabetic Neuropathy

Symmetrical distal polyneuropathy

Symmetrical proximal neuropathy

Asymmetrical proximal neuropathy
  Cranial
  Trunk radiculopathy or mononeuropathy
  Limb plexus or mononeuropathy
  Multiple mononeuropathy
  Entrapment neuropathy
  Ischemic nerve injury from acute arterial occlusion

Asymmetrical neuropathy and symmetrical distal polyneuropathy

Adapted from Dyck PJ, Karnes J, O'Brien PC: Diagnosis, staging, and classification of diabetic neuropathy and associations with other complications. In Dyck PJ, et al (eds): Diabetic Neuropathy. Philadelphia, W.B. Saunders, 1987, pp 36–44.

Symmetrical distal polyneuropathy is the most common presentation of diabetic neuropathy. It commonly affects sensory, motor, and autonomic fibers and is length-dependent in presentation, i.e., typically involving the feet before the hands.

3. Which cranial mononeuropathies occur as complications of diabetes?
Four cranial mononeuropathies are associated with diabetic neuropathy: CN 3, 4, 6, and 7.

Mononeuropathies of CN 3, 4, and 6 are classified under the rubric of **diabetic ophthalmoplegia**. The most dramatic presentation of diabetic ophthalmoplegia is the third nerve palsy. It often begins with a unilateral frontal headache or severe pain in or behind the eye. Over days, the patient experiences profound ptosis and double vision. The examiner detects severe weakness of eye elevation, eye depression, and adduction. The pupil is usually uninvolved, a feature helping to differentiate diabetic third nerve palsy from a compressive lesion such as a posterior communicating aneurysm. Complete recovery is expected within 3–5 months.

Diabetic sixth nerve palsy has a similar presentation with eye pain. Like the third nerve palsy, involvement is unilateral. Patients have double vision primarily on distant gaze. The examiner finds weakness of eye abduction, but no other oculomotor weakness. The least common diabetic cranial neuropathy is a trochlear or fourth nerve palsy.

Bell's palsy (CN 7) occurs more commonly in diabetics than in the normal population. In some studies, the risk for Bell's palsy in diabetics is as high as two-fold.

4. What is diabetic truncal or thoracoabdominal neuropathy or radiculopathy?
This condition is a relatively rare manifestation of diabetic neuropathy. Typically, it presents in patients older than 50 who are non–insulin-dependent. Patients complain of the acute onset of unilateral pain and dysesthesia in a thoracic or abdominal nerve dermatome pattern. The pain is typically severe, often characterized by neuropathic terms such as jabbing, ice pick-like, tearing, sharp, or lightning-type pain. Often patients find that the skin overlying the thoracoabdominal radiculopathy is sensitive and contact by clothing or another individual is extremely irritating.

Physical findings may be normal or may include either increased or decreased sensitivity of the skin to light touch, pinprick, and cold. Frequently, diabetic thoracoabdominal radiculopathy is associated with anorexia and unexplained weight loss of 20 to 25 lbs. If the diagnosis is not considered, patients may undergo costly evaluations for cardiac or intra-abdominal causes, often leading to a delay in diagnosis and treatment. Thoracoabdominal radiculopathy or neuropathy can be the presenting feature of diabetes. Fortunately, the prognosis for recovery is good, and most patients become pain free within 2 years after disease onset.

5. What is diabetic amyotrophy?
Amyotrophy refers to the loss of muscle or atrophy. Diabetic amyotrophy shares some characteristics with diabetic thoracoabdominal neuropathy or radiculopathy. It can be the presenting

feature of diabetes and is commonly associated with weight loss and poor appetite. Diabetic amyotrophy occurs in approximately 0.3–1.0% of diabetics.

The typical presentation is unilateral severe pain in the groin, hip, back, or anterior thigh region. This pain is not precipitated by trauma and is followed after several days by weakness and wasting of muscles innervated by the lumbosacral plexus. In most cases, the brunt of the disease affects the iliopsoas, quadriceps, and thigh adductors and, less frequently, muscles below the knee. The quadriceps phasic stretch reflex is usually reduced or lost. EMG and nerve conduction studies typically show denervation and reinnervation in a larger area than would be predicted by the clinical examination. The paraspinal muscles may be affected.

The term diabetic amyotrophy applies to either a polyradiculopathy, lumbosacral plexopathy, or multiple proximal lower-extremity mononeuropathies. The underlying pathophysiology is felt to be infarction of nerve precipitated by metabolic imbalance. The prognosis for recovery is good. Approximately 60–70% of patients achieve improvement within 30 months of disease onset.

6. How do mononeuropathy multiplex and mononeuritis multiplex differ?

Mononeuropathy multiplex and **mononeuritis multiplex** are interchangable terms and describe the evolution of two or more mononeuropathies over a short period of time. The terms imply a multifocal and asymmetrical process affecting individual peripheral nerves. The condition is commonly caused by nerve infarctions that result from occlusion of the vas nervorum. Mononeuropathy multiplex carries a much graver prognosis than mononeuropathies due to entrapment conditions, such as carpal tunnel syndrome, ulnar neuropathy at the elbow, and peroneal mononeuropathy at the knee.

7. What is the differential diagnosis for mononeuropathy multiplex?

Mononeuropathy multiplex is commonly a complication of vascular, connective tissue, and inflammatory conditions:

Vascular causes: polyarteritis nodosa, vasculitides associated with connective tissue disorders and carcinoma, Churg-Strauss allergic angiitis, Wegener's granulomatosis, amyloid vasculitis

Infectious and inflammatory causes: leprosy, herpes zoster, HIV infection, Lyme disease

Other etiologies: trauma, diabetes, sarcoidosis, tumor infiltration, lymphoid granulomatosis, hereditary neuropathy with liability to pressure palsies

The diagnosis of mononeuritis multiplex demands a thorough investigation for treatable and reversible causes and, in many patients, requires tissue confirmation. The evaluation should be conducted quickly so that the process can be treated during the acute phase and before extensive axon loss ensues. Although multiple compressive mononeuropathies, strictly speaking, can be classified along with other mononeuropathy multiplex disorders, the underlying pathophysiology differs from vascular or inflammatory etiologies.

8. What type of neuropathies can present as a paraneoplastic phenomenon?

The most distinctive of the paraneoplastic neuropathies is the **subacute sensory neuronopathy**. It is more likely to be associated with oat cell carcinoma of the lung than any other neoplasm. The clinical presentation of the neuropathy often precedes the discovery of the malignancy. Neurologic features include areflexia, sensory ataxia, and pseudoathetoid movements of the hands and feet in a patient complaining of distal paresthesia and dysesthesia. Pathology shows inflammation in the dorsal root ganglia and degeneration of dorsal root cell bodies and distal axon loss.

The most common paraneoplastic neuropathy is a **distal sensory and motor axonopathy**. Clinically, this condition manifests as a slowly progressive, symmetrical, distal-to-proximal gradient loss axonopathy involving sensory and motor function. Its pathology is that of a distal dying-back axonopathy.

In rare situations, patients with **chronic inflammatory demyelinating polyneuropathy** are found to have an underlying malignancy. It is often impossible to determine whether the inflammatory neuropathy results from an underlying immunologic process incited by the malignancy or whether it occurs serendipitously. Equally rare is a paraneoplastic vasculitic presentation of a peripheral neuropathy in a patient with an underlying malignancy. Pathology reveals "microvasculitis" of the epineurial arterioles.

9. What peripheral neuropathies are commonly associated with autonomic involvement?

Autonomic neuropathies can be conveniently classified into those in which there is no associated somatic involvement (motor or sensory fibers) and those in which motor and sensory involvement is prominent. In the latter situation, diabetic neuropathy is commonly associated with autonomic involvement. This is also the case in primary or secondary amyloidosis. A small percentage of patients with Guillain-Barré syndrome have autonomic complications. This may manifest as paroxysmal tachycardia or bradycardia leading to loss of vascular stability. Autonomic involvement is one of the primary presentations of Riley-Day syndrome or hereditary sensory neuropathy, type III. Patients with HIV neuropathy, leprosy, and Chagas disease can have autonomic manifestations.

10. What clinical manifestations are commonly seen in patients with autonomic neuropathy?

The most common manifestation is **orthostatic hypotension**. In this complication, patients do not have a sufficient rise in pulse after changing to the standing or sitting position to compensate for a drop in blood pressure. Other manifestations include dry skin, cracked nails, hypertrichosis, impaired sweating, abdominal distention, dry mucus membranes, sluggish pupillary responses, slow adaptation to near vision, impotence, nocturnal diarrhea, constipation, urinary retention, and incontinence.

11. Explain the difference between nociceptive and neuropathic pain.

Nociceptive pain arises from a pathologic process in which tissue damage and inflammation are sources of the primary injury. Osteoarthritis, cholecystitis, cellulitis, and abscess are causes of nociceptive pain. **Neuropathic pain** stems from injury to a peripheral nerve or a central somatosensory pathway. Neuropathic pain is usually chronic and can either be constant or paroxysmal. In neuropathic pain, no obvious nociceptive stimulus or ongoing tissue damage can be identified. Common causes are polyneuropathy, nerve injuries, neuroma, post-herpetic neuralgia, and trigeminal neuralgia.

12. Which drugs can be effective in treating neuropathic pain?

Neuropathic pain can be difficult to manage. Some patients respond poorly to drugs, whereas others seem to develop adverse effects even at low dosages. In many patients, a reduction of pain of 30% to 40% can make a significant difference in their quality of life. Commonly prescribed treatments for neuropathic pain include:

NSAIDs	Antispasticity medications
Tricyclic antidepressants (TCAs)	Tramadol HCl
Anticonvulsants	Antiarrhythmics
SSRIs	Sports cream
Topical capsaicin	Transdermal clonidine
Lidocaince cream	

TCAs can serve as a mainstay of treatment for neuropathic pain. Commonly prescribed drugs within this group include: nortriptyline, desipramine, amitriptyline, and imipramine. The therapeutic dosage range is 25–150 mg/day with most or all of the medication given at night. Relief of pain often does not occur until several weeks after the treatment is initiated. Common side effects are drowsiness, dry eyes and mouth, weight gain, urinary retention, and constipation. Little information from human studies exists comparing the analgesic potency of one antidepressant to another.

13. Discuss the role of anticonvulsants in treating neuropathic pain.

Several anticonvulsants can be effective in managing neuropathic pain. These drugs probably work by modulating sodium channels, stabilizing nerve fiber membranes, and suppressing ectopic discharges arising from peripheral or central nerves. Phenytoin, carbamazepine, gabapentin, lamotrigine, and valproic acid have been studied in uncontrolled and controlled patient populations. **Gabapentin** appears to be the most effective agent in this drug group. Many patients respond to a total dosage of 900–1200 mg/day, whereas others need 3600–4800 mg/day to achieve adequate pain relief. **Topiramate** has recently been studied to treat the pain of diabetic neuropathy. Early results are promising.

14. What is the role of topical agents, tramadol HCL, and antiarrhythmics?

Topical agents such as capsaicin cream and lidocaine gel produce pain relief in a small percentage of patients. Since both agents are topical, they can be useful in patients taking a large number of medications and in whom drug interaction must be avoided.

Tramadol hydrochloride is a unique pharmacologic agent that acts in two ways—as an opioid agonist and as an activator of monoaminergic spinal inhibition of pain. A recent double-blind, placebo-controlled study showed a reduction of pain intensity and greater pain relief in patients taking an average dose of 210 mg/day.

Mexiletine is an antiarrhythmic agent that occasionally produces pain relief in patients with chronic neuropathy. Unfortunately, the medication causes side effects in many patients, resulting in poor patient compliance.

15. What are the most common etiologies for brachial plexopathy?

Dysfunction of the brachial plexus can be caused by many mechanisms. **Trauma**, such as motorcycle accidents, obstetrical paralysis, avulsion, and gunshot wounds, accounts for most of them. Neoplastic infiltration of the brachial plexus from **primary tumors of the lung** or **secondary metastasis** can also produce brachial plexopathy. **Radiation**-induced brachial plexopathy can be a delayed cause of brachial plexopathy in patients with neck, shoulder and lung neoplasia. It is the authors' experience that **neuralgic amyotrophy** or **idiopathic brachial plexopathy** is the most common cause of brachial plexopathy. This condition has many synonyms, including acute brachial neuropathy, acute brachial plexitis, brachial plexus neuropathy, brachial neuritis, cryptogenic brachial neuropathy, and Parsonage-Turner syndrome.

The latter disorder typically begins with pain located in the shoulder region, soon followed by prominent wasting and weakness of muscles in the shoulder girdle and arm. The muscles involved vary from patient to patient. Muscles innervated by the upper trunk are more commonly involved than those in the middle and lower trunk. Physical findings are consistent with those predicted by the area of pathology. Fortunately, idiopathic brachial plexopathy has a good prognosis. More than 80% of patients recover within 2 years of onset and > 90% within 4 years.

16. Which drugs cause peripheral neuropathy?

Peripheral sensory and motor fibers react to toxins (in this case, medications) in a limited manner. Schaumburg and Spencer theorized that toxins cause disease at one of four regions of the peripheral nerve: (1) the distal sensory and motor axon (axonopathy), (2) the Schwann cell, (3) the dorsal root ganglion (gangliopathy or neuronopathy), and (4) anterior horn cell or motor neuron. Most neuropathies caused by medications can be grouped into one of those four categories.

Drug-induced Neuropathies

Axonopathy

Amiodarone	Ethambutol	Nitrofurantoin
Amitriptyline	Ethionamide	Nitrous oxide
Chloramphenicol	Glutethimide	Phenytoin
Chloroquine	Gold	Sulfapyridine
Cisplatin	Hydralazine	Sulfasalazine
Clioquinol	Isoniazid	Statins
Colchicine	Lithium	Thalidomide
Cyanate	Mercury	Vancomycin
Disopyramide	Methaquolone	Vinblastine
Disulfiram	Metronidazole	Vincristine
Enalapril	Misonidazole	

Table continued on following page

Drug-induced Neuropathies (Continued)

Anterior Horn Cell	Schwann Cell	
Dapsone	Allopurinol	Zimeldine
	Amiodarone	L-tryptophan contaminant
Dorsal Root Ganglion	Indomethacin	
Paclitaxel (Taxol)	Perhexiline	
Pyridoxine	Suramin	

17. What tests are helpful to identify the cause of a diffuse polyneuropathy?

In a patient with long-standing diabetes, laboratory evaluation can be limited to a few studies unless clues exist in the history and physical examination that suggest that the polyneuropathy may be secondary to other causes. In a person with diabetes who has rapidly progressive weakness and sensory loss over several weeks to months, chronic inflammatory demyelinating polyneuropathy (CIDP) must be included in the differential diagnosis. A superimposed distal symmetric diabetic neuropathy may also be present, but the tempo of the presentation is atypical for diabetes. In the case of a rapidly progressive polyneuropathy, a more extensive evaluation will be necessary including a lumbar puncture, testing for the presence of a monoclonal protein, bone survey, and possibly a nerve biopsy.

Commonly needed tests for the evaluation of a distal symmetric polyneuropathy are CBC, fasting blood sugar, serum B_{12} level, serum protein electropheresis, urinalysis, metabolic panel, erythrocyte sedimentation rate, and thyroid function studies. If those studies are unremarkable, on subsequent visits the etiology may be identified by testing for HIV status, angiotensin-converting enzyme (ACE) level, rheumatologic studies, chest x-ray or CT scan, a 24-hour urine for heavy metals, and cerebrospinal fluid analysis. In rare instances, patients can be found to be vitamin E or vitamin B_6 deficient. Testing for autoimmune antibodies, such as anti-MAG, anti-GM1 and other autoantibodies may uncover a polyneuropathy treatable with immunotherapy.

Even in conditions where the underlying cause is known, electrophysiologic testing (nerve conduction studies and EMG) can be helpful to confirm the primary pathologic process (demyelinating or axon-loss), determine the severity and duration of the neuropathy, and differentiate whether another neuromuscular condition is present, such as a lumbosacral plexopathy or polyradiculopathy. Electrophysiologic testing can be pivotal in guiding eventual therapy.

BIBLIOGRAPHY

1. Brandenburg NA, Annegers JF: Incidence and risk factors for Bell's palsy in Laredo, Texas. Neuroepidemiology 12:313–325, 1993.
2. Donofrio PD: Diabetic Neuropathy. In Leahy JL, Clark NG, Cefalu WT (eds): Medical Management of Diabetic Mellitus. New York, Marcel Dekker, 2000, pp 479–497.
3. Donofrio PD: Electrophysiologic evaluations. Neurol Clin 18:601–613, 2000.
4. Dyck PJ, Karnes J, O'Brien PC: Diagnosis, staging, and classification of diabetic neuropathy and associations with other complications. In Dyck PJ, et al (eds): Diabetic Neuropathy. Philadelphia, W.B. Saunders, 1987, pp 36–44.
5. Galer BS. Neuropathic pain of peripheral origin: Advances in pharmacologic treatment. Neurology 45(suppl 9): S17–S25, 1995.
6. Kelly JJ: Polyneuropathies associated with malignancies and plasma cell dyscrasias. In Brown WF, Bolton CF (eds): Clinical Electromyography. Boston. Butterworth, 1987, pp 305–327.
7. McLeod JG, Tuck RR: Disorders of the autonomic nervous system: Part 1. Pathophysiology and clinical features. Ann Neurol 21:419–430, 1987.
8. Parry GJG: AAEE Case Report #11: Mononeuropathy multiplex. Muscle Nerve 8:493–498, 1985.
9. Pirart J: Diabetes mellitus and its degenerative complications: A prospective study of 4400 patients observed between 1947 and 1973. Diabetes Care 1:168–188, 1978.
10. Schaumberg HH, Spencer PS: Toxic neuropathies. Neurology 29:429–431, 1979.

25. ELECTROPHYSIOLOGY OF DISORDERS OF NEUROMUSCULAR TRANSMISSION

Thomas E. McGunigal, Jr., M.D.

1. What is the neuromuscular (NM) junction?

It is the specialized synapse between a motor nerve and a muscle fiber consisting of a presynaptic nerve terminal, synaptic cleft, and postsynaptic endplate of the muscle fiber.

2. What are the two types of abnormalities and what is the clinical presentation?

NM transmission abnormalities may be due to **structural** or **chemical** alterations by disease or toxic processes and are characterized clinically by fatigable weakness of skeletal muscles.

3. Which NM disorders are postsynaptic, and which are presynaptic?

The most common disorder is **myasthenia gravis**, which is due to a postsynaptic abnormality. **Myasthenic syndrome**, sometimes associated with bronchial carcinoma and botulism poisoning, is associated with a presynaptic abnormality of the NM junction.

4. What is the neurotransmitter of the NM junction? What are the three physiologic events that occur?

Acetylcholine. The three events are (1) presynaptic storage, synthesis, and release; (2) synaptic transmission and degradation; and (3) postsynaptic coupling with receptors.

5. Describe the presynaptic storage and release of acetylcholine.

Acetytcholine (Ach) storage occurs in three interrelated compartments. In the largest compartment, the main store, Ach is not immediately available for release across the synaptic cleft. It supplies a smaller compartment, the mobilization store, which in turn supplies the smallest compartment, which contains Ach available for immediate release into the synapse. Here, Ach is packaged in vesicles approximately 300–500 A in diameter, each vesicle containing 5000–10,000 Ach molecules (a quantum). The main store contains approximately 300,000 quanta, the mobilization store holds 10,000 quanta, and the immediate-release store holds 1000 quanta. When an action potential reaches the presynaptic nerve terminal, it causes a voltage-sensitive influx of calcium ions, which signals the vesicles to release Ach into the synaptic cleft.

6. What are the common disorders of NM transmission?

Myasthenia gravis
Lambert-Eaton myasthenic syndrome
Botulism
Congenital myasthenia
Tick paralysis
Toxic exposure (e.g., organophosphate insecticide)
Side effects of medications (e.g. aminoglycosides, procainamide, penicillamine)

7. How does a patient with a disease of NM transmission typically present?

With progressive weakness and fatigue, especially with repetitive activities. Strength is often restored with rest.

8. Do the major disorders of NM transmission differ in their clinical presentations?

In more than 90% of cases of **myasthenia gravis**, the levator palpebrae (extraocular muscles) are involved. Drooping of the eyelids and intermittent diplopia result. The muscles of facial expression, mastication, swallowing, and speech are involved in 80% of cases, leading to altered facial appearance and difficulty in eating. Muscles of the neck, shoulder girdle, trunk, and hips may also be involved.

In **Lambert-Eaton myasthenic syndrome**, the muscles of the trunk, shoulder girdle, and lower extremities are more likely to be initially affected. Unlike myasthenia gravis, patients may experience an increase in muscle power during the first few contractions.

Symptoms of **botulism** usually appear within 12–36 hours of ingestion of tainted food. The typical neural symptoms of blurred vision and diplopia may be accompanied by anorexia, nausea, and vomiting. Unlike myasthenia gravis, pupils are often unreactive in botulism. Other bulbar symptoms, such as nasal or hoarse vocal quality, dysarthria, and dysphagia, follow rapidly and are soon joined by weakness of the neck, trunk, and limbs and respiratory insufficiency. This takes place over 2–4 days.

9. Are there any special procedures to help quantify and classify disorders of NM transmission?

Repetitive stimulation and **single-fiber EMG** (SFEMG) are used to evaluate function of the NM junction. SFEMG employs a specialized needle electrode with a recording surface of 25–30-µm diameter located 3–4 mm along the shaft from the tip. It allows recording of two single fibers within a motor unit. SFEMG is one of the most sensitive (not specific) measures of NM transmission defects. SFEMG shows increased *jitter* (variation within consecutive discharges of the interpotential interval between two muscle fiber action potentials) and *blocking* (failure of the action potential to be propagated to one of the two fibers) in diseases of NM transmission. Repetitive stimulation in rapid succession to the same site allows inspection of the resultant compound muscle action potentials (CMAPs) for consistency of amplitude and duration.

10. How do Lambert-Eaton myasthenic syndrome (LEMS) and myasthenia gravis differ electrophysiologically?

Myasthenia gravis is an autoimmune disease primarily affecting older men and younger women. It is often seen in association with other autoimmune diseases, such as rheumatoid arthritis. The defect occurs when antibodies bind to the postsynaptic acetylcholine receptor, resulting in destruction and reduction of surface area of the postsynaptic membrane and fewer acetylcholine receptors. Electrophysiologically, the CMAP amplitudes are usually normal. With 2–5 Hz of repetitive stimulation, there is > 10% decrement in CMAP amplitude. Decrement is typically greatest between the first and second responses, with the maximum occurring between the first and fourth to fifth responses (see figure on following page). With continued stimulation, response amplitudes generally return toward normal. A 10-sec maximum isometric contraction will usually result in an increased responses amplitude, but not > 50% above baseline.

LEMS occurs more often in men than women, usually presenting in the fifth decade. There is a high coexistence of malignancy, most commonly oat-cell carcinoma of the lung. LEMS appears to be due to antibodies directed at the voltage-gated calcium channels of the motor nerve terminal, which interfere with release of acetylcholine. Electrophysiologically, the initial CMAP is usually low in amplitude. With 2–5 Hz of stimulation, there may be a decremental response. With > 10 Hz stimulation or a 10-sec maximum isometric contraction (which approximates a 50-Hz stimulation), there is an increase in the CMAP amplitude that is usually much greater than 50%, often 200–400% above the single-stimulation CMAP (see figure on following page).

11. What is the "safety factor"?

Following depolarization of the terminal axon in normal persons, there is an overabundance of acetylcholine released, more than enough to bind receptors. This redundancy is called the "safety factor." In disease states such as myasthenia gravis, the NM transmission is much more tenuous. With fewer receptors available, a slight drop in acetylcholine concentration may block transmission.

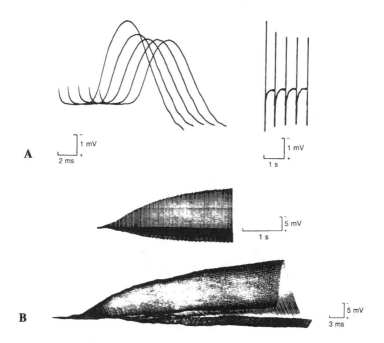

Repetitive nerve stimulation. A, Decrementing response in myasthenia gravis. B, Incrementing response in LEMS. (From Kimura J: Electrodiagnosis in Disease of the Nerve and Muscle: Principles and Practice, 2nd ed. Philadelphia, F.A. Davis, 1989; with permission.)

12. How is the course of events at the NM junction related to findings on repetitive stimulation?

Motor axonal discharge frequency affects NM transmission by modulating acetylcholine availability and calcium concentrations at the synaptic cleft. Depolarization of the nerve terminus causes the immediate release store to dump quanta into the synaptic cleft. Five to 10 sec are required for the mobilization store to replenish the lost acetylcholine. Therefore, volleys arriving faster than every 5 sec progressively deplete the immediate-release store. On the other hand, the calcium that is released with each depolarization requires 100–200 msec (or $\frac{1}{10}$–$\frac{1}{5}$ of a second) to diffuse away from the nerve terminal. Therefore, stimulation that arrives at rates greater than 5–10/sec (5–10 Hz) causes calcium to accumulate.

Thus, in myasthenia gravis repetitive stimulation at rates between 3–5 Hz shows a decremental response as smaller amounts of acetylcholine are released into the NM junction, preventing some fibers from reaching critical threshold. In LEMS, the CMAP may show a decremental response similar to myasthenia gravis at low stimulation frequencies. At frequencies of 20–50 Hz, however, facilitation is observed. Successive CMAPs show increasing amplitude, often exceeding single-stimulation CMAPs by 200% of baseline, because rapid rates of stimulation result in accumulation of calcium at the presynaptic cleft of the NM junction, progressively allowing more acetylcholine to be released.

13. What rate is best for stimulating a motor nerve repetitively?

The most useful information is usually obtained with a relatively low stimulation frequency, 2–3 Hz. Stimulation at faster frequencies (> 5 Hz) may not detect faulty transmission because faulty transmitter release will be enhanced due to residual calcium in the presynaptic terminal. Frequencies slower than this mask a transmission disorder since very low frequencies permit mobilization of acetylcholine into the immediately available store with enhancement of transmission.

The safety factor for NM transmission is at its nadir at relatively slow stimulation frequencies. Stimulation at higher frequencies can sometimes yield additional useful information, especially in presynaptic disorders, but is quite painful. The information can often be obtained much less painfully with brief isometric exercise.

14. What are some of the more common technical errors in repetitive stimulation?

Electrode movement, submaximal stimulation, low temperature, and pseudofacilitation.

15. What is pseudofacilitation?

Stimulation rates > 10 Hz may produce a phenomenon known as pseudofacilitation: an increase in the amplitude of the M-wave accompanied by a decrease in the duration, without any change in the total area under the curve. It is due to synchronization of the action potentials in muscle fibers, not an increase in the number of muscle fibers activated. It can produce an increase in M-wave amplitude of 50%, which should not be mistaken for abnormal pathologic facilitation.

16. Are myasthenia gravis and LEMS due to antibodies?

Yes. In myasthenia gravis, antibodies to the acetylcholine receptor attack and destroy the postsynaptic membrane. In LEMS, autoantibodies against the calcium channels attack the acetylcholine release sites at the active zone on the presynaptic membrane, resulting in failure of acetylcholine release.

17. Classify the NM junction (NMJ) disorders into three categories.

IMMUNE-MEDIATED DISORDERS	TOXIC/METABOLIC DISORDERS	CONGENITAL MYASTHENIC SYNDROME
LEMS Myasthenia gravis	Athropod venom poisoning (e.g., black widow spider) Organophosphates, insecticide poisoning (e.g., malathion, parathion) Botulism Hypermagnesemia Snake venom poisoning	Defective synthesis or packaging of acetylcholine Deficiency of acetylcholinesterase Deficiency of acetylcholine receptors Slow postsynaptic ion channel

18. Which NM disorder presents with a true reduction in reflexes?

LEMS presents with reduced reflexes. Myasthenia gravis, botulism, and congenital myasthenia present with normal reflexes, although they may be reduced in proportion to the degree of muscular weakness.

19. What is the most important aspect of determining the validity of any test used in assessing NMJ function?

Reproducibility. A consistent response is viewed in a more favorable light than a result that varies with each repetitive stimulation.

20. What factors may account for false-positive results?

- Electrodes: stimulating or recording electrode movement.
- Other diseases: reinnervation from axonal loss may cause a secondary NMJ disorder.
- Pseudofacilitation: see question 16 above.
- Edrophonium chloride: a decremental repair after the administration of edrophonium chloride is not diagnostic of mysathenia gravis, although this may occur in prejunctional disorders.

21. What factors may account for false-negative results?
• Muscle selection: proximal muscles have a higher yield.
• Temperature: a cool muscle may mask an NMJ disorder.
• Anticholinesterase medication: stop this 12 hours prior to the study.
• Excluding facilitation and exhaustion: a study is not complete without analysis of the patient's response to exercise and postactivation exhaustion.

22. Describe a repetitive nerve stimulation (RNS) protocol for evaluating the NMJ.
Warm the limb to 33°C and immobilize. When the routine motor nerve conduction study is normal, perform RNS at rest at 3 Hz, supramaximal stimulation, for 5–10 impulses, repeated three times, 1 minute apart. If a > 10% decrement occurs, have the patient perform voluntary exercise for 10 sec and immediately repeat 3-Hz RNS to demonstrate postexercise facilitation and repair of the decrement. If a < 10% decrement or no decrement occurs, have the patient perform voluntary exercise for 1 min and perform 3-Hz RNS immediately and at 1, 2, 3, 4, and 5 min after exercise to demonstrate postexercise exhaustion. If a significant decrement occurs, have the patient perform maximal voluntary exercise for 10 sec and immediately repeat 3-Hz RNS to demonstrate repair of the decrement. If a distal muscle is normal, study at least one proximal muscle, and always try to study weak muscles.

BIBLIOGRAPHY

1. Campbell W: Essentials of Electrodiagnostic Medicine. Baltimore, Williams & Wilkins, 1999.
2. Dumitru D: Electrodiagnostic Medicine. Philadelphia, Hanley & Belfus, 1995.
3. Kimura J: Electrodiagnosis in Disease of the Nerve and Muscle: Principles and Practice, 2nd ed. Philadelphia, F.A. Davis, 1989.
4. Preston D, Shapiro B: Electromyography and NM Disorders. Boston, Butterworth-Heineman, 1998.

26. SENSORY AND MOTOR EVOKED POTENTIALS

Gary Goldberg, M.D., Jeffrey L. Cole, M.D., and Mark A. Lissens, M.D., Ph.D.

1. What is meant by an evoked potential (EP) study?
There are two types of EP studies: sensory and motor. A **sensory EP** is averaged electrical activity recorded on the body surface following delivery of a discrete stimulus via a selected sensory pathway (somatosensory, visual, or auditory). Most commonly, these EPs are recorded as voltage changes at a fixed point on the scalp plotted against time in milliseconds following the stimulus. These voltage changes reflect the activation of bioelectrical sources within different parts of the CNS. A **motor EP** is a compound muscle action potential produced by transcranial stimulation of the motor cortex or stimulation of the motor roots of the spinal cord.

2. What is a somatosensory evoked potential (SEP) study?
An SEP is the electrophysiologic examination of central somatosensory transmission using a peripheral afferent pathway. The SEP pathways can involve the body's longest axons stretching from the feet up to the base of the medulla. SEP can be viewed simplistically as the CNS extension of the peripheral sensory nerve action potential (SNAP) study. The SEP technique traces the afferent impulses through the plexus and root, through to the spinal cord, and into the brainstem and cerebrum, finally arriving at the part of the primary somatosensory cortex that receives input from the stimulated part.

3. Are only electrical stimuli used for eliciting SEP studies?

It is possible to record an SEP with mechanical skin tapping or muscle stretch, as the first peak contains skin mechanoperceptive afferents, but the advantage of using electrical stimulation is that it produces synchronous activation of the majority of low-threshold, large-diameter peripheral nerve fibers, leading to a highly coherent peripheral nerve activation. When a mixed nerve is stimulated, this coherent action potential volley is conducted along the peripheral processes of the large-diameter, rapidly-conducting epicritic sensory system (discriminative tactile and kinesthetic information) and continues along the central processes in the ipsilateral spinal cord dorsal columns to synapse at the cervicomedullary junction in the dorsal column nuclei.

4. How are SEP peaks usually labeled?

There are many variations in nomenclature, but the most typical labels for the upper-extremity SEP studies use the **polarity** (P1 or N1, for positive or negative) and expected normal **latency** (in milliseconds), such as P_{14} or N_{20}.

5. What factors can affect the latency of an SEP component?

In normal individuals, many different factors influence the absolute latency of the SEP components. These include pathway length, a factor that is clearly related to body size. In young children, while central pathways are not yet fully myelinated, the latencies are relatively prolonged due to slower conduction that is partially offset by shorter pathways. Length-dependent variation is greater for studies with stimulation of the lower limbs where a correction for height can be helpful both for absolute latencies as well as for the spinal cord conduction time measured from the lumbar spine peak potential to the peak of the first cortical component at the scalp. Interpeak latencies used for measuring transit times in the CNS tend to be less variable measures.

6. Can the scalp SEP be conclusively interpreted without evaluating peripheral conduction?

No. To ascribe any SEP latency anomaly to a central lesion, it must be established that there is no peripheral nerve conduction slowing. It is helpful to record a peripheral afferent neurogram with electrodes placed between the stimulation site and entry into the CNS or to perform a full nerve conduction study of the pathway being studied. This documents adequate stimulation of the peripheral nerve as well as establishing measurable peripheral nerve conduction.

7. What is the central somatosensory conduction time (CSCT)?

In the SEP recorded after stimulation of the median nerve at the wrist, the CSCT is the time interval between the major negative peak (i.e., N_{13}) identified in the cervical spine response and the initial major negative peak identified in the cortical response (i.e., N_{19}). It is typically between 5 and 6 msec. The CSCT can be helpful in detecting slowed transmission through the central neuraxis between the cervicomedullary junction and the cortex. It is especially helpful for side-to-side comparisons, where the difference in CSCT between sides should not exceed 1.1 msec.

8. How can the abnormalities of the SEP be classified?

Abnormalities of the SEP can be divided into changes in component onset or peak latencies, changes in component amplitude or structure, or loss of specific waveform components. CNS demyelination tends to produce CSCT delays and prolongation of interpeak latencies in segments of the pathway spanning the CNS. Components may be attenuated or absent at proximal recording sites depending on the severity of the demyelination. When there is unilateral or asymmetric extent of pathology, side-to-side comparisons of interpeak latencies or component amplitudes can be helpful.

9. What is the main diagnostic limitation of the SEP?

Abnormalities of the SEP are etiologically nonspecific.

10. When can the SEP be helpful in the intensive care unit?

When the cortical responses of the median nerve SEP are bilaterally absent, a patient in coma is extremely unlikely to recover from their condition. This is especially true for atraumatic (e.g., anoxic) coma in adult patients.

11. What is a visual evoked potential (VEP) study?

A VEP is the occipital cortex potential generated after a discrete visual stimulus. The stimulus can be a bright flash of light or a sudden change in light pattern (as with a reversing black-and-white checkerboard pattern) with constant luminance (40–100 cd/m^2). The latter is referred to as a pattern-shift VEP (PSVEP). Light stimulates the retinal photoreceptors and transmits a signal to the bipolar cells and then to the inner retinal ganglion cells. The ganglion cell axons make up the optic nerve fibers. Through the chiasm, retinal fibers from the nasal halves cross over to the opposite side to join the temporal field's ipsilateral fibers, forming the optic tracts. Each optic tract's fibers synapse in the lateral geniculate bodies in the thalamus. The lateral geniculate body and retinal neurons respond strongly to sharp contrasting borders, opponent colors, and spots of light. The signals are relayed through the geniculocalcarine tract, or optic radiation, to the primary visual cortex in the calcarine fissure on the medial aspect of each occipital lobe. The primary visual cortex response is recorded from electrodes placed over the occipital scalp referenced either to the vertex or a midfrontal electrode.

12. Which VEP component is used primarily for clinical interpretation?

With pattern-shift visual stimulation, the wave usually has a triphasic structure, with three peaks that are labeled by their polarity and position (N_1, P_1, or N_2) or by latency (N_{75}, P_{100}, N_{140}). The most important PSVEP parameter is the P_{100} latency because of its stability and its clinical correlation with lesions affecting the anterior optic pathway.

13. What type of problem is best detected with a VEP study?

The greatest utility of VEP is detection of retrobulbar optic nerve demyelination. This condition is associated with significant prolongation of the P_{100} latency. Each eye is tested separately. An abnormality can be detected as an increase in the P_{100} latency of an affected eye beyond the normal range or by an abnormal increase in the interocular difference between the recorded P_{100} latencies for the two eyes.

14. What are the indications for doing a brainstem auditory evoked potential/auditory brainstem response (BAEP/ABR) in an adult?

In adults, the BAEP has found utility in a variety of **audiologic problems**, including unexplained "central" losses on behavioral audiometry and in the differential diagnosis of a sudden-onset unilateral deafness or severe hearing loss. The test has superb sensitivity in diagnosing **multiple sclerosis** and other demyelinating conditions, looking for **acoustic neuromas**, for **intraoperative monitoring**, and for evaluating brainstem function during a **barbiturate coma** or in those who appear to be "**brain dead**."

15. When is a BAEP/ABR study indicated in a child?

"Objective" audiometry using the ABR can be used in infants and neonates to detect the presence of hearing impairment. These studies should be considered in:

1. Infants and children suspected of hearing loss or hearing problems

2. Families with a history of metabolic or genetic diseases known to cause an early or congenital hearing impairment

3. Orofacial dysmorphic syndromes

4. All premature infants who have been treated in a neonatal ICU and have failed an auditory screening examination

5. Term infants who had hypoxic episodes which resulted in changes in consciousness lasting > 24 hr or unexplained impaired consciousness

6. Congenital infections or neonatal bacterial meningitis

7. After exposure to ototoxic drugs

16. What are the otoacoustic auditory emission (OAE) and BAEP peaks? What are their presumed anatomic correlates?

ANATOPHYSIOLOGIC PROCESSES	WAVES PRODUCED	PEAK LATENCIES
))) → **Tympanic membrane** vibration (sound) ↓	Sound waves	
Auditory ossicle vibration ↓	Sound waves	
Traveling pressure wave in the **basilar membrane** ↓	OAE*	
Stimulation of the sensory **hair cells** ↓	OAE*	
Depolarization (generator potentials) of the **dendrites** and the **spinal ganglion** ↓	ABR–wave I	1.35–2.08 msec
"All or none" **auditory nerve** action potential ↓	ABR–wave I	1.35–2.08 msec
Cochlear nuclei (second-order neuron) in medulla ↓	ABR–wave I	2.54–3.22 msec
Trapezoid body **Dorsal acoustic striae** **Intermediate acoustic striae** ↓	ABR–wave II	2.54–3.22 msec
Superior olivary complex (contralateral and ipsilateral third-order neurons) in pons ↓	ABR–wave III	3.58–4.30 msec
Lateral lemniscus (contralateral and ipsilateral in pons) ↓	ABR–wave IV	5.00–5.60 msec
Inferior colliculus (primarily fourth-order, few third-order neurons; contralateral and ipsilateral) in midbrain ↓	ABR–wave V	5.32–6.16 msec
Medial geniculate body (fifth-order neurons) in thalamus ↓	ABR–wave VI	7.05–7.78 msec
Thalamocortical auditory radiations ↓	ABR–wave VII	8.70–9.45 msec
Primary auditory area ↓	ABR–wave VII	8.70–9.45 msec
Secondary and tertiary auditory area	ABR–wave VII	8.70–9.45 msec

* The OAE is the recordable response from the cochlear mechanism's outer hair cell.

17. What clinical examination should be done before doing an ABR/BAEP?

Gross assessment of hearing prior to establishing threshold values.

Otoscopic examination of the external auditory canal with tympanic membrane visualization to ensure that the canal is not blocked; if the auditory canal shows significant blockage, this should be removed before the studies are performed.

18. Which BAEP/ABR peaks are used for clinical interpretation?

The **I–III interpeak latencies** have shown correlation with lesions in the peripheral auditory mechanism, auditory nerve, and lower pons. The **I–V interpeak latencies** have more widespread use in brainstem, thalamic, and cortical injuries when the I–III interpeak latencies are normal. There can be diffuse involvement both in the I–III and III–V interpeak latencies with multiple sclerosis and other demyelinating processes. Low stimulus intensity or hearing losses are suggested by a **wave I** peak delay.

19. What is a (magnetically or electrically) stimulated transcranial motor evoked potential (MEP)?

MEPs evaluate transmission along a pathway that includes the efferent spinal motor conduction pathway. This complements the afferent dorsal column and spinocerebellar tract information derived from SEP studies. The transcranial MEP involves initiation of an efferent motor volley through activation of the cortical motoneurons in primary motor cortex. Responses are recorded over a targeted peripheral muscle. Cortical and spinal MEP studies were originally applied during intraoperative procedures to document efferent motor conduction through the spinal cord. This was initially accomplished with dipolar electrical stimulation. Magnetic stimulation has generally replaced electrical stimulation techniques. The MEP recording paradigm can be viewed simplistically as an extension of the motor nerve conduction study into the CNS. Instead of stimulating the peripheral nerve percutaneously, stimulation is applied directly to CNS structures, such as the motor cortex or rostral spinal cord, that generate or transmit efferent motor impulses to muscle.

20. Where are transcranial and spinal MEPs helpful diagnostically?

Maximization of the magnetic MEP responses is best obtained on awake cooperative patients who can voluntarily contract the "target" muscle. MEP studies can be used to examine impairment of conduction through central motor pathways traversing the brain and spinal cord. MEPs have proven useful in the study of patients with stroke, multiple sclerosis, motor neuron disease, and myelopathy. They can be used to assess and localize damage to CNS pathways that results in motor impairment.

21. How should the skin-electrode interface be prepared for recording EPs?

Even though the preamplifier input impedances have improved over the years, the skin–electrode interface presents a formidable conduction barrier. Because CNS responses are so small relative to peripheral nerve and muscle responses and ambient electrical noise, the skin at the recording site should be lightly abraded, an electrolyte applied, and the electrode firmly attached to the skin. The resultant impedance from a properly applied cup or disc surface electrode should be 1–5 kΩ. Interdermal pin electrodes have inherently higher impedances because of the nature and small size of their skin-electrode interface. If the tested surface electrode impedance is too low, it may be due to interelectrode conduction bridging by perspired salts and fluids or conductive gel.

22. How should EPs be reported?

An acceptable report should include the relevant aspects of the history and physical examination and the clinical reason for the referral. Signal EP data should be attached. The traces used for analysis and interpretation must show at least two clearly superimposed runs to confirm the recording reliability. The stimulus site (type, intensity), active recording electrode site, reference location, equipment (settings), and recording parameters used for the test should be included with the data as well as a basic summary of the technique employed. Interpretation of latency, amplitude, and waveform morphology should always be based on side-to-side comparisons and statistical analysis (mean ± 2.5 SD) for all the data criteria used to assess normality versus abnormality.

BIBLIOGRAPHY

1. Binnie CD, Cooper R, Fowler CJ, et al (eds): Clinical Neurophysiology: EMG, Nerve Conduction and Evoked Potentials. Oxford, Butterworth-Heinemann, 1995.
2. Chiappa KH (ed): Evoked Potentials in Clinical Medicine, 3rd ed. Philadelphia, Lippincott-Raven, 1997.
3. Cole JL: Central nervous system electrodiagnostics. In DeLisa J (ed): Rehabilitation Medicine: Principles and Practice, 3rd ed. Philadelphia, J.B. Lippincott, 1998.
4. Goldberg G: Clinical neurophysiology of the central nervous system. Evoked potentials and other neurophysiologic techniques. In Grabois M, Garrison SJ, Hart KA, Lehmkuhl LD (eds): Physical Medicine and Rehabilitation: The Complete Approach. Malden, MA, Blackwell Science, 2000.
5. Mauguière F: Clinical utility of somatosensory evoked potentials (SEPs): Present debates and future trends. Electroencephalogr Clin Neurophysiol Suppl 46:27–33, 1996.

V. Rehabilitation of Organ-Based Systems

27. STROKE

Elliot J. Roth, M.D.

1. How many people suffer a stroke? Who is typically affected?

Stroke is a very common clinical problem. Recent estimates have placed the incidence at about 700,000 new strokes per year in the U.S., which is approximately 150,000–200,000/year more than past estimates. It is believed that better epidemiological assessments, rather than a true increase in the number of new strokes, accounts for the recent increase in reported incidence. About 150,000 die each year within 1 month after the stroke, making stroke the third leading cause of death in the U.S. It is estimated that about 4 million people are alive today who sustained a stroke at some time in the past, and a substantial proportion (perhaps one-half to two-thirds) of these survivors have varying degrees and types of neurologic impairments and functional disabilities. Stroke is the second most frequent cause of disability (second only to arthritis), the leading cause of *severe* disability, and the most common diagnosis among patients on most rehabilitation units.

Men have a 30–80% higher incidence than do women, and African-Americans have a 50–130% greater incidence than do whites. The incidence is age-related, with the rate increasing nine-fold between the ages of 55 and 85. About two-thirds of all stroke patients are over age 65.

2. List the risk factors for stroke.

RISK FACTORS MODIFIABLE WITH BEHAVIOR CHANGE	RISK FACTORS MODIFIABLE WITH MEDICAL CARE	UNMODIFIABLE RISK FACTORS
Hypercholesterolemia	Hypertension	Age
Obesity	Diabetes	Gender
Sedentary lifestyle	Heart disease	Race
Cigarette smoking	Transient ischemic attack	Family history
Alcohol abuse	Significant carotid artery stenosis	
Cocaine use	History of prior stroke	

3. How can subsequent strokes be prevented in patients who have survived a first stroke?

Risk factor modification
Antiplatelet agents—aspirin, ticlopidine, and clopidogrel
Anticoagulation—warfarin
Carotid endarterectomy
Surgical procedure to correct cerebral aneurysm or arteriovenous malformation

4. What is a stroke?

A stroke is an acute neurologic dysfunction of vascular origin, with relatively rapid onset, causing focal or sometimes global signs of disturbed cerebral function lasting for > 24 hours.

5. What are the different types of strokes?

Stroke types are generally divided into two broad etiologic categories: ischemic (65–80% of the total) and hemorrhagic (15–25% of the total). The cause of a few strokes (up to 10% of the total) is either unknown or more unusual.

TYPE OF STROKE	% OF THE TOTAL
Ischemic strokes	
Thrombotic brain infarction	45–65%
Embolic brain infarction	10–20%
Hemorrhagic strokes	
Intracerebral (intraparenchymal) hemorrhage	5–15%
Subarachnoid hemorrhage	5–10%
Other strokes	0–10%

6. What are the common impairments caused by stroke and their relative frequencies?

IMPAIRMENT	ACUTE (%)	CHRONIC (%)
Any motor weakness	90	50
Right hemiparesis	45	20
Left hemiparesis	35	25
Bilateral hemiparesis	10	5
Ataxia	20	10
Hemianopsia	25	10
Visuoperceptual deficits	30	30
Aphasia	35	20
Dysarthria	50	20
Sensory deficits	50	25
Cognitive deficits	35	30
Depression	30	30
Bladder incontinence	30	10
Dysphagia	30	10

7. What are lacunar strokes?

Accounting for about 15% of all strokes, lacunar strokes are caused by small deep infarctions located in the deeper portions of the brain and brainstem, resulting from occlusion of the deep penetrating cerebral arteries. Risk factors for lacunar stroke include hypertension and diabetes. Because the cerebral lesions are small, they usually do not cause severe impairment or disability. Because they are caused by deeper cerebral lesions, they usually do not impair higher cortical functions.

The most common lacunar syndromes are pure motor hemiplegia, hemimotor-hemisensory syndrome, pure sensory stroke, dysarthria-clumsy hand syndrome, and hemiparesis-hemiataxia.

8. What is locked-in syndrome?

Locked-in syndrome is a severely disabling condition, characterized by the combination of complete quadriplegia, facial paralysis, and anarthria. It is caused by interruption of the bilateral corticospinal and corticobulbar tracts that occurs with bilateral infarction of the ventral pons.

9. What is pseudobulbar palsy?

Pseudobulbar palsy is the combination of emotional lability, dysphagia, dysarthria, and hyperactive brainstem reflexes.

10. Describe the usual course of natural recovery after the onset of hemiplegia.

Natural spontaneous recovery of motor function follows a relatively predictable sequence of stereotyped movement events for most (but not all) patients who recover from stroke-induced hemiplegia. The pattern of recovery is most consistent in patients with cerebral infarction in the middle cerebral artery distribution. Lower-extremity function recovers earliest and most completely, followed by upper-extremity and hand function. Tone usually returns before voluntary movement, volitional control over the proximal limb before the distal limb, and mass movement (synergy) patterns before specific isolated coordinated volitional motor functions. Most exceptions to these patterns occur in patients with stroke types other than cerebral infarctions and with lesion locations other than middle cerebral artery distribution.

The relative uniformity of these phases of recovery was first studied and documented systematically by Twitchell in 1951 and later formalized into a series of stages by Brunnstrom in 1970.

11. Describe the features of each of the Brunnstrom stages of motor recovery in hemiplegic patients.

Stage I
    Flaccidity
    Phasic stretch reflexes absent
    No volitional or reflex-induced active movement
Stage II
    Spasticity, resistance to passive movement
    Basic limb synergy patterns
    Associated reactions
    Movement patterns stimulated reflexively
    Minimal voluntary movement
Stage III
    Marked spasticity
    Semivoluntary
    Volitional initiates movement of involved limbs, resulting in synergy
    Usually flexion synergy in arm and extension synergy in leg
Stage IV
    Spasticity reduced
    Synergy patterns still predominant
    Some complex movements deviating from synergy
Stage V
    Spasticity declines more, but still present with rapid movements
    More difficult movement patterns deviating from synergy
    Voluntary isolated environmentally specific movements predominate
Stage VI
    Spasticity disappearing
    Coordination improves to near normal
    Individual joint movements possible
    Still have abnormal movement and faulty timing during complex actions
Stage VII:
    Restoration of normal variety of rapid complex movement patterns with normal timing, coordination, strength, and endurance

12. Name the components of the limb synergy patterns.

Synergy patterns are the stereotyped mass movement patterns that characterize limb activity after injury to the cerebral voluntary motor system. The affected upper and lower extremities each can assume a flexion or an extension synergy pattern. In the following list, the predominant movement in each pattern is marked with an asterisk.

Upper Extremity Flexion Synergy Pattern	Upper Extremity Extension Synergy Pattern
Scapular retraction	Scapular protraction
Scapular depression	Scapular depression
Shoulder external rotation	Shoulder internal rotation

Shoulder abduction	*Shoulder adduction
Forearm pronation	Forearm pronation
*Elbow flexion	Elbow extension
Wrist flexion	Wrist extension
Finger flexion	Finger flexion
Lower Extremity Flexion Synergy Pattern	Lower Extremity Extension Synergy Pattern
Pelvic protraction	Pelvic retraction
Pelvic depression	Pelvic elevation
*Hip flexion	Hip extension
Hip abduction	Hip adduction
Hip external rotation	Hip internal rotation
Knee flexion	*Knee extension
Ankle dorsiflexion	Ankle plantarflexion
Foot inversion	Foot inversion
Toe dorsiflexion	Toe plantarflexion
Great toe extension	Great toe extension

13. What are the most common causes of death in stroke survivors?

During the first month after a stroke, the major causes of death, arranged in order of descending frequency, are:

- The stroke itself, with progressive cerebral edema and herniation
- Pneumonia
- Cardiac disease (myocardial infarction, sudden death arrhythmia, or heart failure)
- Pulmonary embolism

After the first month, cardiac disease is the most common cause and stroke is the second most common cause of death in stroke patients.

14. How common are venous thromboemolic phenomena in stroke patients?

Deep venous thrombosis (DVT) has been reported to occur in 22–73% of stroke survivors, with the best estimates of incidence of 40–50%. The incidence of pulmonary embolism in stroke is about 10–15%. Peak incidence is during the first week after stroke, but the risk of venous thromboembolism persists thereafter. Clinical features of DVT or pulmonary embolism are present in less than one-half of patients with these problems, making laboratory diagnosis necessary for most patients suspected of having these conditions.

15. Can venous thromboembolic complications be prevented?

Because of the high risk of venous thromboembolism, DVT prophylaxis is recommended for all patients with stroke who have muscle weakness and who undergo inpatient rehabilitation. Methods of prophylaxis include repeated doses of low-dose subcutaneous heparin or low-molecular-weight heparin compounds, external pneumatic calf-compression boots, and other physical methods. The optimal duration of prophylaxis is not known, but persistence of severe muscle weakness and lack of ambulatory ability are considered indicators of increased DVT risk.

16. How common are dysphagia, aspiration, and pneumonia after stroke, and what can be done about them?

The incidence of dysphagia in stroke patients is between one-third and one-half. Although dysphagia can be associated with cortical, subcortical, or brain stem lesions, the highest incidence is in patients with brainstem strokes.

One third of stroke patients with dysphagia will have aspiration, defined as entrance of material into the airway below the level of the true vocal folds. Of those who aspirate, 40% will do so silently, without cough or other clinical manifestations of difficulty. Aspiration usually results from disturbances in the pharyngeal phase of swallowing related to reduced laryngeal closure, pharyngeal paresis, or reduced pharyngeal peristalsis. In order to establish the dysphagia diagnosis and aspiration risk, a clinical evaluation of swallowing function and videofluoroscopic swallowing study can be done.

Complications of stroke-induced dysphagia include pneumonia, malnutrition, and dehydration. Pneumonia occurs in about one-third of all stroke patients, and the major cause of pneumonia is dysphagia with aspiration. Other factors that increase the risk of pneumonia are cognitive deficits, inadequate hydration and nutrition, impaired cough and gag reflexes, immobility, and the decreased ability to cough resulting from expiratory muscle weakness, altered chest wall movement patterns, chest wall spasticity, and contracture.

Interventions to treat dysphagia include changes in posture and head position; oral motor exercises for the tongue and lips to increase strength, range of motion, velocity, and precision; use of thickened fluids and soft or pureed foods in smaller boluses; tactile-thermal application of cold stimuli; practice in proper eating techniques; and the use of alternative feeding routes such as nasogastric, gastrostomy, or jejunostomy tubes.

17. Describe the major bladder problems caused by stroke. What can be done to treat them?

The incidence of urinary incontinence is 50–70% during the first month after stroke and about 15% after 6 months, a figure comparable to that in the general population. Incontinence may be caused by the brain damage itself (resulting in an uninhibited spastic neurogenic bladder with a synergic sphincter), urinary tract infection, impaired ability to transfer to the toilet or remove clothing, aphasia, or cognitive-perceptual deficits that result in lack of awareness of bladder fullness. Bowel impaction and some medications may exert an adverse effect. Urinary incontinence can cause skin breakdown, social embarrassment, and depression, and it increases the risk of institutionalization and unfavorable rehabilitation outcomes.

The most important therapeutic approach to the stroke-induced neurogenic bladder is the implementation of a timed bladder-emptying schedule. Other important management strategies include treatment of urinary tract infection, regulation of fluid intake, transfer and dressing skill training, patient and family education, and (rarely) medications.

Urinary retention is less common but can occur in the presence of diabetic autonomic neuropathy or prostatic hypertrophy. Urinary retention may cause urinary tract infections requiring treatment with catheterization, medication, and attention to the primary genitourinary cause.

18. What is the incidence of bowel dysfunction in stroke? How can it be treated?

The incidence of bowel incontinence among stroke patients is 31%. While this problem usually resolves within the first 2 weeks after stroke, persistent bowel incontinence may reflect severe brain damage. Bowel continence may be adversely affected by infection resulting in diarrhea, inability to transfer to the toilet or to manage clothing, or inability to express toileting needs. The more common bowel complications are constipation and impaction, resulting from inactivity, inadequate fluid intake, and psychologic disturbances.

Management of bowel dysfunction emphasizes a timed toileting schedule; use of dietary fiber; adequate fluid intake; use of stool softeners, suppositories, or enemas; training in toilet transfers and communication skills; and judicious use of laxatives.

19. Explain the motor facilitation approaches frequently used in physical therapy with stroke patients.

Each of the neuromuscular facilitation exercise approaches commonly used in stroke survivors has a neurophysiologic basis and a somewhat unique focus.

The **neurodevelopmental treatment method**, developed by the Bobaths, is currently the most widely used approach for the treatment of hemiplegia resulting from stroke. This method emphasizes inhibition of abnormal tone, postures, and reflex patterns, while facilitating specific automatic motor responses that will eventually allow the performance of skilled voluntary movements.

The **Brunnstrom treatment method** uses the reflex tensing and synergistic patterns of hemiplegia to improve motor control through central facilitation.

The **Rood method** relies on the peripheral input of cutaneous sensory stimulation, in the form of superficial brushing and tapping, to facilitate or inhibit motor activity.

Proprioceptive neuromuscular facilitation, introduced by Kabat and Knott, uses such mechanisms as maximum resistance, quick stretch, and spiral diagonal patterns to facilitate normal movement.

The more recently-developed **motor relearning program** of Carr and Shepherd emphasizes functional training, practice, and repetition in the performance of specific tasks, and carry-over of those motor skills into functional activities.

Only a few studies have investigated the relative effectiveness of these methods; results are inconconclusive, but no single method has been found to be more effective than any other to improve outcome after stroke. A common clinical practice is to incorporate elements of several methods.

20. What is the "forced-use paradigm" of treatment after stroke?

In the forced-use intervention, also known as constraint-induced movement therapy, the non-hemiplegic limb is restrained in an attempt to force the individual to rely on the use of the hemiplegic limb for functional activities. Based originally on the observation that some of the disability in stroke survivors resulted in part from the patient's lack of use of the affected limb (as opposed to neurologically induced weakness of the limb itself) and also supported by favorable results derived from animal studies, this method was found in recent human studies to improve recovery of ADL function and also brain activity among individuals with hemiplegia resulting from stroke.

21. Describe the common treatment approaches used for spasticity caused by stroke.

Hemispheric strokes affect motor activity in several ways, causing weakness and synergy patterns as well as spasticity. Typically causing more functional impairment in the upper extremity than in the lower limb, spasticity is usually (but not always) less severe in patients with cerebral lesions than in those with spinal cord lesions. Treatment of spasticity relies most heavily on proper positioning, orthotics, and aggressive, consistent stretching exercises to maintain and improve ROM. Other management strategies include casting, pharmacologic injection blocks of motor points or peripheral nerves (using phenol or botulinum toxin), therapeutic exercise other than stretching, casting, oral medications, and surgical release, the latter of which may be very effective in selected patients. The efficacy of medications remains controversial, but dantrolene sodium (Dantrium) is probably the drug of choice for patients with cerebral spasticity. Most recently, selective local intramuscular injection of low doses of botulinum toxin A (Botox) has been found to be effective in reducing local muscle tone for about 3–6 months, resulting in improved function and decreased pain sensation in some patients.

22. Describe common shoulder problems in stroke survivors and what can be done about them.

Approximately 70–80% of patients with stroke and hemiplegia have shoulder pain, contracture, or another form of dysfunction, making it one of the most common secondary complications of stroke. Causes of hemiplegic shoulder dysfunction are many and can include glenohumeral subluxation, adhesive capsulitis (frozen shoulder), impingement syndromes, rotator cuff tears, brachial plexus traction neuropathies, complex regional pain syndrome ("shoulder hand syndrome," present in up to 25% of patients), bursitis and tendinitis, and central pain. Often, there is either a history or radiographic evidence of a preexisting or long-standing shoulder problem, and it is likely that the abnormal mechanical forces resulting from the stroke either exacerbate or make manifest the chronic problem. In some patients, pain and loss of ROM are associated with improper positioning or handling, weakness of the shoulder girdle muscles, or spasticity. Shoulder dysfunction has been found to be present significantly more frequently in patients with spastic upper limbs than in those with flaccid upper limbs. Pain and glenohumeral subluxation may occur together or independently, and the extent to which there is a causal relationship between pain and subluxation is unclear.

Treatment of shoulder dysfunction is individualized and may consist of arm supports, shoulder slings, arm troughs, lap boards, medications, physical modalities, proper positioning and staff handling, and, most importantly, aggressive and consistently performed ROM exercises. The use of shoulder slings is controversial, but if subluxation is the main cause of the shoulder dysfunction, then slings may be helpful. Ensuring consistent performance of stretching exercises is the major clinical task.

23. What is central post-stroke pain syndrome?

Previously known as thalamic pain or Dejerine-Roussy syndrome, central post-stroke pain syndrome occurs in less than 5% of stroke survivors. It causes severe and disabling pain, which usually is described by patients as diffuse, persistent, and refractory to many treatment attempts. The most common descriptions of the pain are "burning and tingling", although many experience "sharp, shooting, stabbing, gnawing," and more rarely, "dull and achy". The dysesthesias are often associated with hyperpathia, which is an exaggerated pain reaction to mild external cutaneous stimulation. Only about 50% of the patients have thalamic strokes; the remainder have cerebrovascular lesions in a variety of locations.

Treatment methods include:
Medical and nursing care
  Prevention and treatment of bladder, bowel, and skin problems
  Prevention and treatment of other medical problems such as infection
  ROM exercises
  Mobility exercises
Psychologic methods
  Relaxation, imagery
  Biofeedback
  Hypnosis
  Psychotherapy
  Preoccupation/distraction
Medications
  Analgesics
  Antidepressants
  Anticonvulsants
Surgical techniques (rarely used)

24. Describe the common types of aphasia that occur after stroke.

Global aphasia: loss of both expression and comprehension abilities. Patients have nonfluent or absent speech.

Broca's aphasia: reduction in expressive, and therefore repetition, abilities, but *with* preservation of comprehension. Speech is nonfluent.

Wernicke's aphasia: reductions in comprehension and repetition, but with preservation of expression. Speech is fluent but often nonsensical.

Transcortical motor aphasia: expressive dysfunction with intact comprehension and repetition.

Transcortical sensory aphasia: loss of comprehension ability with intact expression and repetition.

Conduction aphasia (relatively rare): isolated loss of repetition, while expression and comprehension remain intact.

25. What is melodic intonation therapy? How does it work?

Melodic intonation therapy is a direct form of aphasia treatment that utilizes the patient's relatively unimpaired ability to sing, which can facilitate spontaneous speech in some patients. Therapy starts with the therapist and patient chanting simple phrases and sentences in unison to melodies that resemble natural intonation patterns. This progresses to a level at which the patient is able to chant answers to simple questions, and in some cases, the patient makes the transition off intoned speech and into normal prosodic speech patterns. This method is most successful in patients with good auditory comprehension and limited verbal expression. It is thought that the effectiveness of this method derives from the reliance on the unimpaired musical functions of the right hemisphere to support the damaged motor speech function in the left hemisphere.

26. What is hemispatial neglect and how can it be treated?

Unilateral hemispatial inattention, or neglect, is the lack of awareness of a specific body part or external environment. Neglect usually occurs in patients with right (nondominant) hemisphere cortical strokes; these patients ignore or have muted responses to visual, auditory, or tactile stimuli on the left side of the body or environment. Patients with severe hemi-inattention deny that they have an illness or that neglect is a problem, or they may not recognize their own body parts. Neglect can improve spontaneously but can impede performance of functional tasks and complicate rehabilitation efforts.

Treatment methods emphasize retraining, substitution of intact abilities, and compensatory techniques. Specific treatment strategies include providing visuospatial cues, fostering awareness of deficits, using computer-assisted training, visual scanning skill training, caloric stimulation, Fresnel prism glasses, eye patching, dynamic stimulation, and optokinetic stimulation.

27. What is Gerstmann's syndrome?

Gerstmann's syndrome occurs following damage to the left parietal region of the brain, which causes the four findings of dyscalculia, finger agnosia, right-left disorientation, and dysgraphia.

28. What are the apraxias?

The term *apraxia* is applied to a group of complex cognitive disorders that adversely affect motor function, usually characterized by difficulty in planning, organizing, sequencing, and executing learned voluntary movements, in the absence of weakness, ataxia, or extrapyramidal dysfunction. Several specific types of apraxias have been identified:

Motor or ideomotor apraxia: Patient can perform a particular movement automatically or spontaneously, but cannot repeat the movement when asked.

Ideational apraxia: Failure to hold onto ideas and plans necessary to perform an activity.

Constructional apraxia: Disturbance in the organization of individual spatial elements such that the patient is unable to synthesize the elements into a whole. Inability to put together an object from separate parts or to draw a picture of an object.

Apraxia of speech: Deficit in motor programming of speech. Often associated with Broca's aphasia.

Dressing apraxia: Inability to dress self despite adequate motor ability.

Apraxia of gait: Difficulty in initiating and maintaining a normal walking pattern when sensory and motor functions are otherwise unimpaired. Usually associated with frontal lobe lesions.

29. How common is post-stroke depression? What can be done about it?

The incidence of depression after stroke ranges between 10% and 70%, with the best estimates at around 30%. Major depression is present in about one-third of all of those with depression. Depression may result from a biologic effect of the brain damage itself, a reaction to the losses caused by the stroke, effects of certain medications, manifestations of certain medical conditions, or a combination of these factors. Depression may adversely affect both participation in rehabilitation and functional outcomes.

The choice of treatment depends on the cause and severity of the symptoms. Review of medications and treating intercurrent medical illnesses are important first steps. A rehabilitation program that includes therapy for physical and cognitive disabilities, interaction with others, and attention and encouragement from family and staff is often extremely helpful. Many patients respond favorably to more intensive psychotherapy or to the use of antidepressant medications, which have been demonstrated in at least three randomized controlled clinical trials to be effective in treating post-stroke depression and in improving functional abilities.

30. What are some of the typical functional outcomes after stroke?

It is estimated that only about 1 in 10 stroke patients are functionally independent at the time of stroke and that nearly one-half are independent at 6 months. Results of the Framingham Study provide estimates for the types and frequencies of long-term disabilities in stroke survivors:

TYPE OF DISABILITY	%
Decreased vocational function	63
Decreased socialization outside home	59
Limited household tasks	56
Decreased interests and hobbies	47
Decreased use of transportation	44
Decreased socialization at home	43
Dependent ADL	32
Dependent mobility	22
Living in institution	15

The frequencies for all of these disabilities were significantly greater than those in age- and gender-matched controls in that study. Estimates for disabilities in some specific activities after 6 months post-stroke are as follows:

TYPE OF DISABILITY	%
Unable to walk	15
Needs assistance to transfer	20
Needs assistance to bathe	50
Needs assistance to dress	30
Needs assistance to groom	10

31. List the commonly cited predictors of unfavorable functional outcome after stroke.

Prior stroke
Urinary incontinence
Bowel incontinence
Depression
Visuospatial perceptual deficits
Cognitive deficits
Delayed acute medical care
Delayed rehabilitation
Low functional score on admission
   to rehabilitation program
Poor social supports
Unmarried
Unemployed
Cardiac disease
Coma at onset
Inability to perform ADL (most important)
Poor sitting balance
Large cerebral lesions
Dense hemiplegia
(Homonymous hemianopsia)
(Aphasia)
(Increased age)
(Medical comorbidity)

32. Describe some of the unique considerations in rehabilitation of older adults with stroke.

Because a substantial proportion of stroke survivors are over age 65 years, consideration of issues that tend to be more common among older adults assumes prominence in the care of stroke survivors. Some of the most important of these problems are the increased frequency of preexisting medical conditions and prior stroke, increased risk of secondary post-stroke medical complications, increased likelihood of recurrent stroke, and slower recovery from secondary intercurrent medical illnesses. Many of these problems result from reduced endurance and limited physiologic reserve among older adults. Older adults are at greater risk for falls with injuries, adverse drug reactions, and neurologic changes resulting in altered cognitive, sensory, and motor functioning.

For many older patients, the problem that is more significant than medical comorbidity is a relative lack of family, economic, and social resources. Spouses and other caregivers are often either not available or not able to provide post-rehabilitation care for the older stroke survivor. Institutional discharges tend to be more common among older adults.

These problems may delay or inhibit participation in the therapeutic exercise program, complicate the rehabilitation course, and prolong hospitalization. It is important to note, however, that studies have shown that *older adults are able to make functional improvements in amounts that are similar to those of younger stroke patients.* Compared to younger individuals, older adults tend to have lower functional ratings on admission (and therefore at discharge), primarily because of the greater frequencies of comorbidities and prior strokes and also because of greater stroke severities among older patients.

33. Describe some of the unique considerations in rehabilitation of younger adults with stroke.

Approximately one-third of all strokes occur in individuals who are under age 65 years. The distribution of various diagnostic etiologies of stroke differ for this group. Hemorrhagic strokes tend to be more common in younger adults, accounting for about one-third of all strokes, and infarctions are caused by atherosclerosis (about 20% of all infarctions), cardiogenic embolism (about 20%), cerebral vasculitis with or without systemic collagen vascular diseases (about 10%), coagulopathy (about 10%), and other causes.

Rehabilitation and long-term care issues that are more relevant for younger adults than for others include employment, sexuality, child care, instrumental ADLs (e.g., meal preparation, shopping, housekeeping), psychological aspects of life-role changes, spousal and other relationship changes, financial management, driving, leisure planning and hobbies, and socializing. As a consequence, specialized rehabilitation training efforts focused in these areas for these patients, together with psychological counseling, community reentry training, and social programs, can help to enhance the quality of life for young adults with stroke.

BIBLIOGRAPHY

1. Brandstater ME, Basmajian JV (eds): Stroke Rehabilitation. Baltimore: Williams & Wilkins, 1987.
2. Brandstater ME, Roth EJ, Siebens HC: Venous thromboembolism in stroke: Literature review and implications for clinical practice. Arch Phys Med Rehabil 73:S379–S391, 1992.
3. Brocklehurst JC, Andrews K, Richards B, Laycock PJ: Incidence and correlates of incontinence in stroke patients. J Am Geriatr Soc 33:540–542, 1985.
4. Cailliet R: The Shoulder in Hemiplegia. Philadelphia, F.A. Davis, 1980.
5. Couser JI: Diagnosis and management of pneumonia and ventilatory disorders in patients with stroke. Topics Stroke Rehabil 1:106–118, 1994.
6. Davidoff G, Keren O, Ring H, et al: Assessing candidates for inpatient stroke rehabilitation: Predictors of outcome. Phys Med Rehabil Clin North Am 2:501–516, 1991.
7. Dombovy ML, Sandok BA, Basford JR: Rehabilitation for stroke: A review. Stroke 17:363–369, 1986.
8. Gordon WA (ed): Advances in Stroke Rehabilitation. Boston, Andover Medical Publishers, 1993.
9. Gresham GE, Phillips TF, Wolf PA, et al: Epidemiological profile of long-term stroke disability: The Framingham study. Arch Phys Med Rehabil 60:487–491, 1979.
10. Gresham GE, Duncan PW, Stason WB, et al: Post-Stroke Rehabilitation. Guideline Report, no. 16. Rockville, MD, Agency for Health Care Policy and Research. Public Health Service, U.S. Department of Health and Human Services, 1995, AHCPR Publication No. 95-0662.
11. Hachinski V, Norris JW: The Acute Stroke. Philadelphia, F.A. Davis, 1985.
12. Hoogasian S, Walzak MP, Wurzel R: Urinary incontinence in the stroke patient: Etiology and rehabilitation. Phys Med Rehabil State Art Rev 3:581–594, 1989.
13. Jongbloed L: Prediction of function after stroke: A critical review. Stroke 17:765–776, 1986.
14. Lorish TR, Sandin KJ, Roth EJ, Noll SF: Stroke rehabilitation: 3. Rehabilitation evaluation and management. Arch Phys Med Rehabil 75:S47–S51, 1994.
15. Roth EJ: The elderly stroke patient: Principles and practices of rehabilitation management. Topics Geriat Rehabil 3:27–61, 1988.

16. Roth EJ, Harvey RL: Rehabilitation of stroke syndromes. In Braddom RL (ed): Textbook of Physical Medicine and Rehabilitation. Philadelphia, W.B. Saunders, 1995.

17. Roth EJ, Noll SF: Stroke rehabilitation: 2. Comorbidities and complications. Arch Phys Med Rehabil 75:S42–S46, 1994.

18. Roth EJ: Medical complications encountered in stroke rehabilitation. Phys Med Rehabil Clin North Am 2:563–578, 1991.

19. Teasell RW, Gillen M: Upper extremity disorders and pain following stroke. Phys Med Rehabil State Art Rev 7:133–146, 1993.

20. Wade DT, Langton Hewer R, Skilbeck CE, David RM: Stroke: A Critical Approach to Diagnosis, Treatment, and Management. Chicago, Year Book, 1985.

28. MULTIPLE SCLEROSIS

Brian D. Greenwald, M.D., Jan Lexell, M.D., Ph.D., and Allison Averill, M.D.

1. What are the demographics of multiple sclerosis (MS)?

One-quarter to one-half million people in the U.S. have MS, and about 8,000 new cases are diagnosed each year. Symptoms begin between ages 20–50 in 90% of cases; the peak age is 33. MS is twice as common in whites and females. Residing in a temperate climate is also an associated factor. Identical twin concordance is 30%. The lifetime risk of a female child whose mother has MS is 5% (50-fold higher than general population).

2. Describe the pathophysiology of MS.

MS is a very complex disease characterized by recurrent plaques scattered throughout the brain, spinal cord and optic nerves. Plaques are demyelinated white matter of the CNS with lymphocytic invasion. New evidence suggests there is also axonal damage and brain atrophy. Discrepancies in the numbers of MRI lesions and clinical presentation may exist.

Many environmental and genetic factors have been implicated in the cause of the disease: human herpesvirus 6, *Chlamydia pneumoniae*, and the hepatitis B vaccine have been implicated as possible factors in triggering the disease. In short, the development of MS is determined by a number of genetic and environmental factors.

3. What patterns of disease are seen in MS?

There are typically four patterns. **Relapsing-remitting MS**, the most common pattern (40–60%), involves episodic relapses approximately once per year with recovery and a stable phase between relapse. Recovery may be incomplete, and disability accumulates over time. Ten percent of patients have a benign course with no or mild disability. Half of patients with relapsing-remitting MS change patterns after 10–20 years to **secondary progressive MS** (gradual neurologic deterioration without acute relapses). These two patterns account for 85% of MS patients. Ten to 15% have **primary progressive MS**; this pattern shows gradual but continuous neurologic deterioration. **Progressive relapsing MS** occurs in less than 5% of cases and involves gradual but continuous neurologic deterioration with superimposed relapses. Death may occur in weeks to months.

4. What is a pseudoexacerbation?

An MS patient can have transient worsening of neurologic symptoms that is caused by an acute medical problem, usually a febrile illness. For instance, a urinary tract infection may cause worsening spasticity, which may mimic an exacerbation.

5. What are important prognostic signs in MS?

Unfortunately, a poor prognosis is easier to predict than a good prognosis. Signs associated with **poor prognosis** include being male, over age 35, initial motor or cerebellar dysfunction, a rapid progression of disease, and initial symptoms being polysymptomatic. **Better prognostic factors** include being female, age < 35, initial sensory signs or optic neuritis, sudden onset with good recovery and long remissions, and complete and rapid remission of initial symptoms.

6. Describe the MRI and evoked potential findings that are seen in MS.

Using standard MRI, 80–90% of patients diagnosed with MS have evidence of plaques. These hyperintense lesions are most common in periventricular white matter, corpus callosum, brainstem, optic nerves, and spinal cord. Standard MRI alone cannot make the diagnosis of MS. Enhanced FLAIR MRI promises to improve differentiation of plaques from normal structures. Magnetic transfer imaging (MTI) is more sensitive and specific for MS lesions. MTI may detect white matter lesions in those patients who have a negative MRI.

Interocular latency difference on visual evoked potential testing is the most sensitive indicator of optic nerve dysfunction. The most common somatosensory evoked potential abnormality with MS is increased interpeak latencies.

7. What clinical outcome measures of impairment and disability are used for MS?

Kurtzke introduced a 10-step Disability Status Scale for MS in 1955. It was revised in 1961 to describe more detailed neurophysiologic involvement relative to functional status. Currently, the most widely used MS clinical outcome measure is the **Expanded Disability Status Scale** (EDSS). It divides the original 10 levels in half to increase the sensitivity for functional status. Criticisms of the scale are that it is an impairment scale rather than a measure of disability, it is insensitive to small changes, and it has poor inter-rater reliability. Additionally, it focuses on ambulation as the primary functional activity.

To overcome this limitation, a new outcome measure has been proposed. The **Multiple Sclerosis Functional Composite** (MSFC) consists of three objective quantitative tests of neurologic function, encompassing arm, leg, and cognitive function. Studies have found that MSFC predicted subsequent change in the EDSS, suggesting that the MSFC is more sensitive to change. Other scales developed for MS patients include the Minimal Record of Disability, Inability Status Scale, Environmental Status Scale, and Scripps Neurologic Rating Scale.

8. Is inpatient or outpatient rehabilitation useful in treating multiple sclerosis?

Studies show that **inpatient rehabilitation** has an effect on disability and handicap despite no change in impairment. In addition, there are improvements in health-related quality of life perception. After discharge, as the neurologic status worsens, benefits may last for over 6 months but diminish without ongoing therapies.

Outpatient therapies therefore play an important role in this progressive disease. DiFabrio studied a group of patients with chronic progressive MS treated with an extended outpatient rehabilitation program. After 1 year of outpatient treatment, patients had reduced fatigue and a lower rate of decline in physical function than subjects in a control group not receiving ongoing therapy.

9. Can MS patients benefit from exercise?

Caution must be taken when prescribing physical activity. Symptoms can temporarily worsen on exposure to heat or physical exercise. Programs are designed to activate working muscles but avoid overload. Exercise evaluation and prescription must account for fatigue, spasticity, ataxia and incoordination, as well as neurologic deficits seen in MS. Emphasis should be maintenance of general conditioning. Maximizing passive and active ROM is critical. Aerobic training improves fitness and quality of life. In addition, studies show aquatic therapy in cooler water results in strength gains.

10. How can fatigue be assessed and treated in MS?

Fatigue is the most common symptom impairing ADLs and the most common complaint by MS patients. Several different scales, such as the Fatigue Severity Scale, Fatigue Descriptive Scale, and Fatigue Impact Scale, are used for assessment. In evaluating the patient, ensure that he or she is getting enough sleep, and rule out medical problems such as hypothyroidism or infection.

Nonpharmacologic management is generally the most effective treatment. Both physical and occupational therapists will be helpful to train the patient in energy conservation techniques and work simplification. An evaluation should be made for adaptive equipment needs. Amantadine and pemoline (Cylert) are common pharmacologic treatments used and are each effective in about 50% of patients treated. Other pharmacologic treatments include SSRIs, calcium channel blockers, methylphenidate, amphetamines, and selegeline.

11. What is Uhthoff's phenomenon?

Fatigue worsened by heat. Fatigue is usually less in the morning and more in the afternoon. It is worsened by physical exertion and heavy meals that may increase core temperature. Therapies should be scheduled with this in mind. A cooling vest may decrease core temperature 0.5–1°C which may improve the ability to exercise.

12. How is spasticity managed in MS?

Spasticity is seen in about 55% of MS patients. It can cause pain, disrupt sleep, and impair volitional movement and daily activities. Conversely, spasticity may play a role in ability to transfer, stand, and ambulate, and, therefore, the decision to treat spasticity must consider the problems and benefits. Causes for an increase in tone must be determined prior to initiating treatment. The most common cause of exacerbation of spasticity is a urinary tract infection, but other sources of noxious stimuli must be excluded.

The first line of treatment involves splinting, positioning, stretching, and cooling the muscles. Baclofen is usually used first when oral agents are needed. It is started at 5 to 10 mg/day, with the dose titrated every 5–7 days. Other oral medications include dantrolene, diazepam, clonidine, clonazepam, tizanidine, gabapentin, and cycloheptadine. Botulinum toxin injections and phenol blocks are most effective for focal spasticity. Intrathecal baclofen is an option when other medications are ineffective. It is most effective for lower-extremity spasticity.

13. What types of bladder dysfunctions occur and how can they be treated?

Symptomatic bladder dysfunction occurs in most patients with MS. The severity of dysfunction is not related to the age of the patient or duration of disease, but urologic complaints are strongly related to the degree of disability. Bladder hyper- and hyporeflexia may occur. The most common urodynamic lesion found in MS is detrusor hyperreflexia. Unfortunately, symptoms do not differentiate between failure to store and failure to empty. In addition, bladder dysfunction may change over the course of the disease. Periodic urodynamics should be considered.

Intermittent catheterization is recommended for patients with failure to empty. Nighttime bladder dysfunction can be treated with low-dose intranasal antidiuretic hormone (desmopressin). Detrusor hyperreflexia can be treated with oxybutynin (Ditropan) or tolterodine (Detrol).

14. How is incoordination treated?

Incoordination is a common problem in MS and ranges from mild tremor to severe ataxia. Cerebral outflow tremors are the most common type. Therapy is aimed at compensatory strategies. Weighted cuffs to dampen incoordination may diminish the amplitude of tremor but are not well tolerated. **Frankel's exercises**, originally described to treat tabes dorsalis, are used to treat incoordination and ataxia. They require a high degree of concentration and frequent repetition and therefore may not be appropriate for all MS patients. Carbamazepine has been reported to reduce the severity of tremors at doses of 400–600 mg/day. Isoniazid, propanolol, primidone, and clonazepam have all been used with varying success. Stereotactic ventrolateral thalamotomy has had benefit in select patients.

15. How is ambulation impairment treated in MS?

Seventy-five percent of MS patients have varying degrees of ambulatory impairment. Treatment requires a comprehensive evaluation. Weakness, fatigue, spasticity, and incoordination may all contribute to ambulation impairment and may require treatment. Gait evaluation should be made on varying terrains, elevations, and stairs. Evaluation of deficiencies will guide the therapy prescription. The need for orthotics and assistive devices should be considered. Increasing the width of the ambulatory-base with a cane or lightweight walker often improves the safety of ambulation.

16. What affective disorders are seen in MS?

Affective symptoms range from mania to depression. Depression is an important consideration when patients complain of fatigue. The frequency of depression ranges from one-quarter to greater than one-half of patients. The risk of suicide in the MS population is 7–14 times greater than in the normal population. Incidence of depression appears to be correlated with gender, age, education, and a history of previous depression. Surprisingly, it does not appear to be related to disease severity, or the physical and cognitive status of the patient. Selective serotonin-reuptake inhibitors (SSRIs) are effective but can precipitate spasticity and require close evaluation. Amitriptyline or SSRIs can be used for excessive laughing or crying. Clonazepam and buspirone are useful for anxiety.

17. What cognitive changes are seen with MS?

Jean-Marie Charcot first recognized an association between cognitive deficits and MS over 100 years ago. Varying degrees of cognitive impairment are seen in MS, even early in the disease, and it appears to be more significant in chronic progressive than relapsing-remitting MS. Approximately half of MS patients are affected, and up to 7% are severely impaired. There is no correlation between disease duration or extent of physical disability and cognitive impairment; however, Bone and colleagues demonstrated a correlation between plaques load and dementia. Feinstein documented progressive MR imaging changes correlating with change on several psychometric tests.

The most frequent cognitive deficits seen in MS are in short-term memory, abstract reasoning, executive functions, and delayed processing. Frontal lobe dysfunction is commonly seen, including initiation, insight, and planning. Prefrontal disconnection may exhibit itself as inappropriate behavior, excessive talking, and poor judgment. Neuropsychological assessment should be offered to MS patients with cognitive decline. Subsequent counseling and cognitive rehabilitation are important to reduce the effects of cognitive deficits on ADLs.

18. What speech and language problems are seen in MS?

Voice, articulation, and swallowing disorders are a significant problem in greater than one-third of MS patients, particularly those with brain stem involvement. Aphasia, anomia, and apraxia are seen in less than 1% of patients. Cognitive impairment also plays a significant role in language disorders.

Speech therapists teach compensatory techniques for dysarthria, such as slowing the rate of speech and emphasizing key words. Evaluation for dysphagia often includes a videofluoroscopic swallowing study. Changing food consistency, eating smaller more frequent meals, chin-tuck while swallowing, and monitoring the rate of eating are compensatory strategies.

19. Is GI dysfunction a significant problem in MS?

Bowel dysfunction in MS (especially constipation) is relatively common (> 50%) and poorly studied. Bowel dysfunction has multiple causes. Reduced colonic transit and disorders of defecation can cause constipation. Fecal incontinence can be due to loss of sensation in the rectum and reduced voluntary anal sphincter contractions. MS-related spinal cord involvement seems to be less important for bowel dysfunction than for neurogenic bladder dysfunction. Treatment involves the common medications for constipation but is usually not very successful.

20. What type of pain is seen in MS?

Not very long ago, MS was considered a painless disease! We now know that more than half of all MS patients experience pain, that there are different types of pain, and that all types of pain can be severe. Acute types of pain in MS are trigeminal neuralgia, episodic facial pain, paroxysmal pain in arms and legs, and headache. Two percent of MS patients experience trigeminal neuralgia. It occurs 400 times more often in MS than in the general population. Treatment of trigeminal neuralgia and episodic/paroxysmal pain involves carbamazepine, baclofen, phenytoin, gabapentin, or lamotrigine. Chronic pain of neurogenic origin is common in MS patients and is described as burning, tingling, or tickling. Older tricyclic antidepressants, in particular amitriptyline, are effective in many patients, often in combination with TENS. Gabapentin up to or above 2400 mg is usually well tolerated and effective. Spasms and cramps can also be very painful. Treatment is the same as for spasticity.

21. How does MS affect pregnancy and vice versa?

MS does not appear to affect a woman's fertility, risk of spontaneous abortion, or congenital malformations. However, caution should be taken by women considering pregnancy because many medications taken for MS are or may be teratogenic. The consensus on risk of relapse during pregnancy is that it is not increased and may be decreased in the third trimester. The relapse rates in the 6 months after pregnancy, however, may be two to three times the nonpregnant rate. Pregnancy does not appear to have an adverse effect on long-term outcome and disability.

22. Explain the relationship between optic neuritis and MS.

The Optic Neuritis Study Group followed > 400 optic neuritis patients for > 5 years. Those who were more likely to develop MS were white, female, had a history of vague neurologic symptoms at the time of presentation with the optic neuritis, had a family history of MS, or had a positive MRI. Fifty-one percent of those with three or more lesions on MRI at the time of the original presentation developed MS.

23. What is the scoop on the new MS medications?

Corticosteroids remain the mainstay for the treatment of acute exacerbations of MS. They shorten the duration of exacerbation, but do not appear to affect the long-term course of the disease. ACTH may also be used.

There are many medications used to prevent the exacerbations seen in relapsing-remitting MS. The three most commonly used are interferon-β1b (Betaseron), interferon-β1a (Avonex), and glatiramer acetate (Copaxone). Both of the interferons are well tolerated, with interferon-β1a generally being tolerated better than Interferon-β1b. The most common side effect is flu-like symptoms. Interferon-β1a is the only medication that has been shown to reduce the number of exacerbations and lesions on MRI and to reduce the risk of disability progression. Glatiramer acetate is usually used when there is a treatment failure with the interferons. There is no documented benefit of hyperbaric oxygen or other alternative medicine approaches.

BIBLIOGRAPHY

1. Bone G, Ladurner G, Dinichauser L, et al: Cognitive disturbances and MRI findings in MS. J Neuroimag 3:169–172, 1993.
2. Damek P, Schuster EA: Pregnancy in multiple sclerosis. Mayo Clin Proc 72: 977–989, 1997.
3. DiFabrio RP, Soderberg J, Choi T, et al: Extended outpatient rehabilitation: Its influence on symptom frequency, fatigue, and functional status for persons with progressive multiple sclerosis. Arch Phys Med Rehabil 79:141–146, 1998.
4. Erikson BJ, Noseworthy JH: Value of magnetic resonance imaging in assessing efficacy in clinical trials on multiple sclerosis therapies. Mayo Clin Proc 72:1080–1089, 1997.
5. Feinstein A, Ron M, Thompson AJ: A serial study of psychometrics and MRI changes in multiple sclerosis. Brain 116:569–602, 1993.
6. Filippi M, Rocca MA, Minicucci L: Magnetic transfer imaging in patients with definite MS and negative conventional MRI. Neurology 52:845–848, 1999.
7. Fischer JS, Rudick RA, Cutter GR, et al: The multiple sclerosis functional composite measure (MSFC): An integrated approach to MS clinical outcome assessment. Multiple Sclerosis 5:244–250, 1999.
8. Freeman JA, Langdon DW, Hobart JC, et al: The impact of inpatient rehabilitation on progressive multiple sclerosis. Ann Neurol 42:236–244, 1997.
9. Freeman JA, Langdon DW, Hobart JC, et al: Inpatient rehabilitation in multiple sclerosis: Do the benefits carry over in the community? Neurology 52:50–56, 1999.
10. Gehlsen GM, Grigsby SA, Winant DM: Effect of aquatic fitness program on the muscular strength and endurance of patients with multiple sclerosis. Phys Ther 64: 653–657, 1984.
11. Hinds JP, Eidelman BH, Wald A: Prevalence of bowel dysfunction in multiple sclerosis: A population survey. Gastroenterology 98:1538–1542, 1990.

12. Hunter SF, Weinshenker BG, Carter JL, et al: Rational clinical immunotherapy for multiple sclerosis. Mayo Clin Proc 172:765–780, 1997.
13. Krupp LB, Coyle PK, Doscher C, et al: Fatigue therapy in multiple sclerosis: Results of a double-blind, randomized, parallel trial of amantadine, pemoline, and placebo. Neurology 45:1956–1961, 1995.
14. Krupp LB, Pollina DA: Mechanisms and management of fatigue in progressive neurological disorders. Curr Opin Neurol 9:456–460, 1996.
15. Kurtzke JF: A new scale for evaluating disability in multiple sclerosis. Neurology 5:580–583, 1955.
16. Kurtzke JF: On the evaluation of disability in multiple sclerosis. Neurology 11:686–694, 1961.
17. Kurtzke JF: Rating neurologic impairment in multiple sclerosis: An Expanded Disability Status Scale (EDSS). Neurology 99:1444–1452, 1983.
18. Lublin FD, Reingold SC: Defining the clinical course on multiple sclerosis: Results of an international survey. Neurology 46: 907–911, 1996.
19. Optic Neuritis Study Group: Visual function 5 years after optic neuritis. Arch Ophthalmol 115:1545–1552, 1997.
20. Petajan JH, Gappmaier E, White AT, et al: Impact of aerobic training on fitness and quality of life in multiple sclerosis. Ann Neurol 39:432–441, 1996.
21. Rao SM: Neuropsychology of multiple sclerosis: a critical review. J Clin Exp Neuropsychol 8:503–542, 1986.
22. Rodriguez M, Siva A, Ward J, et al: Impairment, disability, and handicap in multiple sclerosis: A population-based study in Olmsted County, Minnesota. Neurology 44:28–33, 1994.
23. Rudick R, Antel J, Confavreux C, et al: Clinical outcomes assessment in multiple sclerosis. Ann Neurol 40:469–479, 1996.
24. Rudick RA,. Cohen JA, Weinstock-Guttman B, et al: Management of multiple sclerosis. N Engl J Med 337:1604–1617, 1997.
25. Sadovnick AD, Remick RA, Allen J, et al: Depression and multiple sclerosis. Neurology 46:628–632, 1996.
26. Simon JH, Jacobs LD, Campion MK, et al: A longitudinal study of brain atrophy in relapsing multiple sclerosis. Neurology 53:139–148, 1999.
27. Solari A; Filippini G; Gasco P, et al: Physical rehabilitation has a positive effect in multiple sclerosis patients. Neurology 52:57–62, 1999.
28. Stolp-Smith KA, Carter JL, Rohe DE, et al: Management of impairment, disability and handicap due to multiple sclerosis. Mayo Clin Proc 72:1184–1196, 1997.
29. Trapp BD, Peterson J, Ransohoff RM, et al: Axonal transection in the lesions of multiple sclerosis. N Engl J Med 338:278–285, 1998.

29. MOVEMENT DISORDERS

Kenneth H. Silver, M.D., Paul Fishman, M.D., Ph.D., and John Speed, MBBS

Never confuse motion with action.—Benjamin Franklin

1. How can we categorize the involuntary movement disorders into their general types?

Involuntary movement disorders can usually be classified as those characterized by too little (hypokinetic) or too much movement (hyperkinetic):

Hypokinetic	Hyperkinetic
Parkinson's disease	Tremors
Parkinson-like conditions	Tics
Progressive supranuclear palsy	Tourette syndrome
Drug-induced	Dystonia (generalized and focal)
Olivopontine-cerebellar degeneration	Dyskinesia (including tardive dyskinesias)
Multisystem atrophy	Hemifacial spasm
Shy-Drager syndrome	Athetosis
Nigral-striatal degeneration	Chorea (including Hungtington's disease)
	Hemiballismus myoclonus
	Asterixis

PARKINSON'S DISEASE

2. What are the major clinical features of Parkinson's disease?

Parkinsonian patients commonly show a **resting tremor**, **bradykinesia** or slowness of movement, and a form of increased muscular tone called **rigidity**. Other common features include a reduction in movements of facial expression resulting in "**masked facies**," **stooped posture**, and reduction of the amplitude of movements (**hypometria**). Also seen are changes in speech to a soft monotone (**hypophonia**) and small, less legible handwriting (**micrographia**). Walking becomes slower, stride length is reduced, and pivoting is replaced with a series of small steps (**turning "en bloc"**).

3. Who gets Parkinson's disease?

Parkinson's is a disease of older people. Although its incidence is only 20/100,000 in the general population, over 1% of those over age 65 have Parkinson's. The cause of Parkinson's disease is unknown, but people with a history of exposure to pesticides and herbicides (such as farm workers) appear to be at increased risk. Between 5% and 10% of cases may have an inherited basis.

4. How does Parkinson's usually begin?

The most common initial symptom is **resting tremor**, which usually goes away when the limb is in motion. The tremor usually begins in the hand, while head tremor (titubation) is unusual. Activities that involve other limbs, such as walking, usually increase the tremor. Patients may feel clumsy or weak as well as slow and stiff. They will have noticed that certain normal activities such as dressing (particularly buttoning), shaving, cutting food, and writing are more difficult. Family members may notice the patient's appearance and feel that he or she is "depressed" (there *is* an increased incidence of depression among patients with Parkinson's).

5. What other conditions can look like Parkinson's disease?

1. **Drug-induced parkinsonism:** dopamine-blocking medications, including antipsychotics such as haloperidol (Haldol) and thioridazine (Mellaril) and antinausea drugs such as metoclopramide (Reglan) and prochlorperazine (Compazine), can cause a syndrome that appears identical to Parkinson's disease. This type of parkinsonism usually has **prominent tremor** and is related to the dose and potency of medication. It usually develops within days to weeks after starting the medication and resolves within days to weeks of its discontinuation.

Other syndromes may present with the characteristic symptoms of Parkinson's disease (tremor and rigidity) but also include other features. These syndromes generally respond poorly to drug therapy and are less likely to have the isolated resting tremor of Parkinson's disease.

2. **Progressive supranuclear palsy** (PSP): reduction in vertical gaze and slowing of eye movements.

3. **Multisystem atrophy** (MSA) which includes **Shy-Drager syndrome** (autonomic failure with prominent postural hypotension) and corticobasal ganglionic degeneration with dystonia and dementia.

4. **Multiple head trauma (parkinsonism pugilistica):** early dementia with brisk tendon reflexes.

5. **Olivoponto-cerebellar degeneration** (OPCA): prominent intention tremor and ataxia.

6. Which drugs are used to treat early Parkinson's disease?

L-**Dopa** given in combination with **carbidopa** (Sinemet) is the most effective medication for the relief of Parkinson's disease but is usually not the first medication given to a newly diagnosed patient. L-Dopa typically loses its efficacy within 3–5 years after beginning therapy, so an effort is made to manage early disease with other medications.

A guiding principle is to start L-dopa treatment in patients with symptoms that interfere with the performance of ADLS despite other treatment. A resting tremor alone does not *usually* impede function.

Anticholinergic drugs such as trihexyphenidyl (Artane, 2–15 mg) are widely used to treat early Parkinson's patients with tremor as their primary symptom. **Amantadine** (Symmetrel, 100 mg bid) is another useful medication in early disease. Although its usefulness in early disease is controversial, the monoamine oxidase inhibitor **deprenyl**, or **selegiline** (Eldepryl, 5 mg bid), is widely given to newly diagnosed patients.

7. When and how is L-dopa therapy administered?

Within 1–2 years of diagnosis, most patients will have sufficient difficulties with movement and ADLs to require L-dopa. A common starting dose is 25 mg/100 mg twice daily (25 carbidopa, 100 L-dopa). Over time, patients will notice that improvement seen with each dose seems to "wear off" before the next dose. Gradually over the years, the patient's frequency of dosing, total dose needed, and need for other medications will all increase.

Controlled release forms of carbidopa/L-dopa and selegiline are useful to increase the duration of action of L-dopa. The recently introduced COMT inhibitors to **tolcapone** (Tasmar) and **entacapone** (Comtan) can substantially increase the duration of action of L-dopa. Tolcapone's use is limited by reports of serious hepatoxicity, although it is far less toxic than the never-released Alcapone (joke!). Early Parkinson's disease can also be treated with the newer dopamine agonists pergolide (Permax), pramipexole (Mirapex), or ropinirole (Requip). These agents have a longer duration of action and are also useful in patients showing signs of decreased drug efficacy.

8. What are the common side effects of drugs used in treating Parkinson's disease?

Antiparkinson medications work either by replacing dopamine (levodopa), acting as a post-synaptic dopamine agonist (pergolide), or reestablishing the dopamine/acetylcholine balance in the striatum (anticholinergics). The commonest side effects of L-dopa are **nausea, abdominal cramping**, and **diarrhea**. These side effects are significantly reduced when L-dopa is given in combination with carbidopa, a peripheral decarboxylase inhibitor which prevents the peripheral conversion of levodopa to dopamine. Dopamine agonists, in general, cause nausea more frequently than the L-dopa/carbidopa combinations.

All antiparkinson drugs cause **postural hypotension**, which can reach symptomatic levels. This can be treated with salt supplements and salt-retaining mineralocorticoids (fludrocortisone, Florinef). Virtually all antiparkinson drugs can cause **confusion**, hallucinations, and even psychosis. Cognitively impaired patients and those with psychiatric illness are most at risk. Low doses of the atypical antipsychotic clozapine (Clozaril) have been shown to treat such psychosis without worsening the signs of Parkinson's disease; olanzapine (Zyprexa) and quetiapine (Seroquel) are also useful.

9. What are the surgical options for treating or controlling Parkinson's disease?

Patients with moderate to severe motor symptoms despite optimal medical management— particularly those with fluctuating responses to each dose of medication—can benefit from surgery. Three different brain regions which are potential sources of the tremor in Parkinson's disease (thalamus, globus pallidus, and subthalamic nucleus) can be targets for **stereotactic-guided surgery**. A lesion created in these regions inhibits the generation of tremor. Patients can have a lesion created with "a radiofrequency device" (this is in general a better way of informing patients than the lay explanation "we will stick a microwave probe in your head and cook a small part of your brain"). These procedures should be done only by very skilled neurosurgeons. Performing stereotactic surgery is like playing a PGA golf course: the penalties for missing the green even slightly are severe.

For patients who do not want a brain "lesion," an alternative is the implantation of a **deep brain stimulator** (DBS). This high-frequency jamming signal creates the same benefit as destructive surgery but is potentially adjustable and reversible if complications occur. The disadvantage is that the patient will indefinitely have a wire in their brain connected to a pacemaker-like device in their chest, with the need for battery replacement and the potential for device failure. DBS to the thalamus is very effective for relief of severe tremor whether caused by Parkinson's disease or essential tremor.

Another procedure, **fetal nigral cell transplantation**, is an experimental procedure still under development.

10. Describe the usual course of Parkinson's disease.

Parkinson's disease usually begins in one limb, but all limbs eventually become affected. Most patients have increasing disability despite medical treatment within 3–5 years after diagnosis. In moderately affected patients, not only is gait affected, but also postural stability becomes impaired. More advanced patients can also have loss of action of L-dopa at times not simply related to end-of-dose (**on-off syndrome**), which can be very abrupt (freezing). Attempts to improve symptoms by increasing medications seem to overshoot, resulting in the induction of involuntary jerking and twisting movements (**dyskinesias**). Advanced patients move frequently from periods of relative immobility ("off" or akinesia) to normal mobility ("on") to abnormal movements that interfere with voluntary movements ("on" with dyskinesias). **Postural changes** such as stooping with the development of permanent kyphosis can occur after years of disease.

Symptoms that respond poorly to pharmacological treatment include freezing, loss of postural stability (with falling), stooping with kyphosis, and dementia. Depression, commonly seen in Parkinson's patients, improves with standard antidepressants such as tricyclics or serotonin reuptake inhibitors, not usually with L-dopa.

11. What are the causes of disability in Parkinson's disease?

Social isolation, often due to changes in physical appearance, is common in Parkinson's patients. Even in mildly affected patients many physical activities require additional effort to perform. This leads to declining efficiency at work and, in many cases, abandoning many forms of leisure activities. **Manual dexterity** is invariably impaired as Parkinson's worsens, affecting many ADLs such as dressing, cutting food, writing, and handling small objects (e.g., coins).

Walking becomes impaired as the disease progresses. Postural alterations include increased neck, trunk, and hip flexion which, coupled with a decrease in righting and equilibrium reactions, leads to balance deficits and an increased risk of falling. Slowing of gait is typically seen, with difficulty turning and a tendency toward short shuffling steps. Tripping may occur on irregular surfaces. The patient tends to stagger backwards (**retropulsion**) when pushed from the front and forward (**propulsion**) when pushed from behind. Patients have a gait similar to the very elderly, where attempts to increase speed result in more rapid stepping but not in increased stride length. Worsening proximal muscle rigidity signficantly reduces trunk rotation and arm swing.

Speech impairment in Parkinson's results in soft, monotonic, virtually mumbled speech. Advanced patients will have **dysphagia** as well and are at risk of silent aspiration. **Drooling** is more a result of decreased frequency of spontaneous swallowing rather than an increase in saliva production.

12. As rehabilitationists, what is important in evaluating the patient with Parkinson's disease?

First, assess the degree of rigidity and bradykinesia and how these syptoms interfere with ADLs. This can be done objectively using established scales for Parkinson's disease, such as the Unified Parkinson's Disease Rating Scale (UPDRS). It is important to note not only which tasks can be performed but how long is required. The general pattern of gait, including walking speed and distance, should be gauged. Forward and backward stepping as well as the ability to navigate obstacles needs to be checked. Fine motor tasks such as writing should be periodically assessed. Measurements need to be recorded for restrictions in joint mobility, particularly hips, knees, shoulders, and trunk. Analysis of equilibrium is important and should include tandem walking. Because of the difficulty Parkinson's patients have in performing complex movements, evaluation should include the ability to perform simultaneous and sequential tasks.

13. Which physical therapy strategies are useful for the Parkinson's patient?

In general, patients need to be counseled to maintain a reasonable level of activity at all costs, as physical exertion becomes more difficult with disease progression and the risk of deconditioning increases. More complex disability will often require the attention of the rehabilitation team.

The typical habitus of the Parkinson's patient is a stooped posture with flexed upper extremities, minimal trunk rotation, and a shuffling gait with a narrow base of support. Exercises focus on proper body alignment (upright posture) and postural reflexes (response to dynamic balance challenges). Although symptoms caused by the disease itself (rigidity, bradykinesia, and tremor) are not generally amenable to specific physiotherapies, the secondary manifestations of loss of extremity and axial ROM and deconditioning, which in turn contribute to defects in gait, balance, and transfers, are often responsive to PT.

14. Describe PT strategies to help with postural problems in Parkinson's disease.

To offset the tendency toward forward trunk flexion, performing hip extension while standing is stressed. Pelvic-tilt exercises for the low back and stretching the pectoral and iliopsoas muscles will assist in maintaining normal postural alignment. A variety of arm, leg, and trunk stretching exercises performed either by the therapist or at home can offset the tendency to lose joint ROM from the rigidity and bradykinesia. These may include passive and active-assisted stretching combined with relaxation techniques and can include shoulder-girdle exercises with a broomstick handle or a pulley to stretch the arms and trunk. Back flexion and extension exercises can be useful in improving balance and posture in sitting and standing. Quadriceps and hip extensor strengthening also can assist the patient in being able to climb stairs or arise from a sitting surface.

15. Which PT strategies should be considered to help with gait difficulties?

Frenkel exercises for coordination of foot placement are helpful to maintain accurate lower-extremity positioning during the gait cycle. Wobbleboard or balance-feedback trainers can be used to improve body alignment and postural reflexes. The tendency to topple backwards can be addressed with heel-lifts as well as by assistive mobility devices.

Stationary bicycles, arm ergometers, and treadmills can help to restore diminished reciprocal limb motions and increase step length. Proper heelstrike should be emphasized, as should adequate arm swing and trunk rotation during ambulation. The tendency to freeze in narrow and complicated spaces can be reduced with visual targets, such as the tip of a walking stick or markers on the floor. Some patients prevent freezing by counting rhythmically as they walk or humming marching music. When frozen, relaxing back on the heels and lifting the toes as well as raising the arms from the sides with sudden movements can help restore locomotion.

The difficulty in arising from sitting surfaces can be addressed with elevated sitting surfaces (chair, toilet) and strategically placed grab rails/bars (bed, bathtub). Small mats and rugs that can trip the shuffling patient should be removed.

16. Discuss the use of wheelchairs and walkers for these patients.

The patient may eventually need a wheelchair. An effort should be made to keep the person with Parkinson's ambulatory as long as feasible to minimize the development of contracture, stiffness, and deconditioning that attends further immobilization. Although wheeled walkers are useful in assisting ambulation particulary by preventing backward instability, patients with significant postural deficits may prefer more stable devices (such as a supermarket shopping cart or walking behind a wheelchair). Some wheeled walkers have been designed specifically for Parkinson's patients. They have added weight to lower their center of gravity. Handbrakes are essential in such devices to ensure control, and patients must have the arm/hand dexterity and cognition to use them.

17. Which occupational therapy strategies can help the person with Parkinson's?

OTs can provide vital input for maintaining the home, vocational, leisure, and transportation capabilities of the patient. **Adaptive equipment** is provided when deficits in upper-extremity control limit efficient and safe function. For instance, plate-guards or specialized dishes prevent food from sliding off; plates can be weighted or made more adherent to the table. Cups and utensils can have large handles and also may be weighted to dampen excessive motions with tremor. Swivel forks and spoons can help compensate for lost ROM. Buttons on clothing can be replaced with Velcro or zipper closures.

Other **environmental aids** can help keep the person with Parkinson's disease productive at work. Workplace adaptations to accommodate for Parkinson's-related impairments and disabilities may include equipment to support writing (built-up pens and forearm supports) and typing skills (electronic keyboards and computerized scanning and pointing devices), as well as power mobility devices (scooters or wheelchairs).

Manys patients can retain driving ability, although the slowing of motor responses as the disease worsens may place these patients at risk when driving. Occupational therapists (or other qualified therapists) can play a critical role in **assessment and retraining of driving skills**, particularly extremity reaction timing and visual field scanning. Families should be counseled to have the patient undergo driver's testing and training earlier when mobility and ADL performance has begun to suffer, rather than later when accidents will more likely occur.

18. How can the speech therapist intervene in Parkinson's disease?

The hypokinetic dysarthria seen in patients can be addressed with **diaphragmatic breathing exercises** and improved posture and flexibility that increase vital capacity. There is variability in the prevalence and type of swallowing disorder of the Parkinson patient. The patient often has trouble with oral bolus formation, as well as loss of coordination between oral and pharyngeal stages of swallowing. Tongue and mandibular movement and range are commonly limited. After proper **swallowing assessment**, strategies can include using smaller portion size taken more frequently, altering food textures and consistencies to maximize safe oropharyngeal function, optimizing head and neck position during swallow, facilitating oral and pharyngeal movement and reflexes, and performing exercises to increase facial and lingual strength and ROM.

HYPERKINETIC MOVEMENT DISORDERS

19. What is tremor and how can it be classified?

Tremors, the most common form of involuntary movement disorders, are characterized by rhythmic oscillations of a body part. Tremors can be classified as to the situation in which they are most prominent. First, is the tremor most pronounced at rest or with movement?

- **Tremors with movement** are subdivided into those occurring (1) with maintained posture (**postural or static tremor**, tested by holding arms out in front of the patient); (2) with movement from point to point (**kinetic or intentional tremor**, tested by performing finger-to-nose); or (3) only with a specific type of movement (**task-specific tremor**).
- Tremors that are at their **worst at rest** are exclusively associated with Parkinson's disease or other parkinsonian states (such as those produced by neuroleptics).

20. Name the common postural tremors.

Physiologic tremor	Tremor with peripheral neuropathy
Essential (familial, senile) tremor	Post-traumatic tremor
Tremor with basal ganglia disease	Alcoholic tremor
Cerebellar postural tremor	

21. What are the common kinetic tremors?

Cerebellar tremor and rubral tremor.

22. What are the common task-specific tremors?

Primary writing tremor, vocal tremor, and orthostatic tremor.

23. Are physiologic tremors worrisome?

No, they are usually of no clinical significance and often increase or are precipitated by emotional stress, aggravated by fatigue, hypoglycemia, thyrotoxicosis, exercise, alcohol withdrawal, and fever, and can be drug-induced (caffeine, theophylline, lithium). They can be treated by educating the patient to avoid precipitating conditions.

24. How are other tremors treated?

Although **essential tremor** is commonly abbreviated as ET, it is the commonest cause of tremor on earth. The most useful medication in treating ET, task-specific tremor, and action tremor is **propranolol** (40–240 mg). Other beta-blockers have fewer side effects but are less effective. The anticonvulsant **primidone** and the benzodiazepene **clonazepam** are also effective antitremor drugs.

Measures to reduce or alleviate anxiety are useful, as are strategies to control oscillation excursion with weights or other mechanical compensations. Treatment is usually unsatisfactory for intention tremor, but again weighting the limb can be of limited help. Severe, disabling tremor can be significantly, and at times dramatically, improved with stereotactic thalamotomy or implantation of a deep brain stimulator (the only FDA-approved treatment of ET).

25. What is the physiologic basis for tics?

This is largely unknown. Tics are sustained nonrhythmic muscle contractions that are rapid and stereotyped, often occurring in the same extremity or body part during times of stress. Usually, the muscles of the face and neck are involved, with movement of a rotational sort away from the body's midline. They are often seen in otherwise normal children between ages of 5 and 10 and usually disappear by the end of adolescence. Tics have not been known to cause physical impairment but may have obvious social consequences and handicaps.

Tics can be seen as representing a spectrum of disease from **transient** tic disorder (duration < 1 year) to **chronic** tic disorder (duration > 1 year, manifesting as either vocal or motor tics, but not both). **Tourette's syndrome** lies somewhere on that spectrum, characterized by motor and vocal tics lasting for more than 1 year. Tic disorders are commonly familial (predominantly male) and are possibly variable expressions of the same genetic abnormality.

26. What is the most socially disabling aspect of Gilles de la Tourette syndrome?

Probably, the involuntary use of obscenities (**coprolalia**) as well as obscene gestures (**copropraxia**), although such behavior may be mild and transient and occurs only in a minority of afflicted persons. Other unfortunate features of this hereditary disease include vocal and motor tics, echolalia, loud cries, and yips. The tics can begin with the eyes or as a facial grimace, but can involve the head, neck, trunk, or legs. Some affected individuals have few symptoms, while others can be socially disabled. The tics may not always be present, having a waxing and waning quality, and the patient may be able to voluntarily suppress them. Emotional problems during childhood are common in those affected, as are attention-deficit disorders, obsessive-compulsive disorders, and learning problems. Many have behavioral problems later in life.

Neuroleptics, most commonly pimozide and haloperidol, are most predictably effective, but sedation limits their use. Other medications shown to be of use include benzodiazepines, clonazepam, clonidine, reserpine, and calcium channel blockers. Behavioral manifestations can respond to psychotherapy, and anxiety can be addressed with relaxation exercises and biofeedback.

27. What common features of dystonias distinguish them from other movement disorders?

Dystonias are slow, sustained contractions of muscles that frequently cause twisting movements or abnormal postures. The disorder resembles athetosis but shows a more sustained isometric contraction. When rapid movements are involved, they are usually repetitive and continuous. The movements are a result of simultaneous co-contraction of agonists and antagonists and can interfere with speed, smoothness, and accuracy of movements in the affected body part.

Dystonia often increases with emotional or physical stress, anxiety, pain, or fatigue and disappears with sleep. Symptom severity can vary through the day. Patients often develop methods to self-inhibit or diminish the dystonic movements by changing posture or touching the affected body part.

28. How are the dystonias classified?

Usually by the distribution of affected muscles:
Focal
Torticollis (neck)
Blepharospasm (periorbital)
Oromandibular (mouth or jaw)
Writer's or occupational cramp (arm or leg)

Segmental	**Multifocal**
Cranial	Generalized
Brachial	Dystonia musculorum deformans
Crural	

29. What causes dystonias?

The most common dystonias are usually idiopathic. Some patients have inherited or metabolic disorders, such as **dystonia musculorum deformans**, **Wilson's disease** (degeneration of liver and basal ganglia), and **lipid storage diseases**. Patients with certain neurodegenerative diseases can exhibit dystonia, such as Parkinson's, Huntington's, and Leigh's diseases. Dystonias can have acquired causes such as perinatal brain injury, carbon monoxide poisoning, or encephalitis. Focal brain disease involving the basal ganglia, such as stroke, tumor, or local trauma, can cause dystonia on the contralateral body side. Spinal cord disorders such as syringomyelia or tumor can cause segmental or focal dystonia.

30. What is spasmodic torticollis? How is it treated?

Spasmodic torticollis is the most common focal dystonia. It affects most frequently the sternocleidomastoid, trapezius, scalenes, and posterior neck muscles in an asymmetric pattern. The patients are predominantly female in their fourth or fifth decade. The movement can be tonic or intermittent, and the head usually rotates to one side or the other but also can assume a predominantly forward (**antecolic**) or backward (**retrocolic**) position. Improvement of symptoms often occurs with the use of certain gestures of the hands to various head or facial sites (e.g., lightly touching the chin with a finger). Symptoms are worsened by prolonged standing or walking or under conditions of stress or fatigue. Associated pain is common and can either be an initial presentation or develop in time. Complete or partial remissions can occur. Social stigmatization is a major concern as are functional impairments, which can include driving, reading, or activities that involve looking down and using the hands.

Rehabilitation management can include pain control, stretching tight musculature, and trigger point injections. Although some suggest exercises to strengthen contralateral, uninvolved muscles and reciprocally inhibit involved ones, others feel such exercises worsen symptoms. Biofeedback has been used but is not routinely effective. The mainstay of treatment here, as in the other focal dystonias, remains pharmacological intervention, especially intramuscular injection of botulinum toxin.

31. What is blepharospasm?

Blepharospasm is characterized by intermittent contractions of the orbicularis oculi. Its early presentation may be as uncontrolled, excessive blinking from presumed eye irritation, but the condition progresses to irregular and more forceful and sustained closure of the lids. It can stigmatize the patient and even interfere with the performance of some ADLs, particularly driving. Sunlight can make the problem more pronounced.

32. What features are characteristic of writer's cramp?

Writer's or occupational cramp involves the dominant hand and wrist and appears during certain activities, such as writing, typing, or playing a musical instrument. The many appellations referring to the precipitating activity include writer's cramp, pianist's hand, telegrapher's cramp, or "chapter-writer's spasm." It presents with onset of a specific activity as an uncontrollably tight grip, accompanied by flexion of the wrist. It may be associated with jerking or sustained movements. Usually, other coordinated movements of that extremity are normal. Often, the symptoms present in a certain posture or position—for instance, a patient may be able to write at a blackboard, but not seated at a desk.

Therapy is directed at re-educating muscle movement patterns and maintaining ROM. Enlarging or changing the contour of grasped objects, such as built-up pens, are useful. Relaxation exercises are helpful as can be splinting to minimize or inhibit dystonic postures or teaching contralateral hand use.

33. Define oromandibular dystonia.

Oromandibular dystonia involves muscles of the tongue, mouth, and jaw, causing the mouth to pull open or forcibly shut. The mentalis and platysma muscles also may be involved. The jaw can be retracted or deviated to the side. With lingual involvement, the tongue has abnormal movements during speaking or deglutition. The result of such dystonias is impaired speech and eating. Occupational and speech therapy can address these problems in similar ways to Parkinson's disease.

34. Which multifocal dystonia typically presents with spasms of the lower extremities and later progresses to involve other muscle groups?

Dystonia musculorum deformans is a rare hereditary disorder, with symptoms beginning between ages 5 and 15 and consisting of sustained movements with torsional spasms of the pelvis and legs, resulting in abnormal gait. Upper-extremity, neck, and facial muscles become involved later in the course. Unfortunately, the disease is often confused with hysterical or other psychiatric disturbances. In the more severe forms, progression to death within 5 to 10 years occurs. The cause is unknown, but some have described pathological alterations in the basal thalamus.

35. How are dystonias treated?

Detection and correction of an underlying abnormality (drug-induced, structural cause) is the first step. In children particularly, a small group (10–20%) improve with L-dopa therapy. Anticholinergics such as trihexyphenidyl and benztropine are the most effective oral agents for both generalized and focal dystonias. Baclofen, carbamazepine, and clonazepam are sometimes helpful. Focal dystonias are now commonly treated with botulinum toxin.

36. What is the role of botulinum toxin injection in treating the dystonias? How does it work?

Although more commonly used for treating spasticity, the use of botulinum toxin was pioneered in the treatment of focal dystonias. It has proved highly effective for blepharospasm and laryngeal dystonias (spasmodic dysphonia) and cervical dystonias and has also shown benefit in focal dystonias of the upper extremity (e.g., writer's cramp).

For a detailed discussion of botulinum toxin, see chapter 81 of this book. Briefly, the injected toxin interferes with the release of acetylcholine at the presynaptic cholinergic terminal, resulting in a chemical denervation of the treated muscle. The effect begins in several days, is maximal in 1–2 weeks, usually persists for 3–4 months, and requires periodic reinjection. Side effects are transient and almost always mild—usually either additional weakness of the injected muscle, local soreness, hoarseness, or dysphagia, depending largely on the proximity of injected muscles to important structures. Presently, the medication, although used in minute doses, is extremely expensive, and its cost may not be reimbursed by all insurers.

37. What is hemifacial spasm?

This is the most frequent form of the facial hyperkinetic movement disorders, although it still is relatively uncommon. It is seen most often in women in mid life. The disorder can interfere with vision and be socially and psychologically disabling. It is aggravated by stress and fatigue. The spasms, which are tonic, usually begin in the orbicularis oculi and later involve other muscles innervated by CN7.

The etiology is generally unknown but usually involves a region of abnormal electrical impulse generation and transmission in the peripheral facial nerve. Some feel that the disorder is due to vascular compression of the facial nerve, and surgery has often proved effective. It is important to rule out other rare but serious causes such as brainstem glioma.

Although carbamazepine has been suggested as being useful, it has not been shown effective in clinical studies. Treatment options usually boil down to either surgery for facial nerve decompression or botulinum toxin injection.

38. Which movement disorder is associated with chronic neuroleptic therapy?

Tardive dyskinesia (TD) is a condition characterized by involuntary, choreiform movements of the face and tongue associated with chronic neuroleptic medication use. Common movements include chewing, sucking, mouthing, licking, "fly-catching movements," and puckering or smacking (buccal-lingual-masticatory syndrome). Choreiform movements of the trunk and extremities can also occur, along with dystonic movements of the neck and trunk. TD occcurs in up to 20% of patients treated chronically with neuroleptics (dopamine antagonists) and probably represents hypersensitivity of dopamine receptors and overactivity of the dopamine system due to long-term dopamine receptor blockade. Duration of treatment, dose, and age are risk factors for its development. Similar movements can also be seen in the elderly without exposure to dopamine-blocking drugs. Resolution of TD after neuroleptic drugs are withdrawn is slow and incomplete, with half of TD patients still symptomatic a year after drug discontinuation.

39. Can tardive dyskinesia be treated or prevented?

Preventive measures include using minimal doses of neuroleptics and withdrawal of these medications at the onset of TD-like symptoms. The atypical neuroleptics **clozapine** and **risperidone** are useful to control psychosis in TD patients without worsening symptoms. Benzodiazepines such as **clonazepam** are the most useful medication for suppression of the movements. Dopamine depletion with **reserpine** can improve symptoms but is commonly associated with hypotension and depression. Since the symptoms are most prominent at rest, activity (including chewing gum) can be of some value to patients. Some have suggested value in oral desensitization when hyperreactivity to sensory stimuli exists. Other rehabilitation strategies are not of proven utility.

40. What causes ataxia and how can it be treated?

Along with intention tremor and dysmetria (inaccuracy on finger-nose-finger testing), ataxia is usually associated with cerebellar disease. Common causes include stroke, multiple sclerosis, and acute and chronic toxicity (alcohol most commonly). Slowly progressive ataxia may represent a group of hereditary disorders, some of which are diagnosed with genetic testing. Unexplained ataxia can be an autoimmune manifestation of an otherwise occult malignancy (ovarian, breast, small cell carcinoma).

The response to drug therapy has been poor with many agents touted as useful (propranolol, isoniazid, carbamazepine, clonazepam, tryptophan, buspirone, thyroid-stimulating hormone). The mainstay of treatment for ataxia is occupational therapy to help learn compensatory techniques for performing basic self-care and occupational activities, and assessing the benefits of weighted bracelets or similar devices to damp the oscillations. Gait training and education in the use of assistive devices for walking can prevent falls and enhance mobility in the ataxic individual.

41. How do athetosis, chorea, and ballismus differ?

Athetosis is characterized by involuntary, slow, writhing, and repetitious movements. They are slower than choreiform movements and less sustained than dystonia. Athetosis may be seen alone or in combination with other movement disorders and itself leads to bizarre but characteristic postures. Any part of the body can be affected, but it is usually the face and distal upper extremities. The onset may be idiopathic, but the disorder is often secondary to another neurologic disease, such as stroke, tumor, or Wilson's disease.

Chorea presents as nonstereotyped, unpredictable, and jerky movements that interfere with purposeful motion. The movements are rapid, erratic, and complex and can be seen in any or all body parts, but usually involves the oral structures (causing abnormal speech and respiratory patterns). It may occur in almost any disease of the CNS. When seen in Parkinson's disease, chorea is usually secondary to antiparkinson's medication. Treatment approaches with medications aim at decreasing dopamine availability or increasing anticholinergic activity. The most familiar, generalized form is **Huntington's disease** (see below).

Hemiballismus is an uncommon disorder consisting of extremely violent flinging of the arms and legs on one side of the body. It is usually secondary to hemorrhage or infarction of the contralateral subthalmic nucleus. It can also be the result of tumor or abscess. So violent are the movements that they can lead to exhaustion or injury if not controlled. Some success has been noted with neuroleptic agents, and careful weighting of the extremities can help.

42. Is Huntington disease (HD) treatable and who is at risk?

Chorea means "to dance," and the gait in these patients takes on an ataxic, dancing appearance. HD unfortunately is a terminal disorder involving involuntary, choreiform movements that are abrupt and purposeless and is associated with a progressive dementia. It is an autosomal dominant hereditary disorder affecting 4–6 persons/100,000 population. It reached the public's attention as afflicting Woody Guthrie, a well-known American folksinger.

Symptom onset can range from childhood to the eighth decade, although most individuals become affected after age 30. The abnormal movements begin in the fingers, toes, and facial regions, often with dysarthria, teeth grinding, and facial grimacing. Along with the choreiform movement, progressive dementia and emotional/behavioral abnormalities are seen. As the disease progresses, the presentation becomes less choreiform and more parkinsonian and dystonic (i.e., restricted motions, immobility, and unsteadiness of gait). Intellectual impairment and psychosis invariably occur and progress rapidly to become the most disabling features. The rate of suicide is 2000 times the national average. Symptoms progress over a 10–25-year period and death is usually by aspiration pneumonia.

The pathology of HD includes degeneration of the basal ganglia, particularly the caudate nucleus. There is no treatment proven to reduce the progression of disease, but symptomatic relief is indicated, especially for the abnormal movements, depression, and psychosis. Family supportive services and psychosocial and genetic counseling are invariably needed, particularly as recent genetic testing diagnoses the disease in both symptomatic and presymptomatic individuals. Rehabilitation techniques that involve improving coactivation and trunk stability, rhythmical stabilization, and traditional relaxation techniques (including biofeedback) have been mentioned as reasonable strategies.

43. What causes myoclonus, and is it common?

Myoclonus is one of the most common involuntary movement disorders of CNS origin. It is characterized by sudden, jerky, irregular contractions of a muscle or groups of muscles. It can be subdivided into myoclonus that is *stimulus-sensitive* (**reflex myoclonus**), appearing with volitional movement, muscle stretch, or superficial stimuli such as touch, or *non–stimulus-sensitive myoclonus* which occurs at rest (**spontaneous myoclonus**). Myoclonic movements can be either irregular or periodic.

Etiologically, myoclonus can be either **physiologic** (occurring in normals while falling asleep, walking. or with anxiety, e.g., sleep jerks and hiccups); **essential** (increasing with activity, sometimes disabling but without neurologic deficit); **epileptic** (associated with generalized seizures, as in juvenile myoclonic epilepsy), and **symptomatic** (part of a more widespread neurologic disorder such as an encephalopathy or stroke). **Spinal myoclonus** involves a group of muscles innervated by a certain spinal segment (segmental myoclonus) and can be associated with spinal cord disease (i.e. trauma or multiple sclerosis) and tumors.

A number of drugs have been used to treat myoclonus and can be effective in some situations. These include diazepam, clonazepam, valproate, and the new antiepileptic leviracetam. Tryptophan was once considered useful but is no longer prescribed because of an uncommon, severe side effect (eosinophilia-myalgia syndrome).

44. What types of movement disorders can be psychogenic?

Psychogenic movement disorders mimic the entire spectrum of organic movement disorders, including tremor, dystonia, myoclonus, and parkinsonism (in decreasing order of frequency). In one series of 842 patients with movement disorders, 28 (3.3%) were diagnosed as having some type of psychogenic movement disorder. Psychogenic movement disorders can occur in conjunction with organic movement disorders; this occurs in about 25% of patients diagnosed with psychogenic movement disorder.

45. How can psychogenic movement disorders be distinguished from organic disorders?

Psychogenic movement disorders are diagnosed by clinical features inconsistent with the presentation or natural history of organic movement disorders. A careful evaluation should include history and setting of onset; factors that exacerbate or abate the movements; observation at rest, in action, and with distraction; and evaluation of tone, reflexes, and strength. Psychogenic etiologies should be considered when the onset, course, or manifestations are unusual. There is often an association with prior psychiatric disease, particularly depression, and most patients will have other pseudoneurologic symptoms (e.g., weakness or sensory loss). There is often obvious secondary gain and/or litigation involved.

Psychogenic Dystonias

Psychogenic dystonia—usually of abrupt onset, with rapid progression to a fixed dystonic posture, with inconsistent dystonic movements that attenuate with distraction. Intervening periods of normalcy are common. Lower extremities more commonly involved. Pain can be a prominent feature.

Psychogenic tremor—can vary enormously with distraction, and often will assume the frequency of repetitive movements performed by another limb. There is fatigue of the tremor and variable sensitivity to different stimuli.

Psychogenic parkinsonism—characterized by rigidity with features of voluntary resistance that varies with distraction. Arm swing may be reduced or absent, or the arm may be held tightly to the side. Most patients have tremor, present at rest and persisting with action. Tremor frequency may be highly variable. There may be generalized slowness of movement, "overflow" of motor activity to other body parts, grimacing or sighing with effort, and variability of function between tasks.

46. How can psychogenic movement disorders be treated?

As with other types of conversion disorder, the manner in which the suspected diagnosis is discussed is critical. It is best to be nonjudgmental, and stress that careful neurologic evaluation has demonstrated that the brain, spinal cord, nerves, and muscles are intact (when this is true!) and that with appropriate intervention, the movement disorder will resolve. Symptoms of shorter duration, of acute onset occurring in a previously healthy individual, or with an identified stressor are more likely to resolve quickly.

Treatment approaches include psychotherapy, placebo treatment, or behavioral management as used in other types of conversion disorder. Behavioral management involves immobilization of the affected body part(s), except while in physical or occupational therapy, and extinction of the abnormal behavior, with copious praise (reinforcement) given for more normal target behaviors. Psychogenic tremor, dystonia, and parkinsonism have been treated effectively in this manner.

BIBLIOGRAPHY

1. Dombovy M, Pippin B: Rehabilitation concerns in degenerative movement disorders of the central nervous system. In Braddom RL (ed): Physical Medicine and Rehabilitation, 2nd ed. Philadelphia, W.B. Saunders, 2000.
2. Duvaisin R: Parkinson's Disease: A Guide for Patients and Families. New York, Raven Press, 1991.
3. Elbe R, Koller W: Tremor. Baltimore, Johns Hopkins Press, 1990.
4. Factor R, Podskalny G, Molho E: Psychogenic movement disorders: Frequency, clinical profile, and characteristics. J. Neurol Neurosurg Psychiatry 59: 406–412, 1995.
5. Hallett M: Classification and treatment of tremor. JAMA 266:1115, 1991.
6. Jain S, Francisco G: Parkinson's disease and other movement disorders. In DeLisa JA, Gans BM (eds): Rehabilitation Medicine: Principles and Practice, 3rd ed. Philadelphia, Lippincott Williams & Wilkins 1998, pp 1035–1056.
7. Jankovic J, Hallett M: Therapy with Botulinum Toxin, New York, Marcel Dekker, 1994.
8. Johnson R, Griffen J (eds): Current Therapy in Neurologic Disease. St. Louis, Mosby, 1993.
9. Lang A, Lozano A: Parkinson's disease. (two parts) N Engl J Med 339:1044-1053, 1130–1143, 1998.
10. Marjama J, Troster A, Koller W: Psychogenic movement disorders. Neurol Clin 13:283–297, 1995.
11. Pentland B: Parkinsonism and dystonia. In Greenwood R, Barnes M, McMillan T, Ward C (eds): Neurological Rehabilitation. London, Churchhill Livingstone, 1993, pp 474–485.
12. Ranen N, Peyser C, Folstein S: A Physician's Guide to the Management of Huntington's Disease. New York, Huntington's Disease Society of America, 1993.
13. Weiner W, Lang A: Movement Disorders. New York, Futura, 1989.

30. TRAUMATIC BRAIN INJURY

Robert L. Harmon, M.D., M.S., and Lawrence J. Horn, M.D., M.R.M.

1. Why shouldn't I skip this chapter and simply read about stroke rehabilitation?

Although stroke and traumatic brain injury (TBI) both may involve brain lesions due to ischemia or hemorrhage, patients with TBI tend to have more diffuse impairments in brain function. These patients also classically tend to have more cognitive, personality and behavioral impairments than those following stroke. Also, a much larger proportion of younger patients have TBI than stroke. Understanding the issues surrounding TBI and its rehabilitation, however, can add to one's understanding about stroke and its rehabilitation, as well as rehabilitation following other forms of brain injury such as encephalitis.

2. What are the common causes of TBI?

Over half of the TBIs that occur in the United States are related to traffic accidents. Falls are the next most common cause of traumatic brain injury, most often occurring in those under 15 and over 70 years of age. Assaults and failed suicide attempts may also be significant causes in certain regions.

3. How does drug and alcohol use, use of helmets while riding motorcycles, and use of seat belts impact TBI incidence?

Alcohol use is associated with the occurrence of motor vehicle accidents and may also contribute to the occurrence of intracranial hemorrhage following head trauma. Other drugs, both legal and illegal, can impair cognition or reaction time and may also increase the risk of a motor vehicle accident. Illicit drug use in a region may also be associated with an increased risk of head injury from assaults. The use of seat belts and motorcycle helmets has been shown to significantly decrease the number of head injuries for wearers; the presence of air bags in a vehicle may also be found to significantly decrease TBI as more information becomes available. The occurrence of TBI, therefore, can be modified. This point will be important to remember as the consequences of TBI are discussed.

4. How often is TBI associated with spinal cord injury?

It is difficult to know exactly how many patients have a combined traumatic brain and spinal cord injury as many relatively mild brain injuries go undetected. Because motor vehicle accidents cause both types of injury, these lesions may occur together as high as 25–50% of the time. Motor or sensory system abnormalities not explained by a spinal cord lesion or cognitive deficits in a patient with spinal cord injury should trigger an evaluation for a possible associated brain injury.

5. How often is TBI associated with extremity fractures?

This also is difficult to determine. Approximately 10–11% of patients admitted to a rehabilitation service following TBI have previously unrecognized skeletal trauma, including of the spine. This is important because unrecognized fractures or joint dislocations may interfere with the functional restoration of these patients. Skeletal trauma may be associated with peripheral nerve injuries; long bone fractures also may be associated with an increased risk of heterotopic ossification. It has been suggested that radiographs of the spine and pelvis (and knees if the patient was a pedestrian hit by a motor vehicle) should be obtained 10–14 days postinjury in this population, with a whole-body bone scan considered for the skeletally immature patient.

6. What are the principal types of primary injuries resulting from TBI?

Primary injuries to the brain occur as a direct result of the forces involved in the traumatic event upon the brain and are not preventable except by preventing the traumatic event itself. These primary injuries include:

1. Contusions and lacerations of the brain surface (typically occurring on the frontal and temporal lobes inferiorly where the brain contacts the base of the skull)
2. Diffuse axonal injury (related to shearing injury disrupting nerve axons in the brain white matter)
3. Diffuse vascular injury resulting in multiple petechial hemorrhages within the brain
4. Contusion or shearing of the cranial nerves (most commonly the olfactory nerve)
5. Tearing of the pituitary stalk

7. What are secondary types of injury arising from brain trauma?

Secondary damage to the brain results from processes produced by the injuring event but tend to be somewhat delayed in their presentation, suggesting that it may be preventable (at least in theory). The principal types of secondary injuries include:

1. Intracranial hemorrhage (which may be extradural, subdural, subarachnoid, or intracerebral)
2. Brain swelling related to increased cerebral blood volume and/or cerebral edema
3. Increased intracranial pressure
4. Brain damage associated with hypoxia
5. Intracranial infection (particularly with penetrating injuries)
6. Hydrocephalus.
7. Neurochemical sequelae leading to neuronal death

8. What is diaschisis?

The term *diaschisis* refers to one of several general theories that relate to recovery of function following brain injury. Classically, this would appear as functional depression in intact areas of the brain at a distance from, but anatomically linked to, the damaged brain area. The resolution of behavioral deficits would be expected to occur in conjunction with a return of activity in these functionally depressed areas.

There are certainly other theories regarding the recovery of function, such as *vicariation* (where functions are taken over by brain areas not originally handling that function), *redundancy* (where recovery of function is based on the activity of uninjured brain regions that normally would contribute to that function), and *behavioral substitution* (where new strategies are learned to compensate for the behavioral deficit). Additionally, functional recovery would depend on the reversal of ischemia and edema in regions surrounding the areas of neuronal loss, changes in neurotransmitter levels and receptor number, and neuronal sprouting. Because areas involved by diaschisis are still intact, there have been attempts to modulate the rate of recovery from this process experimentally and in the clinical setting.

9. Describe the neurochemical changes following brain injury.

Research suggests that cells die through the processes of necrosis (a somewhat rapid and disorganized loss of cellular homeostasis and viability) and apoptosis (a more prolonged and orderly process of cellular breakdown that is energy-dependent and genetically regulated). In **necrosis** acutely after brain injury, there is a release of large amounts of neurotransmitters, particularly excitatory neurotransmitters such as glutamate. These neurotransmitters bind to receptors in neuronal cell membranes, activating postsynaptic ion channels. Excess amounts of ionized calcium, in particular, are allowed to enter the cell this way, as well as through voltage-activated channels in the cell membrane, activating phospholipases within the cell. This results in increased arachidonic acid metabolism and the production of free radicals that may damage or destroy the neuronal membrane if levels exceed what cellular enzymes can remove. The release of intracellular contents including excitatory amino acids and free radicals may trigger inflammation leading to the damage of neighboring cells. These processes may occur over the course of minutes to hours following brain injury.

In contrast, the cellular degradation through **apoptosis** usually does not lead to the damage of neighboring cells. Necrosis generally occurs in the center of an ischemic area, whereas apoptosis tends to be found more in the penumbra; however, there is overlap of these processes in areas of ischemic injury. The release of toxic chemicals from neurons undergoing necrosis may result in apoptosis of other cells. Post-acute neurochemical changes relate to alterations in the level and turnover of various neurotransmitters and their receptors. These postacute changes may be responsible for diaschisis-like effects which were described in an earlier question.

10. Can we intervene in this neurochemical process to minimize the adverse effects?
In general, drugs that have been used to minimize injury in association with acute TBI include those that may offer neuroprotection, preventing cellular injury before it occurs, and "rescue" of damaged cells, reversing cellular damage before cell death occurs. Various neurotrophic factors have been found that assist in neuronal repair and survival under experimental conditions. Drugs have also been produced that block the N-methyl-D-aspartate glutamate receptor in order to minimize glutamate-mediated calcium influx into neurons. Other drugs can minimize inflammation associated with cellular necrosis, including antioxidants and free radical scavengers. Much of the research in animal models of TBI suggests that these various treatment approaches work best when the animals are pretreated before brain injury or receive treatment concurrently with the brain injury. Clinical efforts in the acute post-brain injury period have focused on using pharmacologic agents to block neuronal calcium channels, particularly the N-methyl-D-aspartate receptor-activated channel. Other work has focused on using agents that inhibit the formation, or increase the clearance, of free radicals. The results so far have been discouraging, but the work continues.

In the postacute period, some limited clinical evidence suggests that amphetamine and methylphenidate may be associated with improved rates of functional recovery after stroke and brain injury. In some case reports and case series, various other medications, including dopamine agonists, catecholamine antagonists, amantadine, and tricyclic antidepressants, have been thought to improve the rate of recovery of patients in low functioning states following TBI. Overall, however, the clinical information available in the post-acute period is limited, with no large controlled trials of these medications.

11. What are the best prognostic indicators for patients following TBI?
Prognostic indicators related to the injury itself include the duration of coma (the shorter the better, but > 4 weeks is extremely bad), the duration of post-traumatic amnesia (again the shorter the better, but > 11 weeks is inconsistent with independent living), and the motor response on the Glasgow Coma Scale (with active posturing, decorticate/decerebrate or worse representing a fairly clear demarcation prognostically from higher levels of motor function). Other clinical findings, including evidence for brain stem involvement, such as dysconjugate gaze or altered pupillary responses, can add power to prognostication. Perhaps the most useful information that can be gleaned is the actual early recovery course that a patient demonstrates. Although site of lesion is not associated directly or very powerfully with outcome, knowing that the language areas, for example, have been damaged or that the patient has hemianopsia does have an impact on predicting ultimate outcome.

Other useful prognostic indicators include a patient's age, with people under 20 years of age generally doing much better than those over 60 if they have sustained the same kind of injury. Between the third and sixth decades, there is not a great deal of variability decade by decade in terms of outcome. The exception to this rule of thumb is for very young children (< 2 years of age). Another variable unrelated to the injury itself is the patient's premorbid psychosocial status; an individual who has had considerable psychological impairment or social disruption can be anticipated to have a relatively poorer outcome from a brain injury than someone without these problems. This is particularly true in the case of significant substance abuse.

Sadly, predicting functional outcome after TBI may never be completely accurate or specific, although work continues towards this goal. When using prognostic indicators for the purpose of counseling family members and/or treatment planning, it is often helpful to divide the indicators into three general stages. The first includes indicators useful in the acute care setting; these have been demonstrated to be most effective in prognosticating life versus death as opposed to long-term functional outcome. The second stage of prognostication would be after the acute phase has passed and the patient has begun involvement in active rehabilitation, whether in the acute care setting or a rehabilitation facility. A "final" prediction regarding long-term outcome is probably best reserved until several months or a year has passed following the injury. It is important to bear in mind that, even with a constellation of factors that may predict poor outcome, there is always a small percentage of patients who do very well. Similarly, there is always a small percentage of patients who, regardless of the accumulation of favorable predictors, have a bad functional outcome.

12. What assessment scales are commonly used to measure function and outcome for TBI patients?

The most frequently used assessment scales include the Glasgow Outcome Scale and the Disability Rating Scale. The **Glasgow Outcome Scale** is divided into five categories: dead, persistent vegetative state, severe disability, moderate disability, and good outcome. It has been criticized as being relatively insensitive, particularly given the span of the "severe disability" category (ranging from near-vegetative to being completely independent except for needing some daily assistance by a caregiver).

The **Disability Rating Scale** includes a reversed Glasgow Coma Scale and additional measurements of basic functional skills, employability, and total level of dependence. This scale has been correlated with evoked potential studies and has been demonstrated to be scientifically valid. It has also been proven to be far more sensitive than the Glasgow Outcome Scale.

Other scales include the Rancho Los Amigos Scale, a descriptive scale with eight categories that has been proven not to be scientifically valid. Its utility is essentially to expedite communication. Additional scales have been used to measure functional status, such as the Functional Independence Measure and Functional Assessment Measure, the latter being more specific for TBI as opposed to general disability. There are also scales that are used to assess patients in a minimally responsive state, such as the Coma/Near-Coma Scale, the Western Neuro Sensory Stimulation Profile, the Coma Recovery Scale, and the Sensory Stimulation Assessment Scale.

13. How should post-traumatic neuroendocrine disorders be managed?

Central dysautonomia may present with hypertension, tachycardia, temperature elevation, or a constellation of these features that may also include periodic perspiration over the face and shoulders. The **cardiovascular problems** may involve a generalized increase in circulating catecholamines or may occur without this. In general, the hypertension and tachycardia have been proven to be effectively treated by beta-blockers, although clonidine, calcium channel blockers, and even dopamine agonists have been anecdotally reported to be effective. Caution must be observed in the acute care setting, however; regional perfusion differences in the brain preclude the overzealous correction of hypertension or tachycardia with these modalities.

Central hyperthermia is typically managed with dopamine agonists. Again, there are anecdotal reports of response to beta-blockers or clonidine. The utility of modalities for hyperthermia should not be underestimated; if necessary, iced saline lavage through a nasogastric tube can rapidly decrease the core temperature. The episodic perspiration may respond to beta blockers but often transdermal scopolamine must be used. When the entire constellation presents as episodic severe dysregulation, it has been called **diencephalic fits**. In addition to the types of medications mentioned above, carbamazapine or valproic acid at times may be effective.

Other neuroendocrine problems that may accompany TBI include feeding and eating disorders (hyper/hypophagia) and disorders of the hypothalamic pituitary axis (including extrahypothalamic regulation). SSRIs may be helpful in the treatment of hyperphagia. For hypophagia, the use of mild psychostimulants may be effective. For disorders of the hypothalamic pituitary axis, treatment typically involves replacement of end-organ hormones (e.g., thyroid hormone, steroids). Correcting the actual hormone deficiency may be a bit complex, especially when dealing with fertility-related issues. Posterior pituitary problems include oversecretion or, less commonly, undersecretion of antidiuretic hormone; these are often transient.

14. How does the occurrence and management of heterotopic ossification in TBI compare to that in spinal cord injury?

Admittedly, as in spinal cord injury, the exact etiology of heterotopic ossification is unknown. One main difference with TBI, however, is in the joint sites involved. Heterotopic ossification involves the upper and lower extremities equally following TBI, whereas the hip and knee are primarily affected following spinal cord injury. The incidence of heterotopic ossification following TBI ranges from 11% to 76%. It most commonly involves the shoulder, elbow, and hip, infrequently occurring at the thigh and knee. Patients at highest risk are those in coma > 2 weeks, with spasticity, and with long bone fractures.

While passive ROM is advocated (as in spinal cord injury) to decrease the risk of heterotopic ossification, controversy exists as to whether these exercises may actually contribute to the ectopic bone formation. One small study of patients with TBI suggested that etidronate disodium may significantly decrease the risk of heterotopic ossification if given early after injury at a dose of 20 mg/kg for 3 months, followed by 10 mg/kg for an additional 3 months. NSAIDs also have been used, although studies supporting their efficacy in this patient population are lacking.

15. How does the management of spasticity associated with TBI differ from that in spinal cord injury?

Historically, there has not been much difference. The use of physical agents, splinting, neurolytic and motor point blocks, botulinum toxin injections, and surgical intervention usually follows the same line of decision-making regarding management in both patient populations. **Dantrolene sodium** has been considered the oral agent of choice in managing spasticity associated with various forms of brain injury; baclofen and diazepam tend not to be advocated as much because they have side effects that may include sedation and impairment of cognitive function. **Alpha-2 adrenergic agonists**, such as clonidine and tizanidine, have been found to be effective in managing spasticity following various forms of brain injury. **Intrathecal baclofen** therapy is now being used in the management of severe spasticity following brain injuries; while tending to have its main effects on the lower limbs, improved upper limb function with reduction in hypertonicity may also be noted.

16. Do TBI patients require anticonvulsants?

While some TBI patients do require anticonvulsants, the general consensus currently is that anticonvulsant prophylaxis has been overused. Approximately 5–7% of all hospitalized TBI patients develop seizures. This number may approach 35–50% in the more critical patients with penetrating injuries. Evidence supports the use of anticonvulsant prophylaxis and treatment of early seizures occurring within the first week after brain injury. Antiepileptics are not recommended after 1 week of injury in the patient following nonpenetrating TBI with no history of seizures, although some recommend treating prophylactically in the case of missile or open injuries, which have an association with seizures of approximately 40%.

17. Which anticonvulsant medications are most appropriate for this patient population?

The choice of anticonvulsant agent continues to be somewhat controversial. Both **phenytoin** and **phenobarbital** can be given parenterally; however, they have a considerable number of side effects. While phenytoin has been shown in studies to be effective for prevention and treatment of early posttraumatic seizures, concern has been raised that phenytoin may be associated with cognitive impairment as well as inhibit learning and brain plasticity following brain injury. Therefore, some have recommended using **carbamazepine** or **valproate**, as these medications may be better tolerated in the brain-injured population. However, carbamazepine may also adversely influence cognitive function following TBI, although animal studies suggest it may not adversely affect neurologic recovery. Of note, some evidence suggests that valproate may be as effective as phenytoin in posttraumatic seizure prophylaxis. Although limited information suggests that **gabapentin** may help in the management of seizures associated with stroke and brain tumor, more information is needed as to how effective this medication might be in patients following TBI.

18. What intracranial complications commonly arise relatively late after TBI?

Intracranial sequelae that occur in the weeks or months following TBI, sometimes overlapping secondary injuries discussed earlier, may slow the functional recovery of or actually lead to a reversal of gains made by a patient. One significant complication is **post-traumatic hydrocephalus**, which should be differentiated from ventricular dilatation due to encephalomalacia or loss of brain tissue associated with the brain trauma itself. **Cerebrospinal fluid fistulas** may also occur as a consequence of head trauma, reaching an incidence as high as 5–11% in patients with basilar skull fractures. **Post-traumatic movement disorders**, such as tremor and parkinsonism, may be significant sequelae of injury, impairing behavioral recovery. While **post-traumatic seizures** have already been discussed, it is important to remember that post-traumatic epilepsy may first occur relatively late (even several years) following injury.

19. What peripheral nervous system injuries are commonly associated with traumatic brain injury?

Plexopathies, particularly involving the upper extremity, may occur as a result of traction, compression, or lacerations arising from the traumatic event itself. These may overlap **radiculopathies** resulting from nerve root avulsions or nerve root compression associated with spine fractures. **Focal neuropathies** may occur as a result of heterotopic ossification (particularly involving the ulnar nerve at the elbow), spasticity producing extremity contractures (particularly affecting the median nerve at the wrist and ulnar nerve at the elbow), fractures (resulting in injury commonly to the peroneal, median, and ulnar nerves), and soft tissue injury associated with the traumatic event. The **polyneuropathy** associated with prolonged alcohol use may be seen as well in that subgroup of patients who ultimately sustain brain injury.

20. What behavioral and personality changes are commonly seen following TBI?

Because the brain is the organ of consciousness and personality, virtually any change in behavior or intellectual function can be observed following its injury. The most common problems **cognitively** are deficits in attention (inability to concentrate, increased distractibility, or even perseveration) and memory. As with stroke, specific cognitive disorders may emerge that include (but are not limited to) aphasias, agnosias, apraxias, temporal sequencing problems, visual-perceptual and spacial dysfunctions, prosodic deficits, and, with frontal lesions, disorders of judgment, planning and other "metacognitive" skills.

Behaviorally, the most common problems have to do with impulse control or disinhibition of the dampening system for an emotional response to a stimulus. This may present as anger and violent behavior or as emotional lability, including crying or even laughing which is out of proportion to a stimulus. Another problem may be "agitation," which in the early stages of recovery is often related to confusion and post-traumatic amnesia; it is not necessarily related to any long-term behavioral changes. More chronic problems include social impropriety, loss of pragmatic skills, low frustration tolerance, and, less commonly, actual violence and aggression.

21. What should be included in the evaluation of behavioral and cognitive changes following TBI?

Most investigations relate to the **environment** and only require common sense. Does the patient have a normal sleep-wake cycle? Is the patient in pain? Is the environment disorienting instead of orienting (e.g., ICU settings)? Does the environment reinforce inappropriate behaviors?

An organized approach should follow to rule out correctable **biological etiologies** for cognitive and behavioral problems. Neurologically, the patient should be evaluated for possible seizures, particularly partial complex seizures, and intracranial space-occupying lesions, such as hydrocephalus or subdural hematoma/hygroma. An endocrine evaluation, particularly of thyroid function, is important as is ensuring electrolyte balance.

All **medications** should be reviewed, including those prescribed and those used for recreational pursuits; pharmacologic agents are a common correctable etiology for cognitive or behavioral deficits. A search for toxins may also be important.

22. Describe some behaviorally based and environmentally based strategies for managing TBI patients with disruptive or aggressive behavior.

It is important to remember that behaviors are defined by the context in which they occur. In some situations, it is tempting to consider sedation for those around the patient rather than to treat the patient's "agitated" behavior. The first step in the approach to management should be to define the undesired behavior in a way upon which all observers can agree. The behavior should then be observed in regards to its frequency of occurrence and associated environmental factors serving as its "triggers." The environment should then be modified to remove triggers if at all possible, and the behavior then monitored to see if its occurrence diminishes. Principles of operant conditioning may also be utilized to help extinguish the undesired behavior.

23. What are some appropriate pharmacologic interventions for patients with disruptive or aggressive behavior?

This area still tends to be more art than science, even among practitioners experienced in the management of TBI. **Carbamazepine** and **amitriptyline** are some of the most commonly used medications. **Beta-blockers** also may have some usefulness in managing posttraumatic agitation, such as in association with central dysautonomia. **Amantadine** and **methylphenidate** may be used when the agitated behavior is felt to be related to attention and concentration deficits. **Neuroleptics** and **benzodiazepines** are less commonly used by persons because of concerns related to cognitive impairment and potential slowing of behavioral recovery; these medications tend to be reserved for acute situations in which the patient endangers himself/herself or others.

24. Can "cognitive remediation" therapy or pharmacotherapy really help improve the cognitive deficits seen following TBI?

Pharmacotherapy seems to have the most clear-cut usefulness for problems of basic arousal and attention. Methylphenidate, amantadine, bromocriptine, and tricyclic antidepressants may improve attentional dysfunction in patients, although studies have tended to have mixed results. There is limited evidence that bromocriptine and amphetamines can be associated with improvements in motor aphasias; dopamine agonists also appear to reduce neglect in some patients. Very limited evidence also suggests that cholinergic precursor and cholinesterase inhibitor medications may improve memory function in some TBI patients, but more work needs to be done in this area.

In general, cognitive remediation programs have not been shown to intrinsically improve the intellectual function of a patient for all situations. Their principal role is in teaching adaptive strategies and compensatory techniques. From this perspective, they are most effective when they are task-specific and site-specific because one of the biggest problems people with brain injuries may have is generalizing performance from one site or one task to another. There is evidence supporting the concept of "bringing the therapy to the patient" (instead of bringing the patient to a hospital or outpatient area), using job coaches at the job site or independent living counselor/therapists in the community to teach adaptive strategies to patients.

25. How can you rule out correctable causes of coma or a minimally responsive state?

As with cognitive and behavioral changes, a search for possible seizures, space-occupying brain lesions, endocrine and electrolyte abnormalities, toxins, and potentially contributory pharmacologic agents is warranted.

26. How is a "coma management" program and pharmacotherapy used in managing patients in low-functioning states following TBI?

At present, there is no clear evidence that any kind of therapy-based program will help end a coma or minimally responsive (or vegetative) state. However, an organized approach to a low- functioning patient permits a quantitative assessment of responses to stimuli and early recognition of changes or improvements in response to intervention or through spontaneous recovery.

There is a clear indication for preventative therapeutic interventions to maintain the body "in readiness" for the hoped-for neurologic improvement, particularly early on. These measures include basic rehabilitation strategies to manage bowel and bladder function, maintain appropriate nutrition, maintain skin integrity, control spasticity, and prevent contracture formation. The rationale is that, if the patient comes out of coma or a minimally responsive state, this intervention will permit more rapid participation in an active rehabilitation program and a shorter total program length of stay. There is also some limited evidence that, for individuals who are "destined" to come out of a transient vegetative or akinetic mute state or coma, this recovery process may be hastened through the use of pharmacotherapy, particularly dopamine agonists (such as combined levodopa/carbidopa or bromocriptine), amantadine, or tricyclic antidepressants.

27. What is the prognosis for patients in a vegetative state following TBI?

There is still no way to accurately predict the amount of functional recovery expected for a TBI patient in a minimally responsive state, although older age tends to be associated with a poorer outcome. While some amount of recovery can occur in up to 50% of patients in a vegetative state for about 1 month, the odds that this will be functionally significant recovery tend to decline with time in that state. Of patients in a vegetative state for 2–4 weeks after injury, 8–18% remain in this state at 1 year. Data suggest a mortality rate of 15–24% for these minimally responsive patients between 1 month and 1 year.

28. List the common symptoms experienced by patients with mild TBI.

The symptoms largely parallel those of patients in the more severe portion of the spectrum of traumatic brain injury:

Headache (the most common complaint and one fairly unique to the more mildly injured patient)

Vestibular or disequilibrium complaints

Fatigue, weakness, numbness, and "tingling"

Sensory deficits relating to hearing, blurred or "changed" vision, smell and taste dysfunction

Attentional and memory problems

Irritability and sleep disturbances (aggression and other personality changes also possible)

29. What are the management strategies available to help patients following mild TBI?

Management of patients with mild TBI, as with other brain injuries, requires a coordinated team approach. The first management issue pertains to identification and possible verification of the organicity of the presenting signs and symptoms. While MRI and other imaging studies should be undertaken, much of this documentation occurs through a neuropsychological assessment. It is important to distinguish individuals who have true organic changes from those with emotional or psychiatric problems and from those who have a combination of both. Of note, some of the physical and secondarily cognitive complaints may be related to injuries of the cranial nerves and craniocervical neurovascular systems. Also, a fair number of complaints can be attributed to musculoskeletal injury of the head and neck; this is particularly true in the case of post-traumatic headache, which nearly always has a musculoskeletal component. While possible, the incidence of overt malingering is not felt to be very high at present.

After a clear idea of a patient's cognitive, emotional, and intellectual state is established along with some clarification as to organicity, evaluation and intervention should target those deficits that are brain-injury related. This may include the use of compensatory strategies and pharmacotherapy as already discussed. There is also a strong role for education and counseling of the patient and family members.

30. Given the wide range of cognitive and functional impairments associated with TBI, how does one decide what level of therapy intensity or type of program is appropriate for a given patient?

Interventions by various therapeutic disciplines, including physical and occupational therapy, speech and language pathology, psychology, social work, therapeutic recreation, vocational counseling, and nursing, may be provided in a variety of settings depending on a patient's medical requirements, need for and potential benefit from specific therapeutic interventions (particularly those requiring equipment that cannot be transported out of a facility), and activity tolerance, as well as the unique skills of the particular health care providers involved.

Often a continuum of services is felt to be optimal to manage the evolving issues of a brain injured patient throughout recovery. The acute care hospital therapies for patients in a low-functioning state focus on maintaining the body "in readiness" while waiting for neurologic recovery. As the level of function improves, therapies may progress to include mobility training, self-care activities, and programs to facilitate communication and cognition. Depending on a patient's needs, additional services may be provided in an extended-care facility with therapies, a subacute rehabilitative facility, an intensive inpatient rehabilitation hospital program, as outpatient therapies either in a standard format or a more specialized community reentry program, or as home-based therapies (if services do not require extensive equipment). Socioeconomic and insurance coverage restrictions play a significant role as well in determining what options will be pursued.

31. What percentage of patients with TBI subsequently return to work?

Reports vary widely, ranging from 12% to 100%. It would be safe to say that the majority of patients can return to work, as about 80% of TBIs are of the mild type. However, for people who have sustained more moderate to severe brain injuries, the incidence of returning to work is considerably less in terms of competitive or gainful employment. For severe injuries, this has been estimated to be under 20%, perhaps even closer to 10%.

32. How much impact does TBI as a disorder really have on society?

A lot. It has been estimated that about 200 TBIs per 100,000 population occur annually in the U. S. (about 40 times the incidence of traumatic spinal cord injury), although study results vary depending on the methods used. Also, about 17–30 deaths due to brain injury per 100,000 population occur annually. The associated economic impact is difficult to determine. A patient with severe brain injury may incur several millions of dollars in lifetime medical care costs, not including lost earnings and indirect costs to the patient or the family. The true costs, however, are not only economic but societal as well, with residual neurologic deficits impacting a patient's ability to cope with life changes, have desired interpersonal relationships, and achieve a level of vocational performance that might have been anticipated prior to the injury. It is worth mentioning again that traumatic brain injury is a potentially preventable disorder. After this discussion, it should be clear why ongoing efforts to minimize its occurrence should be encouraged and applauded.

ACKNOWLEDGMENT

The authors wish to thank Pamela Harmon for her kind assistance in preparing this manuscript.

BIBLIOGRAPHY

1. Boyeson MG, Harmon RL: Acute and postacute drug-induced effects on rate of behavioral recovery after brain injury. J Head Trauma Rehabil 9:78–90, 1994.
2. Cooper PR (ed): Head Injury, 3rd ed. Baltimore, Williams & Wilkins, 1993.
3. Horn LJ (ed): Pharmacology and Brain Rehabilitation. Physical Medicine and Rehabilitation Clinics of North America, vol. 8, no. 4. Philadelphia, W.B. Saunders, 1997.
4. Horn LJ, Zasler ND (eds): Post-Concussive Disorders. Physical Medicine and Rehabilitation State of the Art Reviews, vol. 6, no. 1. Philadelphia, Hanley & Belfus, 1992.
5. Horn LJ, Zasler ND (eds): Medical Rehabilitation of Traumatic Brain Injury. Philadelphia, Hanley & Belfus, 1996.
6. Kushawha VP, Garland DG: Extremity fractures in the patient with a traumatic brain injury. J Am Acad Orthop Surg 6:298–307, 1998.
7. McDeavitt JT (ed): Traumatic Brain Injury. Physical Medicine and Rehabilitation State of the Art Reviews, vol. 15, no. 2. Philadelphia, Hanley & Belfus, 2001.
8. Nance PW (ed): Rehabilitation Pharmacotherapy. Physical Medicine and Rehabilitation Clinics of North America, vol. 10, no. 2, Philadelphia, W.B. Saunders, 1999.
9. Rosenthal M, Griffith ER, Bond MR, Miller JD (eds): Rehabilitation of the Adult and Child with Traumatic Brain Injury, 2nd ed. Philadelphia, F.A. Davis, 1990.
10. Stone LR (ed): Neurologic and Orthopaedic Sequelae of Traumatic Brain Injury. Physical Medicine and Rehabilitation State of the Art Reviews, vol. 7, no. 3. Philadelphia, Hanley & Belfus, 1993.

31. SPINAL CORD INJURY MEDICINE

Steven A. Stiens, M.D., M.S., Barry Goldstein, M.D., Ph.D.,
Margaret Hammond, M.D., and James Little, M.D., Ph.D.

1. What is SCIWORA?

Spinal cord injury without radiologic abnormality. This condition is commonly seen in young children and older adults. Mechanisms of injury in children include traction in breech delivery, violent hyperextension, or flexion. Predisposing factors in children include their large head-to-neck size ratio, elasticity of the fibrocartilaginous spine, and the horizontal orientation of the planes of the cervical facet joints.

The typical presentation of SCIWORA in the elderly is an acute central cord syndrome after a fall forward and a blow on the head. The ligamentum flavum may bulge forward into the central canal and narrow the sagittal diameter as much as 50%.

Essential history in a person with head trauma or neck pain includes identifying any paresthesias or other neurologic symptoms. Flexion and extension films should be done cautiously only after static neck films have been cleared by a radiologist and only if no neurologic symptoms or severe pains are present. Empiric use of a 24-hour cervical collar with repeat films at resolution of cervical spasm is warranted. Delayed onset of paralysis may occur rarely due to vascular mechanisms or edema accumulation at the injury site.

2. What are the key muscles tested to clinically define the spinal cord injury (SCI) motor level?

The American Spinal Cord Injury Association (ASIA) has developed standards for neurologic classification (revised 2000) that quantify impairment through objective recording of sensory and motor findings. Due to the multiple segmental innervations of muscles, antigravity strength (3/5 or greater) is considered enough to define a **motor level** if all muscles above have normal 5/5 strength. The **motor level** is the caudal key muscle group that is graded 3/5 or greater with the segments cephalad graded normal (5/5) strength. A patient is classified as **motor incomplete** if there is there is voluntary anal sphincter contraction *or* he or she has sensory sacral sparing with sparing of motor function more than three levels below the motor level. The index muscles that define each motor level are:

C4—diaphragm	T1—abductor digiti minimi
C5—biceps, brachialis	L2—iliopsoas
C6—extensor carpi radialis (longus and brevis)	L3—quadriceps
C7—triceps brachii	L4—tibialis anterior
C8—flexor digitorum profundus to middle finger	L5—extensor hallucis longus
	S1—gastrocnemius, soleus
	S2—anal sphincter

3. How is sensory level defined and documented with bedside examination of persons with SCI?

It is most effective to work from areas of decreased or absent sensation toward areas of normal sensation. A **pinprick stimulus** (clean, unused safety pin) is presented lightly to the skin starting at S1 (lateral aspect of the fifth toe), then advanced by dermatome until normal perception is documented. Results are recorded as 0 = absent, 1 = present but abnormal, or 2 = normal perception (as compared with areas above the lesion). The same process is repeated for **light touch** (brush or cotton). The **zone of partial preservation** is the area of altered sensation that separates areas without sensation from those with normal sensation. A patient is described as **sensory incomplete** if any anal canal sensation is present.

4. What is the neurologic level of injury?

The neurologic level of injury is the most caudal level at which *both* motor and sensory modalities are intact on both sides of the body. The motor and sensory levels for SCI are the same in < 50% of complete injuries. At spinal cord segments where there is no key muscle that has a sensory dermatone intact (high cervical, thoracic, and sacral levels), the motor level and the neurologic level is determined by the sensory level.

5. Why is sensation most likely to be spared in the perianal area?

Sacral sparing is due to spinal cord somatotopic organization. Sensory and motor fibers are laminated within the tracts of the spinal cord such that fibers that serve caudal regions are located laterally and closer to the surface. Contusions and spinal cord ischemia produce relatively more damage to centrally located spinal neurons and axons than those peripherally located within the spinal cord.

6. What are the most important long tracts in the spinal cord?

Long Tracts in the Spinal Cord

TRACT	LOCATION	FUNCTION
Gracile	Medial dorsal column	Proprioception from the leg
Cuneate	Lateral dorsal column	Proprioception from the arm
Spinocerebellar	Superficial lateral column	Muscular position and tone
Pyramidal	Deep lateral column	Upper motor neuron
Lateral spinothalamic	Ventrolateral column	Pain and thermal sensation

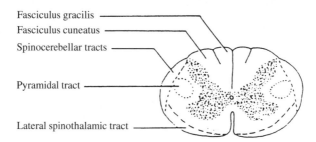

Fasciculus gracilis
Fasciculus cuneatus
Spinocerebellar tracts
Pyramidal tract
Lateral spinothalamic tract

(From Joynt R: Clinical Neurology. Philadelphia, J.B. Lippincott, 1992, with permission.)

7. Where in the cord is each of the major long tracts located?

The figure shows the somatotopic organization of the major long tracts of the spinal cord. The dorsal columns have lower-extremity fibers (sacral and lumbar) lying medially, while the pyramidal and spinothalamic tracts have lower-extremity fibers lying laterally.

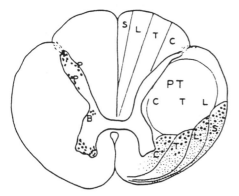

C = cervical, T = thoracic, L = lumbar, S = sacral, PT = pyramidal tract. (From Joynt R: Clinical Neurology. Philadelphia, J.B. Lippincott, 1992; with permission.)

8. What is the artery of Adamkiewicz?

The artery of Adamkiewicz is a major radicular branch that arises from the aorta and enters the cord between T10 and L3. Although radicular arteries supply each spinal root, typically only this one large artery actually supplies the low thoracic and lumbar spinal cord via the **anterior spinal artery**. The anterior spinal artery supplies the anterior two-thirds of the spinal cord. It supplies the lumbar and lower thoracic segments, anastomosing with the anterior spinal artery in the lower thoracic region, which is thus the watershed area of the cord. The diagram shows the blood supply of the spinal cord. The **lumbar radicular artery** is commonly called the artery of Adamkiewicz.

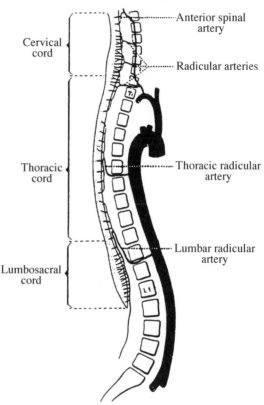

(From Joynt R: Clinical Neurology. Philadelphia, J.B. Lippincott, 1992, with permission.)

9. What is the arterial supply of the posterior third of the cord?

Paired dorsolateral **posterior spinal arteries** extend the length of the cord and supply the posterior third of the cord through circumflex and penetrating vessels. They arise from the vertebral or posterior inferior cerebellar arteries.

10. What is the difference between quadriplegia and tetraplegia?

It is a matter of medical etymology. *Quadra* is a Latin root meaning four. *Tetra* (four) and *plegia* (*plege*, meaning stroke or paralysis) are Greek roots. The compound word *tetraplegia* is more correct because it does not mix Greek and Latin roots.

11. Name the SCI syndromes. What are their lesions, clinical findings, and common causes?

Anterior cord syndrome. The clinical syndrome includes hyporeflexia, atrophy, and variable motor loss, with preservation of position sensation but impaired pin prick (hypalgesia) and temperature sensation. Common causes for these findings are thoracolumbar burst fracture, abdominal aortic aneurysm, and aortic clamping for surgery which compromise segmental spinal cord circulation.

Central cord syndrome. The clinical constellation includes weakness greater in the arms than legs, lower-extremity hyperreflexia, upper-extremity mixed upper-motor-neuron and lower-motor-neuron weakness, and preserved sacral sensation with the potential for preservation of bowel and bladder control. Common causes are spinal stenosis with extension injury, expanding intramedullary hematoma mass, or syrinx.

Brown-Séquard syndrome. This syndrome presents with hemi- or monoplegia or paresis with contralateral pain and temperature sensation deficit. There is a good prognosis for motor recovery progressing from the proximal extensors to distal flexors, although spasticity may compromise total function. Causes include knife wounds to the back and asymmetrically oriented spinal tumors.

Posterior cord syndrome. This uncommon presentation manifests with bilateral deficits in proprioception. The potential causes are vitamin B12 deficiency (subacute combined degeneration) and syphilis (tabes dorsalis).

12. Compare the Frankel classification with the ASIA Impairment Scale as revised for 2000.

The **Frankel classification** was an attempt to separate SCI patients into various functional groups as follows:

Frankel A: motor and sensory function complete without any movement or sensation below the lesion

Frankel B: motor complete with some sensory sparing

Frankel C: motor and sensory incomplete without functional motor recovery

Frankel D: functionally useful movement below the lesion

Frankel E: motor and sensory recovery to normal function but residual clinical evidence of SCI may still be present

The **ASIA Impairment Scale** (2000) further refined distinctions between categories by specifying sensory dermatomes and muscle grades as follows:

ASIA A: complete (no motor or sensory S4 or S5 function)

ASIA B: incomplete sensory but no motor function preserved through S4–5

ASIA C: motor and sensory incomplete with the strength of more than half of the key muscles below the neurologic level having a muscle grade < 3

ASIA D: motor and sensory incomplete (motor functional) with at least half of key muscles below the neurologic level having a muscle grade ≥ 3

ASIA E: normal motor and sensory function

13. What is the highest complete SCI level that is consistent with independent living without the aid of an attendant?

C6 complete tetraplegia. An occasional exceptionally motivated individual with C6 tetraplegia demonstrates the capability and chooses independent living in an accessible environment without the aid of an attendant. A review of outcomes from a subset of people with motor and sensory-complete C6 SCI revealed that the following percentage of patients were independent for key self-care tasks: feeding 16%, upper body dressing 13%, lower body dressing 3%, grooming 19%, bathing 9%, bowel care 3%, transfers 6%, wheelchair propulsion 88%. Feeding is accomplished with a universal cuff for utensils. Transfers require stabilization of elbow extension with forces transmitted from shoulder musculature through the limb as a closed kinetic chain. Bowel care is performed with a suppository insertion wand and Fickle finger for digital stimulation.

14. How much motor recovery is expected in a patient with a stable diagnosis of motor and sensory complete traumatic tetraplegia with central spinal cord edema and hematomyelia on MRI?

Recovery is greatest in muscles supplied within the zone of injury. Less than 30% of SCIs will go from C4 to C5 but > 66% of those at C5–8 gain one root level by 6–12 weeks. The ability to perceive pain from a pin stimulus over the lateral antecubital space (posterior brachial cutaneous nerve) is a good prognostic indicator for eventual recovery of the extensor carpi radialis to 3/5. Eighty-five percent of patients' muscles that demonstrate 1/5 strength initially within the zone of partial motor preservation (myotomes caudal to the neurologic level that remain partially innervated) will achieve > 3/5 strength by 1 year. Below the injury zone, only 3% of patients initially (at 72 hours) Frankel A improve to grade D or E. Negative prognostic indicators on MRI include transection, hematomyelia, and edema, but MRI adds little to the clinical exam for prediction of prognosis.

15. What are the mechanisms of motor recovery after SCI?

Motor recovery after SCI occurs rapidly during the first and second week; then recovery continues at a slower pace for the first 4 months and slows further thereafter. Initially, recovery could be mediated by central mechanisms (cortical reorganization) such as recruitment of latent pathways (unused until injury). At the injury site, edema and hematomyelia may resolve reducing secondary injury, neurapraxic block, and demyelination. Within the anterior horn, central synaptogenesis may occur in response to denervation hypersensitivity of the anterior horn cell. Root impingement may resolve with decompression, spinal alignment, and fixation as needed.

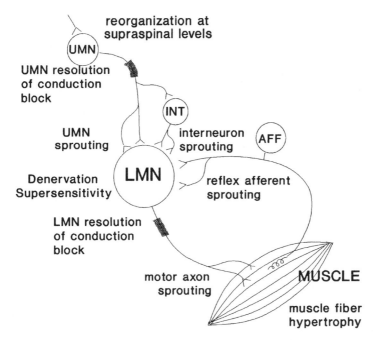

Mechanisms of recovery. (From Little J, Stiens SA: Electrodiagnosis in spinal cord injury. Phys Med Rehabil Clin North Am 6:263–296, 1995, with permission.)

16. Which are the most common and disabling contractures of the upper extremities after SCI?

Adduction of shoulder, flexion of elbow, extension of the MCP, DIP, and MIP. Helpful contractures are mild flexion of the MCP, PIP, and DIP. They provide **tenodesis**, which is finger prehension (opposition of the thumb to the index finger) with active wrist extension. Even greater strength can come from a wrist-driven flexor hinge orthosis, which stabilizes the thumb, index, and middle fingers for a tight pincer grasp.

17. A patient with T4 complete paraplegia complains of a pounding headache and was noted to have a blood pressure of 190/100 mmHg, gooseflesh of his trunk and legs, and a paradoxic bradycardia at 50 bpm. What is the diagnosis, pathophysiology, and treatment?

Autonomic dysreflexia is an acute hypertensive syndrome due to a hyperactive reflex sympathetic discharge often precipitated by viscus distention or noxious stimuli registered below the level of the SCI. The nerve cell bodies for sympathetic outflow are located in the **intermediolateral cell columns**, which run from T1 through L2 bilaterally in the spinal gray matter. Lesions above T6 cut off central modulation of sympathetic discharges. Hypertension often produced by excessive vasoconstriction is registered at the carotid baroreceptors, resulting in corrective parasympathetic outflow via the vagus nerve to reduce heart rate and contractility.

Treatment includes identification and elimination of the cause (commonly urologic obstruction/distention, bowel impaction, skin irritation, ingrown toenail, or intra-abdominal processes). Sit the patient up and administer nifedipine orally or sublingually. Nitropaste can be placed for prevention in situations that may precipitate autonomic dysreflexia.

18. Why is deep vein thrombosis (DVT) a pervasive problem after SCI?

The primary risks were summarized in 1856 as Virchow's triad:

1. **Venous stasis** (paralysis, spinal shock)
2. **Hypercoagulability** (trauma, tumor as cause for increases in circulating thrombogenic factors)
3. **Vessel injury** (primary trauma or secondary injury due to sensory deficits after SCI)

The incidence of DVT after SCI ranges from 47–100% as revealed with various noninvasive surveillance techniques for subclinical disease. The risk is highest during the first 2 weeks to 3 months after SCI, and prevention of clot formation is essential.

19. How is DVT best prevented after SCI?

- Check a baseline activated partial thromboplastin time and platelet count.
- Immediate initiation of subcutaneous heparin, 5000 U every 12 hours or low-molecular-weight (LMW) heparin, once emergency trauma management is complete and hemostasis has been achieved. (Higher heparin doses have an increased effectiveness but also an increased incidence of hemorrhagic complications. LMW heparins do not bind thrombin or inhibit platelet function. Studies indicate that LMW heparin given once daily is also effective.)
- Thigh-high Ted hose and heel protectors are placed and kept on all day to prevent edema and trauma.
- Stasis is reduced by sequential pneumatic compression, which should be continued for a minimum of 2 weeks.

20. What muscle function is typically required to allow community ambulation?

Walking ability is directly related to the proportion of lower-extremity joints that are animated with sufficient muscular force to overcome gravity. At least 3/5 strength in hip flexion bilaterally with at least 3/5 knee extension on one side is required for an effective reciprocal gait pattern to permit community ambulation. Bilateral bracing (ankle-foot orthosis or knee-ankle-foot orthosis) with forearm crutches or a walker maximizes efficiency. The calculation of the sum of bilateral lower-extremity strength measures produces the ASIA Lower Extremity Muscle Score (LEMS, normal 50). LEMS correlates with gait velocity, energy expenditure, and peak axial load by arms on crutches. Values above 30 are associated with community ambulation.

21. A chronic T2 ASIA B SCI patient mentions that he was unable to tell the difference between a cold and a warm beer by grasping the can with his hand at a recent party. What are your thoughts and actions?

This represents a change in temperature perception, which is carried by the superficially located lateral and ventral **spinothalamic tracts**. Afferent fibers enter through the dorsal root and *cross over* to the opposite side of the spinal cord via the anterior commissure just anterior to the central canal. A differential diagnosis might include progressive post-traumatic syringomyelia (an expanding intramedullary cyst that may originate at the injury site), tethered cord syndrome (progressive spinal cord dysfunction due to stretch or traction of the cord), myelopathy, radiculopathy, plexopathy, and peripheral neuropathy.

The patient should be questioned about shooting pain with sneeze or cough, Valsalva, or heavy-lifting, which may all increase subarachnoid pressures. The exam should include neck flexion to assess the presence of **Lhermitte's sign** (a sudden electric-like shock extending down the spine with head flexion), pinprick/touch sensation, reflexes, and strength. Further evaluation includes electrodiagnostic testing and MRI.

22. What is the treatment and outcome for progressive post-traumatic syringomyelia?

Conservative measures include avoidance of high-force isometric contractions, Valsalva, head elevation at night, and maintenance of the neck in a neutral position. Surgical shunting may be associated with shunt obstruction and syrinx reaccumulation.

23 How can an acute abdomen be diagnosed in a person with an SCI?

The diagnosis of abdominal emergencies requires a high index of suspicion, since they often produce subtle and minimal symptoms and poor localizing findings on examination. The most prominent objective finding may be just an elevated pulse rate!

Signs and symptoms depend on the level of injury and degree of completeness, thus dictating the responsiveness of the remaining intact nervous system. A person with an injury level above T6 may experience autonomic dysreflexia, vague nonlocalized abdominal discomfort, increased spasticity, and a rigid abdomen. A level between T6 and T10 may allow for some reflex responses and localization, depending on the specific organ involved. A level lower than T12 spares sympathetic splanchnic outflow and responses are normal.

Key symptoms, although not always present, include anorexia, nausea, restlessness, changes in spasticity, nonlocalized abdominal pain, and shoulder pain in the person with tetraplegia. Signs may include elevated pulse rate (although bradycardia may exist if autonomic dysreflexia is present), fever, and spasticity. Abdominal tenderness is not common in those individuals with a level above T5. Rapid diagnosis with laboratory studies (complete blood count, amylase) and imaging studies is warranted to improve on the all-too-common delays in diagnosis. Beware, there is a resultant 10–15% mortality rate in this population.

24. What is Charcot spine? Why would someone with SCI have it?

Jean M. Charcot was a French neurologist who treated many syphilitics. He described osteoarthropathy from trauma in people with **tabes dorsalis** (syphilitic posterior column deterioration) who lacked protective sensation.

Because of their spinal trauma and analgesia below the level of injury, those with SCI are particularly prone to this insensate joint destruction. After spinal fixation, the fusion mass acts as a lever, contributing to hypermobility at the joint just caudal to the fusion. The joints themselves can be a pain source that triggers autonomic dysreflexia or a nidus of infection after hematogenous spread.

25. A 17-year-old, newly SCI-injured, muscular, C6 incomplete tetraplegic complains of lethargy and abdominal cramping. What could it be?

Immobilization hypercalcemia should be considered. Symptoms of hypercalcemia can be remembered with the mnemonic **stones, bones, and abdominal groans**. Other symptoms include lethargy, nausea, and anorexia.

The diagnosis is made with measurement of the total serum calcium adjusted for the total protein. Serum ionized calcium is also elevated and is a more accurate test. The 24-hour calcium excretion normally should be < 250 mg. Treatment includes mobilization, rehydration with saline, and treatment with furosemide (which enhances Ca^{2+} secretion in the loop of Henle). Calcitonin can be used in resistant cases.

26. A 63-year-old man who has had T7 paraplegia for 37 years presents to your clinic with right shoulder pain of 2 years' duration. He describes the pain as insidious in onset (except for periods of bursitis), located in the posterolateral shoulder, and now interfering with reaching activities. Physical exam reveals significant atrophy of the involved supraspinatus and infraspinatus muscles and severe weakness of external rotation, abduction, and forward flexion. Radiographs reveal upward displacement of the humeral head against the coracoacromial arch. The patient has had approximately six steroid injections into the affected shoulder. He has a 75-pack-year smoking history. **What is the differential diagnosis for shoulder pain in this individual with paraplegia?**

The working diagnosis from his history and physical examination is a **rotator cuff tear**. However, there are other common causes of shoulder pain and weakness in this population, including rheumatologic diseases (glenohumeral osteoarthritis, acromioclavicular osteoarthritis), soft tissue disorders (subacromial bursitis, rotator cuff tendinitis, bicipital tendinitis), post-traumatic syringomyelia, cervical radiculopathy, heterotopic ossification, avascular necrosis, brachial neuritis, and various nerve palsies (long thoracic nerve, suprascapular nerve). Therefore, the physical examination and diagnostic evaluation should confirm the working diagnosis and rule out other etiologies. This is particularly important in individuals who have had paraplegia for many years because shoulder pain and rotator cuff tears are common findings. The diagnosis of rotator cuff tear is supported by the upward displacement of the humeral head and could be confirmed by MRI, arthrography, arthroscopy, or surgery.

27. How is a rotator cuff tear treated in a person with paraplegia such as the 63-year-old man above?

Surgical treatment of rotator cuff tear in persons with SCI is complex. At best, the surgery will be successful with full restoration of shoulder function. The individual will require many weeks of non-weight-bearing, placing great demands on the contralateral shoulder and great stresses on the vocational and home situation. The usual postoperative restrictions for an able-bodied person are much more difficult for the person with SCI to follow. Return to upper-extremity weight-bearing and extreme loading of the newly repaired cuff frequently occur more rapidly than in the able-bodied population because anything less requires assistance from a family member or attendant. It is also important to remember that rotator cuff repairs commonly do not result in full restoration of function. Discouraging prognostic factors include an older age (> 65 yr), insidious atraumatic onset, weakness > 6 months, a long smoking history, repeated steroid injections, previous cuff repair attempts, poor nutrition, severe weakness, and upward displacement of the humeral head. This patient has many negative prognostic factors.

Conservative treatment of rotator cuff tear has not been well studied in the SCI population. However, nonoperative management of tears of the rotator cuff have been examined in the able-bodied population. In general, NSAIDs, stretching, and strengthening programs have been used. People with paraplegia have relatively strong, shortened anterior shoulder muscles and weaker, lengthened posterior muscles. It is particularly important to stretch the anterior musculature and strengthen the posterior shoulder musculature. It is also important to identify and eliminate bad habits (e.g., poor transfer technique), to correct posture and optimize the wheelchair set-up, and to lose weight if obesity is a factor.

28. A 64-year-old with T2 SCI complains of a gradual reduction in endurance for pushing up a long hill to his office that has occurred over the last 3 months.

Evaluation should include blood pressure, objective upper-extremity strength assessment with myometry, EKG, and laboratory studies including CBC and electrolytes. A drop in blood pressure with exercise suggests coronary ischemia. Silent cardiac ischemia is common after SCI due to blocks in cardiac pain perception with lesions above T5. Coronary narrowing can be detected by doing persantine thallium testing of dynamic cardiac perfusion. Patients with SCI are at high risk for coronary artery disease due to inactivity, lower HDL, tendency toward hyperglycemia, and the risk for obesity.

BIBLIOGRAPHY

1. American Spinal Injury Association, International Standards for Neurological Classification of Spinal Cord Injury, rev 2000. Chicago, ASIA, p 24.
2. Bayley JC, Cochran TP, Sledge CB: The weight-bearing shoulder: The impingement syndrome in paraplegics. J Bone Joint Surg 69A:676–678, 1987.
3. Blackwell T, Krause J, Winkler T, Stiens S: A Desk Reference for Life Care Planning for Persons with Spinal Cord Injury. New York, Demos, 2001.
4. Charney KJ, Juler GL, Comarr AE: General surgery problems in patients with spinal cord injuries. Arch Surg 110:1083–1088, 1975.
5. Duchling P, Wilberger JE: Spinal cord injury without radiographic abnormalities in children. J Neurosurg 57:114–129, 1982.
6. Green D, et al: Prevention of thromboembolism in spinal cord injury: Role of low molecular weight heparin. Arch Phys Med Rehabil 75:290–292, 1994.
7. Hussey RW, Stauffer ES: Spinal cord injury: Requirements for ambulation. Arch Phys Med Rehabil 54:554–557, 1973.
8. Ingberg HO, Prust FW: The diagnosis of abdominal emergencies in patients with spinal cord lesions. Arch Phys Med Rehabil 49:343–348, 1968.
9. Little JW, Ditunno JF, Stiens SA, Harris RM: Incomplete spinal cord injury: Neuronal mechanisms of motor recovery and hyperreflexia. Arch Phys Med Rehabil 80:587–599, 1999.
10. Sgouros S, Williams B: A critical appraisal of drainage in syringomyelia. J Neurosurg 82:1–10, 1995.
11. Stiens SA, Johnson MC, Lyman PJ: Cardiac rehabilitation in patients with spinal cord injuries. Phys Med Rehabil Clin North Am 6:263–296, 1995.
12. Waters RL, Adkins R, Yakura J, Virgil D: Prediction of ambulatory performance based on motor scores derived from standards of the American Spinal Injury Association. Arch Phys Med Rehabil 75:757–760, 1994.
13. Yarkony GM: Spinal Cord Injury: Medical Management and Rehabilitation. Gaithersburg, MD, Aspen, 1994.

32. MOTOR NEURON DISEASE

Michael Hatzakis, Jr., M.D., James C. Agre, M.D., Ph.D., and Arthur A. Rodriquez, M.D.

1. What is a motor neuron disease?

A motor neuron disease produces dysfunction of the motor neurons, which results in weakness and muscle wasting. These diseases or conditions include those that affect the upper (corticobulbar and corticospinal) motor neurons and/or the bulbar and spinal lower motor neurons. Motor neuron diseases are classified based on the location of the pathophysiologic involvement.

2. Describe the classification of the motor neuron diseases:

1. *Upper-motor-neuron disorders*
   Primary lateral sclerosis
   Tropical spastic paraparesis
   Lathyrism
   Epidemic spastic paraparesis
   Familial (hereditary) spastic paraplegia
2. *Combined upper- and lower-motor-neuron disorders*
   Amyotrophic lateral sclerosis (ALS)
   Familial ALS
   Western Pacific ALS–parkinsonian dementia complex
3. *Lower-motor-neuron disorders*
   Spinal (bulbospinal muscular) atrophies
   Monoclonal gammopathy and motor neuron disease

Cancer and motor neuron disease
Poliomyelitis and post-polio syndrome

3. What is known about the pathophysiologic causes of the motor neuron diseases?

As is the case in many disorders, the cause of most of the motor neuron diseases is unknown, except in cases of **lathyrism**, which is an upper-motor-neuron disorder that is produced by an excessive consumption of the chickling pea (*Lathyrus sativus*). This "toxic pea" is thought to contain β-*N*-oxalylamino-L-alanine, which is an agonist of the excitatory neurotransmitter, glutamate. The chickling pea is used as an emergency food in times of drought or flooding on the Indian subcontinent.

The pathogenesis of poliomyelitis is also known and is caused by a viral infection of the anterior motor neurons.

4. How is the poliomyelitis virus transmitted?

It usually enters via the oral route. Once in the body, the virus replicates in the lymphoid tissues of the pharynx and intestine and then spreads to the regional lymphoid tissues, resulting in a viremia and nonspecific illness. Viremia is the most accepted mechanism for direct nervous system exposure to the virus. The reason for the selective vulnerability of certain cells, such as the motor neurons, to the poliomyelitis virus is unknown, but it may relate to specific receptors on their cell membranes. It is possible to get polio more than once since the offending virus has three antigenically distinguishable forms.

5. Is it true that most people who had polio in the past didn't even know they had the disease?

The poliovirus is an extremely infectious agent, but only a fraction of those infected have any symptoms. The disease progresses to CNS involvement with paresis or paralysis in only 1–2% of cases. In 4–8%, only a nonspecific illness is noted by the individual, and in the others, the infection is inapparent.

6. How is it that polio caused weakness in the people who experienced paresis or paralysis?

The poliomyelitis viruses, for unknown reasons, appear to have an affinity for the anterior horn cells. In histologic studies of motor neurons of monkeys with acute paralytic poliomyelitis, nearly all (96–97%) of the motor neurons of severely paralyzed limbs were affected by the virus during the acute infection. About one-half of these motor neurons died during the early convalescent period, and the other half survived. A good correlation was found between the proportion of destroyed motor neurons and the severity of paralysis. With death of the motor neurons, wallerian degeneration occurs, and the muscle fibers associated with those neurons become "orphaned," resulting in motor weakness. Some recover by reinnervation of muscle cells by axonal sprouts from neighboring branches of alpha motor neurons.

7. Why is it that polio patients often required several years to plateau in their functional recovery?

Survivors commonly recovered muscle strength gradually in muscles not completely paralyzed. Some lucky individuals ultimately recovered to a point of minimal or no residual dysfunction. Improvements in function often began in the first weeks but could continue for several years after the acute illness. The mechanisms of recovery include both resolution of dysfunction of partially damaged motor neurons as well as reinnervation of denervated muscle fibers by surviving motor units and muscle hypertrophy following reactivation.

8. Which is the most common presenting form of motor neuron disease in adults? Who is the iron man that died of it?

ALS, or **Lou Gehrig's disease**, is the most common adult form of motor neuron disease and was named after the Yankee first baseman who died from this disorder. Lou played first base for the N.Y. Yankees from 1923 to 1939, batting after Babe Ruth with a lifetime batting average of

.340 and a record 23 grand slams. Lou was best known as the "iron man" for playing in 2130 consecutive games.

ALS encompasses two conditions: **progressive bulbar palsy** and **progressive muscular atrophy**, which differ only in their site of onset. Individuals with ALS have varying degrees of these two disorders, with some having more of the upper- or the lower-motor-neuron involvement or maybe equally involved. Initially, progressive bulbar palsy affects the bulbar motor neurons, while progressive muscular atrophy initially affects the spinal motor neurons. These two diseases overlap the longer the patient survives. Death usually results from complications of the bulbar involvement.

9. What is the prevalence and incidence of ALS?

The incidence of ALS is approximately 1.6 to 2.4 cases/100,000 population, but it may increase with age. For instance, in a study in southwestern Ontario, the incidence increased to 7.4 cases/100,000 population by the eighth decade, with an average age at diagnosis of 62 years. Half of patients with ALS are between 50 and 70 years of age. The average survival from time of diagnosis is approximately 2.5 years, with shorter life expectancy with later age of onset. The male-to-female ratio varies from 1.2 to 1.6:1.

10. Describe the typical clinical features of ALS.

The typical complaint is weakness. The most common findings at the time of initial examination include **atrophy, weakness, spasticity** (upper motor neuron), and **fasciculations** (lower motor neuron). Additionally, muscle stretch reflexes can be depressed in regions where there is primarily lower-motor-neuron involvement or where atrophy is so advanced that upper-motor-neuron signs cannot be found. Otherwise, it is common to find brisk muscle stretch reflexes in areas of muscle atrophy. On occasion, the patient may present with only mild spasticity, suggesting a purely upper motor neuron disorder (e.g., spastic dysarthria or facies or both with no detectable lower motor neuron signs). Muscle cramping is also a frequent complaint.

In general, the most striking feature of ALS is the focal, often asymmetrical, onset of **weakness**, which then spreads to adjacent areas of the body. Spasticity can be disabling and make ambulation difficult. The bowel and bladder are spared in this disease, except for constipation related to inactivity or poor nutritional intake. Sensation is generally spared, although paresthesias and decreased vibratory sensation can be found in up to 25% of patients.

11. What are some of the characteristic features that, when present, weigh against the diagnosis of ALS?

Signs that, when present, weigh against a diagnosis of ALS include a lack of sensory symptoms, spared voluntary eye movements and sphincter control, as well as spared cognitive function. These are generalizations, as some research is now finding some cormorbidity with dementia in ALS. Classic ALS includes degeneration and/or complete loss of motor neurons in the brainstem and spinal cord areas corresponding to the muscle atrophy and degeneration of the large pyramidal neurons in the primary motor cortex and the pyramidal tracts, thus leaving intact the ascending sensory tracts. The nucleus of Onuf (the nucleus controlling the striated muscles of the pelvic floor and the bowel and bladder sphincters) is preserved, explaining why bowel and bladder functions are preserved.

12. Are other motor neuron diseases found in children besides poliomyelitis?

Acute infantile spinal muscular atrophy (Werdnig-Hoffmann disease) is an autosomal recessive disorder with an estimated incidence of 1/15,000 to 1/25,000 livebirths. The disease is apparent at birth in one-third of the children and is usually diagnosed by age 3 months. Survival averages 6–9 months from diagnosis and does not exceed 3 years. Severe hypotonia and weakness and resultant delays in motor milestones dominate the clinical picture. The infants characteristically lie motionless with the lower limbs abducted in the frog-leg position. Fasciculations of the tongue are almost pathognomonic for the disease. Death usually results from respiratory failure.

Chronic infantile spinal muscular atrophy (chronic Werdnig-Hoffmann disease) is much more slowly progressive than the acute form of this disease. Clinical signs are usually present by age 3 years, but occasionally as early as 3 months. This disease has variable progression, with the average age of death being over 10 years. It also has an autosomal recessive inheritance.

Juvenile proximal spinal muscular atrophy (Kugelberg-Welander disease) is characterized by slowly progressive weakness and atrophy of the proximal limb and girdle musculature. It is usually transmitted as an autosomal recessive disorder (type III proximal hereditary motor neuropathy) but also has an autosomal dominant form (type IV juvenile proximal hereditary motor neuropathy). The clinical onset can occur anytime between childhood and the seventh decade of life (in the adult form, type V proximal hereditary motor neuropathy) but usually occurs between ages 2 and 17 years. Both the juvenile and adult forms of this disease begin with symmetrical atrophy and weakness of the pelvic girdle and proximal lower limbs, then progress to involvement of the shoulder girdles and upper arms.

Progressive bulbar paralysis of childhood has two forms, Fazio-Londe disease and Brown-Vialettlo-Laere syndrome. Both cause a slowly progressive weakness of the muscles of the face, tongue, and pharynx. Fazio-Londe disease, which has been described rarely since 1925, produces bilateral deafness as the first symptom. This occurs between the ages 18 months and 31 years (average onset, 12 years). Cranial nerve palsies usually appear about 4–5 years later. Survival may exceed 2 decades. Inheritance is apparently autosomal recessive.

Distal spinal muscular atrophy (spinal form of Charcot-Marie-Tooth disease) has several forms with different inheritance patterns: (1) autosomal recessive juvenile mild (onset, 2–10 years of age) and juvenile severe (onset, 4 mo to 20 yr), and (2) autosomal dominant in the juvenile (onset, 2–20 years) and in the adult (onset, 20–40 yr). Life expectancy is normal except in some severe juvenile cases. Clinical features include weakness and atrophy, which usually start distally in the legs.

13. Can cancer cause motor neuron disease?

This possibility has been raised, because some individuals with cancer become extremely weak and appear to have a motor neuron disorder. However, this observation has not yet been substantiated, and there are many other explanations for these neurologic findings, such as metastases to the nervous system and meninges, cachexia, neuropathy, myopathy, mixed neuropathy/myopathy, and other factors included in the spectrum of paraneoplastic syndromes.

14. What is post-polio syndrome?

Post-polio syndrome is essentially a diagnosis made by exclusion in polio survivors. A good definition of post-polio syndrome has been given by Halstead and Rossi (1987) and is based on five criteria:

1. A confirmed history of paralytic poliomyelitis
2. Partial to fairly complete neurologic and functional recovery
3. A period of neurologic and functional stability of at least 15 years' duration
4. Onset of two or more of the following health problems since achieving a period of stability: unaccustomed fatigue, muscle and/or joint pain, new weakness in muscles previously affected and/or unaffected, functional loss, cold intolerance, new atrophy
5. No other medical diagnosis to explain these health problems

15. What are the most frequent complaints of patients with post-polio syndrome?

In general, new musculoskeletal and neuromuscular symptoms. The table lists the most frequent new health and ADL problems of post-polio individuals, whether they were seen in a post-polio clinic or had responded to a national survey. The most prevalent new health-related complaints were fatigue, muscle or joint pain, and weakness. The most prevalent new ADL complaints were difficulties with walking and stair-climbing.

New Health and ADL Problems in Post-Polio Patients

SYMPTOM	HALSTEAD[1] (n = 539)	HALSTEAD[2] (n = 132)	AGRE[3] (n = 79)
New health problems			
Fatigue	87%	89%	86%
Muscle pain	80	71	86
Joint pain	79	71	77
Weakness			
Previously affected muscles	87	69	80
Previously unaffected muscles	77	50	53
Cold intolerance	—	29	56
Atrophy	—	28	39
New ADL problems			
Walking	85	64	—
Stair-climbing	83	61	67
Dressing	62	17	16

1. Halstead LS, Rossi CD: Orthopedics 8:845–850, 1985.
2. Halstead LS, Rossi CD: In Halstead LS, Wiechers DO (eds): Research and Clinical Aspects of the Late Effects of Poliomyelitis. White Plains, NY, March of Dimes Birth Defects Foundation, 1987, pp 13–26.
3. Agre JC, Rodriguez AA, Sperling KB: Arch Phys Med Rehabil 70:367–370, 1989.

16. How many polio survivors have post-polio syndrome?

The answer is not precisely known. One study reported that 41% of respondents to their questionnaire had new complaints compatible with post-polio syndrome, another study reported approximately 25%, and a third study reported 28.5%. One might estimate from these reports that somewhere between 25% and 40% of polio survivors may be experiencing post-polio syndrome at present. As these individuals age, this proportion may well increase significantly.

17. Why do post-polio individuals lose strength as they age?

There is no empirical evidence that the loss of strength is directly related to poliomyelitis. All individuals lose motor neurons and strength with age, and those that have a reduced number of motor neurons due to the poliovirus infection are at greater risk of losing strength. Imagine a normal individual with 100 motor neurons and a post-polio survivor with 10 motor neurons for a given muscle group. If loss is 1 motor neuron per year, it is clear that the post-polio survivor will decline in strength more quickly. Some also suggest that motor neurons damaged by the poliovirus may age prematurely due to the increased metabolic demand.

18. Is it possible for individuals with clinically normal muscles to be affected by the post-polio syndrome?

Yes, it is possible that an individual who had up to 80% of his motor neurons affected by polio in a given muscle to have recovered to full muscle strength and later have this muscle weakened by the post-polio syndrome due to the abnormal number of motor units. This is due to the fact that a smaller percentage of anterior horn cells innervate many more muscle fibers.

19. Outline the evaluation of a patient with a possible motor neuron disease.

As with all diseases, the initial assessment to determine the diagnosis includes obtaining a detailed history, performing a good physical examination, and obtaining appropriate laboratory tests.

History

1. Major complaints of the patient (and/or parents)
2. Pattern of weakness (in general, motor neuron diseases produce proximal weakness, while neuropathic disorders cause distal weakness, often accompanied by sensory abnormalities)
3. Age of onset and rate of progression
4. Family history

Physical examination

1. Visual inspection for areas of muscular atrophy, muscular hypertrophy, and fasciculations
2. Sensory examination (sensory loss is very rare in motor neuron diseases, but common in neuropathic disorders)
3. Muscle stretch reflexes (increased in upper-motor-neuron disorders, decreased in lower-motor-neuron disorders, and increased or decreased in the combined disorders)
4. Manual muscle testing to show the level of residual muscle function and distribution of weakness (proximal, distal, or asymmetrical)
5. ROM testing to detect contractures (including passive ROM)
6. Functional assessment (to determine the patient's level of functional abilities for assistive devices)

Laboratory studies

1. Muscle biopsy
2. Nerve conduction studies
3. Electromyography
4. Other evaluations, depending on the clinical presentation of the patient (to look for specific disorders, e.g., rare disorders, diabetes mellitus, thyrotoxicosis)
5. Urinalysis (to check for heavy metal intoxication, such as lead or mercury)

20. How are electrodiagnostic studies helpful in diagnosiing ALS? What are the classic features of ALS on electrodiagnostic testing?

It is of primary importance in the diagnosis of ALS to ensure that no treatable or nonfatal disorder accounting for the patient's signs and symptoms is overlooked (see question 21 below). Electrodiagnostic studies are used to exclude the presence of an axonal or demyelinating disease, such as chronic inflammatory demyelinating polyneuropathy, or a neuromuscular junction disorder, such as myasthenia gravis. Needle EMG sampling must be performed, especially in the weakest muscles, and be performed in at least three levels (cervical, lumbar, and sacral) or two levels and bulbar musculature (most commonly, tongue). Classic features seen on EMG sampling of muscles are the presence of fibrillations, positive sharp waves, and motor unit action potential changes typical of reinnervation with fasciculations and decreased recruitment.

The El Escorial criteria for a definitive diagnosis of ALS specify electrodiagnostic evidence of upper- and lower-motor-neuron abnormalities (reduced recruitment, large motor unit action potentials, and fibrillations) in at least three of the four possible levels of the neuraxis (bulbar, cervical, thoracic, lumbosacral) in the absence of electrophysiologic or neuroimaging evidence of another explanation for weakness. No major criteria would be without controversy, and the diagnosis of ALS is no exception. Many electromyographers prefer the Lambert criteria, which include fasciculations as a major finding suggesting lower-motor-neuron involvement and specify nerve conduction studies with normal sensory studies and motor conduction not less than 70% below the lower limit of normal in severely affected muscles.

21. List some disorders that must be considered during the electrodiagnostic evaluation for ALS.

Cervical spondylosis	Myositis
Motor polyradiculopathy	Myopathies
Chronic inflammatory demyelinating polyneuropathy	Myasthenia gravis
	Stroke
Multifocal motor conduction block	Paraneoplastic syndromes
Spinal muscular atrophy syndromes	Mononeuropathies
Focal amyotrophy	Parkinson's disease
Primary lateral sclerosis	Syndrome of benign fasciculations
Multiple sclerosis	

22. What are the general principles of rehabilitation management of a patient with a motor neuron disorder?

The management should be divided into prospective care and expectant care. **Prospective care** includes all the usual health measures provided to any individual regardless of their health status and includes such things as appropriate vaccinations and health screening tests. **Expectant care** is focused on the individual's specific situation and disease. It includes anticipation of complications that might occur during the course of the patient's motor neuron disease. Aggressive measures can be made to prevent or minimize complications and maximize function and independence for as long as possible.

23. How should you approach the treatment of a patient with motor neuron disease?

The primary goal in treating patients with motor neuron diseases is to assist the patient in the maintenance of function, independence, and quality of life for as long as possible. With the knowledge of disease progression, many of the complications of this disease may be prevented with good expectant care. Appropriate preventive and therapeutic interventions for the treatment of pain, decline of swallowing function, soft-tissue tightness, deformity, scoliosis, weakness, and respiratory dysfunction can minimize complications and maximize the patient's ability to function. Functional training for locomotion, dressing, eating, and other ADLs can prolong the independent or partial independent phase of disease progression.

Selective surgical procedures (such as tendon transfers, releases, and arthrodeses) may be available at most centers and can improve the patient's ability to function. Gastrostomy and jejunostomy tubes are also recommended when the patient begins to have significant dysphagia to maintain adequate nutrition and to reduce the risk of aspiration. These interventions are best performed within the framework of a coordinated rehabilitation team.

Drug therapy for ALS is limited. A recently developed drug such as riluzole (Rilutek), an anti-glutamate agent, may be effective in slowing the progression of the disease. It has been found to improve survival in patients with *bulbar onset disease* but the effects generally are small compared with its side effects, which include asthenia as well as being costly to administer.

24. What are a few of the prognostic indictors for patients with ALS?

Survival is typically 3–5 years from onset of symptoms. About 10–16% live > 10 years. Poorer prognostic indicators include more severe disease at onset, older age at onset, female sex, and bulbar onset. Electrodiagnostic indicators of poor prognosis include profuse spontaneous fibrillations and sharp waves and low-amplitude compound muscle action potentials.

25. Is pain a common problem in patients with motor neuron diseases?

Pain is uncommon in the early presentation of ALS. Pain also is not often a major problem, except in patients with acute poliomyelitis, who may have severe muscle pain.

Control of pain for the individual with ALS can usually be accomplished by both physical and pharmacologic treatments. The use of hot packs, especially the Kenny hot packs (made from woolen blankets), applied at 5-minute intervals for 20 minutes, can be helpful. The heat treatments along with stretching are useful in the acute stages to control pain and maintain ROM. NSAIDs may also be used. Many patients, however, may have mechanical pain related to weakness, contracture, or deformity. Muscle cramps and stiffness related to spasticity may be treated with baclofen with care taken not to cause fatigue or loss of function.

26. What is your approach to sialorrhea?

Sialorrhea is a significant cause of social distress for the individual with a motor neuron disease, and individuals with motor neuron diseases typically have impaired saliva management. The first priority is to determine if the patient is suffering sialorrhea or thickening of mucus production. Thickening of mucus can be treated by improvement of hydration and with medications. Management of sialorrhea begins with methods to reduce production of saliva. Pharmacologic means include drugs such as glycopyrrolate (Robinul), amitriptyline (Elavil), or benztropin (Cogentin). Individuals with sialorrhea can be given suction machines if saliva production is a problem. For thick mucus production, manually and mechanically assisted techniques can improve mobilization of saliva. One such device is an insufflator-exafflator to extract excess mucus. Individuals with ALS may retain the ability to cough, but it is often ineffective.

27. How is pseudobulbar affect managed in an individual with motor neuron disease?

Pseudobulbar affect is pathologic crying or laughing often triggered by a seemingly innocuous emotional event and one in which the magnitude of the emotional response may be out of proportion with the trigger. It is important to recognize this condition as it contributes to the anxiety and social distress of individuals with a motor neuron disease if poorly understood by the individual and their families. This condition is treated by reassuring and educating the patient and their families. Pharmacologic management is appropriate and recent trials indicate that amitriptyline and fluvoxamine are effective.

28. How are muscle contractures treated?

Muscle contracture is a common problem in patients with motor neuron diseases. The best treatment is **prevention**. Contractures usually first occur at muscles that span two joints with the joints in the flexed position. Common sites include the shoulder adductors, elbow flexors, forearm pronators, finger adductors, hip flexors or internal rotators, knee flexors, ankle plantar flexors, and foot invertors.

Physical treatment includes passive, active assistive and active ROM, depending on the condition of the patient, usually after the application of superficial heat. Prolonged stretching is required to correct contracture. When using orthotics to help prevent contractures, one must carefully assess the kinesiologic factors. When preventing or correcting shortening of a muscle that spans two joints, it is important to ensure that the muscles are stretched at both joints that they cross. Also, splinting and casting can be used to treat contracture. Surgery is only rarely needed. Appropriate positioning can aid in the prevention of deformity.

29. How does one treat deformity in patients with motor neuron disorder?

Malalignment of body segments leads to contracture and deformity; therefore, appropriate **prospective treatment** is needed to prevent or minimize the development of contracture or deformity. Appropriate stretching, bracing, and positioning can help prevent contractures. For instance, in a child sitting in a large wheelchair with a sling-type seat, frequently one hip will be higher than the other, with the hips internally rotated and adducted, and the child leaning on one elbow for support. This position will lead to contracture and subsequent scoliotic deformity. The minimal wheelchair prescription should include a firm seat, with adequate lumbar, truncal, and arm support. Also, thoracolumbosacral orthotic devices can help to prevent progressive scoliotic deformity in patients with significant weakness of the trunk.

Some patients with post-polio syndrome place significant stress upon the knee while ambulating. This can cause either genu valgus and/or genu recurvatum deformity to develop, which is usually treated with a knee-ankle-foot orthosis.

30. How is scoliosis managed?

Prevention and management of scoliosis comprise one of the major goals in the management of neuromuscular disease. Scoliosis occurs with increasing age and with advancing disability. Usually, the paraspinal muscular weakness is symmetrical, and while the child is ambulatory, the development of scoliosis is uncommon; however, once the child becomes nonambulatory, scoliosis develops rapidly. Most children with motor neuron disease develop a collapsing, paralytic type of scoliosis.

The initial approach to managing scoliosis is to order the most appropriate **wheelchair**, which must be measured for each individual. A symmetrical sitting posture with adequate upper- and lower-extremity support must be maintained; the sling seat should be avoided because it permits asymmetrical pelvic rotation. A solid foam-padded seat cushion can be used to level the pelvis during sitting in the early stages. Children tolerate **sitting-support orthoses** until the curve reaches > 40°. At that point, a relatively rapid progression continues that generally cannot be managed orthotically, and surgery may be indicated. Current literature supports using a surgical approach before ventilatory capacity (VC) drops below 50% of age-adjusted expected values. This literature suggests greater postsurgical morbidity and mortality once VC drops below 50%.

31. What is the approach to strengthening and exercise for individuals with motor neuron disease?

Strengthening exercises must be prescribed judiciously and followed carefully. It is generally accepted that vigorous, fatiguing, progressive resistive exercise may cause further weakness and muscle fiber degeneration. Low-intensity, nonfatiguing, and submaximal exercise may be beneficial for maintenance or improvement in muscle strength and cardiorespiratory fitness as well as positive psychological effects. Weakness is also treated with appropriate orthotic devices for support. Post-polio patients with grade 4/5 muscle strength have improved strength with resistive exercise without apparent harm. Exercise should be prescribed carefully in muscles with less than 3/5 strength.

32. How does one treat the patient with respiratory difficulty?

When weakness or deformity sufficiently limits the patient's ability to ventilate, mechanical ventilatory assistance is needed. Early signs and symptoms of hypoxia include difficulty with sleeping, nighttime dyspnea, nightmares, and daytime somnolence. As these signs appear, appropriately prescribed ventilatory aids (such as cuirass or plastic wrap) enhance ventilation in the recumbent position. In the later stages of motor neuron disease, oral positive-pressure ventilation, pneumobelt, or cuirass ventilators can be used throughout the day, energized by the wheelchair battery. Tracheostomy is rarely needed, and its use is somewhat controversial.

33. How is dysphagia in motor neuron disease detected and treated?

Individuals with motor neuron disease and dysphagia are at increased risk of suboptimal caloric and fluid intake as well as worsened muscle atrophy, weakness, and fatigue. Symptoms of dysphagia include jaw weakness, fatigue, drooling, choking on food, and slow eating. Early techniques include modification of food and fluid consistency and coaching and training by a speech therapist guided by barium swallow examination. As dysphagia progresses, gastrostomy or jejunostomy tubes are indicated if conservative management does not maintain a safe level of caloric intake. If dysphagia is developing, placement of a feeding tube should occur before the vital capacity falls to 50% of age-predicted.

34. Discuss the approach to end-of-life issues with the individual with motor neuron disease.

It is important to establish an open environment of communication with patients with progressive motor neuron diseases. It is important that patients and their families understand the progression of the impairments and the potential risks of not treating specific conditions such as dysphagia. It is also vital to discuss plans for end-of-life, such as hospice care and relief of pain and dyspnea. Provide supportive care for depression and anxiety. It is important to review advance care directives with patients and their families well ahead of significant functional impairment.

BIBLIOGRAPHY

1. Agre JC, Rodriquez AA, Tafel JA: Late effects of polio: Critical review of the literature on neuromuscular function. Arch Phys Med Rehabil 72:923–931, 1991.
2. Agre JC: The role of exercise in the patient with post-polio syndrome. Ann NY Acad Sci 753:321–334, 1995.
3. Agre JC, Mathews DJ: Rehabilitation concepts in motor neuron diseases. In Braddom RL (ed): Physical Medicine and Rehabilitation. Philadelphia, W.B. Saunders, 1996, pp 955–971.
4. Daube JR: Electrodiagnostic studies in amyotrophic lateral sclerosis and other motor neuron disease. Muscle Nerve 23:1488–1502, 2000.
5. Dumitru D: Electrodiagnostic Medicine. Philadelphia, Hanley & Belfus, 1995.
6. Francis K, Bach JR, DeLisa JA: Evaluation and rehabilitation of patients with adult motor neuron disease. Arch Phys Med Rehabil 80:951–963, 1999.
7. Grimby G, Einarsson G: Post-polio management. CRC Crit Rev Phys Med Rehabil 2:189–200, 1991.

8. Halstead LS, Grimby G (eds): Post-Polio Syndrome. Philadelphia, Hanley & Belfus, 1995.
9. Hadjikoutis S, Wiles CM, Eccles R: Cough in motor neuron disease: A review of mechanisms. Q J Med 92(9):487–494, 1999.
10. Hudson AJ: The motor neuron diseases and related disorders. In Joynt RJ (ed): Clinical Neurology, vol 4. Philadelphia, J.B. Lippincott, 1991, pp 1–35.
11. Kottke FJ: Therapeutic exercise to maintain mobility. In Kottke FJ, Lehmann JF (eds): Krusen's Handbook of Physical Medicine and Rehabilitation, 4th ed. Philadelphia, W.B. Saunders, 1990, pp 436–451.
12. Matthews DJ, Stempien LM: Orthopedic management of the disabled child. In Sinaki M (ed): Basic Clinical Rehabiliation Medicine. St. Louis, Mosby, 1993, pp 399–411.
13. Miller RG, Rosenberg JA, Gelinas DF, et al: Practice parameter: The care of the patient with amyotrophic lateral sclerosis (an evidence-based review): Report of the Quality Standards Subcommittee of the American Academy of Neurology: ALS Practice Parameters Task Force. Neurology 52:1311–1323, 1999.
14. Sinaki M: Exercise and rehabilitation measures in amyotrophic lateral sclerosis. In Tsubaki T, Yase Y (eds): Amyotrophic Lateral Sclerosis [Excerpta Medica International Congress series 769]. Amsterdam, Elsevier Science, 1988, pp 343–368.
15. Swash M: An algorithm for ALS diagnosis and management. Neurology 53(suppl 5):S58–S62, 1999.

33. FRONTIERS AND FUNDAMENTALS IN NEUROREHABILITATION

Charles E. Levy, M.D., Andrea Behrman, Ph.D., Leslie Gonzalez Rothi, Ph.D., Haim Ring, M.D., and Kenneth Heilman, M.D.

1. With the new therapies that can markedly reduce the damage from stroke, is stroke rehabilitation passé?

Great progress has been made in limiting the damage from stroke. Thrombolytic agents such as tissue plasminogen activator (TPA), applied under favorable conditions, can limit the damage from stroke and may even enable a complete recovery. Neuroprotective agents, such as those that interfere with glutamate-induced cellular depolarization and the resulting uncontrolled calcium entry into neurons, can limit ischemic brain damage in experimental models (although clinical trials of neuroprotective agents administered within 6 hours have failed to replicate the results of animal studies). Unfortunately, the therapeutic window for limiting the extent of primary damage appears to be between 3 and 6 hours. Because the signs and symptoms of stroke usually do not cause pain or external bleeding, their significance often goes unrecognized until after the therapeutic window has closed.

Therefore, most people who experience a significant stroke will sustain a functional deficit. Furthermore, even when TPA is administered in a timely manner, while many may experience complete remission of their symptoms, others may be left with persistent deficits, including those who may have been so impaired as to not have been rehabilitation candidates if not for these new treatments. For these people, rehabilitation holds the greatest hope of improving abilities and adjustment after stroke.

2. What is constraint-induced movement therapy (CIMT)?

CIMT is a physiotherapeutic technique to restore hand function to those with upper limb hemiparesis. Sometimes referred to as **forced use**, it includes time-intensive exercise of the paretic upper limb, usually with restraint of the able upper limb in a mitt or sling.

3. What is the minimum amount of motion a person must be able to generate in the paretic limb before being enrolled into a CIMT protocol?

Typically, the minimum criterion has been set at 20° of voluntary wrist extension and 10° of extension in two fingers at the metacarpophalangeal or interphalangeal joints of the paretic hand.

This criterion has been established because those with less motion respond less robustly. Those with a complete paralysis are unlikely to benefit.

4. Describe a typical CIMT regimen.

Although many variations exist, a generic program would include:

- A mitt worn over the able hand during 90% of waking hours. The mitt prevents use of the able hand and thus encourages use of the paretic hand.
- A series of tasks performed with the paretic hand, such as tossing a bean bag at a target, reaching and grasping objects, stacking blocks, moving blocks from one container to another, turning pages of a magazine, flipping playing cards, writing on and erasing a chalkboard, and feeding.
- Physiotherapy 6 hours/day, 5 days/week, for 2 weeks performing these tasks. The patient is encouraged and expected to use the paretic hand as much as possible throughout the day whether or not he or she is in therapy.

5. What evidence supports the efficacy of CIMT?

Numerous small studies have demonstrated the benefit of CIMT for those with upper-limb hemiparesis due to stroke. Most subjects have been enrolled 6 months to 1 year post-stroke, in a period where conventional physiotherapy has failed to garner further functional improvement. Subjects as great as 18 years post-stroke have benefited in these trials. Significant improvements in strength, range of motion (ROM), and actual use have been documented. These benefits persist long after the treatment.

6. Describe the phenomenon of "learned nonuse" as it might apply to a stroke patient with a right upper limb paresis.

Immediately after the stroke, whenever the patient attempts to use the paretic right limb, he or she experiences failure. The flaccid hand cannot grip, so coffee is spilled on the lap and the toothbrush cannot be grasped. Conversely, when the person employs the able left hand, he or she is successful. This creates a situation in which use of the left hand is rewarded with success, whereas use of the right hand consistently leads to failure. In a relatively short time, the patient stops trying to use the right hand and learns to rely exclusively on the left. In time, a certain amount of neurologic healing necessary for right hand function may take place, but because the individual no longer tries to use the hand, no functional recovery occurs.

7. What is "massed practice," and why is it a treatment for learned nonuse?

Simply stated, massed practice refers to the idea that if one wants to acquire a new skill, one must practice, practice, practice. Performing artists understand that seamless performance demands multiple rehearsals. This apparently is true for relearning a skill as well. CIMT literature builds a case that in order to coax movement from a paretic hand, the person must undergo extensive training.

8. How much training constitutes massed practice?

This is one of the key questions facing rehabilitation medicine. The experience of many who undergo CIMT suggests that the typical acute inpatient stroke program of up to 3 hours/day of unconcentrated therapy followed by outpatient therapy 1 hour/ session, three times per week, does not reach the threshold of massed practice. However, wearing a mitt during all waking hours and receiving 6 hours of therapy per day for 2 weeks does constitute massed practice. We have defined the range, but we still don't know the exact level of the threshold.

9. Does CIMT induce neuroplasticity?

Since the concept of learned nonuse was first proposed, animal studies have shown that after parts of the cerebral cortex representing a limb have been damaged, cortical representations of that limb can develop in immediately adjacent regions of the cortex, but only if the animal is engaged in activity that encourages use of that limb.

Both functional magnetic resonance imaging (fMRI) and transcortical magnetic stimulation studies in humans have documented changes in cortical activation that correspond with improved motor abilities in upper-limb paresis due to stroke following CIMT. In two subjects with cortical strokes, Levy et al. found that tissue around the rim of the infarct that had been had been silent prior to training was activated during finger tapping after 2 weeks of CIMT.

Liepert et al. used transcranial magnetic stimulation to compare cortical maps of motor function in six subjects before and after CIMT for upper-limb paresis due to stroke. Prior to CIMT, the cortical representation of the abductor pollicis brevis (APB) contralateral to the paretic limb was smaller than that ipsilateral to the paretic limb. Following CIMT, subjects experienced improvement in hand function. The motor evoked potentials recorded at the paretic APB increased in amplitude, the location of the cortical representation of the paretic APB migrated, and the extent of the representation expanded to an area greater than the uninjured APB representation. In a follow-up study using the same methodology, Liepert et al. found that the size of the cortical representations of the APB ipsilateral and contralateral to the paretic hand equalized at 6 months. These three studies show short- and long-term alteration in brain function associated with therapy-induced improvement in physical function after neurologic injury.

10. How soon after a stroke can a CIMT therapy be employed?

It is clear that in the postacute phase (approx. 3 months post-stroke), CIMT can be helpful to selected patients. However, how close to the time of the stroke a CIMT program can be implemented is yet unknown. There are theoretical and pragmatic problems with implementing a traditional CIMT program immediately after stroke. It has been hypothesized that CIMT is effective because it overcomes the habit of nonuse at a time when the patient is neurologically prepared to accept the challenge of activity in the paretic limb. Immediately after the stroke, presumably, the patient has not yet acquired the learned nonuse. Second, it may take some time (days or weeks) following a stroke before the CNS has recovered sufficiently to profit from CIMT.

On a practical note, the immediate rehabilitation goals after stroke include acquisition of skills that will allow the patient to resume independence as much as possible. This could include gait training requiring the use of the able hand to grip a cane or walker and learning one-handed techniques with the able hand for dressing, feeding, grooming, and toileting. A 2-week, 6 hours/day program of CIMT would leave little room for other necessary therapy aimed at remediating speech/language, cognition, or mobility, or aiding adjustment to disability, and by definition, would exclude compensation with the able hand. If this were not enough of a hurdle there is even animal data to suggest that CIMT immediately after stroke not only confounds recovery, but also may increase infarct size.

11. What other approaches have shown success in restoring function of the upper limb in stroke hemiparesis?

Electromyography-triggered neuromuscular electrical stimulation (ENES) has helped restore hand function in upper-limb paresis both acutely and chronically (> 1 year) following stroke. In this technique, the EMG signal produced by wrist and hand extensors triggers an external unit that augments the signal, thereby inducing effective muscle contraction. As the person learns to generate higher amplitude signals, the trigger threshold is raised. In a randomized study of 9 hemiparetic stroke survivors undergoing acute rehabilitation, Francisco et al. found that those treated with 1 hour/day of ENES showed significantly greater improvement on the Fugl-Meyer and the Functional Independence Measure than the control group, which received an extra hour per day of traditional physical therapy. Caurraugh et al. found improvements in the Box and Block test and in force generation in 11 hemiparetic subjects who were at least 1 year post-stroke and were treated with ENES for 60 minutes 3 times/week for 2 weeks.

Although both of these studies have many limitations including small sample sizes, they offer an interesting contrast to CIMT. While CIMT seems to"work" by the brute force of the intensity of practice, ENES relies on enhanced sensory feedback and is much less time-intensive than CIMT. Whether these approaches engage different neuronal mechanisms of recovery or could be used in combination has yet to be determined.

12. Do neurons in the mature CNS ever re-grow?

Although neurogenesis in the mature CNS is rare, it occurs in at least two regions:

1. New neurons for the olfactory bulb are generated in the subventricular zone in the wall of the lateral ventricle and then migrate rostrally to their destinations, where they assume the role of interneurons.

2. The subgranular zone of the dentate gyrus gives rise to neocortical granule cells. There is even evidence that damage to granule cells can trigger increased proliferation and recruitment of new granule cells from resident progenitors.

There is as of yet no evidence that these processes play a significant role in functional recovery from brain injury. However, their discovery raises the enticing possibility that the brain has latent capabilities for self-repair.

13. Why is it that injured neurons so rarely regenerate in the CNS?

The failure of CNS neurons to regenerate is not due to an intrinsic deficit of the neuron, but rather to a characteristic of the neural environment that either does not support or actually inhibits regrowth.

14. What strategies are being employed to overcome barriers to regeneration?

Regeneration is a multistep process: (1) Injured neurons must survive or be replaced; (2) the damaged or replacement axons must extend their processes to the original targets; (3) the remyelination of the damaged axons must occur; and (4) functional synapses must form.

Stem cells and **fetal tissue** are possible sources for cellular replacement for the damaged CNS. Stem cells have the advantage that they are multipotent, can be propagated in vitro, genetically tagged with markers or therapeutic genes, and directly grafted into the mature CNS, while lacking the ethical controversy associated with the use of fetal tissue. A second possibility is to stimulate brain self-repair: Both of these strategies require greater knowledge of the molecules and genes that govern neuronal proliferation. The new cells will have to be able to thrive in the altered environment of the injured CNS and be capable of functional integration into the remaining CNS circuitry.

Neurotrophic factor delivery. Neurotrophins, such as brain-derived neurotrophic factor (BDNF), aid in cell survival and promote axon growth. They are usually combined with growth-promoting cells or matrices to provide the needed permissive substrate. Schwann cells engineered to express BDNF facilitated the regrowth of supraspinal axons across a transected spinal cord. However, axons have difficulty leaving the permissive substrate to reach their targets in the injured CNS. There is some evidence that this may be accomplished with induction of neurotrophins in the injured tissue.

Axon guidance and **removal of growth inhibition.** Several growth-promoting molecules have a role in axon guidance, synapse formation, and regeneration and activity-dependent plasticity. The identification of these factors has been relatively recent, and thus there are few studies of their application in repair.

After CNS injury, **gliotic scar** may form. The scar can present both a physical and molecular barrier to regrowth. Growth inhibitory molecules, which are present in the normal CNS, may be re-expressed in the scar. These may include semaphorin III/collapsin I, the proteoglycan NG2, chondroitin sulfate, and keratin.

Bridging is a strategy to be applied when a portion of the CNS is lost, a cyst has developed, or extensive scarring exists. A bridge is used to guide axons across these barriers and reintroduce axons into intact parenchyma. Artificial substrates that can act as a scaffold for axon growth are being developed. In a rat model of spinal cord transection, nerve regeneration has been guided by semi-rigid porous tubes composed of acrylonitrile and vinyl chloride seeded with growth-promoting Schwann cells. Rapidly absorbable substrates such as poly-α-hydroxyacids have also been tested in the rat spinal cord.

15. If central regeneration is so limited, why does recovery happen at all?

While regeneration to the original target by the original axon is rare, other modes of neuronal rearrangement are more common.

Pruning (actually branching) occurs in neurons with highly collateralized axons; an uninjured axon grows a new branch to reinnervate the abandoned target. Animal data suggest that when this process occurs, it takes months to reach completion.

Collateral sprouting involves a neighboring axon that branches to assume the territory of the injured axon. This process is widespread and has been studied in the septal nucleus, hippocampus, and peripheral nervous system. This process can aid in recovery if the contributing neuron is similar to the lost neuron, but may also lead to dysfunction if the new sprout transmits signals of significant variance to the original. In experimental animals, collateral sprouting is evident within 8 hours of injury and is usually complete within 1 month.

Ingrowth, which takes months to complete, differs from collateral sprouting in that the contributing axon is remote to the injured axon. Because of the distance traversed, the contributing neuron innervates a foreign target. An example is sympathetic ingrowth. In this instance, intercranial sympathetic fibers, which normally innervate blood vessels on the surface of the brain, assume territory in the injured forebrain normally supplied by cholinergic neurons. It is easy to imagine that this arrangement would most likely be maladaptive and worsen functional deficits.

16. Explain "unmasking" as it relates to recovery of function after brain injury.

In the hours and days immediately following a brain injury, some amount of recovery may be attributed to the resolution of cerebral edema and arterial spasm. **Unmasking** has also been invoked to explain early recovery. This involves activation of previously "silent" synapses that only begin to express function after injury to primary functional synapses. Bach-y-Rita gives the analogy that if telephone lines direct from New York to San Francisco were irredeemably destroyed, less direct routes from New York to Washington to Denver to San Francisco might be employed. With time and increased demand, the more convoluted route might gain efficiency that rivaled the original. In this way, multisynaptic neural routes might be unmasked and compensate for damaged direct pathways. It has also been postulated that intact primary functional structures inhibit or "mask" the activity of potentially useful parallel synapses; with injury to the primary structures, these parallel routes might be freed to flourish.

17. What is neural plasticity?

Neural plasticity refers to the potential of the CNS to reorganize in terms of structure and function. Plasticity can refer to the normal differentiation and specialization that takes place as the human brain and spinal cord mature from the prenatal period throughout childhood. Plasticity can also refer to changes evoked in the CNS by the effects of environmental exposure and experience (learning) or environmental deprivation. Finally, plasticity often describes the response of the CNS to lesion or other injury. Implicit in all these examples is a responsive, flexible, and dynamic CNS, as opposed to the picture often presented of a fixed CNS incapable of repair or adaptation.

18. Who was Constantin von Monakow?

Von Monakow (1835–1930) was a Russian-born German neurologist described as a "huge bearded figure with a shrill voice" given to boisterous and eccentric behavior in youth. He had witnessed the atrophy of the superior colliculus after the removal of the contralateral eye at birth in experimental rabbits, and he had himself removed the occipital lobes in two newborn rabbits and observed the complete degeneration of the lateral geniculate nuclei. Presumably, from this type of work, he formulated the concept of diaschisis.

19. What is "diaschisis"?

Diaschisis (from the Greek meaning "shocked throughout") is a term coined by von Monakow to explain functional deficit and recovery from a brain injury. In his original German article in 1914, he postulated that following focal brain injury, sites distant from the primary injury might be affected by loss of neural input from the injured portion of the brain. Thus, the original deficit reflects not only loss of function attributable to cell death, but also to dysfunction of distant brain sites dependent on the input of the now dead tissue. Gradually, function returns to the undamaged neural tissue. Von Monakow described an active brain struggling to recover function in a way that somewhat mirrors modern conceptions of dynamic neural recovery and plasticity.

20. What objective data support the existence of diaschisis?

There is an abundance of evidence to support the construct of diaschisis. Patients with cortical strokes have shown ipsilateral thalamic or basal ganglia metabolic depression. Patients with frontal lobe infarcts show decreased blood flow and oxygen metabolism in the contralateral cerebellum on PET scans. In rats, a small thrombotic infarction of the left frontal pole causes a decrement of activity of the ipsilateral ventrobasal thalamus, even when the rat receives stimulation that would ordinarily excite this area. Experimentally induced right middle cerebral artery ischemia in rats causes widespread reduction of brain stem neurotransmitters, particularly norepinephrine. This is accompanied by behavioral hyperactivity, which is diminished when a norepinephrine uptake blocker is administered. Other neurotransmitters that are affected by cerebral ischemia include dopamine, serotonin, and GABA.

21. Diaschisis, miaschisis! How is any of this clinically relevant?

Widespread catecholamine depletion is a consequence of focal brain insult and may be one of the mechanisms of diaschisis. Feeney et al.'s work demonstrated that, at least under certain circumstances, treatment with amphetamines speeds recovery, whereas haloperidol impedes recovery, particularly for motor skills. In a commonly cited experiment, Feeney et al. subjected rats to unilateral sensorimotor cortex ablation, causing pronounced but transient hemiparesis as reflected in a beam-walking task. When the rats were given amphetamines after ablation, their performance markedly improved compared to the saline-treated control animals. However, this improvement was abolished if haloperidol, a catecholamine antagonist, was given 2 minutes after the administration of the amphetamines. In fact, performance was below that of saline-treated animals. Rats given haloperidol alone performed even more poorly than those given both drugs.

Another interesting finding was that neither medication had any significant effect if the rat was confined for 8 hours, unable to attempt to walk the beam. Clearly, recovery in this study was susceptible to both pharmacologic and environmental influence. Thus, Feeney postulated that the combination of physical therapy plus stimulation of the catecholamine systems might facilitate recovery in brain-injured humans.

A second experiment in 1989 subjecting cats to bilateral visual cortex ablation and then treatment with amphetamines, saline, or amphetamines plus haloperidol produced similar results. Amphetamine-treated cats recovered binocular vision as measured by a visual cliff task, whereas the saline- and amphetamine/haloperidol-treated cats continued to perform at a chance level.

22. Which medications are stimulants?

The three stimulants usually discussed as potentially beneficial in a rehabilitation setting are dextroamphetamine (Dexedrine), methylphenidate (Ritalin), and pemoline (Cylert). The stimulant class also includes cocaine and nicotine, drugs more commonly cited for their abuse potential. Caffeine, of course, is a commonly used stimulant. Dextroamphetamine and methylphenidate are often grouped together in terms of mechanism of action and effect.

23. Discuss the history of the three potentially useful stimulants.

1. **Amphetamine** was first synthesized by Edeleano in 1887, but its sympathomimetic effect went largely unappreciated until it was resynthesized by Alles in 1927 as part of an effort to find substitutes for ephedrine in the treatment of asthma. Use of amphetamines to treat a wide variety of illnesses including narcolepsy and depression was common in the 1930s. In 1936, benzedrine was available in tablet form without a prescription. World War II saw the expansion of the use and abuse of amphetamines. German Panzer troops used "huge amounts of methamphetamine" during the invasions of Poland, Belgium, and France. American, British, and Japanese forces also used these substances. After World War II, medical interest waned as the

abuse potential became better understood. The use of amphetamines declined further with the development of tricyclic antidepressants, starting with imipramine in 1957 and amitriptyline in 1961. In the U.S., "recreational" use of amphetamines ("speed") resurfaced as part of the youth drug culture in the 1960s. Currently, dextroamphetamine is a highly restricted drug, for which the only FDA-approved indications are the treatment of narcolepsy and attention deficit hyperactivity disorder. The drug has a half-life of 7–10 hours and reaches peak effect in 2–4 hours.

2. **Methylphenidate** was developed by Ciba Laboratories; in 1954 clinical trials were reported by Drasado and Schmidt and methylphenidate was marketed as a mood elevator. This stimulant was reported to induce less euphoria, addiction, and "rebound letdown" than amphetamines. However, by 1960, cases of abuse and addiction were noted, and by 1962, cases of methylphenidate psychosis were reported. This drug has a half-life of 2–4 hours and reaches peak effect in 1–2 hours.

3. **Pemoline**, developed in 1974, is the least potent stimulant of the three. Its mechanism of action is unclear; it is thought to enhance the release of dopamine and reduces catecholamine turnover. Its half-life is 12 hours, and it takes days to weeks to reach its peak.

24. How do the mechanisms of action of amphetamines and methylphenidate differ?

Of the two, much more is known about dextroamphetamine. Both drugs cause increases in the availability of dopamine and norepinephrine. Dextroamphetamine causes direct release of dopamine and norepinephrine as well as the blockade of catecholamine uptake. Evidence suggests that the release of dopamine is from a newly synthesized pool that is not calcium dependent. Pretreatment of experimental rats with reserpine caused no decrement in dopamine release when dextroamphetamine was applied. This is in contrast to methylphenidate, in which reserpine pretreatment abolishes dopamine release. It is believed that the dopamine released by methylphenidate exists in a calcium-dependent storage pool. Furthermore, there is evidence that both drugs affect serotonin in distinct manners.

25. Dextroamphetamine increases the amounts of dopamine and norepinephrine at the synaptic cleft. Which of these neurotransmitters is responsible for the motor recovery seen when the dextroamphetamine is applied?

Boyeson and Feeney infused norepinephrine alone or dopamine with a dopamine-hydroxylase inhibitor into the ventricles of rats that had previously been subjected to a sensorimotor cortex injury. Only the rats treated with the norepinephrine displayed enhanced motor recovery, suggesting that this neurotransmitter is responsible for the positive effects of amphetamine. However, other studies have shown beneficial effects when dopaminergic drugs are administered to rats.

26. What other mechanisms might account for the behavioral improvement associated with amphetamine?.

Evidence suggests that amphetamine plus appropriate behavioral therapy initially increases neurite growth, which is then followed by increased synaptogenesis. When neocortical ischemia was induced in rats, those treated with dextroamphetamine (experimental animals) displayed improved motor function (forelimb placement) and spatial memory (Morris water maze) as compared to placebo-treated animals. Animals treated with amphetamine showed significant increases in GAP-43, which subsided after 7 days. GAP-43, an indicator of neuronal sprouting, is a membrane-bound protein found in the axonal growth cones of sprouting CNS neurites. Synaptophysin (a presynaptic vesicle protein that can be used to quantify the number of terminals during neuroanatomic remodeling) increased in the experimental animals, but not until day 14. Taken together, this evidence suggests that amphetamine plus a therapeutic environment can promote recovery, and that one mechanism underlying recovery may be increased neural sprouting which then leads to increased numbers of synapses.

27. Is there evidence that amphetamines are actually helpful to patients likely to be encountered in a rehabilitation setting?

Lipper and Tuchman's 1976 case study showing the positive response of a traumatic-brain-injured (TBI) patient to amphetamine treatment marked the beginning of the modern era of use of stimulants for the brain-injured. Their patient demonstrated a diminution in confusion and paranoia and an improvement in short-term memory during treatment. Chrisostomo et al. randomized 8 patients with hemiplegia due to stroke to receive either a single dose of amphetamine or placebo in a double-blinded study. The 4 patients who received amphetamine showed a statistically significant improvement in Fugl-Meyer motor scale scores as compared to the controls. Unfortunately, the small number of subjects, the fact that the controls appear to have been more severely affected, and the fact that the outcome was measured only 1 day after patients received the drug limits our ability to generalize from this study. Blieberg et al. studied a single TBI patient who was treated with amphetamine in a double-blind, placebo-controlled, crossover trial. They reported improved performance and consistency on a neuropsychological test battery when the patient received amphetamine.

28. What is the evidence that methylphenidate is useful in the rehab setting?

Methylphenidate has been useful in treating post-stroke depression. Since the prevalence of depression is as high as 30–60% in the first 2 years following stroke, recognition and proper treatment of this entity are critical. In a retrospective chart review, Lazarus et al. found that methylphenidate was at least as effective as nortriptyline; however, the average response time for the methylphenidate group was 2.4 days as compared to 27 days in the nortriptyline group. This is particularly meaningful for stroke survivors on inpatient rehabilitation units who often must demonstrate continuing gains every week or risk being discharged.

Grode et al. performed a double-blind, placebo-controlled study of methylphenidate in a trial that enrolled 21 consecutive patients admitted to an acute rehabilitation hospital following a stroke. Ten patients were randomized to receive the drug. The dose of methylphenidate was escalated from 5 mg/day to 30 mg/day as tolerated, for a period of 1–3 weeks. The methylphenidate group showed greater improvements in mood (Hamilton Rating Depression Scale and Zung Self-Rating Depression Scale) and motor function (Fugl-Meyer Scale and a modified version of the Functional Independence Measure). This study's limitations include the small number of subjects and unequal distributions of left- and right-hemispheric injury and cortical and subcortical infarcts.

The record of methylphenidate in TBI is mixed. Speech et al. subjected 12 "chronic" TBI patients (with an average time since injury of 4 years) to receive 1 week of methylphenidate treatment or placebo using a double-blind, placebo-controlled, randomized crossover design. At the end of each week, patients received neuropsychological testing and were rated by a close friend or family member on social and personality characteristics using the Katz Adjustment Scale. No significant differences were detected in the neuropsychological test results. Although the authors claim there were no significant differences on the Katz results, subjects on methylphenidate scored higher than controls on 9 of 11 subscales. Furthermore, 8 of 11 observers reported cognitive and personality improvement during methylphenidate treatment. Unfortunately this study may be faulted at a number of levels: none of the subjects was identified before enrollment as having deficits in attention that might be amenable to treatment, no washout period between treatments was provided (improvements due to methylphenidate may have persisted for the placebo group), and no precautions to prevent learning between the tests were evident. Even without these flaws, the results of this study cannot be applied to patients who are in the acute or subacute stage after TBI. In a different study using a multi-baseline design, Kaelin et al. found that methylphenidate was associated with improvement in neuropsychological tests measuring attention and arousal in 10 TBI patients.

29. What other pharmacological agents besides stimulants show potential to enhance cognitive recovery in the post-acute stage?

The **dopamine agonists** levodopa/carbidopa (Sinemet), amantadine (Symmetrel), bromocriptine (Parlodel), pergolide (Permax), and selegiline (Eldepryl) have been used to improve arousal and motor activity. Levodopa/carbidopa has been credited with promoting emergence from coma in case studies and small, uncontrolled trials of TBI patients. Five unblinded trials of 6 or fewer patients have supported the use of bromocriptine to treat nonfluent aphasias.

Early in Alzheimer's disease, changes appear in the cholinergic neurons projecting from the basal forebrain to the cerebral cortex and hippocampus. It is thought that dysfunction in these neurons results in the initial memory and cognitive impairments seen in Alzheimer's disease. This forms the rationale for treatment with centrally active, reversible **acetylcholinesterase inhibitors** such as donepezil (Aricept). Treatment with these agents provides a modest improvement in cognitive function. They may also slow the progression of the disease and delay the need for custodial care. Physostigmine, another acetylcholinesterase inhibitor, improved sustained attention of TBI patients in a double-blind trial involving 16 patients.

A variety of other agents have been employed to promote recovery and enhance cognition in the brain injured. Tricyclic antidepressants, GM1 ganglioside, carbaminol choline, CDP choline, phentaramine, yohimbine, and apomorphine are all medications with promise.

30. Are there any human data to support the contention that benzodiazepines inhibit recovery following stroke?

Goldstein et al. prospectively studied the motor recovery of patients assigned to the control group of a larger study on the effects of GM1 ganglioside on stroke. The control group (which did not receive GM1 ganglioside) was then divided into those who were treated with any "detrimental drugs" (n = 37) during their hospital course versus those who were not (n = 57, the "neutral" group). The detrimental drugs were defined as those implicated in animal trials as inhibitory to recovery following brain injury, specifically benzodiazepines, dopamine receptor antagonists (such as haloperidol), α_1-adrenergic receptor antagonists, α_2-adrenergic receptor agonists, phenytoin, and phenobarbital. Of the 37 subjects in the detrimental group, 27 were treated with a benzodiazepine, while 8 received dopamine receptor blockers (there also was some overlap). Members of the detrimental drug group displayed significantly greater upper-limb motor impairment and lesser recovery in activities of daily living (ADLs).

Certain limitations in the study design should be noted. First, the patients were not randomized to the "detrimental" or "neutral" group. Those in the "detrimental group" may have had more significant medical or behavioral problems that thus warranted treatment with the detrimental drugs. In addition, the study design did not allow determination of the degree to which the individual medications were harmful or whether there was a dosing threshold at which point any of these medications exerted negative effects.

Despite these limitations, the results of this study indicate caution in the use of drugs in the detrimental category. Since benzodiazepines were the most commonly used detrimental drug in this study, they fall under the greatest suspicion.

31. What about using haloperidol after TBI?

Haloperidol is a butyrophenone neuroleptic that depresses the central catecholamine system, producing akinesia and often sedation. It is often used to treat acute agitation, particularly in confused or delirious individuals in danger of dislodging catheters or IV lines, extubating themselves, or injuring staff. In this setting, haloperidol can be employed as a chemical restraint.

Haloperidol is associated with unpredictable development of tardive dyskinesia (automatic stereotyped movements) and has been shown to delay motor recovery in animal studies. Feeney's studies showing impaired motor recovery in brain-injured rats and cats after pharmacologic intervention with haloperidol is in part responsible for the reluctance to use this agent. Further, some believe that agitation is a normal stage in emergence from coma among the brain-injured and that unnecessary suppression of agitated behavior may negatively impact recovery. A clinical trial by Rao et al., in which a favorable outcome was reported after treatment of agitation with haloperidol, may partially explain the continued use of this agent by some TBI rehabilitationists. Rao et al.'s study was, however, neither randomized nor blinded, among other flaws. The consensus among physiatrists specializing in TBI is that use of haloperidol should be avoided.

32. What is limb apraxia?

Limb apraxia is defined as a "neurological disorder of learned purposive limb (hand and/or arm) movement skill that is not explained by deficits of elemental motor or sensory systems." The term *purposive* refers to having a purpose (or meaning), and the term *learned* refers to having experienced it before and established a memory for what the action looks or feels like or how it is produced. This definition excludes "constructional apraxia" (difficulties due to spatial deficits), "swallowing apraxia" (disruption in reflexive motor skill of swallowing), "buccofacial apraxia" (the loss of "volition," i.e., a person can blow out an actual match but cannot pretend to blow out an imagined match), and gait apraxia (a loss of the ability to walk in the absence of weakness or sensory loss).

33. How is limb apraxia classified?

Over 100 years ago, Liepmann described three forms of apraxia: limb-kinetic, ideomotor, and ideational forms. Patients with **limb-kinetic apraxia** display loss of the ability to make finely graded, individual movements requiring movement precision. Patients with **ideomotor apraxia** display particular difficulty when asked to pantomime transitive movements to verbal command and most commonly produce spatial and temporal errors. Patients with **ideational apraxia** are most commonly described as displaying an inability to produce actions in series ("show me how you would make a sandwich"). Action elements are often correctly produced but produced out of sequence or deleted. Ochipa et al. have subsequently described conceptual and conduction apraxias. In **conduction apraxia**, patients are able to pantomime to command better than they are able to imitate pantomimes. In **conceptual apraxia**, patients may produce well-formed gestures to command but are semantically inaccurate (e.g., they produce hornblowing when asked to drum). Finally, Heilman et al. and Derinzi described **dissociative apraxia**, in which patients who are unable to produce gestures in one modality (e.g., command) are able to produce them in another modality (e.g., visual cueing).

34. Do different categories of apraxia have different anatomic bases?

Limb-kinetic apraxia is thought to result from lesions to the primary motor and sensory cortices. Portions of the premotor cortex may also be involved.

Ideomotor apraxia results from lesions in the inferior parietal lobe, the supplementary motor area, and even the corpus callosum. In right-handed people, ideomotor apraxia is most often associated with left hemisphere lesions.

Ideational apraxia is commonly associated with degenerative diseases, especially those that predominantly affect the frontal lobes.

The mechanism of conduction apraxia is unknown but may be similar to that of conduction aphasia such that there is a disconnection between the portion of the left hemisphere that contains the memories of movement images and the parts of the left hemisphere that are important for programming movement production. While conceptual apraxia results more often from left hemisphere rather than right hemisphere lesions, no critical anatomic region has been identified.

Dissociative apraxia results from callosal and left hemispheric lesions.

35. How common is limb apraxia?

The incidence of ideomotor apraxia has been estimated at 30% in those with left hemispheric damage and at 8% of those with right-sided damage. In the U.S., there are 550,000 new cases of stroke each year, leaving 350,000 people surviving with disability. There are a total of 2 million stroke survivors. Of these, it is estimated that 41% (820,000) sustain left hemispheric strokes, while another 30% sustain right-sided damage. Thus, just looking at the U.S. population of left-sided stroke survivors, there are potentially 246,000 (30%) with significant limb apraxia. This is a conservative estimate considering that limb apraxia is generally under-identified.

36. How is limb apraxia diagnosed?

The diagnosis of limb apraxia is a two-stage process. The questions to be answered are: (1) Does this patient display limb apraxia? and (2) What type of limb apraxia? The Florida Apraxia

Screening Test-Revised (FAST-R) contains 30 items involving either a transitive gesture (i.e., the use of a tool) or an intransitive gesture (i.e., a gesture that does not use a tool such as waving hello). Incorrect responses are analyzed for errors of content, temporal aspects of production, and spatial aspects of production. Once it is established that a patient does display apraxia, extensive further testing is required to establish the nature of the apraxia.

37. Does a specific diagnosis of limb apraxia imply that a specific behavioral treatment should be employed?

At this point there are no accepted treatments to effectively remediate limb apraxia. However, a number of studies have examined the teaching of gesture to left hemisphere-damaged patients, particularly those with aphasia, and some have reported that these patients have been able to learn gesture production despite limb apraxia. The few reports of treatment directed at the specific remediation of limb apraxia show that limb apraxia can respond to treatment. Smania et al. randomized 13 patients with aphasia and ideational or ideomotor limb apraxia to receive therapy specific for limb apraxia or additional speech therapy. Those in the limb apraxia group showed improvements in tests of ideational and ideomotor apraxia with some generalization to untreated tasks. These efforts represent the beginning of the establishment of effective rehabilitation strategies to treat limb apraxia, which heretofore has been largely ignored.

38. What is locomotor training?

Locomotor training, using a body weight support system on a treadmill with manual assistance from trainers, is an experimental intervention to facilitate the recovery of walking in humans after CNS injury. This training has been described by various names including treadmill training, body-weight assisted training, and body-weight supported treadmill training. Using the term *locomotor training* emphasizes the intent of the training over the devices to implement it. The treadmill provides an external rhythmical drive and means to adjust the training speed for stepping. A body-weight support system consists of a harness worn by the patient about his or her pelvis and trunk and attached to a system able to precisely adjust the amount of body weight supported by the system (or conversely, the amount of body weight the limbs must support). The trainers facilitate overall trunk and limb kinematics, timing, and limb loading consistent with the pattern of normal walking.

39. What is central pattern generation?

Central pattern generation refers to the rhythmical oscillating activity of segmental neural circuitry in the spinal cord. This repetitive, alternating activation of flexors and extensors can occur independent of supraspinal control.

40. In what patient populations has locomotor training been studied? What are the outcomes?

Locomotor training has been predominantly applied to individuals with chronic, incomplete spinal cord injury (SCI) and in individuals post-stroke. In the SCI population, researchers have reported that individuals with incomplete injury have achieved the ability to walk and have progressed in some instances to stair climbing. To date, individuals with chronic, complete SCIs have achieved the ability to take several, repeated steps on the treadmill, but have been unable to translate this achievement to overground walking. A randomized clinical trial is currently underway to compare the effect of locomotor training to conventional rehabilitation in achieving functional walking after acute, incomplete SCI as defined by American Spinal Injury Association categories of impairment B, C, and D.

In the only randomized clinical trial with individuals post-stroke, researchers found that patients receiving locomotor training with 40% body-weight support (BWS) significantly improved their overground walking speed compared to persons trained without BWS on the treadmill.

41. How does locomotor training differ from current practice for the rehabilitation of walking after SCI?

Current rehabilitation practice for ambulation after SCI is designed to strengthen muscles under voluntary motor control and to compensate for deficits of weakness and paralysis by using orthoses and assistive devices. To achieve ambulation, new movement strategies are taught that require upper limb weight bearing on assistive devices such as canes and walkers to compensate for lower limb strength deficits. The gait pattern used varies according to the degree of lower limb paralysis (e.g., a swing-through gait pattern using bilateral knee-ankle-foot orthoses and forearm crutches or a four-point gait pattern using ankle-foot orthoses and forearm crutches). Achieving ambulation via these compensatory strategies produces different limb and trunk kinematics, timing, and load-bearing as compared to a typical walking pattern. Prediction of the ability to ambulate after SCI and using conventional therapy is based on manual muscle test scores of the lower limbs, the completeness of the lesion, and the neurologic level of injury.

42. Should locomotor training be considered for individuals with walking dysfunction secondary to multiple sclerosis, Parkinson's disease, brain injury, or cerebral palsy?

In general, citations supporting the use of locomotor training in populations besides those with stroke and SCI are rare. The potential of locomotor training to optimize the contributions of the spinal cord to the control of locomotion to facilitate the recovery of ambulation suggests that it will only be a matter of time before this therapy is extended to other neurologic conditions. For example, Miyai et al. found body-weight-supported treadmill training more effective than traditional physical therapy in a prospective crossover trial in 10 patients with Parkinson's disease.

43. How can gesture facilitate speech in nonfluent aphasia?

Functional MRI studies suggest that in normal left-hemisphere-dominant individuals, language production mechanisms are usually located in the left lateral frontal cortex, while language initiation mechanisms are located in the left medial frontal cortex. Functional MRI (fMRI) studies of chronic severe aphasia show a shift of lateral frontal activity from the left to the right hemisphere. It has been hypothesized that some of the difficulty in speech production in nonfluent aphasia is due to a "mismatch" between right lateral frontal cortex language production mechanisms and initiation mechanisms in the left medial frontal cortex.

Naming improves in nonfluent aphasia when American Indian Sign Language (AmerInd) gestures are learned with the left hand and performed simultaneously with oral picture naming. Curiously, neither learning AmerInd alone nor practicing oral naming alone improves oral naming. Although it was presumed that the symbolic nature of AmerInd accounted for its efficacy, it is also possible that performing complex movements with the left hand ""primes" initiation mechanisms in the right medial frontal cortex, bringing right hemisphere initiation mechanisms into register with language-production mechanisms that have shifted to the right.

A pilot study coupling complex, nonsymbolic movements of the left hand with picture naming led to improved speech production in 8 of 10 individuals with chronic nonfluent aphasia due to left hemispheric strokes that included the frontal lobe. This study is an excellent example of the translation of the insights gained through functional imaging to new, more precise, and probably more effective therapies.

44. Characterize unilateral neglect.

Patients affected by this syndrome typically have an impaired ability to perceive or respond to stimuli presented on all or portions of the left side. The lack of perception, recognition, or attention can be intrapersonal (the person's own body), peripersonal, or extrapersonal. This situation must be differentiated from hemianopia, which can be present with or without unilateral neglect.

Although unilateral neglect is common in patients with right parietal lobe strokes, it can appear also in patients with left hemispheric strokes regardless of hand dominance. Various aspects of the neglect syndrome may also result from damage to the midbrain reticular formation, intralaminar thalamic nuclei, premotor cortex, cingulate gyrus and the prefrontal cortex. Unilateral neglect is far less common in traumatic brain injury.

Several explanations of unilateral neglect have been offered including the representational hypothesis, arousal hypothesis, and spatial attention hypothesis. Posner and associates have also suggested that at least some aspects of unilateral neglect following right-sided parietal lesions are due to difficulty in disengaging attention from the right hemi-field.

45. What is the clinical significance of the neglect syndrome?

Unilateral neglect can complicate and frustrate the rehabilitation process and also may jeopardize patient's safety (i.e., collisions with objects in the neglected hemi-field). Incontinence and poor functional outcome have both been associated with moderate- to- severe neglect. Anosognosia, the inability to recognize one's body part as one's own can be a particularly debilitating manifestation.

46. Are there any specific rehabilitation treatments for unilateral neglect?

General therapeutic programs include prompting attention to the left side of the body and space during ADLs and ambulation. Exercises using visuospatial tasks at the desk (e.g., drawing, building cubes) with or without a computer have been employed. Beis et al. have reported encouraging results using glasses patched to obscure the right hemifield. Pizzamiglio et al. and Antonucci et al. have had success using a protocol that included visual scanning training, reading and copying written words, copying of line drawings on a dot matrix, and figure description.

BIBLIOGRAPHY

1. Antonucci G, Guariglia C, Judica A, et al: Effectiveness of neglect rehabilitation in a randomized group study. J Clin Exp Neuropsychol 17:383–389, 1995.
2. Bach-y-Rita P: Central nervous system lesions: Sprouting and unmasking in rehabilitation. Arch Phys Med Rehabil 62:413–417, 1981.
3. Basso MD, Behrman AL, Harkema SJ: Recovery of walking after central nervous system insult: Basic research in the control of locomtion as a foundation for developing rehabilitation strategies. Neurol Rep 24:47–54, 2000.
4. Behrman AL, Harkema SJ: Locomotor training after human spinal cord injury: A series of case studies. Phys Ther 80:688–700, 2000.
5. Beis JM, Andre JM, Baumgarten A, Challier B: Eye patching in unilateral spatial neglect: Efficacy of two methods. Arch Phys Med Rehabil 80:71–76, 1999.
6. Bland ST, Schallert T, Strong R, et al: Early exclusive use of the affected forelimb after moderate transient focal ischemia in rats. Stroke 31:1114–1152, 2000.
7. Bleiberg J, Garmoe W, Cederqist J, et al: Effects of dexedrine on performance consistency following brain injury: A double-blind, placebo case study. NNBN 6:245–248, 1993.
8. Bjorklund A, Lindvall O: Self-repair in the brain. Nature 405:892–895, 2000.
9. Boyeson MG, Harmon RL: Acute and postacute drug-induced effects on rate of behavioral recovery after brain injury. J Head Trauma Rehabil 9:78–90, 1994.
10. Cauraugh J, Light K, Kim S, et al: Chronic motor dysfunction after stroke: Recovering wrist and finger extension by electromyography-triggered neuromuscular stimulation. Stroke 31:1360–1364, 2000.
11. Francisco GF, Chae J, Chawla H, et al: Electromyogram-triggered neuromuscular stimulation for improving the arm function of acute stroke survivors: A randomized pilot study. Arch Phys Med Rehabil 79:570–575, 1998.
12. Feeney DM, Baron JC: Diaschisis. Stroke 17:817–829, 1986.
13. Finkelstein DI, et al: Axonal sprouting following lesions of the rat substantia nigra. Neuroscience 97:99–112, 2000.
14. Goldstein LB, Sygen in Acute Stroke Study Investigators: Common drugs may influence motor recovery after stroke. Neurology 45:865–871, 1995.
15. Grode C, Redford B, Chrostowski J, et al: Methylphenidate in early poststroke recovery: A double-blind, placebo-controlled study. Arch Phys Med Rehabil 79:1047–1050, 1998.
16. Horner PJ, Gage FH: Regenerating the damaged nervous system. Nature 407:963–970, 2000.
17. Hovda DA, Sutton RL: Amphetamine-induced recovery of visual cliff performance after bilateral visual cortex ablation in cats: Measurements of depth perception thresholds. Behav Neurosci 103:574–584, 1989.
18. Kaelin DL, Cifu DX, Matthies B: Methylphenidate effect on attention in the acutely brain-injured adult. Arch Phys Med Rehabil 77:6–9, 1996.
19. Johansson BB: Brain plasticity and stroke rehabilitation. The Willis lecture. Stroke 31:223–230, 2000.

20. Lazarus LW, Moberg PJ, Langsley PR, Lingam VR: Methylphenidate and nortriptyline in the treatment of poststroke depression: A retrospective comparison. Arch Phys Med Rehabil 75:403–406, 1994.
21. Levy CE, Nichols DS, Schmalbrock PM, et al: Functional MRI evidence of cortical reorganization in upper-limb hemiparesis treated with constraint-induced movement therapy. Am J Phys Med Rehabil 80:4–12, 2001.
22. Liepert J, Bauder H, Miltner WHR, et al: Treatment-induced cortical reorganization after stroke in humans. Stroke 31:1210–1216, 2000.
23. Lytton WW, et al: Unmasking unmasked: Neural dynamics following stroke. Progr Brain Res 121:203–218, 1999.
24. Lu J, Waite P: Spine update: Advances in spinal cord regeneration. Spine 9:926–930, 1999.
25. Meyer JS: Does diaschisis have clinical correlates? Mayo Clin Proc 66:430–432, 1991.
26. Miyai I, Fujimoto Y, Ueda Y, et al: Treadmill training with body weight support: Its effect on Parkinson's disease. Arch Phys Med Rehabil 81:849–852, 2000.
27. Nadeau SE, Rothi LJG, Crosson B (eds): Aphasia and Language: Theory to Practice. New York, Guilford Press, 2000.
28. Pizzamiglio L, Antonucci G, Judica A, et al: Cognitive rehabilitation of the hemineglect disorder in chronic patients with unilateral right brain damage. J Clin Exp Neuropsychol 14:901–923, 1992.
29. Rothi LJG, Heilman KM (eds): Apraxia: The cognitive neuropsychology of limb praxis. Hove, England, Psychology Press, 1997.
30. Smania N, Girardi F, Domenicali C, et al: The rehabilitation of limb apraxia: A study in left-brain-damaged patients. Arch Phys Med Rehabil 81:379–388, 2000.
31. Somers MF: Spinal Cord Injury: Functional Rehabilitation, 2nd ed. Englewood Cliffs, NJ, Prentice-Hall, 2001.
32. Sullivan KJ, Duncan PW: New perspectives for locomotor training after stroke: Emerging evidence from basic science and clinical research. Neurol Rep 24:55–59, 2000.
33. van der Lee JH, Wagenaar RC, Lankhorst GJ, et al: Forced use of the upper extremity in chronic stroke patients: Results from a single-blind, randomized clinical trial. Stroke 30:2369–2375, 1999.
34. Witte OW: Lesion-induced plasticity as a potential mechanism for recovery and rehabilitative training. Curr Opin Neurol 11:655–662, 1998.
35. Wroblewski BA: Pharmacological treatment of arousal and cognitive deficits. J Head Trauma Rehabil 9:19–42, 1994.

34. PULMONARY REHABILITATION

John R. Bach, M.D.

1. Describe the two basic categories of respiratory diseases.

All respiratory disease can be categorized as intrinsic versus mechanical, or obstructive versus restrictive. Patients with intrinsic or obstructive disease have lung disease that results in **oxygenation impairment** of the blood. These patients are normally eucapnic or hypocapnic despite hypoxia. Patients with mechanical dysfunction of respiratory muscles, lungs, or chest wall have **ventilatory impairment** causing retention of CO_2 initially and later hypoxia, which occurs secondarily.

2. What are the goals of pulmonary rehabilitation?

- Supporting or improving cardiopulmonary function
- Preventing or treating complications by physical medicine (noninvasive) measures
- Fostering compliance with optimal medical care
- Reducing numbers of exacerbations, emergency room visits, and hospitalizations
- Educating the patient to confront the disease realistically
- Preparing the patient to take responsibility for his or her rehabilitation and well-being
- Optimizing psychosocial functioning and coping mechanisms
- Returning the patient to or enabling the patient to have as active, productive, and emotionally satisfying life as he or she desires

VENTILATORY IMPAIRMENT (CO_2 RETENTION)

3. List the diseases causing primarily ventilatory impairment amenable to respiratory rehabilitation.

Ventilatory impairment can result from any neuromuscular or skeletal disorder that causes respiratory muscle dysfunction. Patients with diagnoses listed in the table are often candidates for physical medicine alternatives to endotracheal intubation or ventilatory support and airway secretion management via indwelling airway tubes.

Conditions Causing Ventilatory Impairment Amenable to Physical Medicine Intervention

Myopathies	Neurologic disorders
Muscular dystrophies	Spinal muscular atrophies
Dystrophinopathies (Duchenne and Becker	Motor neuron diseases
dystrophies)	Poliomyelitis
Other muscular dystrophies (limb-girdle,	Neuropathies (phrenic neuropathies, Guillain-
Emery-Dreifuss, facioscapulohumeral,	Barré syndrome)
congenital, childhood autosomal	Multiple sclerosis
recessive, and myotonic dystrophy)	Traumatic tetraplegia and other myelopathies
Non-Duchenne myopathies (congenital and	Sleep-disordered breathing (including obesity
metabolic myopathies, polymyositis,	hypoventilation
myasthenia gravis	Kyphoscoliosis
	Chronic obstructive pulmonary disease

4. What do patients with primarily ventilatory impairment need in order to benefit from noninvasive respiratory rehab interventions?

Patients who can most benefit from physical medicine and general rehabilitation interventions must (1) be able to cooperate and learn and (2) have adequate bulbar muscle function to use equipment and techniques that can optimize general physical functioning, including the various inspiratory and expiratory muscle aids and oximetry feedback that can optimize pulmonary function. In general, only the bulbar muscle function of patients with advanced, averbal bulbar amyotrophic lateral sclerosis and spinal muscular atrophy type 1 without adequate parental involvement can require tracheostomy to prolong survival.

5. Name the eight most common errors in managing patients with ventilatory impairment.

1. Misinterpretation of symptoms due to hypercapnia and inspiratory muscle weakness
2. Failure to do spirometry with the patient supine
3. Failure to monitor sleep by simple oximetry
4. Use of arterial blood gas analyses instead of oximetry and noninvasive CO_2 monitoring
5. Administration of oxygen, periodic intermittent positive-pressure breathing (IPPB), continuous positive airway pressure (CPAP), or inadequate bi-level positive airway pressure (BiPAP) when noninvasive respiratory muscle aids are indicated
6. Use of methylxanthines and any other respiratory medications on an ongoing basis without evidence of bronchospasm
7. Failure to prevent acute respiratory failure and hospitalization
8. Resort to tracheostomy when peak cough expiratory flows exceed 3 L/sec

6. Name the clinical parameters critical for monitoring patients with neuromuscular disease.

- Spirometry for vital capacity and maximum insufflation capacity
- Peak cough flows, unassisted and assisted
- Oxyhemoglobin saturation via oximetry
- Capnography

7. What are respiratory muscle aids?

The respiratory muscles can be aided by applying manual or mechanical forces to the body or intermittent pressure changes to the airway. The devices that act on the body include the negative-pressure body ventilators (NPBVs) which create atmospheric pressure changes around the thorax and abdomen, body ventilators and forced exsufflation devices which apply force directly to the body to mechanically displace respiratory muscles, and devices that apply intermittent pressure changes directly to the airway.

8. What are the ideal inspiratory muscle aids for daytime use?

Mouthpiece intermittent positive pressure ventilation (IPPV) and the intermittent abdominal-pressure ventilator (IAPV) are the ideal inspiratory muscle aids for long-term daytime ventilatory support. For **mouthpiece IPPV**, a mouthpiece is set up near the mouth, adjacent to the sip-and-puff, tongue, or chin controls of a motorized wheelchair, where the patient can easily grab it about 2 to 10 times a minute as needed for up to full ventilatory support.

The **IAPV** intermittently inflates an air sac contained in a corset or belt worn beneath the patient's outer clothing. Inflation by a positive-pressure ventilator moves the diaphragm upward, causing a forced exsufflation. During deflation, the abdominal contents and diaphragm fall to the resting position, and inspiration occurs passively. Since it depends on gravity, a trunk angle of $\geq$ 30° from horizontal is necessary for the IAPV to be effective. The IAPV augments tidal volumes by 250–1200 ml. Patients with < 1 hr of ventilator-free breathing ability often prefer to use the IAPV when sitting rather than use noninvasive methods of IPPV.

9. What are the ideal inspiratory muscle aids for nocturnal use?

Nasal IPPV delivered via CPAP masks or custom-molded nasal interfaces has become the most popular method of noninvasive nocturnal ventilatory support. At least three or four different nasal interfaces should be tried by each patient to determine which ones will be preferred. Many patients use different styles on alternate nights to vary skin contact pressure.

Mouthpiece IPPV with lip seal retention is a more effective but generally less preferred method of nocturnal ventilatory support. Using the lip seal, mouthpiece IPPV can be delivered during sleep with less insufflation leakage and with little risk of the mouthpiece falling out of the mouth. However, speaking clearly is difficult.

10. How can airway secretions be best eliminated in this population?

At least 3 L/sec of expiratory flow is necessary to bring airway secretions out of the airway and into the mouth. However, whether using a ventilator or not, patients with primarily ventilatory impairment are often unable to generate adequate peak cough flows without assistance. With the use of an insufflation to > 1.5 L and with a properly timed abdominal thrust, peak cough flow can usually be increased to 3–7 L/sec. When scoliosis, abdominal distension, trauma, moderate bulbar muscle dysfunction, or obesity interfere with manually assisted coughing, a mechanical insufflator-exsufflator can be used to provide over 4 L/sec of peak expiratory flow with cough.

11. Which factors decrease blood oxyhemoglobin saturation (SaO_2)?

1. Hypoventilation (hypercapnia)
2. Airway encumberment usually from mucus (can be sudden or chronic)
3. Intrinsic lung disease (such as atelectasis or pneumonia)

Oximeters that measure pulse and blood SaO_2 are increasingly inexpensive, and oximetry should be considered a fourth vital sign. If airway mucus encumberment (especially to the extent that causes oxyhemoglobin desaturation) is not cleared and SaO_2 not returned to normal (> 94%) in a timely manner, pneumonia develops.

12. Discuss the use of oximetry in starting noninvasive IPPV.

Introduction to and use of mouthpiece or nasal IPPV can be facilitated by oximetry feedback. An SaO_2 alarm may be set at 94%. The patient sees that by taking deeper breaths, the SaO_2 will exceed 94% within seconds. The patient is instructed to maintain the SaO_2 > 94% all day and can achieve this by increasing unassisted breathing rate and volumes and supplementing this by mouthpiece or nasal IPPV delivered by a portable ventilator. With time and advancing muscle weakness, the patient requires increasing periods of noninvasive IPPV to maintain adequate ventilation ($SaO_2 > 94\%$). In this manner, an oximeter may also help to reset central ventilatory drive and facilitate optimal daytime use of noninvasive IPPV.

13. How is SaO_2 useful in managing acute respiratory tract infections?

During acute respiratory infections, respiratory muscle weakness is exacerbated which, along with airway mucus encumberment, causes a diminution in the patient's vital capacity. Plugging and hypoventilation, compounded by patient fatigue, cause decreases in SaO_2. The patient is instructed to augment ventilation and maintain a normal SaO_2 by taking mouthpiece-assisted insufflations as necessary. When mucus plugging causes a sudden decrease in SaO_2, manually and mechanically assisted coughing are used until the mucus is eliminated and the SaO_2 returns to normal. When the SaO_2 baseline decreases below 95% despite optimal ventilation and aggressive assisted coughing, at least microscopic atelectasis is present. This generally clears with continued treatment. Lower baseline SaO_2s occur when airway secretion management is inadequate and either pulmonary infiltrations or some other serious pulmonary complications have occurred. This event justifies hospitalization, diagnostic work-up, and intensive measures that may include intubation and oxygen supplementation.

14. What is glossopharyngeal breathing (GPB)?

The patient is instructed to take a deep breath and then augment it by projecting boluses of air past the glottis with the tongue and pharyngeal muscles. The glottis closes with each "gulp." One breath usually consists of 6–8 gulps of 60–200 ml each. During training, GPB efficiency is monitored by spirometrically measuring the milliliters of air per gulp, gulps per breath, and breaths per minute. A GPB rate of 12–14 breaths/ minute can provide patients with little or no vital capacity with normal tidal volumes, minute ventilation, and hours of ventilator-free breathing ability.

15. What is GPB used for?

GPB is most commonly used as a method for providing maximal insufflations and as a noninvasive method for supporting ventilation. It is an excellent back-up in the event of ventilator failure. Deep GPB is also useful for manually assisted coughing and to prevent microatelectasis. GPB can normalize the volume and rhythm of speech and permit the patient to shout. A tracheostomy virtually precludes use of GPB, because even with the tube plugged, gulped air leaks around the tube and out the tracheostomy site.

16. When is endotracheal intubation or tracheostomy indicated?

For **respiratory distress** and:
- When peak cough flows, unassisted or assisted, cannot exceed 2.7 L/m
- A mentally incompetent or uncooperative patient, or one who is using heavy sedation or narcotics
- Severe intrinsic lung disease
- Substance abuse or uncontrollable seizures
- Conditions interfering with the use of IPPV interfaces, such as facial fractures, inadequate bite for mouthpiece entry, or nasogastric tube

17. Does oxygen therapy ease symptoms of hypoventilation?

Although oxygen therapy is routinely given to virtually all ventilator users, whether or not they are hypoxic, for patients with primarily ventilatory impairment, its use is tantamount to putting a bandaid on a cancer! Oxygen therapy depresses ventilatory drive; exacerbates hypercapnia; prevents the use of oximetry feedback; increases hypoventilation symptoms like daytime drowsiness, nightmares, and depression; and can render the nocturnal use of nasal or mouthpiece IPPV ineffective. In addition, hypercapnic patients who are treated with oxygen therapy have a higher incidence of pulmonary complications than patients not treated at all. *A cardinal rule is to always first attempt to normalize SaO₂ by providing adequate ventilation and assisted coughing before considering oxygen therapy along with intubation.*

18. What is the difference between CPAP and BiPAP?

Continuous positive airway pressure (CPAP) delivered via a CPAP mask provides a pneumatic splint that maintains airway patency during sleep and allows the patient with obstructive sleep apneas to breathe using his or her own muscles. **Bi-level positive airway pressure** (BiPAP) permits independent adjustment of inspiratory (IPAP) and expiratory positive airway pressures (EPAP): the greater the IPAP/EPAP difference (span), the greater the inspiratory muscle support. Spans of ≥ 20 cm H_2O are often required to ensure adequate ventilation.

19. Pressure support ventilation, synchronized intermittent mandatory ventilation (SIMV), positive end-expiratory pressure (PEEP), and oxygen administration are necessary for ventilator weaning? Right?

No. In our ventilator unit, virtually every ventilator user arrives using a combination of all of the above. When we turn off the oxygen, the SaO₂ plummets until we exsufflate the patient through the airway tube. This clears airway secretions and often normalizes the SaO₂, and the patient can continue to breathe room air. Once the SaO₂ is normal on room air, the SIMV, PEEP, and pressure support are turned off and the patient is placed on a portable volume ventilator from which he or she can take assisted breaths via a mouthpiece whenever needed to prevent dyspnea and maintain normal SaO₂ and alveolar ventilation. Thus, the patient takes fewer assisted breaths and weans himself or herself without resort to complicated and unnecessary technology.

20. List five maxims regarding use of intubation and tracheostomy in the rehabilitation of ventilatory failure.

1. Intubation and tracheostomy are neither needed nor desired by most patients with primarily ventilatory impairment who require 24-hour/day ventilatory support.

2. Oxygen should never be used as a substitute for assisted ventilation and assisted coughing.

3. Rehabilitation is not complete for any ventilator user who has not been evaluated for tracheostomy tube removal and had the tube removed when peak cough flows permit, irrespective of the extent of ventilatory failure.

4. Endotracheal intubation is unnecessary for managing many cases of uncomplicated acute ventilatory failure.

5. Endotracheal suctioning is often less effective than insufflation-exsufflation via an endotracheal tube (exsufflation creates high expiratory flows to clear both lung fields, preventing pneumonia).

Physical medicine alternatives to the invasive measures of endotracheal intubation, tracheostomy, and airway suctioning are cheaper, safer, more comfortable, and greatly preferred by patients with primarily ventilatory impairment. They deserve wider application.

OBSTRUCTIVE DISEASES (OXYGENATION IMPAIRMENT)

21. What causes chronic obstructive pulmonary disease (COPD)?

Chronic bronchitis, emphysema, asthmatic bronchitis, and cystic fibrosis are the most common causes. COPD often results from a combination of genetic predisposition and environmental factors in which allergic diseases (e.g., asthma), respiratory infections (e.g., bronchopneumonitis), chemical inflammation (e.g., cigarette smoke, asbestosis), and metabolic abnormalities (e.g., α_1-antitrypsin deficiency) can play a role. Cigarette smoking is the main cause of chronic bronchitis-emphysema. Smokers are 3.5–25 times more likely (depending on the amounts smoked) to die of COPD than nonsmokers.

22. What is the difference between emphysema and bronchitis?

Emphysema is characterized by distention of air spaces distal to the terminal nonrespiratory bronchiole with destruction of alveolar walls. There is a loss of lung recoil, excessive airway collapse on exhalation, and chronic airflow obstruction. Chronic **bronchitis** and cystic fi-brosis are characterized by enlargement of tracheobronchial mucus glands and chronic mucus hypersecretion and chest infections. Chronic bronchitis is distinguished from asthmatic bronchi-tis by its irreversibility, lack of bronchial hyperreactivity, lack of responsiveness to bronchodila-tors, and distinctive abnormalities in ventilation-perfusion.

23. How can you determine the prognosis for patients with COPD?

The extent of pulmonary function abnormalities correlates with prognosis: 30% of COPD patients with $FEV_1 < 750$ ml die within 1 year and 50% within 3 years. However, pulmonary function abnormalities do not predict the extent of the patient's functional impairment.

24. Who are candidates for pulmonary rehabilitation?

Any motivated nonsmoker or patient who has quit smoking, whose activities are limited by dyspnea due to COPD, and who has adequate medical, neuromusculoskeletal, financial, and psy-chosocial resources to permit active participation. Patients who benefit the most usually have a respiratory limitation to exercise at 75% of predicted maximum oxygen consumption and irre-versible airway obstruction with a $FEV_1 < 2000$ ml or FEV_1/FVC ratio $< 60\%$. Ventilator users should be weaned in inpatient programs.

25. Why use clinical exercise testing?

Clinical exercise testing, whether done with a treadmill, stationary bicycle, or upper extrem-ity ergometer, includes monitoring of oxygen consumption, CO_2 production, minute ventilation, and metabolic rate. It permits the differentiation of impairment due to cardiac disease or exercise-induced bronchospasm from pulmonary disease. It indicates the reasons for exercise-related symptoms and documents the patient's progress during rehabilitation by demonstrating changes in symptom-limited oxygen consumption and other physiologic parameters.

26. When do you terminate a clinical exercise test?

The test should continue until oxygen consumption fails to increase, maximum allowable heart rate for age is reached, or electrocardiographic changes, chest pain, severe dyspnea, or fa-tigue occur. A minute ventilation 35 times the patient's FEV_1 is often attainable.

27. What medical strategies are used to manage patients with lung disease and primarily oxygenation impairment?

Pulmonary function should be optimized medically and by facilitating airway secretion elimination. Hypoxic ($PaO_2 < 60$ mmHg) patients benefit from oxygen therapy with de-creased dyspnea, enhanced performance, and prolonged survival. Medications such as bron-chodilators (β_1-adrenergics, anticholinergics, and methylxanthines) and, occasionally, glucocorticoids, expectorants, mucolytics, antibiotics, and mast-cell membrane stabilizers may also be helpful.

28. Outline a sample rehab prescription for a COPD patient. Name its seven major compo-nents.

1. **Goals**
   Improve endurance
   Optimize medication delivery, oxygen utilization, and airway secretion elimination
   Increase walking capabilities and independent functioning
   Reduce anxiety and improve self-esteem
2. **Precautions**
   Maintain oxyhemoglobin saturation (SaO_2) $> 90\%$
   Discontinue exercise and notify physician if chest pain, severe dyspnea, or ventricular premature beats > 6/min occur during exercise
   Maintain heart rate < 120 bpm

3. **Respiratory therapy**

   With oximetry, titrate oxygen flows to maintain SaO2 > 90% during exercise

   Instruct in diaphragmatic and pursed-lip breathing

   Instruct in inhaler use

   Evaluate and instruct in methods to eliminate airway secretions

   Instruct in home portable oxygen use

   Instruct in respiratory muscle resistive exercise training and log use

4. **Physical therapy**

   Assess baseline 12-minute walk, instruct in using log

   Supervise incremental exercise program with stationary bicycle or treadmill three times daily, instruct in making log entries

   Review body mechanics and coordinate with breathing patterns

   Supervise use of diaphragmatic and pursed-lip breathing as appropriate

5. **Occupational therapy**

   Assess upper body mobility, strength, and endurance

   Develop an upper-extremity exercise program

   Evaluate and facilitate ADLs and use of adaptive aids as appropriate

   Train in energy and work conservation

   Evaluate the home, recommend modifications and equipment to improve safety, efficiency, and independence

   Relaxation exercise training

6. **Nutrition**

   Assess nutritional intake, advise modifications as appropriate

7. **Psychology**

   Evaluate cognitive status and adjustment issues, intervene as needed

29. What methods can be used to assist the patient in airway secretion elimination?

Inexpensive methods: huffing, chest percussion and postural drainage, autogenic breathing, positive expiratory pressure masks, use of flutter valves that create positive back pressure and oscillate airflow.

Expensive methods: vibrating vests, vibrating air under chest shells, high-frequency oscillations (40–200 times/minute) of the air column delivered via mouthpiece or endotracheal tube. The expensive methods have not been shown to be more effective than the less-expensive approaches.

30. Should the respiratory muscles of COPD patients be rested?

Diaphragm rest can be achieved by assisting ventilation noninvasively with the use of body ventilators, mouthpiece or nasal intermittent positive-pressure ventilation (IPPV), or tracheostomy IPPV. Although assisting ventilation can exacerbate air trapping in COPD patients, the benefits of resting respiratory muscles and decreasing oxygen consumption may outweigh this in importance. Some studies suggest that use of ventilatory assistance daily, usually delivered overnight, can improve daytime blood gases, vital capacity, dyspnea, 12-min walking distance, respiratory muscle strength and endurance, functional activities, and quality of life, while decreasing hospitalizations. Patients with some combination of maximal inspiratory force < 50 cm H_2O, FEV_1 < 25% of predicted normal, PCO_2 > 45 mmHg, respiratory rate > 30/min, and chest/abdomen dyssynchrony might be considered for nocturnal ventilatory assistance.

31. When should supplemental oxygen therapy be used?

For patients with PO_2 < 55–60 mm Hg, whether daytime or nighttime. Home oxygen therapy, when indicated, decreases reactive pulmonary hypertension, polycythemia, and perception of effort during exercise and prolongs life. Cognitive function may be improved, and hospital needs reduced. It should be given with caution to patients who retain CO_2.

32. Should supplemental oxygen be used by COPD patients on commercial airlines?

It should not, unless it is already being used on a regular basis, and then an increase of 0.5 L/min is generally sufficient.

33. Are nutritional supplements necessary?

As many as 50% of inpatients with COPD are malnourished. Inadequate or inappropriate nutrition (e.g., increased carbohydrate intake can increase PCO_2) can impair lung repair, surfactant synthesis, pulmonary defense mechanisms, control of ventilation and response to hypoxia, respiratory muscle function and lung mechanics, water homeostasis, and the immune system. Patients with significant nutritional impairment have more tracheal bacteria and are more frequently colonized by *Pseudomonas* species. Malnutrition can lead to hypercapnic respiratory failure, difficulty in weaning from mechanical ventilation, and infection. Short-term refeeding of malnourished patients leads to improved respiratory muscle endurance and, in some patients, increases in respiratory muscle strength in the absence of demonstrable changes in peripheral muscle function.

34. Can respiratory muscles be trained?

Maximum sustained ventilation exercises and inspiratory resistive exercises, including inspiratory resistive loading and inspiratory threshold loading, have been shown to improve respiratory muscle endurance. With a few exceptions, studies have not shown improvements in other pulmonary function parameters, and respiratory muscle exercise does not appear to carry over to improve general exercise tolerance or ADL capabilities. However, the combination of respiratory muscle exercise and rest, which appears to be especially effective for ventilator weaning, has not been adequately explored for the COPD patient.

35. How should reconditioning exercises be prescribed?

The intensity of reconditioning exercises may be guided by clinical exercise testing, e.g., 80–85% of maximum achievable heart rate or heart rate at ventilation levels of 35 times FEV1. Walking, stair climbing, calisthenics, bicycling, and pool activities may be used. Upper-extremity reconditioning should also be part of the program. A stationary bicycle should be purchased for the patient's home and used twice a day. In addition, a daily 12-minute walk can be used as well as several 15-minute sessions daily of inspiratory muscle training. A log should be kept of time and distance bicycled, distance walked, and possibly inspiratory resistance tolerated during 15-minute inspiratory training sessions. Shorter periods of higher-intensity exercise are more effective in increasing exercise tolerance than longer periods of lower-intensity exercise. In general, the pulse should increase at least 20–30% and return to baseline 5–10 minutes after exercise. The program should consist of weekly re-evaluations for several months, after which the patient should continue the home program and maintain the logs.

36. Should exercise reconditioning be used for advanced patients with marked hypercapnia?

There is evidence that even advanced patients with hypercapnia can benefit from an exercise reconditioning program, showing significant improvement in walking distance, ADLs, and, possibly, certain pulmonary parameters.

37. What are the benefits of pulmonary rehabilitation?

1. Reduction in dyspnea and respiratory rate
2. Increased exercise tolerance, symptom-limited oxygen consumption, work output, and mechanical efficiency
3. Improvement in ADLs
4. Decreased anxiety and depression
5. Increased cognitive function and sense of well-being
6. Decreased frequency of hospitalizations for respiratory impairment

BIBLIOGRAPHY

1. Aldrich T: Respiratory muscle training in COPD. In Bach JR (ed): Pulmonary Rehabilitation: The Obstructive and Paralytic Conditions. Philadelphia, Hanley & Belfus, 1996.
2. Bach JR: A comparison of long-term ventilatory support alternatives from the perspective of the patient and care giver. Chest 104:1702–1706, 1993.
3. Bach JR: Guide to the Understanding and Management of Neuromuscular Disease. Philadelphia, Hanley & Belfus, 1999.
4. Bach JR, Alba AS, Saporito LR: Intermittent positive pressure ventilation via the mouth as an alternative to tracheostomy for 257 ventilator users. Chest 103:174–182, 1993.
5. Bach JR: Update and perspectives on noninvasive respiratory muscle aids: Pt 1. The inspiratory muscle aids. Chest 105:1230–1240, 1994.
6. Bach JR: Update and perspectives on noninvasive respiratory muscle aids: Pt 2. The expiratory muscle aids. Chest 105:1538–1544, 1994.
7. Bach JR (ed): Pulmonary Rehabilitation: The Obstructive and Paralytic Conditions. Philadelphia, Hanley & Belfus, 1996.
8. Bach JR, Ishikawa Y, Kim H: Prevention of pulmonary morbidity for patients with Duchenne muscular dystrophy. Chest 112:1024–1028, 1997.
9. Casaburi R, Petty TL (eds): Principles and Practice of Pulmonary Rehabilitation. Philadelphia, W.B. Saunders, 1993.
10. Dail CW, Affeldt JE: Glossopharyngeal Breathing [video]. Los Angeles, College of Medical Evangelists, 1954.
11. Webber B, Higgens J. Glossopharyngeal breathing—what, when and how? (video) Horsham, UK, Aslan Studios Ltd., 1999.

35. CARDIAC REHABILITATION

Yehoshua A. Lehman, M.D., Steven A. Stiens, M.D., M.S., and Eugen M. Halar, M.D.

1. Define cardiac rehabilitation (CR).

A series of definitions should provide perspective:

The **American Association of Cardiovascular and Pulmonary Rehabilitation** defines CR as "the application of rehabilitative services to improve and maintain a patient's physiologic, physical, psychosocial, and vocational functioning at an optimal level."

The **U.S. Department of Health and Human Services** defines CR services as comprehensive, long-term programs involving medical evaluation, exercise prescriptions, cardiac risk-factors modification, education, and counseling to *limit* the physiologic and psychological adverse effects of cardiac illness.

We define CR similarly but emphasize the person as the center for rehabilitation goals and the key to success. CR is a patient-participative interdisciplinary process that seeks to enhance the patient's personal effectiveness through education, cardiac risk prevention, cardiovascular and psychosocial adaptation and lifestyle changes, functional improvement, and reintegration into community functions.

2. Who can benefit from CR?

Patients who have physiological, functional, and psychosocial deficits related to impairments of the cardiovascular system can benefit from CR. This includes patients with the following diagnoses or cardiovascular conditions: ischemic heart disease, recent myocardial infarction, post-coronary artery bypass graft (CABG) surgery, post-percutaneous transluminal coronary angioplasty (PTCA), post-cardiac transplant, post-heart valve replacement, stable angina and congestive heart failure.

3. What is the incidence and significance of coronary artery disease (CAD) in the U.S.?

The 1993 statistics indicate that CAD affects 13.5 million Americans. Seven million suffer from stable angina and could benefit from CR. One and one-half million suffer myocardial infarction each year, and almost 1 million survive. Forty-five percent of all myocardial infarctions are in persons under age 65. In 1999, over 600,000 CABG and over 600,000 PTCA procedures were performed, and these numbers are increasing. All of these people could benefit from CR services, but only 11–20% of them do participate.

4. What are the overall goals of the CR process?

To reduce myocardial ischemia and the risk of infarction or sudden death
To prevent and reverse atherosclerosis
To maximize cardiovascular capacity and fitness
To maximize exercise tolerance and ADL performance
To establish a patient-controlled and safe aerobic exercise program
To provide guidelines for safe activities and work
To control risk factors for CAD
To help patients cope with perceived stressors
To utilize energy conservation and work simplification
To improve quality of life

5. Describe the phases of the CR process.

The CR intervention sequence integrates into the classic medical continuum of care and management of any illness: prevention, acute care (medical/surgical), and rehabilitation. The typical patient referred for CR has sustained a myocardial infarction and/or undergone CABG. CR has therefore typically been divided into three sequential phases that bring the patient out of acute care:

Phase I—Inpatient phase from hospital admission to hospital discharge.

Phase II—Outpatient training phase includes aerobic conditioning, reacquisition of full activity, risk factor management, and lifestyle changes.

Phase III—Maintenance phase, with patient-monitored continuation of the aerobic exercise program, risk-reduction strategies, and activity/work modifications.

These phases represent a timeline for the process of intervention. It is important to recognize that many interventions continue through the phases on an ongoing basis and that the application of CR interventions should be tailored to the need of each individual.

6. How is cardiovascular impairment estimated by the rehabilitation team ?

The history, physical examination, and review of cardiac enzymes, EKG, coronary catheterization, cardiac images, and other pertinent tests may reveal the severity of CAD and help to determine the patients who are at low, moderate, or high risk for complications upon application of activity and exercise program. The following components are to be included in each evaluation.

History: angina (typical, atypical, nocturnal, progressive, as well as activity limits and intensity required), modifiable risk factors (smoking, hypertension, hyperlipidemia, diabetes mellitus, sedentary life style), dyspnea (exertional), paroxysmal nocturnal dyspnea (1–5 hr after recumbent), fatigue level (exercise tolerance), and premorbid level of physical and psychosocial functioning.

Physical exam: vital signs, orthostatics (pulses and BP while supine, sitting, and standing up, if possible), pulses, jugular venous distention, cardiac auscultation (murmurs, gallops), pulmonary assessment (rales), abdominal exam (hepatojugular reflux, bruits), edema, and tolerance of functional activities. Musculoskeletal and neurologic exams are also essential to determine any associated impairments that may affect functional and exercise training.

Functional clinical evaluations (to assess tolerance): grooming, bathing, dressing, bed mobility, transfers, ambulation, stairs, aerobic exercises, work capacity. The intensity and extent of functional testing depend on how many days the patient is after the cardiac invent. Measure heart rate and BP before and perceived rate of exertion after the functional test. This is specifically important to do during the implementation of the Phase I program.

Laboratory tests (to review): total creatine kinase-MB, hematocrit, EKG (arrhythmias, Q waves, estimate MI severity, and ST-T wave changes during subsequent testings), BUN/CR ratio, echo/MUGA (ejection fraction), cardiac exercises stress tests, or other cardiac imaging tests or studies.

From the patient's history and above findings, each patient is stratified as low, moderate, or high risk in order to determine the level of required supervision. The patient's intensity of aerobic exercises for the Phase II program could be obtained from exercise tolerance test.

7. What are possible contraindications for entry into inpatient or outpatient exercise programs?

According to the American College of Sports Medicine, they are:

Unstable angina

Resting systolic BP > 200 mmHg

Resting diastolic BP > 100 mmHg

Orthostatic BP drop or drop during exercise training of ≥ 20 mmHg

Moderate to severe aortic stenosis

Acute systemic illness or fever

Uncontrolled atrial or ventricular dysrhythmias

Uncontrolled sinus tachycardia (120 bpm)

Uncontrolled congestive heart failure

Third degree A-V block

Active pericarditis or myocarditis

Recent embolism

Thrombophlebitis

Resting ST displacement (> 3 mm)

Uncontrolled diabetes

Orthopedic problems that prohibit exercise

8. What are the foci of intervention during phase I, the inpatient phase of CR?

Early ambulation and ADL training under supervision

Alleviation of anxiety and depression

Reassurance to reestablish patient's control of self

Patient education regarding rationale for treatment and exercises

Medical evaluation of cardiac injury, EKG and enzyme changes, imaging

Development of a team knowledge base of the patient's previous activities and work, and life roles as well as current personal goals that he or she wants to achieve during CR.

Establish modifiable risk factor reduction strategies

Assessment of cardiovascular function and impairments

Establish level of the risk for development of complications; risk stratification

Prescription and education with guidelines for activity and work after discharge

9. Describe the relationship between heart rate, stroke volume, cardiac output, aerobic capacity, and the anginal threshold.

The **maximum heart rate** (HR) is defined as the maximum HR obtained on an exercise stress test. It decreases with age and can be estimated for the normal population by subtracting the patient's age in years from 220. **Stroke volume** (SV) is the amount of blood ejected with each ventricular contraction and increases with exercise to become maximum at 50% over the basal HR (resting HR). **Cardiac output** (CO) equals HR × SV and relates directly to the total body oxygen consumption (VO_2) because all O_2 consumed is delivered to the body tissues via the blood. **Maximum aerobic capacity** (VO_2 max) is the greatest rate (VO_2 ml/kg body mass/min) of O_2 consumption a person is capable of metabolizing, and it relates directly to maximum work output in watts. One way to understand and calculate VO_2 max is to use the formula SV × HR × (arterial–venous O_2 difference), which integrates the delivery and extraction of O_2. Thus, an increase in CO, the product of SV × HR, and/or increase in arteriovenous O_2 difference increases in VO_2 maximum. It decreases with age, inactivity and after MI. The **anginal threshold** is defined as the CO at which myocardial O_2 demand exceeds O_2 delivered. An ischemic myocardium is not capable of maintaining the same cardiac work load, which results in a fall in CO, VO_2max, and/or BP.

10. What are the modifiable risk factors for atherosclerotic coronary artery disease?

The significant **risk factors** for developing CAD are age, male sex, elevated total cholesterol, elevated low-density lipoprotein (LDL) cholesterol, low level of high-density lipoprotein (HDL) cholesterol, elevated systolic or diastolic BP, diabetes, obesity, sedentary lifestyle, cigarette smoking, stress, family history of premature coronary disease, and EKG evidence of left ventricular hypertrophy. From the risk factors reported in the Framingham study of 1984, one can define the **modifiable risk factors** as hypertension, cigarette smoking, hypercholesterolemia (> 200 mg/dl), inactivity, low HDL cholesterol (< 35 mg/dl), obesity, hypertriglyceridemia, diabetes mellitus, and stress. There is strong evidence that risk factor modification can cause regression of the atherosclerotic process. For example, a prospective study of patients randomized to a control group and monotherapy with simvastatin, lovastatin, colestipol, or niacin for cholesterol control demonstrated coronary atheroma regression, lower rates of CABG, and reduced mortality rates. Meta-analysis studies of randomized control trials of CR programs consisting of exercise training and risk factor management have demonstrated a 10% reduction in the 3-year mortality rate.

11. Which types of cardiac stress tests are used to evaluate for cardiac ischemia or dysrhythmias?

EKG stress test stratifies risk and determines exercise and work capacity in METS. The test includes EKG monitoring for heart rate, arrhythmia, ischemia (ST depression > 1 mm), and monitoring for symptoms and BP. Exercise tesing increases METS (intensity) by varying the speed and percent grade of the exercise for selected minutes of testing. Treadmills, bicycles, or ergometers are used for testing. Upper extremity ergometry (increase work by increasing arm crank resistance), wheelchair ergometry, or arm-leg ergometry are utilized by hemiplegics or paraplegic individuals.

Nuclear medicine stress testing such as thallium-201 scintigraphy uses exercise or vasodilators (dipyridamole, adenosine), which increases the **cardiac steal phenomenon** (stiff, narrowed vessels dilate less), to evaluate CAD. Immediate perfusion studies indicate myocardial blood flow in various vessel territories. Changes in delayed images 2 to 24 hours later demonstrate viable myocardium.

Dobutamine HCl echocardiography assesses areas of cardiac ischemia by determining regions of wall motion abnormalities. The cardiac demand is increased by dobutamine, which increases both HR and BP. Therefore, in contrast to the dipyridamole thallium tests, dobutamine stress echocardiograms not only identify coronary ischemia (sensitivity 95%, specificity 82% vs catheterization) but also reveal the ischemic anginal threshold and the maximum HR and BP, or rate-pressure product. This additional information helps prescribe the patient's cardiac guidelines for exercises, activities, and work.

12. What are the major goals of phase II, the outpatient phase of CR?

Besides continuing the goals of phase I CR, the major goals of phase II are:

1. To achieve cardiovascular conditioning and fitness via an aerobic exercise training program

2. To achieve control of modifiable risk factors using psychosocial and pharmacologic interventions and lifestyle changes

3. To achieve an early return to work.

During phase II of the CR program, the patient will be educated to self-monitor for the appropriate level of exercise, work, or activities via HR monitoring and/or rating of perceived exertion and receive psychosocial support to reduce anxiety and depression. The CR phase II should result in improvements in VO_2 max, lowering of HR for a given exercise or workload, and reduced systolic BP and have beneficial peripheral effects on improvement of O_2 extraction/utilization by skeletal muscle. It will also result in reduction of anxiety and depression and improved coping mechanisms.

13. List the five major parts of a CR exercise prescription.

1. **Modality**—The American College of Sports Medicine recommends that the exercise modality be "any activity that uses large muscle groups, that can be maintained for a prolonged period, and is rhythmic and aerobic in nature."

2. **Intensity**—Either prescribed by target HR, rating of perceived exertion, or metabolic equivalents. It is usually 60–70% of VO_2max for healthy patients.

3. **Duration**—Depends on the mode and intensity of exercise. Usually it is 20–45 minutes initially and later may increase to 60-minute sessions.

4. **Frequency**— while in the hospital daily and at least three times weekly while in the aerobic training and maintenance phases, usually skipping a day between intensive sessions.

5. **Rate of progression**—Depends on the patient's individual tolerance, progress, endurance, needs, and goals.

14. What is the purpose of a warm-up period?

The warm-up period, usually lasting 5–10 minutes, increases the intensity of exercise gradually from rest to the desired intensity level and also stretches the major muscles that will be used. This warm-up decreases the risk of cardiovascular problems (i.e., delay in onset of angina) and prevents sprain or strain injuries. Some patients, such as those with cardiac transplants and congestive heart failure, need longer periods of warm-up before proceeding to the more intensive aerobic exercises.

15. What is the purpose of a cool-down period?

It allows gradual reduction of cardiac work and redistribution of blood from muscles and extremities to internal organs. A gradual reduction of exercise intensity with continued body movements maintains venous return; prevents pooling of blood in the lower limbs, post-exercise hypotension, and end-organ insufficiencies; and promotes continuous dissipation of heat.

16. What are the major interventions of phase III, the maintenance phase of CR?

Phase III has the same goals as phase II (the training phase), except that the program is monitored by the patient and/or family. The program continues outside the CR center, in a community-based setting or wherever the patient feels comfortable. The members of the CR team (i.e., physician, therapist, nutritionist, psychologist, social worker) then may be available to assist and advise the patient as needed. The patient continues the level of exercise program achieved and self-monitors his or her own exercises and activities to avoid overexertion. Periodic evaluations should be done to monitor the patient's progress and tolerance and maintenance of previously achieved goals. Before beginning or changing the exercise program, the patient should check with his or her doctor.

17. Which changes in lifestyle for CAD are beneficial?

Aggressive lifestyle changes in respect to control of hypertension and smoking, dieting with < 10% of total calories from fat, combined with 3 hours of aerobic exercise per week as well as stress management have been demonstrated to produce clinically significant regression in coronary atherosclerosis as documented by coronary arteriography. In the Lifestyle Heart Trial Study, patients on the American Heart Association–recommended diet of < 30% fat showed progression of their coronary atherosclerosis on repeat catheterization. Such studies suggest that conventional recommendations for patients with CAD are not sufficient to abate or reverse the disease process.

A CR dietary program should provide the metabolites needed for muscle adaption with exercise, reduce risk factors associated with lipids and body fat content, and establish a body habitus that minimizes cardiac work, thus maximizing functional independence. In an attempt to approach this dietary ideal, the amount as well as the content of the diet need to be calculated. The incidence of myocardial infarction in depressed patients is significantly greater, and depression after myocardial infarction increases morbidity and mortality; thus, pharmacologic and psychological intervention are both important components of CR. Adequate social support enhances recovery of patients and is a buffer against stresses.

18. What factors cause reduced cardiovascular capacity after spinal cord injury (SCI)?

Reduced exercise capacity in SCI patients is multifactorial. These factors include impaired autonomic nervous system control of the cardiovascular system; altered hormonal effects on the cardiovascular system; loss of the muscle pump causing decreased venous return, muscle weakness, and/or atrophy; altered respiratory system; small size of cardiac chambers; greater use of type II over type I muscle fibers; and sedentary lifestyle.

19. What modes of aerobic exercise training can be used in SCI patients?

Wheelchair propulsion, arm ergometry, wheelchair cycling using an arm crank, functional electrical stimulation (FES), and hybrid exercise (arm ergometry combined with lower-extremity FES).

20. Should patients with congestive heart failure be excluded from CR?

No, stabilized and compensated patients with congestive heart failure are capable of achieving an increase in functional capacity up to 20%. Slow progression in the intensity and duration of each exercise session, applied at least for 3 months and thereafter continued with a maintenance program, has demonstrated a significant improvement in function capacity in these patients.

21. What about cardiac transplant?

Due to denervation of the heart, the HR increases only in response to changes in circulating catecholamines. Intervention in transplant recipients includes a longer warm-up, slowly progressive endurance exercise at 50–60% of maximum HR, followed by longer cool-down periods. Cardiac transplant patients are characteristically very deconditioned and need conditioning and CR programs.

22. What about other patients under rehabilitative care who may have risk factors for coronary disease and cardiac complications?

The list of patients is enormous and includes geriatric patients, those with stroke, those with a previous history of cardiac abnormalities, etc. These patients should be rehabilitated within the guidelines of cardiac precautions.

BIBLIOGRAPHY

1. Agency for Health Care Policy and Research: Cardiac Rehabilitation Guidelines Panel: Cardiac Rehabilitation. Clinic Practice Guidelines no. 17. Rockville, MD, AHCPR, 1995, AHCPR publication no. 96-0672.
2. American Association of Cardiovascular and Pulmonary Rehabilitation: Guidelines for Cardiac Rehabilitation Program. Champaign, IL, Human Kinetics Books, 1991.
3. Franklin B: American College of Sports Medicine: Guidelines for Exercise Testing and Prescription, 6th ed. Indianapolis, ACSM, 2000.
4. Halar EM (ed): Cardiac Rehabilitation. Physical Medicine and Rehabilitation Clinics of North America, vol. 6, no. 1. Philadelphia, PA, W.B. Saunders, 1995.
5. Lakkat T, Venalainen J, Rauramma R, et al: Relation of leisure-time, physical activity, and cardiorespiratory fitness to the risk of acute myocardial infarction in men. N Engl J Med 330:1549–1554, 1994.
6. Oldridge NB, Guyatt GH, Fischer NE, et al: Cardiac rehabilitation after myocardial infarction: Combined experience of randomized clinical trials. JAMA 260:945–950, 1988.
7. Ornish D, Brown S, Scherwitz L, et al: Can lifestyle changes reverse coronary heart disease? The Lifestyle Heart Trial. Lancet 336:129–133, 1990.
8. Pashkow F, Dafoe W (eds): Clinical Cardiac Rehabilitation: A Cardiologists Guide, 2nd ed. Baltimore, Williams & Wilkins, 1999.
9. Pederson TR, et al: Randomized trial of cholesterol lowering in 4444 patients with coronary heart disease: The Scandinavian Simvastatin Survival Study. Lancet 344:1383–1389, 1994.
10. Skerker R: Review and update. The aerobic exercise prescription. Crit Rev Phys Med Rehabil 2:257–271, 1991.

36. PERIPHERAL VASCULAR DISEASE REHABILITATION

Marvin M. Brooke, M.D., M.S.

1. What are the three organ systems most commonly affected by peripheral vascular disease?

1. **Arteries and arterioles** frequently are affected by atherosclerosis, especially the coronary arteries, carotid bifurcations, and aortoiliac and femoral arteries. In diabetics, the popliteal and tibial arteries and small vessels are affected more frequently than the aortoiliac arteries. Peripheral arterial disease in the lower extremities is one of the best predictors of coronary and carotid atherosclerosis.

2. The **venous system** is most frequently affected by lower-extremity deep vein thromboses (which can lead to fatal pulmonary emboli) and chronic venous insufficiency.

3. The **lymphatic system** drains high-protein lymph fluid from the interstitial space through lymphangions, lymph nodes, the lymphatic trunk, and lymphatic duct into the subclavian veins. Lymphedema is a high-protein edema, most often caused by cancer surgery involving the lymph nodes or by parasites in underdeveloped countries.

2. How frequent is atherosclerotic peripheral vascular disease?

The incidence, if determined by claudication and clinical examination, increases from 1% between 40 and 44 years of age to 7.5% between 60 and 64 years of age. Of patients with claudication, 15–20% develop rest pain or gangrene and 1–2% require amputation. The incidence is higher when measurements are done using arterial Doppler test, because they are more sensitive than relying on symptoms.

3. What patient groups and risk factors predict atherosclerotic peripheral vascular disease?

- **Lipid disorders**—especially low-density lipoproteins and cholesterol.
- **Smoking**—the strongest predictor of peripheral atherosclerosis.
- **Hypertension**—exacerbates atherosclerosis by damaging endothelial cells
- **Diabetes mellitus**—associated with earlier, more frequent, and more rapid development of atherosclerosis
- **Family history, obesity, lack of exercise, and hyperuricemia**—also predictors for atherosclerosis

4. What causes intermittent claudication and rest pain?

Intermittent claudication is caused by atherosclerosis and mechanical muscle action preventing an adequate increase in blood supply to the calf muscles during exercise. This increases muscle metabolites and causes calf pain relieved by rest. Many other conditions can mimic these symptoms.

Rest pain occurs because the blood supply is inadequate for resting muscle. This can be exacerbated by edema, and if the leg is elevated to decrease edema, the arterial pressure may decrease further.

5. What are the signs of atherosclerotic peripheral vascular disease?

- Decreased peripheral pulses, even if no bruit
- Delayed capillary filling
- Rubor (rubor of dependency is a dusky red color occurring within 3 minutes)

- Pallor on elevation: Elevate the leg, and press the sole of the foot for 25 seconds. The capillaries should refill in < 9 seconds.
- Asymmetric temperature (cooler or warmer)
- Trophic changes or early gangrene

Noninvasive Doppler studies are now very effective at confirming the diagnosis, localizing the lesion, and measuring severity. It may be helpful to compare the ankle to the brachial pressure (ankle-brachial index).

6. When should an emergency evaluation and surgery consultation be obtained?

The signs of emergency are rapid onset of the "6 Ps": **p**ain, **p**allor, **p**aresthesia, **p**olar (asymmetric cooling), **p**aralysis, and **p**ulselessness. These signs may indicate an acute thrombosis or embolus needing emergency surgery. Vascular surgery also may help salvage a limb if there is a gradual progression from intermittent claudication to rest pain and then trophic changes.

7. What are the components of good foot care?

- Wash in lukewarm water (< 92°F) and soap daily.
- Apply skin cream such as Eucerin, lanolin, or Alpha Keri.
- Check for red spots, cuts, ingrown toenails, or infections.
- Cut nails straight with corners out, not digging in.
- Wear clean cotton socks each day.
- Wear well-fitted shoes, custom modified when needed.
- Involve a podiatrist when appropriate. Many skin breakdowns, if caught early and treated appropriately, can be healed without progression to amputation.

8. Can medications help?

Aspirin decreases platelet function and clotting. In acute cases, anticoagulants may be indicated. Some feel that pentoxifylline (Trental) decreases blood viscosity, improves microcirculation, and may increase walking distance before claudication. Controlling diabetes is important, and use of a multivitamin with antioxidants seems logical.

9. Can exercise help?

Exercise helps many patients by improving the efficiency of muscle metabolism and walking, improving collateral flow, increasing tolerance, and improving emotional outlook. Other benefits include improvements in lipids, diabetic control, and coronary artery disease. Because of the high incidence of cardiac atherosclerosis, patient should be screened for this. Walking up to tolerance for 30–45 minutes, three times a week, for several months may be needed before a difference is seen on re-evaluation.

10. What are the different types of venous disease?

Venous disease is a component of peripheral vascular disease and includes a spectrum of disorders increasing in severity from varicose veins, chronic venous insufficiency, superficial thrombophlebitis, recurrent deep vein thrombosis, acute deep vein thrombosis, and pulmonary embolism.

11. What is Virchow's triad and why is it important to the rehabilitation patient?

Virchow's triad consists of:
1. Stasis (reduced blood flow velocity)
2. Injury (venous endothelial damage)
3. Hypercoagulable state

During rehabilitation, 9.2% of cases have a thromboembolic complication. Deep vein thrombosis is very common after spinal cord injury, brain injury with hemiparesis, total joint replacement, multiple trauma, cancer, and obesity. It can largely be prevented with a high index of suspicion and prophylactic anticoagulation. Any patient with venous thrombosis without a clear cause deserves a work-up for one of the newly recognized inherited, hypercoagulable states. Noninvasive venous Doppler tests can often clarify or rule out lower extremity deep vein thromboses.

12. Why is it so important to look for pulmonary embolism coming from deep vein thrombosis?

As many as 50,000 patients a year have pulmonary embolism in the United States. Ten percent to 15% of these patients will die. Pulmonary embolism is often called the silent assassin, because it can occur with few warning signs or symptoms and be rapidly fatal. It should be considered in any patient with new cardiac, pulmonary, malaise, or fever problems. It may need to be diagnosed with a ventilation perfusion lung scan, special CT scan, or pulmonary arteriogram.

13. What are the most common prophylactic treatments for deep vein thrombosis?

Risk factors can be reduced by mobilizing patients early, actively moving the ankles, wearing venous compression stockings, elevating the legs, or using intermittent venous compression devices. Subcutaneous low-dose heparin, 5000 units every 12 hours, is often used. Low-dose oral warfarin and the newer low–molecular-weight heparins are also options.

14. What is chronic venous insufficiency?

Chronic venous insufficiency occurs when there are congenital or acquired injuries to valves, obstruction of the veins, or valve obstruction and recanalization by deep vein thrombosis. As many as 67–80% of patients develop postphlebitic syndrome after deep vein thrombosis.

15. How is chronic venous insufficiency treated?

Elevation of the leg higher than the heart and venous compression garments can be of assistance. If there is no congestive heart failure or deep vein thromboses that may be dislodged, venous compression pumps and leg wraps may be helpful. After edema stabilizes, custom compression garments of 30–40 mmHg are essential. In a few cases, venous surgery is useful. Superficial spider veins and other very superficial venous incompetence is sometimes helped with sclerotherapy.

16. How are nonhealing ulcers treated?

In addition to prevention, it is important to determine if the ulcer is caused by nerve, arterial, small vessel, or venous insufficiency. Cultures, x-rays, and bone scan may be important when osteomyelitis is a possibility. Debridement with wet to dry dressings, enzymes, or surgery is sometimes needed. A multidisciplinary approach can sometimes heal chronic ulcers and prevent amputation. Sometimes, modified or custom shoes, extra depth shoes with Plastizote inserts, and a podiatrist consultation are very helpful.

There are many types of dressings and wound care products. An Unna boot is a compression dressing with gauze impregnated with zinc oxide and glycerin that is left on for a week. Hydrocolloid dressings, such as Duoderm, and hydrophilic polyurethane foam dressings often help a clean wound heal. Regranex is an expensive new topical cream to increase regranulation in the base of a clean wound.

17. What is the lymphatic system?

The lymphatic system is a set of one-way tubes that take water, proteins, and waste products from the interstitial space back to the circulatory system. The lymph flows through lymph capillaries into lymphangions, through lymph nodes that fight infection and cancer, the lymphatic trunk, the lymphatic duct, and into the subclavian veins.

18. What is lymphedema?

Lymphedema is a high-protein edema caused by obstruction to the lymphatic system. It is most often caused by cancer or cancer surgery, radiation, trauma or very long-standing venous insufficiency. In undeveloped countries it can be caused by parasites. When it is long-standing, lymphedema produces a firm nonpitting edema, which may lead to tremendous enlargement of the limb.

19. How is lymphedema treated?

Treatment includes prevention and activity, elevation, diuretics, external pneumatic compression devices, custom-fitted compression garments, massage, and surgery. Pneumatic compression is followed by massage, isometric muscle contraction, and then wrapping with bandages. Pneumatic compression is contraindicated if there is a deep vein thrombosis, congestive heart failure, active infection or metastasis of cancer, bilateral mastectomy, pelvic surgery with bilateral proximal edema, primary lymphedema, general lymphedema, or multiple areas.

20. How are compression stockings worn?

Compression stockings are worn with significant effort and commitment on the part of the patient, after the condition has stabilized. Two pairs of custom elastic stockings are usually prescribed at 30–40 mmHg. They are removed at night when the extremity is elevated and before a venous compression treatment.

BIBLIOGRAPHY

 1. Bick RL, Haas SK: International consensus recommendations. Summary statement and additional suggested guidelines (European Consensus Conference, November 1991. American College of Chest Physicians consensus statement of 1995. International Consensus Statement, 1997). Med Clin North Am 82:613, 1998.
 2. Boris M, Weindorf S, Lasinski B, Boris G: Lymphedema reduction by noninvasive complex lymphedema therapy. Oncology 8:95, 1994.
 3. Ernst CB, Stanley JC (eds): Therapy in Vascular Surgery, 2nd ed. Philadelphia, B.C. Decker, 1991.
 4. Gans BM, Burke DT, Merli GJ, Muntz JE: Advances in the prevention and treatment of thrombotic complications in the rehabilitation patient. Am J Phys Med Rehabil 79(suppl 5):1, 2000.
 5. Gardner AW, Poehlman ET: Exercise rehabilitation programs for the treatment of claudication pain. JAMA 274:975, 1995.
 6. Jonason T, Jonzon B, Ringqvist I, et al: Effect of physical training on different categories of patients with intermittent claudication. Acta Med Scand 206:253, 1979.
 7. Lippman HI, Fishman L, Farrar R, et al: Edema control in the management of disabling chronic venous insufficiency. Arch Phys Med Rehabil 75:436, 1994.
 8. Morgan RG, Casley-Smith JR, Mason MR, Casley-Smith JR: Complex physical therapy for the lymphedematous arm. J Hand Surg 17:437, 1992.
 9. Orchard TJ, Strandness TE: Assessment of peripheral vascular disease and diabetes: Report and recommendations of an international workshop sponsored by the American Heart Association and the American Diabetes Association, 18–20 September 1992, New Orleans. Diabetes Care 16:1199, 1993.
10. Papas CJ, O'Donnell TF: Long-term results of compression treatment for lymphedema. J Vasc Surg 16:555, 1992.
11. Pillar NB, Swedborg I, Norrefalk JR: Lymphedema rehabilitation program: An application of anatomical, physiological and pathophysiological knowledge. Eur J Lymphol 3:57, 1992.
12. Sioson ER, Crowe WE, Dawson NV: Occult proximal deep vein thrombosis: Its prevalence among patients admitted to rehabilitation hospital. Arch Phys Med Rehabil 69:183, 1988.
13. Spittell JA: Conservative management of occlusive peripheral arterial disease. Cardiovasc Clin 22:209, 1992.
14. Stillwell GK, Redford JWB: Physical treatment of postmastectomy lymphedema. Proc Staff Meet Mayo Clin 33:1, 1958.
15. Tunis SR, Bass EB, Steinberg EP: The use of angioplasty, bypass surgery and amputation in the management of peripheral vascular disease. N Engl J Med 325:556, 1991.
16. Wittlinger G, Wittlinger H: Textbook of Dr. Votter's Manual Lymph Drainage, 5th ed. Brussels, Haug International, 1992.

VI. Musculoskeletal Rehabilitation

37. NECK PAIN

Rene Cailliet, M.D.

1. What functional anatomy of the cervical spine must be understood to evaluate pain in the neck and from the neck?

The cervical spine is composed of two segments. The upper consists of the occiput, atlas (C1), and axis (C2). The lower comprises functional units C3–C7. The movement of the occiput and C1 causes flexion-extension, the movement of C1 on C2 is rotation, and the movement of C3–C7 causes all ranges of motion.

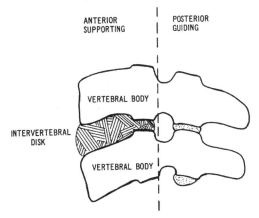

From Cailliet R: Neck and Arm Pain, 3rd ed. Philadelphia, F.A. Davis, 1991, with permission.

2. Describe a functional unit.

A functional unit is two adjacent vertebrae separated by an intervertebral disc and posteriorly two laminae, two pedicles, and zygapophyseal joints termed **facets.**

3. A "pain in the neck" is a common complaint. Where in the cervical spine does pain originate?

The tissue sites where nociception occurs are the posterior longitudinal ligaments, nerve roots and their dural sheaths, the facet capsules, and the neck muscles. Nociception occurs from injury, irritation, inflammation, or infection of these sites.

4. "Disc pain" is a common complaint. Is there such a thing?

The intervertebral disc consists of annular fibers within a mucopolysaccharide matrix with no blood supply and no nerve endings other than minimal unmyelinated nerve endings in the outer peripheral annulus fibrosus. Consequently, only damage to the outer annular fibers can conceivably cause pain.

5. In evaluating pain from the cervical spine, what are the most important factors to consider?

The nerve roots emerge from the cervical spine through the foramina, which contain the dorsal root ganglion and their dural sheath, both sites of nociception. Flexion opens the foramina, and extension closes them. Rotation and lateral flexion of the neck close the foramina on the concave side and open those on the convex side. Passive and active movement of the neck trigger pain by nerve compression.

6. In a clinical evaluation from history, what are the major factors to be determined?

Every chief complaint can be elucidated using the mnemonic PQRST:

P   Palliative—determine the precise position or alleviating and exacerbating factors

Q   Quality of symptoms

R   Radiation of symptoms

S   Severity as experienced throughout the day and with various activities

T   Temporal factors—onset, duration, time the pain is worse, any movement(s) that cause or aggravate the pain

7. What is the Spurling test?

The test defined by Spurling is reproduction of radicular pain by extending the neck, rotating it to one side, and pressing down on the head toward the side of complaint. A positive test reproduces the radicular pain. The site of referred pain indicates which nerve root has been compressed: arm/forearm, C5; thumb, C6; middle finger, C7; fifth finger, C8.

8. Is it radicular pain or radiculous pain?

Radicular pain indicates that a radicle (nerve root) has been compressed and referred to a dermatomal area. Radiculous pain is pain complained of without anatomic basis, pathophysiologic pattern, or consistent findings. For example, a C5–6 intervertebral disk protrusion will encroach on the C6 spinal nerve emerging through the C5–6 intervertebral foramen (see Figure).

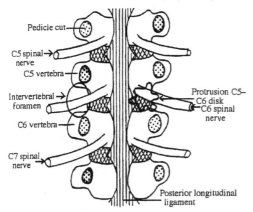

From Schneck CD: Functional and clinical anatomy of the spine. In Young MA, Lavin RA (eds): Conservative Care and Spinal Rehabilitation. Spine: State of the Art Reviews. Philadelphia, Hanley & Belfus, 1998, pp 525–558, with permission.

9. Are x-ray studies of the cervical spine of precise diagnostic value?

No. X-rays often show "pathology" that is irrelevant to the complaints. X-rays are only of value if they confirm the presence and indicate the site of pathology that can explain the symptoms and physical signs.

10. What are the most common causes of neck pain or pain from the neck?

Trauma. The trauma can result from an accident (often vehicular), postural position (e.g., poor ergonomics such as prolonged computer working), or emotional tension.

11. Is posture an important factor in causing neck pain?

Yes. An exaggerated dorsal kyphosis (round back) places the head ahead of the center of gravity increasing the cervical lordosis. The weight of the head in this position is borne by the zygapophyseal joints (facets) and causes pain.

12. Has one tissue site of the cervical spine been considered the prevalent site of neck pain?

The zygapophyseal joints (facets) have been so designated because injection of an irritating substance in them reproduces the pain and injecting an analgesic relieves the pain.

13. What is a whiplash injury?

In a rear-end motor vehicle accident, the impact acutely forces the entire body forward, but the head does not move at the same time and undergoes translation forces with initial extension then reflex flexion. Normal flexion-extension does not occur, but translatory forces cause disc annular fiber damage and facet capsule excessive stress.

14. What is a stinger?

This acute cervical injury in athletes may result in a transient paresis (paraplegia/quadriplegia).

15. Degenerative disc disease of the cervical spine is considered a cause of neck pain and arm pain from the neck. Is this a valid assumption and what are the causative factors?

Degenerative disc disease occurs from age 30 on as a result of the aging process but is aggravated and accentuated by trauma. As the disc dehydrates with age, it narrows allowing the longitudinal ligaments to be separated from the vertebral bodies. The blood that seeps in between the ligament and the body gradually ossifies and forms osteophytes (spurs). These spurs narrow the foramen and can entrap the nerve roots.

16. Can headaches be caused by injury to the cervical spine?

A condition termed **cervicogenic headache** occurs after an injury and responds favorably to neck therapy. Its pathoanatomic basis is not clear.

17. What is a "computer headache"?

Although not yet an official disorder, computer headache occurs in people who spend much time at the computer especially if they wear bifocal glasses. The dorsal kyphotic posture with head forward and up increaes the cervical lordosis. That and emotional tension from intensity cause neck and head pain.

18. What is thoracic outlet syndrome?

The thoracic outlet is the space between the first rib, the clavicle, and the two scalene muscles. The nerves of the brachial plexus and the subclavian blood vessels pass through this space. Acute contraction or chronic contraction of the scalene muscles can compress the nerves and blood vessels causing paresthesia of the arm and hand. Diagnosis is made by the **Adson sign**— diminished radial pulse produced by having the patient take a deep breath with her head turned all the way to the side.

19. What causes the headache from greater superior occipital neuralgia?

The greater superior occipital nerve contains roots from C1 and C2 and a branch from C3. It emerges through the extensor capitis muscles and supplies the dermatomes of C1, C2, and C3 of the posterior occiput. When entrapped or traumatized, it causes a vertex occipital headache. An injection of an anesthetic agent around the nerve at the occiput confirms the diagnosis and relieves the headache.

20. Is cervical traction a viable therapeutic modality?

Properly applied cervical traction has great value in cervical problems. It must comfortably pull the head upward and forward at a 30° angle and be applied twice daily and for periods of 30 minutes.

BIBLIOGRAPHY

1. Cailliet R: Neck and Arm Pain, 3rd ed. Philadelphia, F.A. Davis, 1991.
2. Malanga GA (ed): Cervical Flexion-Extension/Whiplash Injuries. Spine: State of the Art Reviews, Vol. 12, no. 2. Philadelphia, Hanley & Belfus, 1998.

38. LOW BACK PAIN

Maury Ellenberg, M.D., and Joseph C. Honet, M.D., M.S.

1. Is low back pain (LBP) a common problem?

Yes. Epidemiologic studies show that by the age of 20, 50% of the population has experienced LBP. By age 60 years, the incidence may be as high as 80%. LBP is second only to the common cold when it comes to symptoms prompting a physician visit.

2. What are the most common diagnoses of back pain?

In a number of studies, the most common diagnoses are actually nondiagnoses, such as "nonspecific LBP" or "degenerative disease." More specific diagnoses include compression fracture, spondylolisthesis, malignancy, ankylosing spondylitis, and infection. Approximately 2% are diagnosed with "radiculopathy" or "sciatica."

3. Does back pain have a natural history?

Yes. LBP is usually self-limited. Because the incidence is over 50% and point prevalence in the 10–20% range, it is obvious that most individuals are able to deal with their pain for the period of time until resolution. However, in certain populations, the pain, complaints, and subsequent disability become significant and difficult to resolve. Recurrence over time, which is not predictable, is also part of the natural history.

4. Is there a way to prevent recurrences?

There are ways to try to prevent recurrence, but few have proven effective. It makes sense to learn proper back care, exercises including back, abdominal, and back stabilizer strengthening, and stretches for the back and hamstrings. Patients can be educated to respond to acute episodes with nonsteroidal anti-inflammatory drugs (NSAIDs), ice or heat, and activity maintenance and to expect resolution in 3–7 days.

5. Are there really no abnormalities in people with so-called nonspecific LBP?

There are many abnormalities in the spine of people with LBP. However, there is no conclusive evidence that these abnormalities are responsible for the patient's complaints. Clinical studies have shown a poor correlation between spinal x-ray abnormalities and LBP. Nonetheless, past generations of medical practitioners have told patients that their LBP was due to "arthritis" of the spine. More recently, as computed tomography (CT) scanning and magnetic resonance imaging (MRI) evolved and more abnormalities became visible, surgery has been recommended to remove architecturally observable but nonoffending discs. Even today, degenerative discs are blamed for LBP. BAK fusion, IDET (heat dissolution of discs), and a variety of other procedures are being performed to fix the problem.

A number of structures can potentially cause LBP. Anatomic studies have determined which structures have free nerve endings that transmit pain sensations, and irritating material has been injected into structures to determine if and where pain is caused. Newer techniques claim to distinguish some of these structures by differential injection, specifically into the facet joint, the sacroiliac joint, or disc (discogram). These remain controversial and are generally only effective in a reliable patient without psychological, legal, or monetary reinforcers.

6. What is the most important tool to assess patients with LBP?

Believe it or not, the history and physical examination remain the mainstays for evaluating LBP, despite the new expensive technology.[1]

7. What factors of the history are most important?

The history is vital and may be more important than physical examination. Determine the onset and duration of the problem; the reason it occurred; its relation to work, automobile, or other injury; if litigation is involved; and if there is financial remuneration. Define the pain carefully: its location, relationship to position and activity, and time of day it is most prominent. Determine if there are associated symptoms such as pain in an extremity, numbness, or tingling. "Red flags" that may indicate serious pathology include bowel or bladder dysfunction, history of cancer, and generalized disorder such as end stage renal disease, osteoporosis, Paget's disease, AIDS, or drug use. These red flags warrant further testing such as laboratory tests or imaging studies. In acute back pain without red flags, treatment usually only requires a history and physical examination.

Low Back Pain "Red Flags"

Fever	Significant trauma	Failure to improve with treatment
Unexplained weight loss	Osteoporosis	Alcohol or drug abuse
Cancer history	Age > 50 years	

8. Which structures should be examined in a patient with LBP and how is the examination performed?

The physical examination requires demonstration and lots of practice. Keep in mind that few physical exam techniques have been proven to identify the specific structure or disorder that is the cause of pain. The examination should address the low back, pelvis, hips, lower limbs, and gait and should include a neurologic examination for nerve root involvement. Examination points include back motion to look for asymmetric movement, re-creation of pain, and areas of mechanically limited motion or guarded motion (so-called spasm). Examine for tenderness, especially percussion tenderness over bony areas in the back and pelvis; the gait and balance including heel- and toe-walking and squat and return to upright; range of motion (ROM) of the lower extremities; and any muscle tightness, especially the hamstrings and quadriceps. Pay particular attention to hip ROM, which is best examined in the prone position. LBP and hip pain with limited hip range may indicate osteoarthritis or other hip abnormality. A full peripheral neurologic examination should be performed, including testing of reflexes, strength, and sensation.

9. Even though laboratory and imaging studies are not always accurate for diagnosing low back problems, should any tests be performed?

Imaging studies can be used to exclude severe disease. They are indicated only if red flags are present or if there is no improvement after several weeks of treatment. The initial study may be a plain x-ray. Other tests include bone scan, cross-sectional imaging (e.g., CT and MRI), and special tests, such as single photon emission CT (SPECT) scanning and discography. Remember that "abnormal" findings are expected on cross-sectional imaging. If leg pain is present, EMG, which is more specific than imaging, can be performed.

10. Is disability from LBP common?

Patients with disability from LBP present a very different picture from those with acute, acute recurrent, or even chronic LBP who are still functioning. Despite improvements in diagnostic and treatment techniques, disability from LBP has risen astronomically in the last couple of decades (as much as 2500%). We must look beyond pure physical explanation for this rise. Patients with diability from LBP that occurred either spontaenously or, more commonly, from an injury must also be assessed from a psychoemotional, social, and vocational viewpoint.

11. What are signs to look for in identifying the "disability syndrome"?

The most common associations that indicate disability from an injury are *not* physical ones. The best predictors are history of prior injury with time off work, high Minnesota Multiphasic Personality Inventory (MMPI) scale 3 (hysteria), and high work dissatisfication scales. History and physical examination features that may help identify this syndrome include past episodes of back pain that led to disability, a long history of tests and surgical procedures, and a very detailed description of the event that generated their problem. Usually the patient reports that someone or something is at fault (e.g., oil on the floor, extra work that the patient was not supposed to do). Pain is often rated as very severe, such as 9 or 10 on a 0–10 scale, with 10 being excruciating pain. The patient may indicate a 10-level pain while sitting comfortably in no apparent distress. Patients may be very demonstrative, grimace, position their bodies in unusual ways, complain of pain with minor movements, and have bizarre gait patterns. Check for Waddell's signs, which indicate that organic abnormality is not the primary factor in the patient's disability. These signs do not prove malingering but merely show that factors other than physical issues are significant contributors.

Signs (Waddell and Others) that LBP Is Not Organic

- Simulated axial loading—pressure on the neck leading to LBP
- Simulated rotation—neck extension or rotation with back motion leading to LBP
- General overreaction to physical examination
- Superficial tenderness
- Regional weakness (not following anatomic patterns)
- Widespread nonanatomic distribution of pain
- Regional sensory deficient (not following anatomic patterns)
- Distracted straight-leg raising (e.g., sitting position vs. supine)

12. How do you treat the patient with acute LBP?

The offending structure is not known, and the natural history is to improve regardless of (or despite) treatment. Few treatments have proven to be beneficial, but several things may hasten the healing process. **Reassurance** can be very beneficial. Advise the patient that the process is "benign," will not lead to long-term impairment, and most likely will not need major intervention. **NSAIDs** can give the double benefit of pain relief and decreased inflammation. **Educate** the patient on proper back care and exercises. Other treatments for acute LBP are usually not necessary. Several studies suggest that **manipulation** during the first 3 weeks decreases painful episodes, but this is controversial. Mild exercise may be helpful.

13. Is bed rest helpful?

Bed rest was the mainstay of treatment at one time. However, a number of studies show that patients are better off doing as many normal activities as possible. This seems to shorten the course of disability and allow an earlier return to work. Thus, it is recommended that patients be up and about as much as tolerable and avoid anything that significantly increases pain.

14. What if the pain persists for several weeks after the initial treatment?

If pain persists, it is reasonable to do some minor investigations, starting with lumbosacral spine x-ray. Additional treatment depends on the severity of discomfort and degree to which it interferes with function. More tests and treatment can be performed, but the risk-benefit and cost-benefit ratios should be considered. If the pain remains severe, a regular therapy program can be instituted. Other treatments include trigger point injections with lidocaine (Xylocaine) or lidocaine with steroids; injections are easy to perform.

If pain does not resolve in several months and the individual is not disabled but is distressed, repeat reassurances because patients may fear severe illness. If not already performed, imaging studies are appropriate. Bone scan and MRI should be interpreted cautiously and correlated clinically. Determine the severity of pain perception and how it interferes physically, psychosocially, and psychoemotionally with function. Treatment options include medications such as NSAIDs, tricyclic antidepressants, and acetaminophen; injections including sacroiliac joint, facet joint, and local myofascial trigger points; and alternative medicine techniques such as acupuncture.

15. What about the patient who is disabled by the pain?

Other factors contributing to the pain must be identified. There has been a large movement toward treating "benign" or "nonmalignant" pain problems with opioid medications and various injections, disc dissolution techniques, device insertion (spinal stimulation, morphine pumps), and surgery. However, they are unlikely to treat the entire problem. When etiology is not clearly defined and there are multiple inorganic signs, treat the functional loss and disability. This type of patient is best served by an interdisciplinary team approach (not multicisciplinary) such as a functional restoration program.

16. Who should treat patients with LBP?

A variety of clinicians can initiate treatment, and it is appropriate for a primary care physician to start the process. Unfortunately, by the time patients see a specialist, they may have undergone an MRI and been told the pain is due to disc problems or other misinformation. It is difficult to "unteach" the patient, especially because the general population places such credence on MRI findings. Physiatrists (physical medicine and rehabilitation physicians) are the best next line of treatment. Ideally, a physiatrist would be the best primary physician as well.

17. Should neurosurgeons or orthopedic surgeons be consulted first?

Definitely not! If an internist has a patient with a gastrointestinal or cardiac problem that he cannot solve, does he send the patient to a GI surgeon or thoracic surgeon? No! The patient is referred to a gastroenterologist or cardiologist. After an expert evaluation and treatment, these specialists can make any appropriate surgical referrals. The same should occur with LBP, especially because internists receive less training in rehabilitation than in internal medicine subspecialities. In addition, a surgeon's primary training is in surgery. They will not have the knowledge of the total armamentarium that physiatrists have at their disposal.

18. What is the bottom line for LBP?

- LBP is ubiquitous in the human race and not a disease.
- Degenerative disc disease and some of the anatomic sequelae of facet arthropathy or spurring are usual consequences of aging.
- The natural history of LBP is to improve with or without treatment, but certain treatments can hasten the process and are worthwhile.
- There is little or no correlation between anatomic abnormalities seen on imaging studies and the patient's clinical symptoms or signs.
- It is the physiatrist's job to discover serious problems presenting as LBP by identifying the red flags outlined in the AHCPR guidelines. This guideline is worth requesting (remember that the guideline only applies to acute LBP).
- Treatment comprises reassurance, NSAIDs, and having the patient stay out of bed and be active.
- Disability from LBP is a different disorder than acute LBP, and a host of factors contribute to it. It must be evaluated and treated differently than acute LBP.
- Special injection techniques are sometimes indicated in patients with LBP.

BIBLIOGRAPHY

1. Agency for Health Care Policy and Research: Clinical Practice Guideline 14: Acute Low Back Pain in Adults. Rockville, MD, U.S. Department of Health and Human Services Public Health Service, 1994.
2. Cutler R, Fishbain D, Rosomoff H, et al: Does nonsurgical pain center treatment of chronic pain return patients to work? Spine 19:643–652, 1994.
3. Deyo R, Tsui-Wu Y: Descriptive epidemiology of low-back pain and its related medical care in the United States. Spine 12:264–268, 1987.
4. Deyo R, Rainville J, Kent D: What can the history and physical examination tell us about low back pain? JAMA 268:760–765, 1991.

5. Dreyfuss P, Michaelsen M, Pauza K, et al: The value of medical history and physical examination in diagnosing sacroiliac joint pain. Spine 21:2594–2602, 1996.
6. Frymoyer J, Ducker T, Hadler N, et al (eds): The Adult Spine: Principles and Practice, Volume 1. New York, Raven Press, 1991.
7. Haldeman S: Diagnostic tests for the evaluation of back and neck pain. Neurol Clin 14:103–117, 1996.
8. Jensen M, Brant-Zawadzki M, Obuchoswki N, et al: Magnetic resonance imaging of the lumbar spine in people without back pain. N Engl J Med 331:69–73, 1994.
9. Leboeuf-Yde C, Kyvik K: At what age does low back pain become a common problem: A study of 29,424 individuals aged 12–41 years. Spine 23:228–234, 1998.
10. Malmivaara A, Hakkinen U, Aro T, et al: The treatment of acute back pain: Bedrest, exercise, or ordinary activity. N Engl J Med 332:351–355, 1995.
11. Sobel D, Schwartz T: Oh, Your Aching Back: A Sufferer's Guide to the Best Treatment. New Yorker Magazine (Mar):41–45, 1986.
12. Van Tulder M, Assendelft W, Koes B, Bouter LM: Spinal radiographic findings and nonspecific low back pain: A systematic review of observational studies. Spine 22:427–434, 1997.

39. THE SHOULDER: ANATOMY, PATHOLOGY, AND DIAGNOSIS

Rene Cailliet, M.D.

1. Name all the joints involved in the shoulder girdle complex.

Glenohumeral joint   Sternoclavicular joint
Suprahumeral joint   Sternocostal joint
Acromioclavicular joint   Costovertebral joint
Scapulocostal joint

These numerous joints indicate why the term *shoulder girdle complex* is better than *shoulder joint*.

2. Which tissues within the complex can be the site of nociception?

Although many structures in the shoulder can have pain, the main ones are the tendon, the biceps tendon, the subdeltoid bursa, and the glenohumeral capsule. Nonshoulder structures that may cause pain include radicular pain from the cervical spine, cardiac ischemic pain, diaphragm irritation, lung inflammation, and various upper abdominal pathologies.

3. What muscles comprise the rotator cuff?

One way of remembering them is by using the mnemonic **SITS** (**s**upraspinatus, **i**nfraspinatus, **t**eres minor and **s**ubscapularis). At rest, their function is glenohumeral stabilization. All contract isometrically in the dependent arm to prevent subluxation. Dynamically, all contract to abduct and forward flex the arm. All except the subscapularis contract in external rotation of the arm (see figure on following page).

4. Is there a difference between subdeltoid bursitis and supraspinatus tendinitis?

The synovial linings of both the subdeltoid bursa and the glenohumeral capsule are contiguous with the supraspinatus tendon. Inflammation of the sheath inflames both.

5. Is it possible to differentiate a rotator cuff tendon partial tear from tendinitis by clinical means?

No. A partial tear of the rotator cuff tendinopathy (RTC) causes segmental swelling that becomes entrapped under the coracoacromial ligament similar to tendinitis.

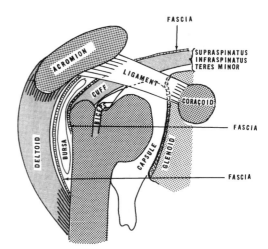

Contents of the glenohumeral joint. (From Cailliet R: Shoulder Pain, 3rd ed. Philadelphia, F.A. Davis, 1991, with permission.)

6. Is there a clinical test that confirms the diagnosis of a torn rotator cuff?

No test on physical examination confirms the diagnosis of a complete tear, but clinically a complete tear is indicated by inability to abduct the arm from dependency, inability to externally rotate the arm, and the patient has a positive drop arm test. Magnetic resonance imaging (MRI) studies are useful in confirming tears and the extent of tendon damage.

7. What is the mechanism of the "drop arm test"?

The arm cannot abduct but once abducted to horizontal can be briefly held there by the deltoid muscle. Because the supraspinatus muscle is not seating the humeral head into the glenoid fossa, the arm gradually or with minimal weight "drops."

8. Aside from faulty shoulder abduction, is there another test to determine the presence of a complete rotator cuff tear?

Yes. Because a portion of the rotator cuff is represented by the tendinous insertion into the tuberosity of the supraspinatus and infraspinatus muscles, in a complete tear, active external rotation of the arm is not possible.

9. Besides rotator cuff disease, what other differential diagnostic possibilities must be considered in evaluating shoulder pain?

Suprascapular nerve entrapment	Thoracic outlet syndrome
Shoulder instability	Cervical radiculitis
Acromioclavicular degenerative joint disease	Bicipital tendinitis

10. Is posture a factor in evaluating shoulder pain?

Yes. An exaggerated dorsal kyphosis causes the scapula to rotate downward. This changes the alignment of the glenoid fossa and the proximity of the acromium, making impingement more possible.

11. Suggest a convenient way of initiating active-passive shoulder movement.

Pendulum (Codman's) exercises are a simple way of instituting active-passive motion of the glenohumeral joint. This is best achieved with the patient bent forward, with the arm in the dependent (pendular) position and the body "actively" moving to "passively" move the pendular arm.

12. What is a "frozen shoulder"?

A frozen shoulder is capsular limitation that prevents full range of motion of the glenohumeral joint. It is essentially adhesive capsulitis and adhesive bursitis in which the synovial tissues become adherent.

13. Name the three most common anatomic structures of the shoulder involved in shoulder impingement syndrome.
1. Subacromial bursa
2. Supraspinatus
3. Biceps tendon

14. What are the components of the scapulohumeral rhythm?
This term indicates the movement of the humerus within the glenoid fossa and the scapula upon the rib cage when the arm abducts or forward flexes. At rest they are vertical, but as the humerus abducts (flexes), the scapula initially remains static then rotates to permit overhead elevation. The "rhythm" implies that for every degree of scapular rotation there are 2° of glenohumeral movement. The ratio 2:1 is not totally accurate for the entire 180°.

15. How is complex regional pain syndrome (CRPS) managed?
Prevention by early intervention is the best treatment. Intervention includes early active range of motion exercises and anti-inflammatory medications. Meaningful explanation to the patient allays fear of aggravation and recurrence with movement. Steroids and stellate ganglion blocks have value as well.

16. What is the mechanism, diagnosis, and management of shoulder subluxation?
Subluxation is partial dislocation. Subluxation can result from direct trauma but also occurs after acute stroke. The head of the humerus is held within the glenoid fossa by the glenohumeral capsule and the rotator cuff muscles. The supraspinatus muscle is predominant in support. In acute stroke, the supraspinatus muscle becomes flail and allows the head of the humerus to sublux. Management entails positioning the patient to avoid downward traction on the glenohumeral joint from gravity. Glenohumeral positioning can be maintained by contraction of the supraspinatus muscle mechanically or electrically.

17. Is bicipital tendinitis an entity?
The biceps tendon acts passively (mechanically) upon the humerus during abduction and forward flexion as the bicipital fossa passes over the tendon. Inappropriate glenohumeral friction that occurs over the tendon, which is contiguous to the subdeltoid bursa and glenohumeral capsule, results in tendinitis.

18. What structures other than the glenohumeral joint can cause pain in the shoulder region?
Because of the number of joints in the shoulder girdle complex (a better term than "shoulder joint"), any or all can cause shoulder pain. These include the acromioclavicular joint and the sternoclavicular joint. Pain can be referred to the shoulder region from the neck, chest, or abdomen as well. This indicates the need for a careful history and examination that includes a musculoskeletal evaluation.

19. Can shoulder pain occur from a nonshoulder structure?
Radicular pain from the cervical spine, cardiac ischemic pain, diaphragm irritation, lung inflammation, and various upper abdominal pathology all can refer pain to the shoulder.

20. In the setting of a complete brachial plexus disruption, what is the ideal (most functional) way of performing a shoulder fusion procedure?
Generally, it is agreed that fixation of the shoulder in flexion, abduction, and internal rotation will facilitate function, although the precise degree is debated.

21. Why does shoulder dislocation occur?
The shoulder dislocates because of its unusual anatomy, including lax ligaments, shallow glenoid cavity, and redundant capsule. Anterior dislocation is more common than posterior dislocation

(sometimes seen in electrocution and seizures). The coracoclavicular ligament is usually torn in forcible dislocation of the shoulder.

22. How is acromioclavicular (AC) pain manifested?

Usually, there is a history of trauma, and pain and tenderness are located at the AC joint. Crepitation is elicited by circumduction of the shoulder. Diagnosis and possible relief are gained by intra-articular injection of an analgesic agent. AC joint separation is diagnosed by taking an upper chest radiograph while the patient stands holding ≥ 10 pounds of weight in each hand as arms dangle to the sides.

BIBLIOGRAPHY

1. Andren L, Lundberg BJ: Treatment of rigid shoulders by joint distention during arthrography. Acta Orthop Scand 36:45, 1965.
2. Cailliet R: Shoulder Pain, 3rd ed. Philadelphia, F.A. Davis, 1991.
3. Grey RG: The natural history of "idiopathic" frozen shoulder. J Bone Joint Surg 60A:564, 1978.
4. MacNab I: Rotator cuff tendinitis. Ann R Coll Surg 53:271, 1973.
5. Neer CS: Impingement lesions. Clin Orthop 173:70, 1983.
6. Stiens SA, Goldstein BA: Rehabilitation after overuse injuries of the shoulder. In Gordon S (ed): Overuse Injury of the Upper Extremity. Rosemont, IL, American Academy of Orthopedic Surgeons, 1995, pp 517–537.
7. Stiens SA, Haselkorn JK, Peters DJ, Goldstein B: Rehabilitation intervention for patients with upper extremity dysfunction: Challenges of outcome evaluation. Am J Ind Med 29:590–601, 1996.

40. REHABILITATION OF SHOULDER DISORDERS

Edward G. McFarland, M.D., Timothy C. Shen, M.D., Tae Kyun Kim, M.D., Ph.D., and Gregory E. Lutz, M.D.

1. What principles are important in rehabilitation after shoulder surgery?

Rehabilitation requires a balance between tissue healing and early range of motion (ROM). It is important to understand what has been repaired and what the limits of motion are, as defined by the surgeon. The type of procedure also affects rehabilitation. For example, operations for instability (either subluxations or dislocations) can be done through an arthroscope or larger open incisions. Although recovery from an arthroscopic procedure may be shorter due to less soft tissue dissection, the surgical repairs are the same. Consequently, rehabilitation is similar for these procedures.

2. What therapeutic factors must be considered in the treatment of the painful shoulder?

Elimination of pain is needed to assure early mobilization. This is available with nonsteroidal anti-inflammatory drugs (NSAIDs) and even intra-articular injections of a steroid. Pendular exercises should be initiated early to prevent capsular adhesion.

3. How does one treat a stiff shoulder?

Nonoperative treatment consists of stretching, decreasing inflammation, and pain relief. To increase motion, aggressive passive ROM is recommended. NSAIDs, pain relievers (narcotic or non-narcotic), and oral steroids are given for pain relief. Operative options include manipulation, arthroscopic evaluation, and release of adhesions. Hospitalization, an indwelling scalene catheter, and aggressive physical therapy may be recommended. Another option is to send the patient home after surgery with immediate physical therapy and nonoperative treatments. Recovery takes 6–12 months.

4. What is the treatment for rotator cuff tendinitis?

Treatment of rotator cuff tendinitis begins with frequent applications of ice, particularly after activity or before bedtime, NSAIDs for 6–8 weeks, avoidance of painful motions, and physical therapy. Exercises should be performed in a pain-free ROM. Focus on stretching to avoid loss of motion and to strengthen muscles. If this does not work, cortisone shots in the subacromial space are recommended. If there is still no improvement, further studies are indicated (e.g., MRI or arthrogram). If there is no rotator cuff tear, surgical treatment involving arthroscopic evaluation with partial acromioplasty should be performed.

5. What does rehabilitation after acromioplasty entail?

Most patients go home the same day with an arm sling and can write or feed themselves in 1–2 days. Lifting anything heavier than a coffee cup is prohibited. The most common complication is a frozen or stiff shoulder. Motion of fingers, wrist, and elbow begins immediately. Structured rehabilitation and physical therapy begin in 7–10 days. If the deltoid muscle was removed and reattached, active motion above table level is not allowed for 4–6 weeks. Otherwise, full motion is allowed as pain permits. The goal is full motion in 2–3 months. An acromioplasty with muscle reattachment may take longer.

6. What about patients with rotator cuff repair?

Rehabilitation after Rotator Cuff Repair

DURATION	TREATMENT	PRECAUTIONS
Phase 1		
0–3 weeks	Elbow, wrist, finger ROM	No weight bearing
	Passive ROM in abduction in scapular plane	No active ROM
	Passive ROM in forward flexion	Sling or immobilizer at all times except exercise
	Pendulum exercises	Avoid arm adduction across body; avoid shoulder extension, internal and external rotation as dictated by surgeon
	Begin scapular retraction and depression exercises	
Phase 2		
4–6 weeks	Start active-assisted ROM in flexion and abduction	Start active ROM
	Active ROM of flexion less than 90°	No lifting of objects causing axial traction
6–8 weeks	Continue active-assisted ROM	Patient allowed to use arms in front of body, below shoulder level
	Isometric strengthening as tolerated by pain in flexion, extension, and internal and external rotation	
8–10 weeks	Progressively more vigorous isometrics	
	Progressive isotonic exercises	
Phase 3		
10–12 weeks	Active ROM exercises, progressive resistance, strengthening	Discontinue ROM precautions
	Stretching in flexion, abduction, and rotation	

7. How do you treat patients with severe arthritis of the shoulder?

Treatment is aimed at maintaining ROM with a home stretching program. Additional therapies include ice or heat for symptomatic relief, NSAIDs, and avoidance of painful activities. Cortisone injections are recommended if there is impingement or rotator cuff tendinitis. When nonoperative treatment fails, joint replacement is the best surgical option. Either the humeral head (hemiarthroplasty) or the humeral head and socket/glenoid (total shoulder replacement) can be replaced. A 1–2-night hospital stay is typical. Rehabilitation begins the day after surgery (see Table).

Rehabilitation after Total Shoulder Replacement

DURATION	TREATMENT	PRECAUTIONS
Phase 1		
0–3 weeks	Gentle passive and active ROM flexion to full flexion as tolerated, abduction to 90°, internal rotation to 45°, external rotation as dictated by surgeon Pendulum exercises Isometric strengthening as tolerated by pain in flexion, extension, and internal and external rotation One-handed ADL	No weight bearing Sling worn at all times except exercise Avoid active abduction, extension > 0°, external rotation as dictated by surgeon
3–6 weeks	Vigorous isometrics as tolerated Active-assisted progressing to active ROM "Wall-walking" with hand used as stabilizer	Continue sling and non-weight bearing May begin active abduction
Phase 2		
6–12 weeks	Vigorous isometrics Progressive isotonics (e.g., elastic tubing exercises) Active-assisted ROM and active ROM past 90° Two-handed ADL encouraged	May lift objects up to 2 lbs. Discontinue sling Discontinue ROM precautions in external rotation Can begin to work on external rotation
Phase 3		
> 12 weeks	Active ROM exercises, progressive resistance, strengthening Stretching in flexion, abduction, and rotation	Discontinue ROM precautions

8. What is the optimum treatment of a frozen shoulder?
• Prevention by early mobilization by pendulum exercises
• Avoidance of splinting
• Minimization of pain and inflammation
Once there is adhesion, active and passive mobilization exercises are effective.

9. Describe brisement treatment for a frozen shoulder.
Brisement is French for "break." This implies breaking the adhered capsule. This can be done by manipulation, but brisement includes injection into the glenohumeral joint of a large quantity of an analgesic agent and long-acting steroid in an amount exceeding that permitted by the adhered capsule. The normal capsule admits 30 ml of fluid, and the frozen shoulder admits approximately 3–5 ml.

10. Discuss rehabilitation after shoulder replacement.
External rotation should be avoided for 6–8 weeks. Interestingly, elevation in front of the body does not stress the subscapularis in most cases and can be instituted soon after surgery. Strengthening is important. The most serious complication is infection. Drainage from the wound after 4–5 days is abnormal. If the subscapularis tendon repair fails, dislocation of the prosthesis can occur. Stiffness is common, and most patients do not entirely regain normal motion.

11. How do fractures of the shoulder affect rehabilitation?
Because treatment often requires immobilization, stiffness and loss of motion may occur. Fractures that do not require surgery are usually stable, and finger, wrist, and elbow motion can begin when pain subsides. Physical therapy including passive, active-assisted motion, active motion, and strengthening should wait until the fracture is healed.

Fractures requiring incision and fixation with pins, plates, or screws can begin motion of the fingers, wrist and elbow in a few days. When the fracture can withstand stress, pendulum exercises should be started, followed by active-assisted motion and active motion. Pain, loss of motion, and poor function should be evaluated with radiographs to check for hardware failure, avascular necrosis of the humeral head, and proper location of the humeral head in the socket. Sometimes the bones heal in a position that will not allow full motion. Re-evaluation by the surgeon may be necessary.

12. When is a prosthesis used for shoulder fractures?

A hemiarthroplasty (which replaces only the humeral head) is used for severe fractures where the proximal humerus and humeral head are broken into many pieces. The rotator cuff tendons or bones are sewn into holes in the prosthesis. It is critical to allow the tendons or bones to heal before too much stress is applied. A 2–3-day hospital stay is typical. The day after surgery, finger, wrist, and elbow motion can be started. When repair of the tendons is secure, pendulum exercises and passive motion of the shoulder should be instituted. Once the structures heal, more aggressive motion exercises can begin. Loss of strength and motion is common, and many patients do not regain full motion. In this case, an evaluation with radiographs and a neurologic examination are warranted.

13. What is the treatment for shoulder instability?

In some cases, instability can be controlled with muscle strength and careful positioning. Rehabilitation is particularly effective in patients with signs of instability but no history of trauma. Patients with a traumatic dislocation, younger patients (< 25 years old), and athletic individuals have a greater chance of recurrence.

Surgery for instability involves repair of the torn labrum to the glenoid rim (Blankart repair) and shortening of the ligaments (capsular shift). Rehabilitation is similar for both procedures (see Table). Repair of the labrum can be done arthroscopically or with a larger incision. Capsular shifts have been done via an open incision, although some surgeons use arthroscopic techniques. Recently, an arthroscopic thermal technique performing capsular shrinkage or shifting has been described. A probe heats the ligaments and causes them to shrink and tighten the shoulder. The arm is put in a sling for 3 weeks while the ligaments become tight, then rehabilitation is similar to the open procedure.

Rehabilitation after Bankart and Capsular Shift (Open), Bankart and Shift (Arthroscopic), and Thermal Capsulorrhaphy*

DURATION	TREATMENT	PRECAUTIONS
Phase 1		
0–3 weeks	Passive ROM in abduction in scapular plane	No weight bearing
	Passive ROM in ER to operative limit	No active external rotation
	Pendulum exercises	Wear immobilizer to sleep and most
	Begin scapular retraction and depression exercises	of the day for 2 weeks, then just to sleep
	Active flexion as tolerated	
	After 1 week, add assisted active ROM for ER to operative limit	
	Gradually progress to isometric flexion and ER without weights below shoulder level	
Phase 2		
3–6 weeks	Progressive isotonic exercises (e.g., elastic tubing exercises) as tolerated	May lift objects up to 2 lbs.
	Full ROM forward flexion, abduction	
	Progression external rotation as tolerated after 4–6 weeks	
6–9 weeks	Progress isotonic exercises as tolerated	Discontinue night bracing
	Emphasis on gently regaining ER	May lift objects up to 5 lbs.

Table continued on following page

Rehabilitation after Bankart and Capsular Shift (Open), Bankart and Shift (Arthroscopic),
and Thermal Capsulorrhaphy* (Continued)

DURATION	TREATMENT	PRECAUTIONS
Phase 3		
9–12 weeks	Begin isokinetic IR/ER/FF, abduction	
> 12 weeks	Active ROM exercises, progressive resistance, strengthening	Discontinue all ROM precautions
	Stretching in flexion, abduction, and rotation	

* In thermal shift, motion of the shoulder is not begun for 3 weeks.
ER = external rotation; IR = internal rotation; FF = forward flexion.

BIBLIOGRAPHY

1. Brander VA, Hinderer SR, Alpiner N, Oh TH: Limb disorders in rehabilitation in joint and connective tissue diseases. Arch Phys Med Rehabil 76:S52, 1995.
2. Bruzga B, Speer K: Challenges of rehabilitation after shoulder surgery. Clin Sports Med 18:769–793, 1999.
3. Cofield HR, Tanner WM: Prosthetic arthroplasty for fractures and fracture-dislocations of proximal humerus. Clin Orthop 179:116–128, 1983.
4. Donatelli RA: Physical Therapy of the Shoulder, 3rd ed. New York, Churchill Livingstone, 1997.
5. Kirkley A, Grifin S, Richards C, et al: Prospective, randomized, clinical trial comparing the effectiveness of immediate arthroscopic stabilization versus immobilization and rehabilitation in first traumatic anterior dislocations of the shoulder. Arthroscopy 15:507–514, 1999.
6. Kibler WB: Rehabilitation of the shoulder. In Kibler WB, Herring SA, Press JM, Lee P (eds): Functional Rehabilitation of Sports and Musculoskeletal Injuries. Gaithersburg, MD, Aspen Publishers, 1998, pp 149–170.
7. McFarland EG, Cosgarea AJ, Krabak BJ: Rehabilitation protocols from Johns Hopkins Medical Institute Sports Medicine and Shoulder Surgery Website: http://www.med.jhu.edu/ortho/sports/protocols.
8. Neer CS, Foster CR: Inferior capsular shift for involuntary inferior and multidirectional instability of the shoulder. J Bone Joint Surg 62A:897–908, 1980.
9. Rockwood CA, Matsen FA: The Shoulder, 2nd ed. Philadelphia, W.B. Saunders, 1998.

41. THE ELBOW: ANATOMY, PATHOLOGY, AND DIAGNOSIS

Edward Magaziner, M.D., and Francisco Santiago, M.D.

1. Name the articulations of the elbow and where the movements occur.
  • The humeroradial joint between the radial head and capitulum of the humerus
  • The humeroulnar joint between the trochlear notch of the ulna and the humerus
  • The radioulnar joint

Flexion and extension occur at the axis of the trochlear and capitulum. Supination-pronation occurs through the longitudinal axis of rotation at the radial head and the radial ulnar notch of the ulna (see figure on following page).

2. What is the carrying angle of the elbow?
The normal anatomic valgus angulation, or carrying angle, is the angle between the upper arm and forearm when the elbow is fully extended. The normal angle for males is 5–10° and for females is 10–15°. Greater than 20° is considered abnormal.

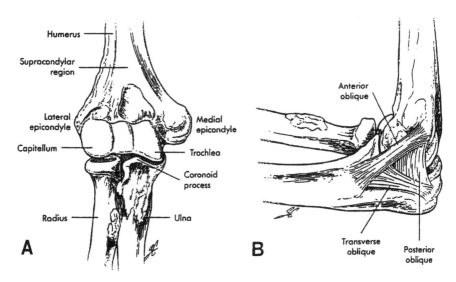

A, Anterior view of the elbow. *B*, The three components of the ulnar collateral ligament. (From Nicholas JA, Hershman EB: The Upper Extremity in Sports Medicine. St. Louis, Mosby, 1990, with permission.)

3. What are the main muscles of the elbow, what movements are they responsible for, and what tricks can be used to isolate them?

MUSCLE	MOVEMENT	TRICKS FOR ISOLATION
Biceps	Flexion, supination	
Brachioradialis	Flexion	Elbow in the neutral position
Brachialis	Flexion	Elbow in full pronation allowing brachialis isolation
Triceps	Extension	
Anconeus	Extension	
Supinator	Supination	Elbow in extension
Pronator quadratus	Pronation	
Pronator teres	Pronation	Least effective as a pronator when elbow in full flexion

4. What is unique about the brachioradialis muscle?

It is the only muscle that attaches from the distal end of one bone to the distal end of another bone and the only muscle producing flexion of the elbow that is supplied by the radial nerve instead of the musculocutaneous nerve. It can also act as pronator or supinator depending on position.

5. What is draftsman's elbow and how is it treated?

This inflammation of the olecranon bursa usually causes pain and swelling at the posterior elbow. It can be associated with trauma or systemic conditions such as gout, rheumatoid arthritis, pseudogout, tuberculosis, chondrocalcinosis, xanthomatosis, or infection. A septic bursa is ruled out by Gram stain and culture. Radiographs rule out osteomyelitis and bone spurs. Treatment of nonseptic olecranon bursitis includes protective padding, nonsteroidal anti-inflammatory drugs (NSAIDs), maintenance of functional range of motion (ROM), a trial of aspiration (often unsuccessful), or local cortisone injection. Surgical intervention may be required.

6. What is a pushed or pulled elbow on a child and how is it treated?

In a **pulled elbow**, the head of the radius is dislocated from the annular ligament, usually caused by a forceful pull on a child's extended arm. Supination is limited. If it cannot be reduced by flexion and supination, the following manual maneuver can be used to correct it. The child stands against the wall with the upper arm abducted and the elbow flexed at 90°. The examiner grasps the lower forearm with the ipsilateral hand, pushes the radius upwards toward the humerus by pressing the elbow against the wall, and rapidly rotates the forearm in both directions. Usually, on full supination, the radial head will click back into place.

A **pushed elbow** describes subluxation of the radial head in a proximal direction, often seen when a person falls on an outstretched hand. The radial head impinges on the capitulum. It is occasionally associated with Colles' fracture. Treatment consists of traction and repetitive stretching.

7. How does myositis ossification occur and where is it common about the elbow?

It occurs after injury to muscle fibers, connective tissue, and blood vessels underlying the periosteum and presents with a triad of symptoms: pain, a palpable mass, and flexion contracture. It is most common in the brachioradialis of the elbow and in males 15–30 years of age.

8. What is tennis elbow?

Tennis elbow is an overuse syndrome caused by repetitive microtrauma to the musculotendinous unit along the radial extensors of the wrist in the lateral epicondyle region. It causes inflammation and degenerative tissue damage and presents as pain in the lateral elbow that can radiate down the forearm to the wrist. Pain worsens with grasping or wrist extension. Less than 5% of patients get tennis elbow by playing tennis. The four sites of occurrence from proximal to distal are supracondylar, tenoperiosteal, tendinous, and muscular. A point of tenderness is usually palpated in one of the four locations. Diagnosis should not be confused with radioulnar or radiohumeral bursitis, annular or collateral ligament sprains, osteoarthritis of the radioulnar joint, or radial nerve entrapment at the supinator or arcade of Frohse.

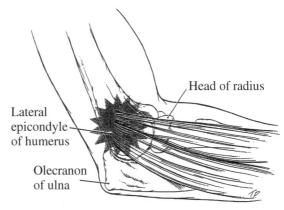

Extensive performance of certain activities such as gripping or twisting can cause microscopic tears of muscle tendons where they are attached to bones in the elbow. Inflammation and pain can then develop. (From Klag MJ, et al: Johns Hopkins Family Health Book. New York, Harper Collins, 1999, with permission.)

9. What is golfer's elbow?

This repetitive strain injury usually affects the flexor pronator musculature such as pronator teres, flexor carpi radialis, flexor carpi ulnaris, and rarely the flexor digitorum superficialis. Pain is present with resisted wrist flexion or pronation with the elbow extended. Causes include an improper serve in tennis, throwing a baseball, a golf swing, or use of hand tools.

10. What is Monteggia's fracture?

A fracture of the upper third of the ulna and dislocation of the head of the radius. It is classified based on location and displacement of the radius.

11. What is a Galeazzi's fracture?

A fracture of the distal radial shaft with a dislocation or subluxation of the inferior radioulnar joint.

12. What is little leaguer's elbow?

This injury in children and adolescents is due to repetitive valgus stress where the medial epicondyle is inflamed. Partial separation of the apophysis can occur. A common symptom is pain when throwing. Radiographs are important in diagnoses and may show widening of the apophyseal line or an avulsion fracture, which needs surgical correction.

13. Describe pronator syndrome.

This entrapment neuropathy affects the median nerve distal to the antecubital fossa. In most cases, the nerve pierces the two heads of the pronator teres muscle where hypertrophy or an anomalous band may injure the nerve. Presentation includes pain in the anterior elbow that increases by resisted pronation, numbness in the hand, and weakness of the wrist and finger flexors. Compression over the median nerve at the pronator teres often reproduces symptoms within 30 seconds. Other sites of compression can be at the lacertus fibrosus or in the flexor digitorum superficialis muscle. Median nerve compression proximal to the pronator teres can occur at the ligament of Struthers at the medial epicondyle.

14. What is cubital tunnel syndrome?

Entrapment of the ulnar nerve along the cubital tunnel at the medial aspect of the elbow associated with a Tinel's sign. Paresthesia and numbness can occur in the fourth and fifth fingers. Over time there may be weakness in grasp and pinch and loss of dexterity. The three zones of compression are:

Zone I   Proximal to the medial epicondyle
Zone II   At the level of the medial epicondyle
Zone III   Distal to the medial epicondyle (cubital tunnel)

Overuse injuries can cause entrapment with a tight flexor carpi ulnaris muscle in zone III. Treatment is with NSAIDs, an elbow pad to protect the nerve, avoidance of aggravating activities, and exercises in the pain-free range. Surgical release or transposition may be required.

15. What is posterior interosseous nerve syndrome?

It is an entrapment neuropathy of the posterior interosseous nerve branch of the radial nerve at the fibrous arch of the supinator or within the muscle belly. Symptoms may include pain with resisted pronation or supination, Tinel's sign over the nerve, resisted pronation or supination, and weakness in wrist or finger extension. There is no associated numbness. Diagnosis is made with electromyography (EMG). Muscles involved can be the extensor carpi ulnaris, extensor digitorum communis, extensor indicis, abductor pollicis longus, and extensor pollicis longus and brevis. The extensor carpi radialis longus and brevis muscles are spared.

16. Is there a boxer's elbow and what causes it?

Yes. Also known as **hyperextension overload syndrome** or **olecranon impingement syndrome,** it is caused by repetitive valgus extension of the elbow in the boxer's jab or in sports that involve throwing.

17. Describe Panner disease.

Osteochondrosis of the capitulum. The etiology is unclear, but it is seen most often in young boys. Patients present with tenderness and swelling over the lateral aspect of the elbow with limited extension. Radiographs show patchy areas of sclerosis and lucency, which may appear fragmented. Treatment includes immobilization with a long arm cast followed by protected motion.

18. What is osteochondritis desiccans of the elbow?

This idiopathic condition affects the capitulum of the humerus, with ensuing avascular necrosis. It is usually seen in the dominant arm of teenage boys involved in throwing sports. It is characterized by poorly localized elbow pain. The radial head is sometimes involved. Treatment includes immobilization followed by gentle ROM.

BIBLIOGRAPHY

1. Bisschop P (ed): The Elbow. Philadelphia, W.B. Saunders, 1995.
2. D'Ambrosia: Musculoskeletal Disorders, Regional Examination and Differential Diagnosis, 2nd ed. Philadelphia, J.B. Lippincott, 1986.
3. Greenman P: Principles of Manual Medicine, 2nd ed. Baltimore, Williams & Wilkins, 1996.
4. Plancher K (ed): Compressive Neuropathies and Tendinopathies in the Athletic Elbow and Wrist. Clinics in Sports Medicine. Philadelphia, W.B. Saunders, 1996.
5. Shankar K: Functional anatomy of the upper extremities. Phys Med Rehabil State Art Rev 10:594, 1996.
6. Wilder R: The elbow. J Back Musculoskel Rehabil 12:145, 1994.
7. Windsor R, Lox D (eds): Soft Tissue Injuries: Diagnosis and Treatment. Philadelphia, Hanley & Belfus, 1998.

42. REHABILITATION OF THE ELBOW

Douglas Sheppard, M.D., Howard Choi, M.D., Matthew Shatzer, D.O., Harry Brafman, P.T., Mark A. Young, M.D., and Henk J. Stam, M.D., Ph.D.

1. What are the treatments for lateral epicondylitis?

Lateral epicondylitis, or tennis elbow, is treated by avoiding repetitive flexion-extension and pronation-supination stresses on the elbow. Physical therapy may be aimed at stretching and strengthening exercises. Nonsteroidal anti-inflammatory drugs (NSAIDs) and local steroid injections may relieve inflammation at the lateral epicondyle region. Occasionally, lateral counter-force braces offer relief. Rarely, patients require surgical intervention to remove inflammatory tissue and reattach the extensor carpi radialis brevis.

2. Explain the mechanism of the lateral epicondyle brace.

The lateral epicondyle brace essentially changes the attachment site of the radial extensors of the wrist, which takes pressure off the inflamed lateral epicondyle.

3. What are the indications for total elbow arthroplasty?

Elbow replacement is an option for any condition causing pain or loss of stability of the elbow resulting in inability to perform activities of daily living. Most commonly, it is performed on patients with rheumatoid arthritis, but it may also be used for post-traumatic arthritis or a distal humerus fracture with malunion or nonunion.

4. When is elbow arthroplasty contraindicated?

- **Absolute** contraindications—active or latent infection of the elbow, active systemic infection, elbow joint arthrodesis.
- **Relative** contraindications—soft tissue contracture about the elbow, biceps or triceps paralysis, young active patients.

5. What are the complications of an elbow replacement?

Infection, neurapraxia, triceps insufficiency, fractures, loosening, and instability.

6. Name and briefly describe the two types of elbow replacement prosthesis.

1. **Constrained.** Original, custom-designed, hinged implants. Provides immediate stability.
2. **Semiconstrained.** Allows 8–10° of varus-valgus. This allows the capsule and ligaments to transmit some forces and decrease the risk of loosening.

7. How may weight bearing be advanced following elbow replacement surgery?

Active elbow flexion and extension begin 4–5 days after surgery. Lifting greater than 1 lb for 3 months is prohibited, and the affected limb may never be used to carry more than 5 lbs.

8. What is the etiology of elbow contractures?

- **Traumatic**—extra-articular (from hemarthrosis resulting from soft tissue injury) or intra-articular (direct injury)
- **Congenital**—muscle or nerve deficiency
- **Acquired**—inflammatory process (Still's disease, septic arthritis)

9. True or False: Elbow contractures cause a great deal of functional disability.

False. Mild-moderate elbow flexion contractures occur in a functional position (i.e., the patient will still be able to feed himself).

10. How may elbow contractures be treated nonoperatively?

Proper positioning, active-assisted range of motion (ROM) exercises, static splinting, dynamic splinting, nerve blocks, and serial casting.

11. What is the most common mechanism of injury in elbow dislocation and what direction does it most commonly occur?

A dislocated elbow is commonly secondary to a fall on an outstretched arm. It is usually dislocated in a posterior direction, but it may occurly anteriorly, particularly in children.

12. What other injuries are associated with elbow dislocation?

Fractures, arterial injury, and median or ulnar nerve injury.

13. Do elbow dislocations require surgery?

No. This type of dislocation can usually be treated with a closed reduction and splinting in a flexed and pronated position.

14. When is surgical intervention of an elbow dislocation required and what follows?

Surgical intervention is necessary if soft tissue interposed in the joint or other intra-articular fractures is present. Postoperatively, the elbow is splinted in full pronation and at 90°. After 3–10 days, unprotected flexion-extension exercises are encouraged; if instability continues, a cast brace is applied. If ROM is still a problem at 6–8 weeks after surgery, flexion-extension splints are used.

15. What are the treatment options and potential complications of fractures and dislocation around the elbow?

Elbow Fractures and Dislocations (Adults)

INJURY	TREATMENT	COMPLICATIONS
Supracondylar	Undisplaced: immobilize 1–2 wks Displaced: ORIF with bone grafting Early ROM exercises	Neurovascular injury, nonunion, malunion, contracture, pain, decreased ROM
Transcondylar	ORIF if displaced	Decreased ROM
Condylar		
Lateral	Undisplaced: immobilize in supination Dispalced: ORIF	Cubitus valgus
Medial	Undisplaced: immobilize in pronation Displaced: ORIF	Cubitus varus (gunstock deformity)
Capitellar	Undisplaced: splint 2–3 wks Displaced: ORIF Comminuted: excise fragment	

Table continued on following page

Elbow Fractures and Dislocations (Adults) (Continued)

INJURY	TREATMENT	COMPLICATIONS
Olecranon	Undisplaced: immobilize 45–90° of flexion for 3 weeks	Decreased ROM, post-traumatic arthritis, ulnar nerve
Neurapraxia	Displaced: ORIF with tension band wiring Comminuted: excision, reattachment of triceps Fracture-dislocation: ORIF with intramedullary device Rehabilitation started once postoperative pain has subsided (usually after 3–7 days) Extremes of motion should be avoided Strengthening exercises delayed until union achieved (usually 8 wks)	Instability
Coronoid process	If fragment < 50%, excision with early ROM If fragment > 50%, ORIF	Instability and post-traumatic arthritis
Radial head	Undisplaced: early motion Displaced: use "rule of 3's" → 30° angulation, 3 mm of displacement, or ⅓ of radial head involved → ORIF Comminuted: excision	Posterior interosseous nerve injury
Elbow dislocation	Usually posterior dislocation; closed reduction, stabilize in a splint for 2–7 days, then gentle active ROM If irreducible: may require open reduction	Median, ulnar nerve injury Brachial artery injury Flexion contracture Heterotopic ossification

ORIF = open reduction and internal fixation.

16. When is elbow fusion indicated and what is the most appropriate position?

Fusion is indicated in cases of chronic osteomyelitis, tuberculosis, and failed total elbow arthroplasty. Positioning is as follows:

- **Unilateral fusion**—place elbow at 90°
- **Bilateral fusion**—one elbow at 110° (for feeding) and the other at 65° (personal hygiene)

17. When is elbow disarticulation indicated and what are the surgical and prosthetic advantages?

Disarticulation is indicated in trauma and neoplasm. In comparison to transhumoral amputations, pronation and supination, it is much easier to control, surgery time is shorter, and there is less blood loss. From a prosthesis standpoint, there is improved suspension with less rotation but there is some sacrifice in cosmesis due to the required external elbow mechanism.

18. What are the causes of ulnar neuropathies at the elbow?

Bony deformity (old fractures, rheumatoid arthritis, osteoarthritis, Paget's disease), trauma, external pressure, tumors or masses, ulnar nerve prolapse, fibrous bands, supracondylar spurs, and diabetes mellitus.

19. What is the goal of night splinting in ulnar neuropathy at the elbow?

Avoidance of greater than 60° of elbow flexion has been shown to improve symptoms.

20. What are the types of surgical intervention for ulnar compression at the elbow?

Decompression—splitting of the flexor carpi ulnaris aponeurosis
Transposition of the ulnar nerve anterior and medial to the epicondyle
Epicondylectomy

21. True or false: Cubital tunnel syndrome is the same thing as ulnar entrapment at the elbow.

False. Cubital tunnel syndrome refers to compression within the flexor carpi ulnaris aponeurosis.

BIBLIOGRAPHY

1. Donatelli RA, Wooden MJ: Orthopaedic Physical Therapy. New York, Churchill Livingstone, 1994.
2. Gould JA, Davies GJ (eds): Orthopaedic and Sports Physical Therapy. St. Louis, Mosby, 1985.
3. Jobe FW, Kvitne RS: Elbow instability in the athlete. In AAOS Instructional Course Lectures, vol. 40. Park Ridge, IL, American Academy of Orthopaedic Surgeons, 1991, p 17.
4. Jobe FW, Nuber G: Throwing injuries of the elbow. Clin Sports Med 5:621, 1986.

43. THE WRIST AND HAND: ANATOMY, PATHOLOGY, AND DIAGNOSIS

Francisco H. Santiago, M.D., and Jaywant J. P. Patil, MBBS, FRCPC

1. Name the carpal bones.

A "handy" mnemonic is "scared lovers try positions that they cannot handle."

S = Scaphoid   T = Trapezium
L = Lunate   T = Trapezoid
T = Triquetrum   C = Capitate
P = Pisiform   H = Hamate

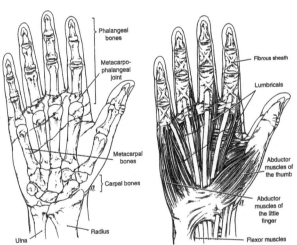

From Klag M, et al: Johns Hopkins Family Health Book. New York, Harper Collins Publishers, 1999, with permission.

2. Describe the key actions of the interossei muscles.

Remember **dab** and **pad**:

Dab = **D**orsal interossei—**ab**duct and assist in metacarpophalangeal (MCP) flexion
Pad = **P**almar interossei—**ad**duct and assist in MCP flexion

3. What structures are found in the dorsum of the hand?

The **extensor tendons** of the hand are divided into six dorsal compartments. From radial to ulnar, they are:

1. Abductor pollicis longus, extensor pollicis brevis
2. Extensor carpi radialis longus, extensor carpi radialis brevis
3. Extensor pollicis longus
4. Extensor digitorum communis, extensor indices proprius
5. Extensor digiti minimi
6. Extensor carpi ulnaris

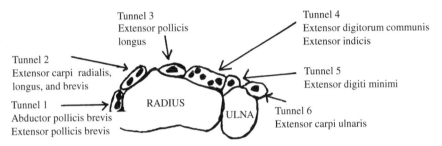

The extensor tunnels on the dorsum of the wrist. (From Emel TJ: Wrist and forearm problems. In Mellion MB (ed): Sports Medicine Secrets. Philadelphia, Hanley & Belfus, 1994, pp 256–260, with permission.)

4. What are the borders of the anatomic snuff box?

Floor: scaphoid bone
Radial border: abductor pollicis longus and extensor pollicis brevis
Ulnar border: extensor pollicis longus

5. Where is "no man's land" in the hand?

This is the area of the hand where the flexor tendons (i.e., the flexor profundus and sublimis) are tightly enclosed within the tenosynovium. It is located in the palm between the distal palmar crease and the crease of the proximal interphalangeal (PIP) joints. Generally, primary repair of the tendons in this region is contraindicated.

6. Explain how lumbrical muscle function is related to its anatomy.

Because the lumbrical muscles originate from the tendons of the flexor digitorum profundus and insert into the extensor hood tendons, their main action is flexion of the MCP joints and extension at the interphalangeal joints.

7. How do you test the flexor digitorum profundus muscle?

Ask the patient to bend the distal interphalangeal (DIP) joint while you stabilize the PIP joint in extension.

8. How do you test the integrity of the flexor digitorum superficialis tendon?

With the superficialis test. The flexor digitorum superficialis flexes the PIP joint. While the examiner holds the adjacent fingers in full extension, the patient flexes the finger. If there is no injury or tear in the flexor digitorum superficialis tendon, the patient is able to flex the PIP joint, but the DIP joint remains in extension or neutral.

9. How can you test the integrity of the flexor digitorum profundus tendon to one particular finger?

By the profundus test. The MCP and PIP joints are held in extension by the examiner, and the patient flexes the DIP joints. If the patient can do this, then the long flexor, or the profundus tendon, to that finger is intact.

10. What does the absence of an okay sign mean?

Absence of flexion of the interphalangeal joint of the thumb and the DIP joint of the index finger, and therefore inability to make an okay sign, may signal a deficit in the anterior interosseous innervated muscles of the median nerve.

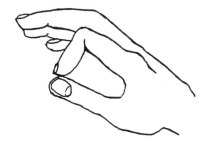

Abnormal OK sign. The patient cannot flex the interphalangeal joint of the thumb. (From Emel TJ: Wrist and forearm problems. In Mellion MB (ed): Sports Medicine Secrets. Philadelphia, Hanley & Belfus, 1994, pp 256–260, with permission.)

11. How is the Finkelstein's test done?

With the patient's thumb flexed into the palm of the hand while the fingers are "fisted" over the thumb, the examiner twists the wrist inward (ulnar deviation). This maneuver maximizes tension on the abductor pollicis longus and extensor pollicis brevis tendon. In deQuervain's disease (stenosing tenosynovitis), pain is reproduced over the radial wrist.

12. What is the Froment's sign?

Although the adductor pollicis is paralyzed in ulnar nerve lesions, the movements of palmar and ulnar adduction can still be performed. Grasping an object such as a piece of paper between the thumb and the edge of the palm is accomplished by flexing the thumb at the interphalangeal joint by means of the flexor pollicis longus, supplied by the median nerve. This is described as a positive Froment's sign.

13. Name the two different types of grips in the hand.

1. **Prehension**, which includes pinch, tip, and lateral grip
2. **Power**, which includes hook, grasp, and palmar grip

14. Describe the Bunnell-Littler test.

This test reviews the tightness of the intrinsic muscles of the hand (lumbricals and the interossei). To test the tightness of the intrinsic muscles, hold the MCP joint in a few degrees of extension and try to move the PIP joint into flexion. If the PIP can be flexed in this position, then the intrinsics are not tight. If the PIP joint cannot be flexed, either the intrinsics are tight or there are joint capsule contractures.

15. Define deQuervain's disease.

Tenosynovitis of the extensor pollicis brevis and abductor pollicis longus tendons can result from direct injury or repetitive activity and may be associated with arthritis. Thickening of the tendon sheath often results in stenosis of the tenosynovium and inflammation. Pinching, gripping, and wrist and thumb movements are associated with pain, and there is tenderness over the tendon on the radial side of the wrist. The patient's symptoms often can be reproduced by the Finkelstein's test. There may also be swelling over the involved tendon on the radial side of the wrist.

16. What is a trigger finger?

Trigger finger occurs secondary to tenosynovitis involving the flexor tendon sheaths. The usual presentation is a fusiform swelling around the area of the flexor sublimis tendon in the vicinity of the metacarpal head. A constriction of the tendon sheath results in locking or obstruction of finger flexion.

Finger locking often occurs in the morning. At times, a popping sensation is perceived when the fingers go from the flexed to the extended position. This type of trigger finger could be associated with trauma, osteoarthritis, or inflammatory arthritis, such as rheumatoid arthritis.

17. Name the three common deformities associated with rheumatoid arthritis in the hands. Describe the mechanism of the deformities.

1. **Boutonnière deformity.** There is hyperextension at the MCP joint, flexion at the PIP joint, and extension at the DIP joint. Often in the rheumatoid process, there is weakness and tearing of the terminal portion of the extensor's hood, which tends to hold the lateral band in place. In this deformity, the lateral bands tend to slip down and flex the PIP joint and exert tension to hyperextend the DIP joint.

2. **Swan-neck deformity.** This often occurs as a result of contractures and shortening of the intrinsic muscles causing flexion at the MCP joint, hyperextension at the PIP joint, and flexion at the DIP joint. Contractures and spasm of the intrinsic muscles cause dorsal subluxation of the tendons, resulting in hyperextension of the PIP joint. This hyperextension is further aggravated by synovitis that causes laxity of that joint. Flexion and tension on the long flexor result in flexion of the DIP joint.

3. **Ulnar deviation of the fingers.** This deformity is often associated with ulnar deviation of the wrist. Basically, the flexor tendons enter the tunnel of the flexor pulley. In rheumatoid arthritis, the mouth of the tunnel becomes more relaxed, and this results in the flexor tendons' deviating more toward the ulnar side.

18. Where are Heberden's nodes usually found?

These discrete but palpable bony nodules are found on the dorsal and lateral surfaces of the DIP joint and may be features of osteoarthritis. The nodules found in the PIP joint are called Bouchard's nodes.

19. What happens to the flexor pollicis longus in rheumatoid arthritis?

Usually, the flexor tendon ruptures as it rubs over an osteophyte on the volar aspect of the scaphoid trapezial joint.

20. How does a mallet finger occur?

This injury, also called baseball finger or cricket finger, occurs when the extensor tendon is under tension and a sudden unexpected passive flexion of the DIP joint avulses a fragment of the bone from the base of the distal phalanx into which the tendon is inserted. Alternatively, the extensor tendon may rupture just proximal to its insertion. In either case, the DIP joint remains flexed and can no longer be actively extended. Treatment usually involves splinting the finger with the DIP extended.

21. What is a boxer's fracture?

This injury is more appropriately considered a street fighter's fracture, because it results from an unskillful blow with a clenched fist. It fractures the neck of the fifth metacarpal bone.

22. Describe a Bennett's fracture.

In adults, a longitudinal force along the axis of the first metacarpal in the flexed thumb may produce a serious intra-articular fracture-dislocation of the carpometacarpal joint. A small triangular-shaped fragment at the base of the metacarpal remains in proper relationship to the trapezium, but the remainder of the metacarpal, which carries with it the major portion of the joint surface, is dislocated and assumes a position of flexion.

23. Who usually gets a scaphoid fracture?

Fracture of the carpal scaphoid is relatively common in young adults, particularly males. The responsible injury is usually a fall on the open hand, with the wrist dorsiflexed and radially deviated. This fracture is frequently overlooked at the time of injury and is usually dismissed as a sprain. Scaphoid fracture can be associated with serious complications, including avascular necrosis, delayed union, nonunion, and post-traumatic degenerative joint disease.

24. Who gets Kienböck's disease?
Osteochondrosis or avascular necrosis of the lunate occurs most frequently in young adults and may be secondary to trauma. Workers such as carpenters and riveters are often affected.

25. How could a gamekeeper and a skier possibly develop the same sort of thumb injury?
Both gamekeeper's thumb and skier's thumb are caused by forcible abduction of the thumb associated with injury to the ulnar collateral ligament of the first MCP. Gamekeeper's thumb earned its name from British gamekeepers who sustained this injury when shooting rabbits. A skier who falls is at risk for an injury through a similar mechanism.

26. What is bowler's thumb?
Traumatic neuropathy of the thumb's digital nerve can be caused by repeated friction or compression by the edge of the thumb-hole in the bowling ball. The digital nerve also can be compressed in racquet sports or by direct injury from playing handball.

BIBLIOGRAPHY

1. Cailliet R: Neck and Arm Pain, 3rd ed. Philadelphia, F.A. Davis, 1991.
2. Cailliet R: Hand Pain and Impairment. Philadelphia, F.A. Davis, 1995.
3. Hoppenfeld S: Physical Exam of the Spine and Extremities. Norwalk, CT, Appleton & Lange, 1999.
4. Hunter JM, Mackin EJ, Callahan AD: Rehabilitation of the Hand: Surgery and Therapy, 3rd ed. St. Louis, Mosby, 1994.
5. Skinner H: Current Diagnosis and Treatment in Orthopedics. Norwalk, CT, Appleton & Lange, 1995, pp 453–511.

44. REHABILITATION OF WRIST AND HAND DISORDERS

Richard A. Rogachefsky, M.D., and Barry D. Stein, M.D.

1. What are the goals of hand and wrist therapy?

Prevent and decrease edema

Assist tissue healing

Pain relief

Relaxation

Prevent overuse/misuse/disuse of muscles and tendons

Avoid joint injury

Skin or scar desensitization

Sensation reduction

Redevelop sensory and motor functions

2. Explain primary and secondary repair. Why is this important for rehabilitation?
Primary repair is surgical repair within 10 days of injury, especially within 12–24 hours. Surgery on days 2–10 after injury is delayed primary repair. Secondary surgical repair occurs 10–14 days after injury. After 4 weeks, it is late secondary repair. Early, primary repair usually means less fibrous tissue, and fewer contractures and other complications.

3. Describe the primary repair and rehabilitation of the flexor tendons of the fingers.
Early passive range of motion (ROM) activities reduce the risk of excessive stress and is the only motion allowed for 3–4 weeks. Active finger flexion follows.

4. What are the two most frequent causes for failure of primary repairs of tendons?
Formation of adhesions and rupture of repaired tendons.

5. What is an early motion protocol for flexor finger injuries?

It is a method to regain ROM and strength. Passive motion starts 1–3 days after surgery of the digits and 1–2 weeks at the base of hand and wrist, combined with passive splinting. Active ROM begins in 3–5 weeks, resistant exercises around 8 weeks, and full lifting and activities at 10–12 weeks. ROM plateauing may occur in 6–8 weeks, with maximal ROM in 12–14 weeks.

6. What is a delayed mobilization program and when is it appropriate?

Delayed mobilization is avoidance of ROM for 3 weeks. It allows more healing to occur before early stresses that the patient may not properly control. It is appropriate for:
- Significant crush injuries (primary repair may not be anatomically accurate because of crushing or bursting)
- Sufficient soft tissue
- Young children who cannot comply with an early motion protocol
- Those with impaired intelligence or psychiatric problems who cannot comply

7. Why do many patients have difficulty flexing the fingers after repair of severe distal radius fractures?

Difficulty is caused by trauma from the injury, muscle atrophy, and weakness. Weak contraction of the finger forearm muscles results in decreased pull through of the fingers and poor flexion. Aggressive active, active assisted, and passive ROM, electrical stimulation of the extrinsic finger flexor musculature, and biofeedback are beneficial.

8. A patient has his long finger surgically amputated through the middle phalanx. When he tries to make a fist, the finger stump goes into extension at the proximal interphalangeal (PIP) joint. What is this called?

This lumbrical plus deformity is due to laxity in the retracted flexor digitorum profundus (FDP) tendon. The lumbrical muscle originates at the FDP and inserts at the extensor hood. When the FDP tendon contracts, it pulls on the lumbrical muscle, which pulls on the extensor hood of the finger causing the finger to go into extension at the PIP joint. Treatment is surgical release of the lumbrical muscle from the FDP tendon.

9. Postoperative rehabilitation is made easier when what law is followed for tendon transfer surgery?

The law of synergy. Muscle-tendon donors that normally contract with the deficient muscle require minimal retraining. For example, the flexor carpi radialis (wrist flexor) muscle can be used as a donor for the extensor digitorum communis (deficient finger extension). Normally, the flexor carpi radialis contracts during finger extension, placing increasing resting tension on the finger extensor muscles augmenting finger extension.

10. What is the Kleinert rehabilitation (dynamic extensor assist) protocol after extensor tendon repair?

Active flexion to 45° at metacarpophalangeal (MCP) joints and dynamic extension of the fingers through the pull of rubber bands allow protected gliding of the extensor tendon repair without excessive stress, risking rupture. This protocol increases tendon gliding and decreases adherence of the repair in the scar limiting motion.

11. What is short arc motion protocol after central slip extensor tendon injury?

The central slip is part of the finger extensor tendon over the PIP joint and inserts at the base of the middle phalanx. The patient is placed in a volar static splint and allowed active motion from 0° to 30° for 2 weeks and full active ROM at the MCP and distal interphalangeal (DIP) joints. At 2 weeks, increased flexion of 10° per week is done. At 4 weeks, full active flexion is instituted.

12. What is the intrinsic tightness test and in what situations can it be demonstrated?

The intrinsic tightness test involves extending the MCP joints and flexing the PIP joints. The PIP joints will not flex in a positive test. This is indicative of tight intrinsic muscles such as found with Volkmann's contracture of the hand from a hand compartment syndrome.

13. After burns to the hand, how should the hands be splinted to decrease the chance of contractures?

The hand is splinted with the fingers in extension at the PIP and DIP joints, placing the collateral ligaments at maximum stretch and preventing PIP joint flexion contracture. The MCP joints should be in 90° of flexion, which keeps the collateral ligaments at maximum stretch (preventing shortening of the ligaments), PIP and DIP in full extension, and thumb in palmar abduction.

14. What is the most common reason patients develop reflex sympathetic dystrophy after placement of an external fixator for treatment of a distal radius fracture and how is it treated?

When the external fixator is applied and left on with excessive distraction across the wrist, increased tension is placed across the median nerve. Resulting nerve irritation or compression may lead to reflex sympathetic dystrophy. Initial treatment is to release traction of the external fixator. If dystrophy persists, medical treatments for reflex sympathetic dystrophy may start. Rehabilitation modalities including active, active assisted, or passive ROM exercises, desensitization, and splinting to prevent contractures.

15. What is the postoperative rehabilitation protocol for a volar plate arthroplasty for a patient with a proximal interphalangeal fracture dislocation with dorsal displacement of the middle phalanx?

For the first 3 weeks, a pin across the PIP joint maintains the reduction. A splint is used for 3 weeks, but DIP and MP motion may be done. At 3 weeks, the pin is removed, and active and passive ROM of the PIP joint begins. If by 5 weeks full extension is not obtained, an extension splint or extensor assist splint is used.

16. What is a mallet injury, its repair, and rehabilitation?

A mallet injury is an avulsion of the extensor tendon to the distal phalanx. The bone may also be avulsed, sometimes involving the DIP. The resulting unopposed flexion of the DIP joint is a "mallet finger." Treatment is splinting the DIP in extension for 6–8 weeks. Surgical pinning may be required. Then, a 3–4-week DIP flexion program starts with nighttime splinting. A chronic mallet injury is one that does not respond to splinting, or is present more than 3–6 months. Further splinting or surgical correction depends on pain and cosmetic appearance. If an avulsion fracture involves more than half of the DIP articular surface and the joint is subluxed, many surgeons will perform open reduction with pin fixation.

17. How is deQuervain's tenosynovitis treated, what mimics it, and how is it treated?

deQuervain's tenosynovitis is an inflammatory stenosing of the first dorsal compartment at the wrist. The tendons are the abductor pollicis longus (APL) and the extensor pollicis brevis (EPB). Commonly noted in women ages 30–50, it presents as pain at the radial aspect of the wrist that worsens with thumb motion. In the Finkelstein's test, the patient flexes the thumb into the palm, and makes a fist around the thumb. The wrist is then bent in ulnar deviation. Duplication of the patient's complaint is a positive test for deQuervain's tenosynovitis. Conditions that mimic this condition include arthritis of the thumb carpometacarpal (CMC) joint (a positive grind test and x-rays will diagnose arthritis), intersection syndrome, a scaphoid fracture, and arthritis of the carpal joints or radiocarpal joints.

Conservative management includes a thumb spica splint, corticosteroid injection, nonsteroidal anti-inflammatory drugs (NSAIDs), activity modification, therapeutic modalities (Coban wrap for edema, ice massage over the radial styloid, phonophoresis with 10% hydrocortisone), and gentle passive and active ROM. If surgical decompression is required, IP joint motion starts immediately after surgery. At dressing removal, gentle active ROM of the IP joint and wrist begins. The presurgical spica splint may be worn for 2 weeks. Postoperative hypersensitivity sometimes occurs at the distal thumb. If sufficiently irritating, desensitization may be needed.

18. What is the difference in rehabilitation for open release versus endoscopic release for Carpal tunnel syndrome?

The smaller amount of tissue cutting in endoscopic release results in faster recovery. Postsurgical dressing may last 2 days instead of 7 with open surgery. Similarly, tolerance of daily activities may be attempted within days, instead of 2–3 weeks, and patients can return to work in approximately 14 days. Open release surgery includes postoperative scar remodeling with elastomer or silicon gel, deep scar massage, and possible scar desensitization, which are not major issues in endoscopic release. However, sometimes recovery for endoscopic release is delayed. Pillar tenderness (pain over the divided radial and ulnar portions of the transverse carpal ligament) may occur with either procedure and can delay return to heavy work activities for 6–10 weeks.

19. What is the goal of splinting in median nerve palsies?

Lesions of the median nerve result in decreased opposition and adduction. There is less sensory input from the thumb, index, middle, and ring fingers. A splint is aimed at reducing the chance of first web contractures and maintaining passive motion of the thumb CMC joint.

20. What is the goal of splinting in ulnar nerve palsies?

Lesions of the ulnar nerve result in decreased pinch and grip strength and thumb stability. Clawing of the ring and little fingers is common. Splinting of the hand prevents clawing while allowing full digital flexion and IP extension.

21. What is the goal of splinting in radial nerve palsies?

Lesions of the radial nerve result in loss of active extension of the wrist, thumb, and fingers, thumb abduction weakness, and decreased grip strength. Splinting provides wrist stability and maintains thumb position.

22. What clinical situation is best suited for consideration of thumb CMC joint arthroplasty?

Arthroplasty is best for patients in whom the joint has a low demand, typically in those with rheumatoid arthritis. Implants have a 25% failure rate, so nonsurgical treatments should be exhausted first.

BIBLIOGRAPHY

1. Calandruccio JH, Jobe MT, Akin K: Rehabilitation of the hand and wrist. In Brotzman SB (ed): Handbook of Orthopaedic Rehabilitation. St. Louis, Mosby, 1996.
2. Derebery VJ, Kasdan ML (eds): Injuries and Rehabilitation of the Upper Extremity. Physical Medicine and Rehabilitation: State of the Art Reviews. Vol. 12, no. 2. Philadelphia, Hanley & Belfus, 1998.
3. Evans R: Early active short arc motion for repaired central slip. J Hand Surg 19A:991–997, 1994.
4. Hunter JH, Mackin EJ, Callahan AD (eds): Rehabilitation of the Hand: Surgery and Therapy, 4th ed. St. Louis, Mosby, 1994.
5. Katarincic JA: Fractures of the wrist and hand. Phys Med Rehabil State Art Rev 12:263–282, 1998.
6. Schutt A, Bengston KA: Hand rehabilitation. In DeLisa JA (ed): Rehabilitation Medicine: Principles and Practice, 3rd ed. Philadelphia, Lippincott Williams & Wilkins, 1998, pp 1717–1732.

45. THE HIP: ANATOMY, PATHOLOGY, AND DIAGNOSIS

Howard Choi, M.D., David Fish, M.D., Mark A. Young, M.D., and Peter Disler, Ph.D., MBBCh

1. Why is the hip joint so stable?

It is a multiaxial ball-and-socket joint comprising a femoral and acetabular component. The femoral head forms about two-thirds of a sphere and inserts deeply into the acetabulum, which is about half a sphere. The fibrocartilaginous labrum of the acetabulum contributes to the depth of the "socket." A tough joint capsule surrounds the articulating surfaces and provides further stability. Muscles play less of a role in providing joint stability at the hip than they do at other joints.

2. What is the price of this joint stability?

The hip joint has a high degree of stability at the expense of some movement. In contrast, the glenohumeral joint has greater freedom of movement but less stability.

3. What are the named ligaments of the capsule of the hip joint?

The three named ligaments (or thickenings) of the capsule are the **iliofemoral** (Y-ligament of Bigelow), which is considered the strongest ligament in the body, the **ischiofemoral**, and the **pubofemoral** ligaments.

4. In which direction is the hip most likely to dislocate?

Posterior. The patient typically presents in severe pain with a hip fixed in adduction, flexion, and internal rotation. It is associated with sciatic nerve injury in 8–20% of cases. Evaluation should include testing of toe and ankle movement and sensory exam of the foot.

5. What about anterior dislocations?

Anterior dislocations present as painful hips that are fixed in abduction, flexion, and external rotation. There may be an associated femoral nerve injury.

6. What is the innervation and blood supply to the hip joint? Why is this clinically important?

The hip joint is supplied by multiple nerves, including the femoral nerve, obturator nerve, superior gluteal nerve, and the nerve to the quadratus femoris. Pain in the true hip joint frequently refers to the groin and other sensory distributions of these nerves. Blood supply to the head of the femur comes from the branch of the obturator artery that passes through the ligament of the head of the femur as well as from multiple branches that pierce the capsule, originating from the femoral circumflex arteries, superior gluteal artery, and obturator artery. These arteries are often damaged during fracture, making healing difficult.

7. What is Legg-Calvé-Perthes disease?

Avascular necrosis of the femoral head. It usually occurs in children aged 5–12 years and may be due to interruption of the vascular supply of the hip leading to ischemic necrosis.

8. What are the most common known causes of avascular necrosis of the hip in adults?

Alcohol abuse and systemic steroid use.

9. Why and how is the Thomas test performed?

The Thomas test is performed to assess flexion contracture of the hip. The patient lies supine on the examining table. To test the right hip, the left hip and knee are maximally flexed. A positive result or (flexion contracture) is present if the right thigh elevates above the table passively. If the right thigh is pushed down to the table and excessive passive lordosis of the spine occurs, this is also positive.

10. What is the FABER test?

FABER stands for **f**lexion, **ab**duction, **e**xternal **r**otation. This nonspecific test (also known as the Patrick test) helps detect pathology in the hip and sacroiliac (SI) joint. The patient is in the supine position and the foot of the tested side is placed on the knee of the opposite side. The tested hip is then lowered to a flexed, abducted, and externally rotated position (the "frog leg" position). Inguinal pain is suggestive of hip pathology. Increased pain elicited by increasing the ROM by placing pressure on the opposite anterior superior iliac spine suggests SI joint pathology.

11. Why and how is the Ober test performed?

The Ober test is used to evaluate contracture of the tensor fasciae latae (TFL) and iliotibial band. The patient lies on his or her side with the lower leg flexed at the hip and knee for stability. The examiner flexes and abducts then extends the patient's upper leg with the knee flexed to 90°. The examiner then releases the upper leg. If a contracture is present, the upper leg will remain abducted and will not fall to the table.

12. What is Ely's test?

Ely's test assesses tightness of the rectus femoris, which is the only quadriceps muscle that crosses both the hip and knee joints. The patient is placed prone on a flat surface, and the examiner flexes the knee. Flexion of the ipsilateral hip suggests rectus femoris tightness.

13. What changes in the physical exam are noted in hip osteoarthritis?

The typical first sign is loss of internal rotation, followed by loss of flexion and extension, and eventually contracture. An antalgic gait and abductor lurch (swaying of the trunk over the side of the affected hip) also may be noted.

14. Why should a patient with unilateral hip osteoarthritis carry a cane on the unaffected side?

It decreases pelvic drop on the side of the cane. This decreases the load on the affected hip and the amount of work the gluteus medius-minimus complex has to accomplish. (A cane on the ipsilateral side does not effectively reduce either of these.) This is consistent with a normal physiologic gait because the upper limb will be moving in concert with the opposite and advancing lower limb.

15. What are common causes of a "snapping hip"?

Snapping in and around the hip (coxa saltans) is sometimes felt when ligamentous structures about the hip travel over bony prominences during movement of the joint. The most common cause is a tight iliotibial band or gluteus maximus tendon riding over the greater tuberosity of the femur. This may happen during hip flexion or extension and is worsened if the hip is held in internal rotation or in the setting of trochanteric bursitis. Other sources of coxa saltans include the iliofemoral ligament riding over the femoral head, or the iliopsoas tendon snapping over the pectineal eminence of the pelvis, over an osseus ridge of the lesser trochanter, or over the anterior acetabulum. Snapping hips also can be associated with intra-articular pathology, including acetabular labral tears or loose bodies. With intra-articular pathology, pain is localized to the groin and anterior thigh when pivoting movements occur. Clicking is felt and heard in hip extension and adduction with lateral rotation.

16. Discuss the symptoms and treatment of trochanteric bursitis.

Classic symptoms include gradual onset pain in the bursa region, pain upon arising in the morning, aggravation of pain during ambulation, and an antalgic gait. Pain can radiate down the lateral aspect of the leg and into the buttock. Thus, the syndrome is sometimes confused with sciatica. Physical exam will reveal point tenderness over the greater trochanter, which can be exacerbated by external rotation and abduction of the hip. Conservative treatment includes anti-inflammatories and an iliotibial band stretching program. Injection of local anesthetic and corticosteroids into the bursa may relieve symptoms.

17. What is a hip pointer? In which sports do they most commonly occur?
A hip pointer is caused by a fall directly on the iliac crest. There will be a contusion of the crest with a subperiosteal hematoma. It commonly occurs in football, basketball, gymnastics, and volleyball.

18. What is SCFE?
A slipped capital femoral epiphysis is typically seen in overweight adolescents, more commonly in males. Hormonal effects on epiphyseal plate development have been suggested as an etiologic factor. Onset is often insidious. There may be some initial hip stiffness, which is followed by a limp and then hip pain. The affected leg may become externally rotated. A true leg-length discrepancy may be noted. In later stages, blood supply to the head of the femur may be compromised and avascular necrosis may result. Anteroposterior (AP) and lateral "frog-leg" x-rays may show widening of the epiphyseal line or displacement of the femoral head. Orthopedic consultation is critical because SCFE is typically progressive, and surgical correction is often warranted.

19. Name the most common cause of a painful hip in children under 10 years of age.
Acute transient synovitis, which is usually nonspecific and self-limited.

20. What is the most common pediatric tumor involving the hip?
Osteogenic sarcoma.

21. A patient presents with a history and physical exam consistent with a hip fracture, yet plain radiographs are negative. What next?
Magnetic resonance imaging (MRI) may demonstrate acute occult hip fractures missed on plain radiographs.

22. What is the Garden classification of fractures?

Garden Classification of Femoral Neck Fractures

GRADE	DESCRIPTION
I	Incomplete or impacted fracture Trabeculae of the inferior neck are still intact
II	Complete fracture without displacement Fracture lines across entire femoral neck Slight varus deformity Displacement will occur unless internally fixed
III	Complete fracture with partial displacement Needs a reduction Shortening and external rotation of distal fragment often occurs Incomplete displacement between femoral fragments
IV	Complete fractured with total displacement No continuity between proximal and distal fragments Acetabulum and the femoral head are aligned

Adapted from Wheeless CR: Wheeless' Textbook of Orthopaedics. 1996.

23. What are treatment options for femoral neck fractures?
For patients under age 65, fractures that are impacted, nondisplaced, or adequately reduced should be fixed internally with screws or pins. For patients over 65, a fixed unipolar or bipolar endoprosthesis may be used when satisfactory reduction and fixation cannot be achieved.

Endoprosthesis is favored if rheumatoid, degenerative, or malignant disease has caused preexisting articular damage.

24. What is an intertrochanteric fracture?

An intertrochanteric fracture occurs between the greater and lesser trochanters along the intertrochanteric line and outside the hip joint capsule. Treatment of choice is a sliding hip screw.

25. What are some significant complications after total hip replacement and how often do they occur?

The most common complication is usually thromboembolic disease, including deep venous thrombosis and pulmonary embolism (PE). PEs are the leading cause of death after hip replacement. Aside from death, the most significant long-term complication is aseptic loosening of the prosthesis (either the femoral or acetabular component). Heterotopic ossification can occur in up to 50% of cases, but only a small percentage will experience loss of motion.

26. How does loosening of the hip prosthesis present? How is it usually detected?

Loosening at the cement–bone or cement–prosthesis interface presents with new onset of thigh or groin pain that worsens during transfers and early ambulation. Plain x-rays may pick up a bone cement lucency > 2 mm wide.

27. What is meralgia paresthetica and how does it present? What are some causes?

Pathology of the lateral femoral cutaneous nerve is commonly called meralgia paresthetica. Patients complain of pain, burning, or hypoesthesia over the anterolateral thigh. Common causes include entrapment under the inguinal ligament, surgical injury, acute blunt injury, and external pressure from belts or clothing. Pregnancy may worsen symptoms by changing the angle between the nerve and the inguinal ligament. Less common causes include hematomas and tumors.

BIBLIOGRAPHY

1. Allen WC: Coxa saltans: The snapping hip revisited. J Am Acad Orthop Surg 3:303–308, 1995.
2. Hoppenfeld S: Physical Examination of the Spine and Extremities. Norwalk, CT, Appleton & Lange, 1976.
3. Hoppenfeld S: Treatment and Rehabilitation of Fractures. Philadelphia, Lippincott Williams & Wilkins, 2000.
4. Magee D: Orthopedic Physical Assessment. Philadelphia, W.B. Saunders, 1997.

46. REHABILITATION OF HIP DISORDERS

Gracia Etienne, M.D., Ph.D., Amar D. Rajadhyaksha, M.D., Harpal Khanuja, M.D., and Michael A. Mont, M.D.

1. Define weight bearing.

Body weight supported through the affected limb is measured by placing the limb on a weight scale and applying force on the scale.

None	0% of body weight
Toe-touch weight bearing	Up to 20% of body weight
Partial weight bearing	20–50% of body weight
Weight bearing as tolerated	50–100% of body weight
Full weight bearing	100% of body weight

2. What is the difference between total hip arthroplasty (THA) and hemiarthroplasty?

A THA resurfaces the femoral head and neck and acetabulum. A hemiarthroplasty replaces the femoral head and neck only.

3. What are the indications for hip arthroplasty?

The goal of hip arthroplasty is to relieve pain, correct deformity, and restore range of motion (ROM) and function. Indications include severe degenerative changes and failure of nonoperative treatment for 3–6 months. Occasionally, THA is chosen when a fracture of the femoral head or neck cannot be repaired or repair has little chance for clinical success (e.g., an 80-year-old with a severely displaced femoral neck fracture).

4. What causes of osteoarthritis in the hip may lead to a THA?

Idiopathic primary osteoarthritis	Developmental dysplasia of the hip
Slipped capital femoral epiphysis	Osteonecrosis (avascular necrosis [AVN])
History of trauma leading to joint incongruity	Other inflammatory arthritides
Rheumatoid arthritis	

5. What nonsurgical modalities are used in management of noninfectious arthritis of the hip?

Many patients respond to a conservative program consisting of weight loss, assistive devices for ambulation, and gentle ROM or strengthening exercises. Pharmacologic agents such as non-steroidal anti-inflammatory drugs (NSAIDs), corticosteroids, glucosamine supplements, and viscosupplements can be used.

6. How many hip arthroplasty procedures are performed in the United States annually?

Approximately 300,000 each year.

7. How successful are these operations?

One year after surgery, approximately 95% of patients can expect minimal to no pain, ability to walk more than 1 mile, increased hip ROM, increased independence with daily activities, satisfaction with the procedure, and good to excellent clinical results at 6–10 years after the procedure.

8. How are the components fixed to bone?

They can be cemented with polymethylmethacrylate or fixed with press-fit or biological ingrowth prostheses. In a press-fit prosthesis, the component is placed in direct contact with the bone. It is finely machined for an exact fit. In biologic ingrowth prostheses, components have a porous or meshed surface that allows bone to grow into the interstices, achieving true biologic fixation.

9. How does mode of fixation affect rehabilitation?

Patients with cemented prostheses are capable of bearing full weight immediately after surgery because the cement reaches 90% of its strength 10–15 minutes after mixing. Patients with a porous ingrowth prosthesis should be on protected weight bearing up to 12 weeks.

10. Why should physiatrists be aware of the surgical approach used in a hip arthroplasty?

Because muscle groups should be targeted according to approach. The lateral approach involves splitting the hip abductors (gluteus medius and minimus) with repair back to the greater trochanter or trochanteric osteotomy with repair of the osteotomy. The hip abductors should be a target of strengthening. The posterior approach involves splitting the gluteus maximus and releasing the short external rotators, which are repaired. The hip extenders and the short external rotators are targeted.

11. How long will patients have significant pain after hip surgery?

Arthritis pain is typically eliminated immediately. Surgical pain can last 2–3 weeks. Pain may be elicited by activities and ambulation for several months depending on various factors, such as preoperative deformity and degree of muscle atrophy. It may take months to rebuild muscle mass and strength to reduce activity-related pain.

12. Can patients return to playing sports after hip replacement surgery?

Most patients can return to low-impact sports (e.g., golf, doubles tennis, bowling, walking, and using exercise machines). High-impact exercises (running, singles tennis, basketball, volleyball, and football) should be avoided, because they may lead to excessive wear of the prosthesis.

13. What are some of the risk factors associated with a dislocated total hip arthroplasty?

1. **Component design**—primarily head-neck ratio
2. **Component alignment**—the femoral stem should be in about 10–15° of anteversion. On the acetabulum (socket), the anteversion of the cup should be 15-20°, and the lateral opening 35–45°.
3. **Soft-tissue tensioning**—the major key is the abductor complex
4. **Soft-tissue function**
5. **Patient factors**—such as alcoholism and noncompliance

14. What is the most common cause for failure in a patient with total hip arthroplasty?

Loosening. There is a 5–30% rate at 10 years. Young, very active, and obese patients are at high risk.

15. When will the patient receive full benefit after hip arthroplasty?

Typically by 3 months, the patient will have regained most of his or her strength across the joint and ROM. By 1 year, the patient usually will have achieved full benefit from the operation.

16. Describe a general management approach in a patient with total hip arthroplasty.

SCHEDULE	MANAGEMENT
Day of surgery	Deep breathing exercises, incentive spirometry, active ankle ROM exercises
Postop day 1	Quadriceps isometric exercises, gluteus muscle isometrics (depending on surgical approach), maintain hips in abduction, active assisted and knee flexion exercises as tolerated
Postop day 2–6 Cemented THA Bony ingrowth THA Trochanteric osteotomy	Begin ambulation with a walker or crutches, progressive gait training WBAT Toe-touch weight bearing for 6 wks; advance to weight bearing as tolerated If secure reattachment, start WBAT; if tenuous, partial weight bearing Instruct on hip precautions, energy conservation, and work simplification techniques Active assisted exercise; progress to active ROM motion and strengthening exercises Teach adaptive ADLs
Postop 7–3 months	Progressive strengthening and ranging of the trunk, hip, and knee Closed kinetic chain exercises Improve endurance and gait pattern Eliminate the use of assistive devices Pool therapy, bicycling, long-distance walking, progressive stair climbing, and isotonic exercises with weights are encouraged
Postop month 3	Follow-up visit Focus on level and location of pain, daily walking distance, sitting or standing duration, use of assistive devices, stair climbing method, analgesics, and community reintegration

ROM = range of motion; WBAT = weight bearing as tolerated; ADLs = activities of daily living.

17. How long should a patient maintain total hip precautions?

12 weeks. This allows for a pseudocapsule to form and soft tissue to heal. Incidence of dislocation is reduced by greater than 95% after 12 weeks.

18. How should a patient negotiate stairs after hip surgery?

"Up with the good and down with the bad." When going up stairs, the patient should lead with the nonoperative extremity and follow with crutches and operative extremity. When descending, he or she should lead with crutches and the operative extremity and follow with the nonoperative extremity.

19. What are the most common causes of falls after hip surgery?

Decreased visual acuity and balance sensation in the elderly population. Accident prevention tips should be stressed. An in-home visit for safety should be considered. Throw rugs, thick carpets, and poor lighting may cause stumbling and should be avoided. All rooms must be well-lit. The path from the bed to the bathroom is especially important, because many falls occur when trying to get to the bathroom at night.

20. Do patients need prophylaxis for deep venous thrombosis (DVT) after hip replacement?

The incidence of DVT after hip surgery is greater than 50% in most reports. It is standard to give some form of prophylaxis, which can include mechanical adjuncts such as support hose and pneumatic compression devices, and should be continued throughout hospitalization. Pharmacologic prophylaxis includes warfarin, heparin, and aspirin.

21. What patients are at risk for heterotopic ossification (HO) and what preventative measures can be taken?

Patients with ankylosing spondylitis, previous HO, diffuse idiopathic skeletal hyperostosism (DISH), and Paget's disease are at risk for HO. Low-dose radiation (a single dose of 700 rads at 24–72 hours after surgery) and indomethacin are the most common prophylactics.

22. What positions are dangerous after THA?

Four basic positions should be avoided after THA, particularly for the first 3 months:
1. Flexion of the hip past 90° with respect to the axis of the body
2. Adduction of the leg past the midline of the body
3. Combined extension of the hip joint with external rotation of the lower extremity
4. Flexion with internal rotation

23. Why should abduction pillows be utilized? When? For how long?

An abduction pillow prevents dislocation of the hip prosthesis (adduction, internal rotation) while the patient is sleeping or resting in bed. It is used for the first 6–12 weeks.

24. What ranges of motion of the hip are allowed after THA?
- 80–90° of hip flexion and full hip extension
- Gentle (20–30°) internal and external rotation of the hip
- Passive abduction as tolerated

Active abduction should be avoided the first 6 weeks in patients who have undergone a lateral approach.

25. What is the sequence of ambulatory aids usually given to patients after THA?

Parallel bars (days 1–2), crutches or a walker (first 6 weeks), and one crutch or cane (next 6 weeks). Greater than 70% of patients are ambulatory without an assistive device at the end of 3 months.

26. Give four goals of occupational therapy after THA.
1. Reestablish basic activities of daily living (ADLs) with modifications that keep the patient's ROM within the restricted limits.
2. Teach joint protection.
3. Review fall risks.
4. Provide equipment with training.

27. Are resisted concentric exercises important after hip or knee surgery?

For the first 6–8 weeks, the patient can perform isometrics and active ROM exercises against gravity. Concentric exercises against resistance should be avoided. After 6–8 weeks, resisted open kinetic chain strengthening with 1–10 lbs. can begin. Heavier weights cause undue wear on the prosthetic components.

28. How do you assess flexion contracture of the hip?

The Thomas test. The patient tries to lower the extremity flat on the examination table, while holding the opposite thigh against the abdomen. The test is positive if the hip does not extend fully.

29. For a patient requiring ipsilateral hip and knee replacements, in which order should the surgeon proceed?

The **hip** should be replaced first because (1) it may rule out a source of referred knee pain from the hip, (2) it is easier to rehabilitate a hip arthroplasty with a diseased knee than the other way around, and (3) some orthopaedists believe there is less chance of damage to a prosthetic hip when replacing a knee than to a prosthetic knee when replacing a hip.

30. What about sex after joint replacement?

Many people express concern about dislocation or damage to the prosthesis while having intercourse. After 10–12 weeks, the risk of a dislocation or damage to the prosthesis is negligible.

31. Where are the most frequent sites of hip fracture in the elderly?

Femoral neck and the intertrochanteric and subtrochanteric areas.

32. What are the surgical indications and rehabilitations for the various hip fracture types?

Surgical Procedures and Rehabilitation for Hip Fractures

FRACTURES AND TYPE	SURGICAL PROCEDURE	WEIGHT-BEARING STATUS
Femoral neck		
Displaced fracture (Garden III and IV)	Hemiarthroplasty; ORIF (in younger patients)	WBAT
Undisplaced and impacted fractures (Garden I and II)	ORIF	Depends on the stability of surgical fixation
Intertrochanteric		
Undisplaced, displaced two-part fractures, or unstable three-part fractures	Treated operatively with multiple pins or screws and side-plate devices	Depends on degree of fracture stabilization, bone stock, patient's frailty, and risks of immobility. Most patients are WBAT
Subtrochanteric		
Simple, fragmented, or comminuted	ORIF with a blade plate and screws or an intramedullary nail	Delayed until fracture demonstrates evidence of healing

ORIF = open reduction and internal fixation; WBAT= weight-bearing as tolerated.

33. What are the negative predictors of ambulation after hip fracture?

Lack of social support, lower-limb contractures, age over 85, and poor prefracture functional status. Generally, a patient will lose one level of function after a hip fracture. Inability to transfer or ambulate, incontinence, dementia, fewer hours of physical therapy, and lack of family involvement may require institutionalization.

34. How can osteoporosis be prevented?

Proper calcium intake, weight-bearing exercise, hormonal replacement at menopause, and reducing the risk factors (i.e., smoking, alcohol use, and caffeine intake). For more progressive osteoporosis, one might consider calcitonin, calcitriol, and/or biphosphonates therapy.

35. What factors are associated with an increased risk of falls in the geriatric population?

Factors that increase the incidence of falls include lower-limb impairment such as weakness and ankle or foot problems, gait abnormalities, use of multiple medications, balance disorders, dementia, visual impairment, previous history of falls, and Parkinson's disease.

36. How does an intertrochantric osteotomy affect the leg length?

Open valgus osteotomy generally lengthens the limb; varus osteotomy usually shortens the limb.

37. Who is the ideal patient for hip arthrodesis?

Young adults or older adolescents with unilateral end-stage arthritis who are engaged in heavy labor.

38. What are the most common effects of hip arthrodesis on adjacent joints?

Pain is the most common problem and is seen in the contralateral hip (25%), the ipsilateral knee (60%), and the lower back (60%). There is also a high incidence of ipsilateral knee laxity or instability (75–80%).

39. How commonly does osteonecrosis occur?

Osteonecrosis annually afflicts about 5000–10,000 adults under age 45 years old.

40. What are the causes or associated factors for osteonecrosis?

Steroid use and alcohol use account for about 90% of known causes of avascular necrosis in the patient population under age 45 years. Other conditions associated with osteonecrosis include myeloproliferative disorders, Gaucher disease, trauma, chronic pancreatitis, Caisson disease, sickle cell and other anemias, and radiation.

41. What is the incidence of bilaterality for osteonecrosis?

Literature shows there is an 80% risk of bilateral involvement. One side may be entirely asymptomatic.

42. What is the most common site of osteonecrosis?

The femoral head. However, the humeral head and distal femur are involved in 10–15% of cases.

43. What are the different methods of evaluating osteonecrosis of the femoral head?

Adequate anteroposterior (AP) and lateral radiographs are the first step. Magnetic resonance imaging (MRI) is the most sensitive and specific modality. Computed tomography (CT) scan can be used to assess femoral head collapse. Invasive modalities include direct pressure measurements, venography, and biopsy. *Note:* Technetium scans have recently been shown to be less sensitive and specific.

44. Propose an algorithm for the management of osteonecrosis based on the University of Pennsylvania classification.

Treatment Plan According to the University of Pennsylvania Staging Systems

RADIOGRAPHIC STAGE	SYMPTOMS	PROCEDURE
1, 2	Asymptomatic	Observation, pharmacologic treatment
1a, 1b, 2a, 2b	Symptomatic	Core decompression
1c, 2c, 3a, 3b, 3c, 4a	Symptomatic	Vascularized or nonvascularized bone grafting, osteotomy
4b, 4c	Symptomatic	Limited femoral resurfacing
5, 6	Symptomatic	Total hip replacement

45. Describe a rehabilitation program for a patient with osteonecrosis.

Exercise, pain control, and joint-protection techniques. Isotonic exercises, such as straight-leg raising, that distribute stress through the hip joint must be avoided. Gravity-eliminated active assistive exercise, such as pool therapy and isometric exercises, can improve hip ROM and strength.

46. What is the prognosis for patients with avascular necrosis treated with nonoperative modalities that restrict weight bearing?

Most studies report greater than 90% progression of collapse and total hip replacement within 4 years.

BIBLIOGRAPHY

1. Callaghan JJ, Dennis DA, Paprosky WG, Rosenberg AG (eds): Orthopedic Knowledge Update: Hip and Knee Reconstruction. Rosemont, IL, American Academy of Orthopaedic Surgeons, 1995.
2. Evarts CM (ed): Surgery of the Musculoskeletal System, 2nd ed. Volume 3. New York, Churchill Livingston, 1998.
3. Kasser J (ed): Orthopedic Knowledge Update 5. Rosemont, IL, American Academy of Orthopaedic Surgeons, 1996.
4. Mont MA, Hungerford DS: Non-traumatic avascular necrosis of the femoral head. J Bone Joint Surg 77A:459–474, 1995.

47. THE KNEE: ANATOMY, PATHOLOGY, AND DIAGNOSIS

Michael E. Frey, M.D., and Warren Slaten, M.D.

1. What joints are in the knee?

Tibiofemoral, patellofemoral, and tibiofibular.

2. What anatomic structures cause referred pain to the knee?

Lumbar spine, hip, sacroiliac joint, and the ankle or foot.

3. Does a positive Lachman's test always mean anterior cruciate ligament (ACL) injury?

No, laxity may be symmetric in the other knee. It is important to compare both knees.

4. What is the camel's sign?

Double hump of a high-riding patella and an uncovered infrapatella fat pad seen in the lateral view of the knee.

5. What is the Q angle?

The quadriceps angle or patellofemoral angle is the angle formed between a line drawn from the anterior superior iliac spine (ASIS) to the midpoint of the patella and a line drawn from the tibial tubercle to the midpoint of the patella with the hip and foot in neutral position. Normally, the angle is 13–18° (although if the quadriceps is contracted the normal angle is 8–10°). The angles in men tend to be lower than in women.

6. What causes increased Q angle?

Chondromalacia patella, subluxed patella, genu valgus, increased tibial torsion, and malalignment of the quadriceps.

7. What causes increased Q angle?
Patella alta and chondromalacia patella.

8. Name three types of knee effusions.
Synovial, hemarthrosis, and purulent.

9. What is genu recurvatum?
Hyperextension or excessive backward knee joint mobility.

10. What is patella alta?
A high-riding patella.

11. What is genu varum?
Bowleg or excessive outward (lateral) deviation of the leg.

12. What is genu valgum?
Knock-knee or excessive medial deviation of the leg.

13. What is O'Donoghue's triad?
Injuries to the medial meniscus, medial collateral ligament (MCL), and ACL caused by a valgus force to a flexed, rotated knee.

14. What is the purpose of the knee menisci?
Lubrication, nutrition, shock absorption, and prevention of cartilage wear.

15. Why do meniscal injuries cause gradual swelling and nonbloody effusions?
The menisci are primarily avascular, especially the inner two thirds.

16. Name the common tests for meniscus injury.
McMurray's, Apley's, Steinmann's, and Bragard's.

17. Can meniscal injuries be treated without surgery?
Yes. Initially, the PRICE (**p**rotect, relative **r**est, **i**ce, **c**ompression, and **e**levation) acronym is prescribed.

18. When is surgical treatment indicated for meniscal tear?
- Locking, or inability to fully extend the knee because of mechanical blockage
- Motion restricted despite a trial of physical therapy
- Instability, which may predispose to further intra-articular damage
- Baker's cyst resulting from a meniscal tear
- Refractory pain not improving with physical therapy and symptomatic treatment

19. Describe the typical signs and symptoms of patellofemoral pain.
- Anterior knee pain with gradual onset that worsens with repetitive knee flexion
- Pain with prolonged sitting or upon arising after sitting (positive **theater sign**)
- Pain with squatting or with descending stairs

20. What is the purpose of the ACL?
To prevent anterior displacement of the tibia over the femur.

21. Name the most common tests for ACL injury.
Lachman, anterior drawer sign, and pivot shift test.

22. Name the most common tests for posterior cruciate ligament (PCL) injury.
Reverse Lachman, Slocum, Godfrey, and posterior drawer sign.

23. Name the acute signs of ACL injury.
Rapid developing effusion, and "pop" sign.

24. What are the degrees of MCL strains?
Grade 1 (first degree)—valgus stress results in medial pain but no increased laxity.
Grade 2 (second degree)—valgus stress demonstrates increased laxity, and an endpoint is appreciated.
Grade 3 (third degree)—valgus stress demonstrates increased laxity with no appreciable endpoint. This indicates rupture of the ligament and the surrounding capsular structures.

25. How much laxity is there in MCL and lateral collateral ligament (LCL) injuries?
Grade 1   0–5 mm
Grade 2   6–10 mm
Grade 3   11–15 mm

26. When can the patient resume sports activities after an MCL injury?
When the patient's strength is near normal (90%) and the valgus instability is reduced to a point no longer requiring a brace. The patient should be able to perform one-legged hopping, jumping rope, and climbing stairs before returning to the playing field.

27. What is osteochrondritis dissecans?
Fragmentation of the articular cartilage with subchondral bone, most commonly the medial femoral condyle or patella, from trauma, predominantly in adolescent males. The usual presentation is stiffness and aching with an effusion.

28. What is Sinding-Larsen-Johansson disease?
Osteochondritis of the inferior pole of the patella in the pediatric age group.

29. What is jumper's knee?
Jumper's knee is insertional tendinopathy of the quadriceps or the patellar tendons.

30. Where is the most common location of jumper's knee?
The site of involvement is most commonly the inferior pole of the patella in 20–40-year old patients. In patients over 40, the quadriceps tendon is affected more frequently.

31. What is Baker's cyst?
A herniation of synovial tissue through a weakening posterior capsular wall causing swelling in the popliteal fossa (popliteal cyst).

32. What is Osgood-Schlatter disease?
Apophysitis at the insertion of the patellar tendon into the tibial tubercle.

33. What is adiposis dolorosa (Dercum's disease)?
Medial knee pain in women with fat knees. Squeezing the fat causes pain.

34. What is plica?
The extra synovium ("remnants") present in the knee joint. It has been implicated as a source of pain in the knee (plica syndrome).

35. How do patients with iliotibial band syndrome (ITB) present?
Lateral knee pain after excessive running or hiking.

36. What is housemaid's knee?

Prepatellar bursitis.

37. What is vicar's knee?

Superficial infrapatellar bursitis.

38. If kneeling in prayer causes vicar's knee and housework causes housemaid's knee, what causes a Baker's cyst?

In children, Baker's cyst is usually congenital. In adults, it is usually secondary to underlying pathology or trauma. The general population is susceptible. Development of the cyst has nothing to do with kneading bread; the cyst was named for William Morrant Baker, a British surgeon.

39. Name causes of anterior knee pain.

Osteoarthritis	Lateral pressure syndrome	Patella tendinitis
Rheumatoid arthritis	Quadriceps muscle imbalance	Quadriceps tendinitis
Patellar femoral syndrome	Tight lateral retinaculum	ITB syndrome
Bursitis	Synovial plica	(anterolateral)

40. What is pes anserinus syndrome?

Anterior medial knee pain caused by friction of the sartorius, gracilis, and semitendinosus tendons at the medial border of the tuberosity of the tibia.

41. Describe the Lachman's test.

This is a test for anterior knee stability. While the patient is supine, the knee is held at 30° flexion. The examiner stabilizes the femur and applies pressure to the back of the tibia below the knee. Increased laxity is indicative of an ACL injury.

42. Describe the Apley maneuver.

This is useful for diagnosing meniscal injury. The patient lies prone with the knee flexed 90°. While the examiner stabilizes the thigh, the tibia is rotated medially and laterally, with downward pressure. Joint line tenderness with this movement is considered positive.

43. Describe McMurray's test.

The patient is supine, and the knee is examined at neutral and at 30°. Valgus and varus stress is applied at both degrees. Valgus stress examines the MCL and varus stress examines the LCL. The posterior capsule is relaxed at about 30° of knee flexion.

BIBLIOGRAPHY

1. Eisle MA: A precise approach to anterior knee pain. Phys Sports Med 19:127, 1991.
2. Ellen MI, Young JL, Sarni JL: Musculoskeletal rehabilitation and sports medicine. 3. Knee and lower extremity injuries. Arch Phys Med Rehabil 80:S59–67, 1999.
3. Magee DJ: The knee. In Orthopedic Physical Assessment, 2nd ed. Philadelphia, W.B. Saunders, 1992, pp 372–447.
4. Sheon RP, Moskowitz RW, Goldberg VM: Soft Tissue Rheumatic Pain: Recognition, Management, and Prevention, 3rd ed. Baltimore, Williams & Wilkins, 1996.

48. REHABILITATION OF KNEE DISORDERS

Harpal Khanuja, M.D., Oliver Perez, B.S., Gracia Etienne, M.D., Ph.D.,
Amar D. Rajadhyaksha, M.D., and Michael A. Mont, M.D.

1. What are the surgical options for osteoarthritis of the knee?
Total knee arthroplasty is used for severe arthritis. Other options depend on the location and severity of the arthritis and include:
Arthroscopic debridement. This includes irrigation and removal of loose bodies from the knee.
Cartilage transplantation. For small isolated areas, portions of autologous articular cartilage can be grafted into the defect.
Osteotomies of the distal femur or proximal tibia are used for arthritis that is limited to the lateral or medial compartment of the knee.
Unicompartmental knee arthroplasty can be performed for isolated lateral or medial compartment arthritis.

2. What is a total knee arthroplasty?
In total knee arthroplasty, the surfaces of the distal femur, proximal tibia, and, often, the patella are replaced. This is performed with a femoral component and a tibial base plate made of a metal alloy, usually cobalt-chromium or titanium. The tibial component has a polyethylene plastic piece that is fixed to the metal base plate and articulates with the femur. The undersurface of the patella is replaced with polyethylene.

3. How are the components of a total knee arthroplasty held in place?
With cement or a rough coating on the surface of the component into which bone can grow (cementless).

4. What are the indications for total knee arthroplasty?
The primary indication is to relieve pain caused by arthritis. Secondary goals are to restore function and correct deformity. Candidates should have degenerative changes on radiographs and failed other methods of nonoperative and occasionally other types of operative care. Nonoperative modalities include anti-inflammatory medications, assistive devices, weight loss, and intra-articular steroid injections. In select cases, surgical options prior to total knee arthroplasty include arthroscopy and osteotomies.

5. What happens to the ligaments in a total knee arthroplasty?
In uncomplicated primary knee replacements, collateral ligaments are preserved. Because these structures can tighten and scar with arthritic deformity, they may need to be "released" to a certain degree. This helps to balance the soft tissues to equalize tension in the collateral ligaments and provide stability throughout the range of motion. Most prostheses require removal of the anterior cruciate ligament. The posterior cruciate is left intact or removed, depending on the type of prosthesis. Prostheses that require removal of the posterior cruciate ligament are designed to substitute for its function in flexion.

6. How successful are total knee arthroplasties?
Usually greater than 90% success rate at 10-year follow-up. Recent reports have shown that this is improving with newer prosthetic designs.

7. How long does pain last after this procedure?

This is extremely variable. Each patient needs to be managed individually. In general, pain management can be summarized as follows:

1–2 days postoperatively—Patients will have significant pain, and most need intravenous or intramuscular narcotic analgesia. Most patients can distinguish between postoperative pain and their preoperative arthritic pain.

3 days postoperatively—The pain is usually controlled with oral analgesics.

2–3 weeks postoperatively—Some patients continue to require analgesics, whereas others may be weaned off their medication.

It can take up to 6 months to a year before the patient feels that the knee is fully recovered.

8. What is the weight-bearing status immediately after total knee arthroplasty?

There are different protocols, and it is important to discuss this with the operating physician. When cement is used to fix both the femoral and tibial components, the patients are routinely allowed to bear weight as tolerated. If fixation requires bony ingrowth, partial weight bearing is usually utilized.

9. What other operative factors govern postoperative rehabilitation?

It is important to consider the operative approach when determining the weight-bearing status and the range of motion (ROM) that will be permitted. The surgeon may need to osteotomize the tibial tubercle or cut the extensor mechanism to gain adequate exposure. In these instances, the rehabilitation protocol needs to be modified to allow the areas to heal.

10. Do all patients need deep venous thrombosis (DVT) prophylaxis after total knee arthroplasty?

All patients should receive some type of DVT prophylaxis postoperatively. DVT prophylaxis has been shown to decrease the incidence of fatal pulmonary embolism. However, there is controversy over the best regimen. Different regimens include warfarin (Coumadin) and low–molecular-weight heparin. Aspirin and sequential pneumatic compression devices can be used. Aspirin may also be combined with hypotensive epidural anesthesia.

11. How should knee ROM be measured and recorded?

ROM should be measured from the lateral side of the patient's leg with a goniometer. Full extension, an angle between the femur and tibia of 0°, should be recorded as 0°. Full flexion is recorded as a positive number, somewhere between 0° and 135°. If the patient's leg cannot be fully extended, the number of degrees possible short of full extension is recorded as a positive number. For example, the patient who lacks 10° of full extension who is able to flex to 100° should be recorded as having a ROM +10–110°. If the patient's knee comes to hyperextension, then the amount past 0° should be recorded as a negative number. For example, if the subject hyperextends approximately 5° and flexes to 100°, the ROM is recorded as –5–100°.

12. What is the benefit of continuous passive motion (CPM) machines?

Although CPM may improve the amount of flexion a patient is able to attain initially, there is no evidence of any long-term benefit. Most surgeons do not use these machines in their rehabilitation protocols.

13. When should knee manipulation be seriously considered after total knee arthroplasty?

If the patient has only 70° of flexion by 14 days postoperatively or less than 90° by 6 weeks.

14. What is the most reliable predictor of the ROM a patient will have after total knee arthroplasty?

The best predictor of ROM after total knee arthroplasty is preoperative ROM. In general, the better the ROM before surgery, the better it will be after surgery. On average, patients can achieve 105–120° of flexion. At least 90° of flexion is desired for a good outcome, and this should be obtained within the first 2 weeks after surgery.

15. Outline a rehabilitation program for the patient with a total knee replacement.

SCHEDULE	REHAB PROGRAM
Day of surgery	Deep breathing exercise, active ankle ROM
Postop day 1	Lower limb isometric exercises (quadriceps, hamstrings and gluteal sets), passive and active ROM exercises
Postop day 2	Active assisted ROM
Postop day 3	Progressive isotonic and isometric knee and hip muscle strengthening Concentrate on terminal knee extension through active knee extension exercises

16. What muscles should be targeted after total knee arthroplasty?

The quadriceps muscles are significantly weaker after total knee arthroplasty. This is, in part, related to the exposure required. Tourniquet and ischemic time also may play a part in muscular weakness. The quadriceps is important for stability during the stance phase of gait. Isometric strengthening and active ROM should begin immediately after surgery and be continued for the first 6 weeks. Resisted isokinetic or isotonic strengthening should be added. Other muscles that should be strengthened include the hamstrings, gastrocsoleus, and ankle dorsiflexors.

17. List the usual sequence of ambulatory aids after a total knee replacement.

1. Parallel bars in inpatient physical therapy
2. Crutches or a walker, depending on patient stability and comfort
3. One crutch or cane

Most patients do not require assistive devices by 3 months

18. How should a patient ambulate stairs after a total knee arthroplasty?

When **ascending** the stairs, the patient should lead with the nonoperative leg following with crutches and the operative limb, one step at a time. When **descending** the stairs, the patient should lead with crutches and the operative extremity, following by the nonoperative extremity.

19. What are the four goals of occupational therapy after total knee arthroplasty?

1. To reestablish basic activities of daily living (ADLs), with modifications that keep the patient's ROM within restrictions
2. To teach joint protection
3. To review the risks for falls
4. To provide equipment with training

20. How long is it before a patient will receive full benefit of total knee arthroplasty?

By 3 months postoperatively, patients usually have regained most of their strength and ROM. It may be up to 1 year before the patient receives full benefit from the procedure.

21. Can a patient return to sports after total knee arthroplasty?

Yes. It is recommended that they refrain from high-impact sports, such as running, singles tennis, and football because these may lead to greater wear of the prosthesis. Low-impact activities include golf, doubles tennis, walking, and riding a stationary cycle.

22. Can a patient return to sex after total knee arthroplasty?

Yes. As with the return to sports, high-impact sexual activities that load the knee directly or indirectly may lead to undue wear of the prosthesis.

23. What is an "extensor lag"?

This refers to the inability to fully extend the knee actively, although passively full extension is possible. This results from lengthening of the extensor mechanism or weakening of the quadriceps. Component malposition may also produce this problem.

24. How does a flexion contracture differ from an extensor lag?

A knee with a flexion contracture cannot be fully extended either actively or passively. This is due to a mechanical block of which there are numerous causes, including scarred posterior capsule or other soft tissue structures, including the hamstrings, or retained osteophytes that may cause structures to tighten and thus block full extension. Component malposition also can cause this problem.

25. How does one test the stability of a total knee arthroplasty?

Medial/lateral (varus/valgus). The knee is stressed at 0°, 30°, 60°, and 90° of flexion. An opening of greater than 5° to varus and valgus stressing is considered excessive.

Anterior/posterior. The knee is tested with an anterior drawer throughout the ROM. The position of greatest instability is noted. Normally in a total knee arthroplasty there is 5–8 mm of displacement in this plane, because the anterior cruciate ligament is sacrificed during the procedure.

26. Who is at risk for peroneal nerve palsy after total knee arthroplasty?

The peroneal nerve is at risk when a retractor is placed on the lateral side of the knee during surgery. However, injury from this is not a common occurrence. Neuropraxias more often result from stretching of the nerve with correction of the limb deformity. The valgus knee with a fixed flexion contracture is most at risk.

27. What measures should be taken in the immediate postoperative patient who is found to have new weakness or absence of the foot and ankle dorsiflexors?

All dressings should be removed, and the knee should be flexed to relieve tension across the peroneal nerve. If there is no resolution of the palsy by 2 months, surgical exploration and decompression should be performed.

28. What patient-related factors have a negative impact on results following a total knee arthroplasty?

Total knee arthroplasty is technically difficult after high tibial osteotomies, and the results are not as good as routine primary total knee replacements. Diabetics and patients with rheumatoid arthritis are at an increased risk for infection. Patients on Workmen's Compensation do not do as well as others.

29. Do obese patients have higher wear rates?

Although the forces across the knee are higher in obese patients, wear rates are not increased in this population. This may be because these patients tend to be less active.

BIBLIOGRAPHY

1. Callaghan JJ, Dennis DA, Paprosky WG, Rosenberg AG: Orthopaedic Knowledge Update. Hip and Knee Reconstruction. Rosemont, IL, American Academy of Orthopaedic Surgeons, 1995.
2. Fu FH (ed): Surgery of the Knee. Baltimore, Williams & Wilkins, 1994.
3. Healy WL, Iorio R, Lemos MJ: Athletic activity after total knee arthroplasty. Clin Orthop 380:65–71, 2000.
4. Insall JN, Kelly M: The total condylar prosthesis. Clin Orthop 205:43–48, 1986.
5. Insall JN, Windsor RE, Scott WN, et al (eds): Surgery of the Knee, 2nd ed. New York, Churchill Livingston, 1993.
6. Krackow KA (ed): The Technique of Total Knee Arthroplasty. St Louis, Mosby, 1990.
7. Lombardi AV Jr, Mallory TH, Eberle RW: Constrained knee arthroplasty. In Scott WN (ed): The Knee. St. Louis, Mosby, 1993, pp 1305–1323.
8. Mont MA, Antonaides S, Krackow KA, Hungerford DS: Total knee replacement following high tibial osteotomy. Clin Orthop 299:125–130, 1993.
9. Mont MA, Alexander N, Krackow KA, Hungerford DS: Total knee arthroplasty after failed high tibial osteotomy. Orthop Clin North Am 23:515–525, 1994.
10. Mont MA, Mathur SK, Krackow KA, et al: Cementless total knee arthroplasty in obese patients: A comparison to matched control group. J Arthroplast 11:153–156, 1996.
11. Mont MA, Mayerson JA, Krackow KA, Hungerford DS: Total knee arthroplasty in patients receiving Workers' Compensation. J Bone Joint Surg 80A:1285–1290, 1998.
12. Rand JA (ed): Total Knee Arthroplasty. New York, Raven Press, 1993.
13. Sema F, Mont MA, Krackow KA, Hungerford DS: Total knee arthroplasty in diabetic patients: A comparison to a matched control group. J Arthroplast 9:375–380, 1994.

49. THE ANKLE AND FOOT: ANATOMY, PATHOLOGY, AND DIAGNOSIS

C. Christopher Stroud, M.D., and Lew C. Schon, M.D.

1. Describe the three areas of the foot and the joints that make up each area.
Hindfoot—talocalcaneal (subtalar), calcaneocuboid, and talonavicular joints
Midfoot—metatarso-cuneiform joints
Forefoot—toes and metatarsals

2. How many bones are in the foot and ankle?
Twenty-six.

3. What are clinical indicators of generalized ligamentous laxity?
Indicators include ability to oppose the thumb to the forearm, recurvatum at the elbow or knee, and greater than 90° of hypertension at the metacarpophalangeal (MCP) joint.

4. Describe three types of toe deformities.
 1. **Hammertoe**—flexion deformity at proximal interphalangeal (PIP) joint, often with extension deformity at the distal interphalangeal (DIP) and metatarsophalangeal (MTP) joints
 2. **Mallet toe**—flexion deformity at DIP joint
 3. **Claw toe**—hyperextension at MTP joint, flexion deformities at the PIP and DIP

5. Define bunion and bunionette deformities.
When the great toe deviates laterally and develops a prominent medial eminence, it is termed a **bunion** or a **hallux valgus deformity**. A prominent eminence about the fifth metatarsal head laterally is a **bunionette** deformity.

6. Describe two types of pathologic foot alignment.
A **pes planus**, or flatfoot deformity, is loss of the longitudinal arch of the foot. Causes include rupture or dysfunction of the posterior tibial tendon, arthritis of the hind- or midfoot, or tarsal coalition. A **pes cavus** is a high arch foot. Causes include physiologic and genetic factors, Charcot-Marie-Tooth disease, and spinal cord lesion.

7. What is a Haglund's deformity?
This painful prominence of the posterolateral aspect of the heel is commonly referred to as a "pump bump."

8. What are the causes of a painful heel?
Plantar fasciitis, central heel fat pad atrophy, Achilles tendinosis, and irritation of the first branch of the lateral plantar nerve.

9. What is hallux rigidus?
It is arthritis that limits motion at the first MTP joint and causes pain.

10. Which area of the foot and ankle is most commonly affected in rheumatoid arthritis and how does rheumatoid arthritis typically present?
The forefoot is the most common and presents with pain, swelling, and deformity. Typically, the great toe deviates laterally, and the lesser toes contract and form hammer or claw toe deformities. There are often prominent metatarsal heads plantarly that may cause pain and ulcerate

overlying skin. If the hindfoot is involved, it usually assumes a flatfoot posture with collapse of the longitudinal arch.

11. When are radiographs indicated in a patient with an ankle injury?
- Inability to bear weight immediately following injury or during the examination
- Tenderness directly over fibula or about the fifth metatarsal base

12. What is a Jones fracture?
This fracture is located at the metaphyseal-disphyseal junction of the fifth metatarsal and often results in delayed healing if untreated. Fractures about the base of the fifth metatarsal are termed **avulsion-type fractures** and will usually heal with a stiff-soled shoe.

13. What are the most common locations of stress fractures in the foot?
Calcaneus, navicular, and metatarsals.

14. What are some common reasons for patients presenting with pain several months after an ankle sprain?
Common undiagnosed causes include peroneal tendinitis, synovitis of the ankle joint, ankle or subtalar instability, an osteochondral defect of the talus, stress (or occult) fractures of the calcaneus, cuboid or lateral talar process, and superficial peroneal neuritis.

15. What are some risk factors for foot ulceration in patients with diabetes?

Neuropathy	Nail disease (ingrown, thin nails)
Vascular disease	Poor hygiene
Foot deformity, bony prominence, or tendon contracture	Inappropriate footwear
	Malnutrition
Previous ulceration or amputation	

16. What are the stages or grades of ulcer presentation?
Wagner classified five grades of ulcer presentation:

Grade 0	Risk of ulcer development
Grade I	Superficial skin breakdown
Grade II	Deep ulceration
Grade III	Infected, deep ulceration
Grade IV	Ulcer with partial foot gangrene
Grade V	Entire foot gangrene

17. How is the vascular status of the foot and ankle assessed?
Skin temperature, turgor, warmth, capillary refill, and presence or absence of pulses are useful for assessment. Noninvasive studies used to assess blood flow include arterial segmental pressure (i.e., ankle-brachial index [ABI]), pulse volume recordings (index of vessel patency, test of noncompressible vessels), duplex scanning, and continuous-wave Doppler (wave forms).

18. What is an acceptable ABI level for wound healing?
A ratio of lower extremity arterial pressure to upper extremity arterial pressure of 0.45 or greater is commonly used as a positive predictor of healing. Readings may be falsely elevated due to arterial calcifications.

19. What foot deformities cause ulcerations?
A varus or supinatory deformity can cause lateral midfoot ulceration. A valgus, rockerbottom, or pes planus deformity can cause medial midfoot ulceration. An equinus deformity can cause forefoot ulceration.

20. What is Charcot neuroarthropathy?

It is the rapid onset of painless, severe joint destruction and dissolution associated with fractures and dislocations in patients with neuropathy. Only 1–2.5% of diabetics develop neuroarthropathy. The most common areas of the foot include the midfoot, hindfoot, and ankle.

21. What factors are thought to be involved in the pathogenesis of Charcot neuroarthropathy?

Factors involved in development include limited sensation and increased vascular perfusion combined with arthritis, avascular necrosis, or fracture. Repetitive or single stresses above the threshold of the foot's biomechanical capacity can initiate the Charcot process.

22. Given areas of the foot, list the tendons in descending order of power.
- Plantar flexors—gastrocsoleus, posterior tibialis (PT), flexor hallucis longus (FHL), flexor digitorum longus (FDL)
- Dorsiflexors—tibialis anterior tendon, extensor digitorum longus, extensor hallucis longus, peroneus tertius
- Evertors—peroneus brevis, peroneus longus
- Invertors—posterior tibialis, FHL, FDL

23. What foot and ankle deformities are common sequelae of a stroke?

Equinus (initially from spasticity, later from spasticity and myostatic contracture), varus deformity, equinovarus deformity (most common), and footdrop. A well-molded, padded ankle-foot orthosis (AFO) can accommodate mild to moderate deformities.

24. In an equinus contracture, how does one differentiate between a gastrocnemius and soleus contracture?

The gastrocnemius muscle crosses the knee joint. If an equinus contracture is present when the knee is extended and improves or disappears with knee flexion, this structure is primarily involved. If contracture is present in knee flexion and extension, the gastrocnemius and soleus muscles are involved.

25. What is a common sequela of a fixed equinovarus foot deformity?

Painful callosities of the lateral plantar foot.

26. What muscles are involved in producing a varus deformity of the ankle and hindfoot?

Tibialis anterior, FHL, FDL, soleus, and tibialis posterior muscles.

27. Name the components of the deltoid ligament and the mechanism involved with injury to this structure.

The deltoid ligament is made up of superficial and deep components and is usually injured with an eversion, or valgus, stress to the ankle.

28. What ligaments are involved in the common ankle sprain?

An inversion moment of the ankle can injure the anterior talofibular ligament (ATFL), most commonly, followed by involvement of the calcaneofibular ligament (CFL), and, least commonly the posterior talofibular ligament (PTFL).

29. Name and describe the two tests used to detect injury and instability of the lateral ankle ligament complex.

The **anterior drawer test** evaluates the ATFL and is performed by applying a forward stress to the ankle while stabilizing the tibia, with the ankle in slight plantar flexion. The **talar tilt test** evaluates the CFL and is performed by applying an inversion stress to the ankle while stabilizing the tibia, with the ankle in neutral flexion. The quality of the endpoint and the amount of translation are noted.

30. How are ankle sprains commonly graded?

Ankle sprains are most commonly graded by the amount of ligament damage:

Grade I—ligament sprain or strain and no increase in translation on stress testing

Grade II—partial ligament tearing and minimal increase in translation on stress testing

Grade III—complete tearing of one or both of the lateral ligaments and no end point noted on stress testing

31. How do most patients with plantar fasciitis present?

The most common complaint is pain about the plantar, inner heel (sharp or bruising) associated with the first step in the morning, arising from a seated position, and toward the end of the day.

32. How is plantar fasciitis treated?

Nonoperative treatment is successful in more than 95% of cases and involves Achilles and plantar fascial stretching exercises, anti-inflammatory medication, a night splint, and occasionally an injection.

33. What is the Maissoneuve fracture?

The Maissoneuve fracture involves either a rupture of the deltoid ligament or a fracture of the medial malleolus associated with a high fibula fracture. It is produced by an extreme external rotation stress at the ankle.

34. What causes a hammertoe deformity?

A hammertoe deformity is the result of a muscle or tendon imbalance between the toe flexors and extensors and results from trauma, inflammatory conditions, neurologic disorders, and poorly fitting shoes in the toe box.

35. Is a heel spur the cause of pain in patients with plantar fasciitis?

A heel spur when noted radiographically is actually present within the substance of the flexor digitorum brevis and is present in only 50% of patients with plantar fasciitis. It occurs as a normal finding in 15–30% of asymptomatic individuals and therefore is not thought to be the cause of pain in these patients.

BIBLIOGRAPHY

1. Myerson MS (ed): The Diabetic Foot. Foot and Ankle Clinics. Vol. 2, no. 1. Philadelphia, W.B. Saunders, 1997.
2. Myerson MS (ed): Foot and Ankle Disorders. Philadelphia, W.B. Saunders, 2000.

50. REHABILITATION OF FOOT AND ANKLE DISORDERS

Mooyeon Oh-Park, M.D., and Dennis D.J. Kim, M.D.

1. What is the correct technique of the Achilles tendon stretching exercise?

It should be called "lengthening of gastrocsoleus muscle," because the Achilles is not quickly stretchable. Perform this exercise with a slightly supinated foot to avoid stretching of the foot. Avoid painful or bouncing movement to prevent stretch reflex (maintain lengthening for 15–30 seconds). Ask patients to demonstrate their technique and reinstruct them on each visit. Lengthening may take several weeks or months.

2. What is the aggressive, conservative treatment of posterior tibial tendon (PTT) insufficiency?

Conservative treatment of PTT insufficiency or rupture had been considered ineffective and surgical intervention was widely recommended. Recently, experts reported successful outcome with **early aggressive** conservative treatment addressing the biomechanics using the University of California Biomechanics Lab orthosis (UCBL) or ankle-foot orthoses (AFOs) instead of simple foot orthoses. UCBL and AFOs align the subtalar joint by direct control of the calcaneus, allowing the healing of PTT. In patients with excessive obesity, fixed deformity of the subtalar joint (STJ), and tight heel cord, UCBL is not effective.[3,9]

3. In which foot or ankle conditions can Unna's boot be useful?

It can be used for chronic venous ulcers and any edematous conditions of the lower leg and ankle, such as congestive heart failure, lymphedema, tendinitis, trauma (ankle sprain), or arthritis. In contrast to cast immobilization, an Unna boot provides support to the ankle, hindfoot, and midfoot, while allowing some movement. It can be used in conjunction with a controlled ankle motion walker.

4. What are the roles of the metatarsal pad, neuroma pad, and wedge?

The metatarsal pad is usually placed proximal to the metatarsal head, with the apex of the pad under the midshaft. The mechanism of relief is not well understood. A neuroma pad is placed between the metatarsal shaft to widen the intermetatarsal space and is useful for interdigital neuritis (Morton's neuritis). Wedges are often called "posting" and can be placed medially or laterally under the hindfoot or forefoot.

5. What is low dye taping?

This simple taping method is designed to support the forefoot and midfoot and is useful for plantar fasciitis, heel spur bursitis (with heel cup), fat pad atrophy, and cuboid subluxation (with cuboid pad). It includes lateral circumferential taping from the metatarsal head around the heel to the other side of the metatarsal head and provides broad support to fat pad and plantar fascia.

6. What is recalcitrant plantar fasciitis? How do you approach it?

Plantar fasciitis is self-limiting. Treatment options include fascial taping in acute stage, mobilization, lengthening exercise of the gastrocsoleus and plantar fascia, roomy footwear, mild heel elevation with soft heel cups, and night splinting. Avoid repeated injections because of complications (fat pad atrophy, rupture of fascia, hematoma, or abscess). The following are common reasons for unsuccessful treatment:

1. Wrong diagnosis. Plantar fasciitis can be confused with heel pad atrophy, Baxter's nerve entrapment, interdigital neuritis, peroneus longus tendinitis, and seronegative spondyloarthropathies

2. Lack of systematic approach in management (not using night splint, trying "quick fix" with injection or foot orthosis alone)

3. Ignoring underlying pathologic biomechanics such as excessive pronation related to forefoot or hindfoot varus, heel cord tightness, or excessive supination (cavus foot).

4. Failure of behavioral modification (over-enthusiastic sports activities, overweight, tight shoes)

7. How are hallux rigidus (HR) and hallux limitus (HL) treated?

First, determine if it is primary or secondary. Secondary HL is commonly caused by:

1. Dorsiflexed first ray in excessive pronation, collapsed medial longitudinal arch from neuroarthropathy, foot orthosis with excessively high medial arch support, or surgery.

2. Tethering the flexor hallucis longus (FHL) after an ankle fracture, deep posterior compartment syndrome of the leg, or diabetes mellitus Charcot joint.

Treat underlying cause (e.g., lengthening exercise of gastrocsoleus muscle, lowering the arch of foot orthosis). Footwear modifications (rocker sole with steel shank, toe-spring, or Springlite carbon plate) are often helpful.

8. Describe sinus tarsi syndrome and its treatment.

This syndrome is characterized by a history of frequent ankle sprains, swelling of sinus tarsi area with pain or feeling of instability, and prompt relief with local anesthetic injection. This is often explained by disruption of the interosseous ligaments in the STJ with associated inflammation and soft tissue proliferation. Often local steroid injection provides only temporary relief. Physiatric management includes UCBL or supramalleolar AFO to provide stability to the STJ.

9. What is the first line of management of Morton's interdigital neuritis?

Because tight shoes are the main culprit of interdigital neuritis, wearing roomy footwear is the first step. Often this is enough to resolve symptoms. Other treatment options (metatarsal pads, neuroma pads, injection, or surgery) are adjunctive.

10. What is the best method for choosing the right size sneakers?

If insoles are removable, place them on the floor and stand on them. Check the space between the toes and insole tip, there should be enough space for the width of your thumb. The widest part of your foot should coincide with the widest part of the sneaker. Your feet should not spread beyond the border. Size and width marked can be used as a guideline, but there is great variability between brands and styles.

11. How can you make sneakers "snug" or "roomy"?

You can wear more socks, insert 3-mm thickness of Poron, PPT, or rigid Plastazote under the sockliner (insole), or provide tongue pads. To make sneakers bigger, stretch with a shoe-stretcher or "shoemaker's swan" or remove sock-liners. Also, sneakers stretch when dampened. The best solution, however, is **buy new sneakers!**

12. What are the features of "walking " and "running" sneakers?

In general, walking sneakers are roomy and better for foot pain or deformity or foot orthosis.

CHARACTERISTIC	RUNNING SNEAKERS	WALKING SNEAKERS
Last (shape)	Semi-curved or curved	Semi-curved or straight
Last (construction)	Slip last or combination last	Board last or combination last
Upper material	Combination of leather and fabric	Mostly leather
Height of toe box	Mostly low	High
Midsole	Firm	Firm
Outsole	Rough grain for better grip	Fine grain
Weight	Light weight	Slightly heavier
Toe spring	Usually very high	High
Color	Various colors	Conservative and simple colors
Designed for	Sprinting and running	Stability and control on walking

13. What is the multidensity insole?

Insoles are usually made of multiple layers of materials with different densities (durometer). The top layer is made of soft materials for comfort, the bottom layer is a rigid material for structural stability, and a medium density middle layer is used for durability. Frequently, Poron or PPT sheets are used as cover material to reduce sliding and shear. Leather is an inferior cover material because of increased sliding and shear.

14. What are the biomechanical principles for treatment of foot and ankle disorders?

The **subtalar-midtarsal joint complex.** It consists of three joints: the talocalcaneal (STJ), talonavicular, and calcaneocuboid. They work as a functional unit as the foot pronates or supinates during the gait cycle. When the STJ pronates after heel strike, the axes of midtarsal joints (MTJ; talonavicular and calcaneocuboid) become parallel, allowing midfoot flexibility (for shock absorption, adaptation to uneven terrain). As the STJ supinates in the late stance phase, the axes of the MTJ cross, resulting in locking of the midfoot (rigid lever for propulsion).

2. **Biomechanical effect of pronation or supination.**

	PRONATION RESPONSE	SUPINATION RESPONSE
Hindfoot (coronal)	Eversion	Inversion
Fore/midfoot (sagittal)	Dorsiflexion	Plantar flexion
Forefoot (transverse)	Abduction	Adduction
Ankle	Dorsiflexion	Plantar flexion
Tibia	Internal rotation	External rotation
Knee	Flexion, valgus	Extension, varus
Femur	Internal rotation	External rotation
Hip	Flexion	Extension
Leg length	Shortened	Lengthened
Effect during gait	Absorbs impact, adapts to uneven terrain	Provides solid leverage for push-off

Adapted from Wernick J, Volpe RG: Lower extremity function and normal mechanics. In Valmassy R (ed): Clinical Biomechanics of the Lower Extremities, St. Louis, Mosby, 1996, pp 2–57.

3. The difference between **equinus deformity and equinus state.** The "equinus state" is the inability to achieve 10° of passive ankle dorsiflexion with the knee extended and STJ neutral. Ten degrees of dorsiflexion is required for reciprocal gait pattern, uphill walking, and proper balance. "Equinus deformity" means that the ankle has passive dorsiflexion less than 0° with knee extended and STJ neutral. Equinus state without equinus deformity can cause significant problems such as excessive pronation or hyperextension of the knee.[9]

4. The **biomechanical consequence of ankle equinus state and deformity.** Pronation at the STJ with dorsiflexion at the MTJ or hyperextension of the knee may compensate for lack of dorsiflexion. The oblique axis of the MTJ is called a **secondary ankle joint** and provides most of the dorsiflexion of the forefoot. Because pronation is a compensatory mechanism, attempts to correct it by foot orthoses (FOs) or UCBL will not resolve the problem and can aggravate the situation. Treatment involves stretching the gastrocsoleus muscle to restore dorsiflexion or heel lifts for equinus.

5. The **biomechanical consequence of the forefoot equinus.** The forefoot equinus is a plantar flexed forefoot. This is commonly observed in cavus foot with limited motion of MTJ (secondary ankle joint). To obtain plantigrade foot on the ground (put the heel down), the patient needs to use maximum dorsiflexion of the ankle or excessive hyperextension of the knee. As a result, pain develops at the anterior of the ankle by degenerative changes or posterior knee by overstretching. A simple remedy is to elevate the heel to accommodate the forefoot equinus. Gastrocsoleus lengthening exercises common for the treatment of cavus foot may aggravate symptoms, becasuse the problem is in the forefoot not the hindfoot. The gastrocsoleus is already stretched to maximum.

6. The **biomechanical effect of soft heel, beveled heel, SACH, and flared heels.**

	BIOMECHANICAL EFFECT	CLINICAL USE
Soft heel/ SCAH	Simulating plantar flexion of ankle	Ankle pain with motion, solid AFO, ankle fusion, arthritis of ankle, prosthesis, anterior shin splint (decrease stress on tibialis anterior)
Beveled heel	Delayed heel strike, decrease the leverage from ankle axis and plantar flexion momentum; similar to barefoot	Similar to soft heel/SACH, no need for additional material for the heel, modification is simpler than SACH
Rocker sole	Simulating dorsiflexion of forefoot, helping toe clearance, relieving stress on forefoot	Hallux rigidus, metatarsalgia, forefoot plantar ulceration, frequently used in combination with SACH

SACH = solid ankle cushioned heel.

15. What are the characteristics of cavus foot in Charcot-Marie-Tooth (CMT) disease?

A high arched foot is called cavus foot. The cavus foot in CMT disease is characterized by hindfoot varus and forefoot valgus with plantar-flexed first ray (medial cuneiform and first metatarsal). This is primarily the result of overpull of the peroneus longus muscle (first ray plantar flexor) against a weakened anterior tibialis muscle (first ray dorsiflexor). The peroneus brevis becomes weakened out of proportion to its antagonist (tibialis posterior), resulting in inversion of the calcaneus.[1] The forefoot valgus is usually flexible initially but becomes rigid later. The fixed combination deformity of hindfoot varus with forefoot valgus has been called **torque foot** with excess stress to the midfoot due to peculiar pronation-supination response on walking.

16. What are the causes of lingering foot or ankle pain after ankle sprain?

Syndesmosis (distal tibiofibular ligament) injury
Peroneal tendinitis
Talar dome injury
Subtalar ligament injury with sinus tarsi syndrome
Calcaneofibular ligament rupture
Recurrent subluxation of the cuboid
Hidden fracture of the calcaneocuboid joint

17. What are the abnormal biomechanical problems of the foot in diabetic patients?

Stiffness of foot tissues (skin, ligament, tendon, and muscles) is common due to nonenzymatic glycation of collagen fibers. This includes heel cord tightness and hallux limitus. Heel cord tightness does not allow the tibia to roll over the foot during the stance phase, contributing to excessive flexion stress (nutcracker effect) and collapse of the midfoot. Surgical correction of ankle equinus is often required for midfoot Charcot neuroarthropathy, in addition to immobilization and non–weight bearing.

18. How do plantar callus and warts differ?

	CALLUS	PLANTAR WARTS
Localization	High shear/friction area	Any location
Skin lines	Cross through the lesion	Pass around the lesion
Satellite lesion (mother/daughter)	No satellite lesions	Multiple daughter lesions
Local tenderness/pain	Pain on direct compression	Pain on side-to-side squeeze
Punctuate hemorrhage at base on shaving	None	Central core with punctate hemorrhages at the base
Age	Common in elderly	Rare in elderly

19. What are useful views of plain radiograph for foot and ankle disorders?

- **Anteroposterior (AP)/axial** projection—to define forefoot pathologies
- **Lateral** projection—for hindfoot and longitudinal arch
- **Medial oblique** projection—for metatarso-cuneiform alignments, lateral midfoot/hindfoot articulations
- **Lateral oblique** projection—for medial midfoot articulations[5]

BIBLIOGRAPHY

1. Alexander IJ, Fleissner PR Jr: Pes cavus. Foot Ankle Clin 3:723–735, 1998.
2. Alexander IJ: Examination of specific systems. In Foot Examination and Diagnosis, 2nd ed. New York, Churchill Livingstone, 1997, pp 17–18.
3. Chao W, Wapner KL, Lee TH, et al: Nonoperative management of posterior tibial tendon dysfunction. Foot Ankle Int 17:736–741, 1996.
4. Kim DJ, Oh-Park M: Foot problems related to functional impairment in the elderly. J Musculoskel Rehabil 12:7–24, 1999.
5. Myerson MS: Foot and Ankle Disorders. Philadelphia, W.B. Saunders, 2000.

6. Park TA, Del Toro DR: Electrodiagnostic evaluation of the foot. Phys Med Rehabil Clin North Am 9:871–896, 1998.
7. Reily MA: Guidelines for Prescribing Foot Orthotics. Thorofare NJ, Slack Inc., 1995.
8. Tollafield D, Merriman L: Clinical Skills in Treating the Foot. New York, Churchill Livingstone, 1997.
9. Wapner KL, Chao W: Nonoperative treatment of posterior tibial tendon dysfunction. Clin Orthop 365:39–45, 1999.
10. Wernick J, Volpe RG: Lower extremity function and normal mechanics. In Valmassy R (ed): Clinical Biomechanics of the Lower Extremities. St. Louis, Mosby, 1996, pp 2–57.

51. MANAGEMENT OF FRACTURES

Arun J. Mehta, M.B., FRCPC

1. How common are musculoskeletal injuries?

Fractures are the fifth leading diagnosis in hospital discharges.

2. Why does a patient with a fracture need rehabilitation?

Treatment of a fracture usually involves prolonged immobilization, which may lead to deconditioning. Even if the fracture does not require manipulation or operation, rehab is an essential component for restoration to the premorbid condition.

3. Describe the mechanisms of injury that lead to fracture.

- **Direct injury**—Direct blow fractures bone at site of impact
- **Indirect injury**—Force applied at one point, fracture occurs at a remote site
- **Transverse or oblique fracture**—Force bends a long bone
- **Spiral fracture**—Result of twisting force
- **Compression fracture**—Compressive forces crush soft spongy bone (e.g., vertebral body)

4. Name the factors that predispose a patient to fractures.

Age. Risk increases due to increases of osteoporosis and falls. Children usually break bones because they are more active and take more risks.

Osteoporosis. Bone loss is a major contributing factor in fractures of the femoral neck and compression fractures of the spine. It is seen 10–15 years earlier in women than men.

Falls. The elderly are more likely to fall and break a bone because of neurologic disorders, such as peripheral neuropathy, cerebrovascular accidents, visual impairment, Parkinson's disease, dementia, or cardiac factors (orthostatic hypotension, arrhythmias, or syncope).

5. What is an open fracture? Why is it important to treat it differently than a closed fracture?

In a closed fracture, the skin is intact. A laceration or puncture wound near the fracture site makes it an open fracture. Infection, external bleeding, and blood loss may delay healing of an open fracture.

6. What systemic complications can occur after a fracture?

Urinary tract infections (indwelling catheter)	Fat embolism
Constipation (opioid analgesics)	Deep venous thrombosis (DVT)
Pressure ulcers (pressure of the cast or bedrest)	Pneumonia
Anemia (injury-related or perioperative blood loss)	

7. How does a fracture heal?

When blood vessels are injured, blood accumulates in tissues and forms a hematoma, which is replaced by new blood vessels and fibroblasts. Later, osteoblasts from the periosteum and endosteum proliferate and form the intercellular matrix in which calcium salts are deposited to form a **callus**. Mechanical loading generates electrical potentials, known as the **piezoelectric** property of the bone. These electrical potentials are recognized by osteoblasts and guide new bone formation. Increasing compression force or stress at the fracture site signals formation and orientation of collagen fibers, deposition of minerals, and strengthening of callus.

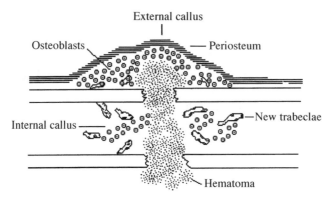

Fracture repair.

8. What do you look for on plain x-rays?
- Fracture location
- Involvement of diaphysis, metaphysis, epiphysis, or articular surface
- Fracture line—transverse, oblique, or spiral
- Deformity—alignment, angulation, rotation
- Number and location of bony fragments, displacement, direction, and distance from normal location, distance between fragments
- Dislocation or effusion of adjacent joints
- Swelling or blood loss

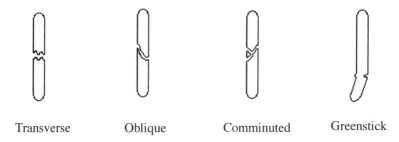

Types of fractures.

9. When do you suspect pathologic fracture?
A pathologic fracture occurs after a minor trauma that would not ordinarily break a bone. The patient may have had pain before the fracture, especially night pain. If a patient has a malignant tumor and later develops a fracture, it may be due to metastatic disease. Pathologic fractures also can occur with hormonal deficiency states (estrogen and testosterone).

10. Which malignant tumors commonly metastasize to bone?
Malignant tumors of the breast, lung, prostate, colon, rectum, kidney, thyroid, and bladder.

11. When should you order a bone scan?

If the initial x-rays do not show a fracture but there is a strong clinical suspicion (especially in suspected stress fractures). Also, fracture of the scaphoid may not be visible on initial x-rays.

12. Is magnetic resonance imaging (MRI) useful in the diagnosis and management of fractures?

Yes. MRI is useful for early diagnosis of infection, tumor, fracture, bone and muscle hematomas, partial and complete tears of ligaments, hematomas within ligaments, and avascular necrosis.

13. What are the goals of treatment after fracture?

Control pain, correct deformity, protect injured tissue, prevent complications and secondary impairment, and regain function. Significant deformity is corrected by closed reduction, traction, or open reduction.

14. What are the different methods of immobilization?

- **Traction** (prolonged continuous force is applied to align and maintain fracture fragments): skin traction, skeletal traction
- **External fixation:** plaster cast, external fixator, splints
- **Internal fixation:** pins, plates, screws, and intramedullary rods

15. What are some local complications of a fracture?

Nerve and **blood vessels** are damaged during injury, manipulation, or orthopedic procedures.

Compartment syndrome is suspected when the patient complains of very severe pain, numbness of toes or fingers, inability to move toes or fingers, and poor capillary circulation under the nails.

Delayed union occurs if a fracture is not healed after a reasonable time.

Nonunion occurs when bone ends look sclerotic and smooth on x-rays.

Malunion occurs when a fracture unites in an altered alignment.

Stiffness and **atrophy** of muscles are very common because of immobilization.

Early **degenerative joint disease** may result from incongruous and rough joint surfaces.

16. Which fractures are likely to be redisplaced after reduction?

Fracture of both forearm bones, comminuted fractures with third fragment or oblique fractures, and when swelling decreases and the cast becomes loose.

17. What is cast disease?

Cast disease comprises muscle atrophy, weakness, osteoporosis, and joint stiffness.

18. What are the general principles in the rehabilitation management of fractures?

1. The physiatrist should have knowledge of the mechanism of injury, type of fracture, orthopedic treatment received, normal course of healing, complications, and outcomes expected.

2. Pain management is very important from the patient's point of view. Analgesic administration before therapy is helpful. Use of narcotics should be reduced as soon as possible.

3. Good, on-going, personal communication with the orthopedic surgeon is essential. Details of operative findings may be missing in the written operative report. The surgeon also can help in deciding progression through rehabilitation (clearance for weight-bearing status).

4. Rehabilitation includes progression through various stages of ROM and strengthening exercises, ambulation training, bracing, home evaluation, adaptive equipment, and coordination of care.

19. Which patients require a systematic, holistic approach to fracture rehabilitation?

Patients at risk for significant functional impairment or complications:

1. **Geriatric patients** at risk for falls and with multiple medical problems. Deconditioning secondary to prolonged bedrest or inactivity makes it difficult to achieve independent ambulation.

2. **Multitrauma patients** with more than one fracture and/or injury to other systems.

3. **Special fractures** (e.g, fractures of the scaphoid) are notorious for a high incidence of nonunion.

4. **Preexisting medical conditions** such as osteoporosis, metastasis, osteogenesis imperfecta, or cardiorespiratory disease.

20. How do you determine when the patient is ready for weight-bearing?

There is no specific timetable. Decisions are based on type of fracture, method and quality of fixation, condition of the bone, patient's ability to control weight-bearing, and if there is bony union.

*Weight-bearing Status for Upper Limb Fractures (after Hoppenfeld)**

FRACTURE	WEIGHT BEARING STATUS
Clavicle	Gradual WB: 6–8 weeks FWB: 8–12 weeks
Proximal humerus	
Rodding	Limited WB: 2 weeks FWB: 12 weeks
Internal fixation	WB: 4–6 weeks FWB: 12 weeks
Distal humerus	NWB: min. 6 weeks FWB: 12 weeks
Olecranon	Gradual WB: 6–8 weeks FWB: 8–12 weeks
Radial head	
Nonoperative fixation	PWB: 4–6 weeks FWB: 8–12 weeks
Internal fixation	NWB: min. 6 weeks FWB: 8–12 weeks
Mid-forearm	FWB: 8–12 weeks
Colles' (including postop external fixation)	WBAT 6–8 weeks
Scaphoid	FWB: after 12 weeks
Metacarpal	FWB: 6–8 weeks
Phalangeal	WBAT: 4–6 weeks FWB: 6–8 weeks

* These are general guidelines for fractures that have been casted or fixed internally except where noted. All fractures begin with NWB.
WB = weight bearing; NWB = no weight bearing; PWB = partial weight bearing; FWB = full weight bearing; WBAT = weight bearing as tolerated.

Weight-bearing Status for Lower Extremity Fractures (after Hoppenfeld)

FRACTURE	WEIGHT BEARING STATUS
Calcaneal	
Up to 1 week	Bedrest with foot elevated
1–4 weeks	NWB
4–6 weeks	Rigidly fixed (internal fixation)-TTWB–PWB Nonrigid: NWB
6–8 weeks	Rigidly fixed: PWB Nonrigid fixed: NWB
8–12 weeks	Rigidly fixed: PWB–full WB Nonrigid: NWB–PWB (do not start WB until approx. 16 weeks)

Table continued on following page

Weight-bearing Status for Lower Extremity Fractures (after Hoppenfeld) (Continued)

FRACTURE	WEIGHT BEARING STATUS
Ankle	
Up to 1 week	NWB (except isolated distal fibula fractures: WBAT)
Up to 2 weeks	Isolated distal fibula fracture: WBAT
	Rigidly fixed fractures: TTWB
	All others: NWB
4–6 weeks	Internal fixator: TTWB
	External fixator: fixator removed but remains NWB
6–8 weeks	Consolidation and fx site nontender or nondisplaced distal fibular fx: progressive PWB
	Open fxs with tendinous soft tissue: TTWB–PWB
	Cast: PWB if nontender
8–12weeks	Progressive increase to FWB
Femoral neck	
Closed or ORIF	
Immediate–1 week	Impacted/rigidly fixed: PWB–FWB with crutches or walker with 3-point gait
	Unstable: NWB
2 weeks	Impacted/rigidly fixed: PWB–FWB with crutches or walker with 3-point gait
	Unstable: NWB–TTWB
4–6 weeks	Impacted/rigidly fixed: PWB–FWB with crutches or walker with 3-point gait
	Unstable: NWB
8+ weeks	WBAT, assitive devices as needed
Endoprosthesis	Immediate WBAT
Intertrochanteric	Most commonly treated with sliding hip screw; WBAT may occur immediately
	Exception is in reverse oblique, pathological, and severely comminuted fractures. Patient begins with NWB–TTWB and advances to WBAT at 8 weeks.
Femoral shaft	
IM nail fixation	Statically locked nail: TTWB–PWB during ambulation and transfers; FWB avoided
	Dynamically locked nail: WBAT encouraged during ambulation and transfers
ORIF	NWB–TTWB up to 8 weeks; PWB until 12 weeks
External fixator	NWB until callus formation
Subtrochanteric	Full WBAT within the first few days if medial bone contact has restored
	Extensive comminution or tx with ORIF: TTWB–PWB
	By 8 weeks all fxs should be FWB unless there is no callus present and bone grafting is being considered
Supracondylar	NWB for 3 months, if proper bone healing, advance WB slowly
Forefoot	
First week	NWB except phalangeal is WBAT
2–4 weeks	Phalangeal and undisplaced 2nd–4th metatarsal: WBAT
	Sesamoids, first phalanx, first metatarsal, Jones fx: NWB
4–6 weeks	Same as above
8–12 weeks	FWB
Midfoot	Earliest PWB: Lisfranc (tarsometatarsal): 6–8 weeks
Navicular	Cortical avulsion and tuberosity: immediate WBAT
	Stress: 6 weeks
	Displaced intra-articular with OR: 6–8 weeks
	Body: 7–10 weeks
Cuboid	Avulsion: WBAT
	Nondisplaced: 4–6 weeks
	Displaced with ORIF: 6 weeks
Cuneiform	Nondisplaced: 4–6 weeks
	Grossly displaced with ORIF: 6 weeks

Table continued on following page

Weight-bearing Status for Lower Extremity Fractures (after Hoppenfeld) (Continued)

FRACTURE	WEIGHT BEARING STATUS
Patellar	FWB with cast or knee immobilizer. At 4–6 wks, immobilizer may be removed for level ground walking and FWB at 8 weeks.
Talar	
First week	NWB with foot elevated
2 weeks	Rigidly fixed: TTWB with an assisted device
	Nonrigid: NWB
4–8 weeks	Rigidly fixed: PWB
	Tx with closed reduction: NWB
8–12 weeks	Rigidly fixed: PWB–FWB
	Nonrigid: NWB–PWB
Tibial plafond (distal tibia)	
0–6 weeks	NWB
6–8 weeks	If appears to be healing: PWB
8–12 weeks	TTWB–FWB
Tibial plateau	
0–6 weeks	NWB
6–12 weeks	Advance to full FWB at the end of 12 weeks
Tibial shaft	Stable: WBAT immediately
	Unstable: NWB until 4 weeks; advance to TTWB at 4–6 weeks; then WBAT

NWB = no weight bearing; WB = weight bearing; PWB = partial weight bearing; FWB = full weight bearing; WBAT = weight bearing as tolerated; TTWB = toe touch weight bearing; ORIF = open reduction internal fixation; fx = fracture; tx = traction.
Table compiled by Dr. Howard Choi from Hoppenfeld S, Murthy V: Treatment and Rehabilitation of Fractures. Philadelphia, Lippincott Williams & Wilkins, 2000.

21. Why would you consider a brace in the treatment of a fracture?

The brace protects the fracture site, allows ROM exercises and wound dressings, and may even facilitate some weight-bearing activities.

22. What are some problem fractures in children?

Supracondylar fracture of the humerus is notorious for complication of Volkmann's ischemic contracture. Dislocation of the head of the radius may be missed initially or recur in cases of Monteggia fracture-dislocation (fracture of the shaft of ulna with dislocation of the head of radius). Metaphyseal and epiphyseal fractures, which involve the growth plate, can lead to premature closure of the epiphysis and a shorter extremity. Osteoporosis from eating disorders and amenorrhea can lead to stress fractures.

23. How are fractures in children different from those in adults?

In children, tissues heal well and more rapidly, joints do not get stiff as easily, and the remodeling process commonly corrects deformity. Greenstick fractures, in which the cortex buckles on only one side of the shaft of a long bone, are seen only in children, and epiphyseal injuries may affect growth of a long bone.

24. What are some common fractures seen in the elderly?

- Compression fracture of the spine—due to flexion injury, common in the osteoporotic spine
- Fracture of the femoral neck
- Fracture of distal radius—Colles' fracture, often associated with osteoporosis and a fall onto an outstretched arm
- Fracture of the neck of humerus—may lead to marked limitation of movement in shoulder joint

25. What is the role of a physiatrist in the management of a pathologic fracture?

A physiatrist can help in management of severe pain and reducing risk of pathologic fracture during rehabilitation. Concentrate on transfers, ambulation, and other functional activities so the patient can be discharged.

26. What are the risk factors for prolonged stay in a nursing home after acute treatment for hip fracture?

Incontinence, patient living alone prior to injury, cognitive impairment, and dependence in ambulation.

27. Where do stress fractures commonly occur?

Stress fractures are caused by small, repeated stresses. A stress fracture of the 2nd, 3rd, or 4th metatarsal is called a **march fracture** because it was described in poorly conditioned soldiers after long marches. Long distance running and ballet dancing also may lead to march fractures. Other frequent sites for stress fractures include proximal tibia, fibula, neck of femur, and pubic ramus.

28. Which fractures are missed more often than others on initial evaluation?

Hairline fractures of the scaphoid may not show on initial x-rays. A history of a fall on an outstretched hand, with pain and tenderness over the anatomic snuff box (radial side of wrist), should be treated as a scaphoid fracture (splinting or casting for 10–15 days) with a repeat x-ray. If fracture is still suspected but not evident, a bone scan or MRI is warranted. A fracture of the neck of the femur may be difficult to visualize on initial x-rays. Management is similar to suspected fracture of the scaphoid.

29. What about fractures with joint dislocation?

In **dislocation**, the articular surfaces are totally separated from each other with no contact at all. In **subluxation**, there is partial contact between articular surfaces. A good example is the shoulder joint after stroke: the head of the humerus slides downward due to gravity and weak muscles unable to maintain normal position. Fracture-dislocations occur in the shoulder, ankle, elbow, and hip.

30. What goals do you want to achieve for your patient during rehabilitation?

1. **Prevent complications** such as joint stiffness, disuse atrophy, contractures, complex regional pain syndrome, pressure sores, and re-displacement of fracture fragments.

2. **Restore** ROM, muscle strength, function of the extremity, and vocational and avocational activities.

BIBLIOGRAPHY

1. Browner BD, Jupiter JB, Levine AM, Trafton PG (eds): Skeletal Trauma, 2nd ed. Philadelphia, W.B. Saunders, 1998.
2. Hoppenfeld S, Murthy V: Treatment and Rehabilitation of Fractures. Philadelphia, Lippincott Williams & Wilkins, 2000.
3. McFarland EG, Young MA: Biomechanical principles in rehabilitation of fractures. Phys Med Rehabil State Art Rev 9:269–283, 1995.
4. Mehta AJ (ed): Rehabilitation of Fractures. Physical Medicine and Rehabilitation: State of the Art Reviews. Vol. 9, no. 1. Philadelphia, Hanley & Belfus, 1995.
5. Mehta AJ (ed): Common Musculoskeletal Problems. Philadelphia, Hanley & Belfus, 1996.
6. Mehta AJ, Nastasi AE: Rehabilitation of fractures in the elderly. Geriatr Clin North Am 9:717–730, 1993.
7. Salter RB: Textbook of Disorders and Injuries of the Musculoskeletal System, 3rd ed. Baltimore, Williams & Wilkins, 1983.
8. Young MA, O'Young BJ, McFarland EG: Rehabilitation of the trauma patient: General principles. Phys Med Rehabil State Art Rev 9:185–201, 1995.

52. REHABILITATION OF SOFT TISSUE AND MUSCULOSKELETAL INJURY

Howard J. Hoffberg, M.D.

1. What are the soft tissues involved in musculoskeletal injuries?

The term *soft tissue* refers to the muscles, tendons, ligaments, supporting vascular and lymphatic structures (myofascial tissue), periarticular and synovial tissue, and subcutaneous fat and skin. The central nervous system and visceral organs also may be included. It does not include discs, bones, joints, or peripheral nerves.

2. What is the difference between a strain and sprain?

A strain is a stretch injury to muscles and tendons resulting in three degrees of severity (from microtrauma to complete tear). A sprain is a stretch injury to ligaments that causes tearing, hemorrhage, and joint instability.

3. What is the most common cause of musculoskeletal trauma?

The most common cause is motor vehicle accidents. Other causes include sports injuries, industrial accidents, repetitive overload activities, and lifting.

4. What is whiplash?

It is an acceleration-deceleration mechanism of energy transfer from the relatively immobilized torso to the head. Whiplash can occur at an impact of 4–5 mph and commonly affects the cervical facet joints and the trapezius, levator scapulae, paraspinal, scalene, and sternoncleidomastoid muscles. Disc disruptions, vertebral fractures, and neurologic deficits such as cervical radiculopathy and myelopathy also may occur.

5. What is the classification of whiplash-associated disorders?

The Quebec Task Force Classifications for the Severity of Cervical Sprains

GRADE	SYMPTOMS
0	No neck pain complaints, no physical signs
1	Neck pain complaints, stiffness or tenderness only, no physical signs
2	Neck complaints, muscoloskeletal signs (decreased ROM and tenderness)
3	Neck complaints, neurologic signs (weakness, sensory and reflex change)
4	Neck complaints with fracture and/or disclocation

ROM = range of motion.

Other symptoms for grades 1–4 include hearing, visual, and cognitive changes; dysphagia; headache; and temporomandibular joint dysfunction.

6. What is the most common x-ray finding following a cervical sprain?

A flattening or reduction of the cervical lordosis indicates a paraspinal spasm, which is a protective mechanism to restrict cervical spine motion. C1–C2 images are used for acute trauma, lateral flexion-extension views identify instability concerns, and oblique views are used to evaluate the neural foramina if radiculopathy is suspected.

7. When should you recommend a soft cervical collar?

A cervical collar is recommended for patients with an acute cervical strain or sprain who need to maintain function (work or driving). The collar supports the neck and prevents painful extremes of neck motion. It should be used no more than 2 weeks. Otherwise, muscle weakness and a head forward posture may result.

8. What are the sources of headaches following trauma?
Postconcussion syndrome (vascular origin)
Referral from jaw muscles (craniofacial dysfunction)
Referral from cervical facet, discs (radiculopathy), or myofascial origins
Muscle tension secondary to stress or tonic activity
Combination of the above

9. What types of disability may result from injuries to the torso?
Pelvic-girdle dysfunction, including effects on the quadratus lumborum, glutei, piriformis, and iliopsoas may occur following pelvic or lumbosacral injury. This may result in functional leg length discrepancy and scoliosis. **Lumbar sprains** may affect the quadratus and paraspinal muscles. **Thoracic and rib cage sprains** may affect the paraspinal, shoulder girdle, intercostals, trapezius, and levator scapulae muscles. **Shoulder injuries** may affect the rotator cuff, pectoralis, biceps, deltoid, latissimus dorsi, levator scapulae, rhomboid, trapezius, and triceps muscles. **Piriformis** involvement may simulate lumbosacral radiculopathy, and involvement of the **upper ribs, scalene, and pectoralis muscles** may cause a functional thoracic outlet syndrome.

10. What is the relationship between myofascial pain and joint dysfunction?
The relationship can be characterized by the mnemonic **ART**:
Asymmetries of related musculoskeletal structures
Restriction of motion
Soft tissue **t**exture abnormalities
Also referred to as **somatic dysfunction**, the myofascial and joint dysfunction is caused by an imbalance in the joint-ligament-tendon-muscle-fascia complex resulting in pain generators from sensitized small myelinated and free nerve endings or alteration of the large myelinated spindle and Golgi tendon organs afferents (joint proprioception). Somatic dysfunction may affect posture and recruitment, tonus, coordination, and balance of muscles.

11. What is the difference between subluxation and dislocation of a joint?
In **subluxation**, there is some contact with the articular surfaces as a result of second degree stretching of the ligaments. Conservative techniques and manual medicine restore balance and alignment by stretching to the anatomic barrier. **Dislocation** occurs when the articular surfaces completely separate, usually a result of ligamentous injury leading to joint instability. Surgical reduction followed by prolonged immobilization may be necessary. Hypermobile joints should be stabilized with exercise, adaptive equipment, and avoidance of joint mobilization.

12. What variables affect prognosis following an injury?
Age, sex, medications, symptom duration, mechanism of injury, restraint usage, delay in treatment, and premorbid level of conditioning and illness affect prognosis.

13. What are the objective findings in musculoskeletal trauma?
Abrasions, lacerations, contusions, ecchymosis, hematoma, edema, temperature or color changes, altered joint range of motion (ROM), joint instability or somatic dysfunction, spasm, weakness with imbalance of the muscles, postural findings, and associated neurologic deficits. Myofascial trigger points may contain a taut band or nodule, twitch response to palpation, and histamine release phenomena. Myofascial tissue biopsy may reveal micro-hemorrhages, tears, and inflammatory cell infiltration, which can result in chronic fibrosis. Diagnostic testing includes thermography, surface electromyography, tissue impedance, compliance and algometry, quantitative sensory testing, electrodiagnostics, postural analysis, soft tissue, magnetic resonance imaging, ultrasonography, and radiographs.

14. What are the subjective findings in musculoskeletal trauma?

Pain, including somatic and autonomic referral patterns, sensory disturbances, fatigue, and a sensation of fullness or swelling. Common referral patterns of neck pain include headache radiating into the upper extremity or scapula. Shoulder pain may refer into the upper extremity, and forearm pain may refer into the wrist and hand. Low back, buttock, and pelvic pain may refer into the lower extremity, hip pain into the knee, knee pain into the calf, and ankle pain into the foot.

15. What is complex regional pain disorder (CRPD)?

Formerly known as reflex sympathetic dystrophy, CRPD usually presents in acute extremity injuries (crush or sprain) with cold, swollen, discolored, sweating limbs, sensitivity to light touch, intolerance of weight-bearing motion, and perceived pain disproportionate to objective findings. **Type 1** occurs with musculoskeletal trauma without neurological deficit. **Type 2** has associated neurologic injury, often described as **causalgia**.

16. Is there a "post-traumatic fibromyalgia"?

Yes. It is a chronic multifocal myofascial pain syndrome from a traumatic injury. These patients may have a predisposition for fibromyalgia, and symptoms become amplified from a lowered pain threshold or psychosocial factors associated with chronic pain and dysfunction.

17. What is a myofascial pain syndrome?

Pain generated from regional myofascial trigger points resulting in restrictions in motion, muscular imbalances with weakness, characteristic referral patterns, and autonomic dysfunction (usually histamine release with increased skin temperature over the trigger points). It often occurs following trauma but can occur as a result of overload and postural, metabolic, and nutritional factors. This syndrome may occur due to other pathologies or injuries (e.g., fractures, neurological deficits, CRPS) and should be treated conservatively in conjunction with other generators of pain.

18. How long does it take for musculoskeletal injuries to heal?

An underlying microtrauma may take 6 weeks to heal. However, a minority of patients continue to experience signs and symptoms including muscular imbalance with weakness, restricted ROM, and consistent pain patterns with palpation, stretch, and activity. Perpetuating factors include persisting active trigger point, fibrotic changes in myofascial tissues, preexisting morbidity, metabolic, nutritional, and postural, activities, temperature, humidity, and psychosocial stressors.

19. What rehabilitation techniques can be used in musculoskeletal trauma?

In acute injuries, use the PRICE (**p**rotection, **r**elative **r**est, **i**ce, **c**ompression, and **e**levation) method. This can be supplemented by analgesics or nonsteroidal anti-inflammatory drugs (NSAIDs), splints or supports, soft tissue injections, and physical and manual medicine modalities. Conservative treatments are performed in conjunction with an active exercise program, consisting of active ROM with a gentle stretch and isometric strengthening with postural training. Once stabilized, exercises to restore flexibility, isotonic and isokinetic strengthening, dynamic stabilization, body mechanics and reconditioning are recommended. In resistant or chronic cases, one should consider psychosocial aspects, particularly if the condition affects functional status (activities of daily living, mobility, work, recreational, sexual activities, and sleep).

20. Once "resolved," can musculoskeletal pain recur?

Yes. Predisposing factors include inadequate rehabilitation resulting in reinjury or overload due to tightness, muscular imbalance, and "pain memory" (altered neuroanatomic pathways in the central nervous system as a result of peripheral trauma). Patients should be told that symptoms may recur, and they should be given guidelines indicating when formal treatment is needed (i.e., when symptoms affect function). A daily exercise program including stretching and postural exercises with adequate reconditioning supplemented by medications and adaptive equipment is necessary.

BIBLIOGRAPHY

1. Allen ME, Weir-Jones I, Motiuk DR, et al: Acceleration perturbations of daily living: A comparison to "whiplash." Spine 19:1285–1290, 1994.
2. Brault JR, Wheeler JB, Siegmund GP, Brault EJ: Clinical response of human subjects to rear-end automobile collisions. Arch Phys Med Rehabil 79:72–80, 1998.
3. Cailliet R: Soft Tissue Pain and Disability. Philadelphia, F.A. Davis, 1977.
4. Gunzburg R, Szpalski M: Whiplash Injuries. Philadelphia, Lippincott-Raven, 1997.
5. Rosen NB, Hoffberg HJ: Conservative management of low back pain. Phys Med Rehabil Clin North Am 9:435–472, 1998.
6. Snider R: Essentials of Musculoskeletal Care. Rosemont, IL, American Academy of Orthopaedic Surgery, 1997.
7. Spitzer WO, Skovron ML, Salmi LR, et al: Scientific monograph of the Quebec Task Force on Whiplash-Associated Disorders: Redefining "whiplash" and its management. Spine 20:1S–73S, 1995.
8. Travell J, Simons D: Myofascial Pain and Dysfunction: The Trigger Point Manual, Vol. 2. Baltimore, Williams & Wilkins, 1992.
9. Young MA, O'Young BO, McFarland EG: Rehabilitation of the orthopedic trauma patient. General Principles. Phys Med Rehabil State Art Rev 8:185–201, 1995.

VII. *Rehabilitation after Systemic Disease and Injury*

53. REHABILITATION OF THE TRANSPLANT PATIENT

Mark A. Young, M.D., M.B.A., and Steven A. Stiens, M.D., M.S.

1. Why should physiatrists know about rehabilitating organ transplant survivors?

As the number of organ transplants performed each year rise, there is an increasing need for rehabilitation of these patients. PM&R is in a unique position to deliver these services because of the specialty's multidisciplinary emphasis on exercise, physical restoration, and improving quality and quantity of life. Rehabilitation units in large academic and tertiary care hospitals are a natural recovery milieu where physiatry-directed, team-oriented programs can be carried out. Rehabilitation after transplantation can enhance functional outcome, improve quality of life, and bolster psychosocial functioning of the transplant recipient.

2. What factors have contributed to the rise in the number of transplantation surgeries?

Transplant surgery has gained widespread acceptance as a therapeutic intervention for patients with hematologic and end-stage solid organ disease. The establishment of organ procurement protocols, refinement of an HLA registry for enhanced transplant matching, and improvement in surgical, antirejection, and infection control strategies have allowed the number of surgeries performed to increase.

3. Who are the members of the transplantation rehabilitation team?

Optimally, the transplant rehab team should include a physiatrist, physical therapist, case manager, occupational therapist, nurse, clinical pharmacologist, nutritionist, transplant surgeon, internist, and social worker. The physiatrist, with his or her skills in coordinating large interdisciplinary teams, should assume a yeoman's role in the postoperative rehab process.

4. How many different transplantable organs are there?

Although the number is increasing, currently 22 organs are transplantable.

5. What are the two major categories of organ transplantation?

Solid organ and hematologic.

6. Name two outcome measures useful for quantifying functional improvement after transplantation.

Life Satisfaction Index (LSI) and Transplant Care Index (TCI).

7. What are the major components of rehabilitation after transplantation?

A therapeutic plan should be based on presurgical functional survey and an indepth analysis of the medical, socioeconomic, and psychological needs of the patient. It is helpful to evaluate the patient's functional status prior to surgery with a thorough musculoskeletal, neurologic, and functional assessment to determine a baseline for rehabilitation. Focus should be placed on maintaining body functions, which may be affected by immobilization. Examples include contracture prevention, skin maintenance, deep vein thrombosis and pulmonary embolism prevention, muscle atrophy prevention, and maintaining bowel and bladder functions. Also, comorbidities and potential complications should be anticipated. Clearly defined precautions in the rehabilitation program should be established.

8. What psychological issues need to be addressed during rehabilitation?

Psychosocial and emotional stress can significantly affect rehabilitation. Coping with chronic disease, waiting for a donor organ, and other socioeconomic issues can significantly impact the patient. For this reason, it may be difficult to motivate the patient. The social worker and psychologist play an important role in dealing with these issues.

9. When should mobilization begin and why is it important?

Mobilization should begin as soon as possible. Bedrest can lead to a significant loss in muscle size and strength and cause cardiovascular deconditioning and deterioration of bone structures.

10. How do you prevent muscle weakness?

The first muscle groups to weaken are the legs and trunk. A strength program of daily contractions of 20% or more of maximal tension sustained for several seconds or vigorous contractions at 50% of maximal tension can help maintain strength. Quadriceps sets and ankle pumps improve strength in the legs and decrease venous stasis.

11. What are the common side effects of antirejection drugs that physiatrists need to know?

Cyclosporine—interstitial edema, ankle swelling, renal dysfunction, hypertension, tremor, sexual dysfunction, liver disease, death

Azathioprine—leukopenia, pancytopenia

Prednisone—edema, hypertension, skin fragility, Cushing's syndrome, myopathy, aseptic necrosis of femoral and humeral heads

12. What are the most common post-cardiac transplant complications?

Allograft failure	CNS infection
Hypertension	Seizures
Neuromuscular deficits	Psychosis
Nutritional limitations	Compression fractures
Metabolic encephalopathy	Cyclosporine-related hypertension
Stroke	Stress fractures of weight-bearing extremities due to steroid-induced osteoporosis

13. Why is pulmonary hypertension an issue after transplantation and what strategies exist?

Following transplantation, the transplanted right ventricle is unable to cope with preexisting pulmonary hypertension. Also, pulmonary hypertension is associated with chronic left-sided heart failure, requiring the patient to use ionotrophic support.

14. What happens to cardiovascular health after transplantation?

Bedrest and inactivity lead to cardiac deconditioning. The resting heart rate of a bed-bound patient increases by about 0.5 bpm. This is called **immobilization tachycardia**. Two weeks of bedrest can reduce stroke volume by 15%. Postural hypotension also may occur due to the body's inability to adjust to upright positioning. Oxygen consumption (VO_2) or maximal oxygen consumption (VO_{2max}) also decrease dramatically.

15. How do you increase cardiovascular fitness?

While the patient is in intensive care, low-intensity bedside exercises can be prescribed. Exercise therapy should begin within a month after surgery. Benefits include improved strength, increased aerobic capacity, improved physical capability, and increased bone mineral density. Most often, it is not necessary to stop therapy when episodes of graft rejection occur. However, therapy may need to be changed when new arrythmias, hypotension, or fever occur.

Cardiovascular fitness can be improved with upright positioning on a tilt table. This increases orthostatic tolerance and strengthens antigravity muscles. Other measures to reduce orthostatic hypotension include early mobilization, conditioning exercises, increasing fluid and salt intake, elevating leg rests, abdominal binders, use of reclining backs, compression stockings, and pharmacologic agents such as ephedrine and phenylephrine.

16. What are the leading indications for lung transplant?

End-stage pulmonary disease, congenital disease, chronic obstructive pulmonary disease (COPD), pulmonary hypertension, cystic fibrosis, α_1-antitrypsin deficiency, sarcoidosis.

17. What are the preoperative considerations for lung transplantation rehab?

Prior to transplant surgery, patients need to be prepared for the operation itself with exercises that improve ventilation, mucociliary clearance, aerobic conditioning, flexibility, and strength. Interval training rather than continuous training puts less stress on patients with end-stage lung disease. Diaphram and segmental breathing increase lung volume and gas exchange. Target heart rates can be used to gauge the level of intensity. There are also helpful monitoring tools for patients with dyspnea, such as the "dyspnea index," dyspnea scale, or Borg Rating Scale of Perceived Exertion (RPE).

18. What are the post-lung transplant considerations?

Following transplantation, the lung is denervated, which causes an impaired cough reflex. Chest physical therapy is needed to produce effective clearance of airway secretions. Diaphragmatic dysfunction is also an issue. Rehabilitation can be complicated by intubation, mechanical ventilation, immunosuppression, pain, and restricted mobility. Bedrest can lead to orthostatic intolerance, reduced ventilation, increased heart rate, and decreased oxygen uptake.

Patients can use the active-cycle breathing technique or a flutter valve after extubation. Begin an exercise program with ROM exercises on the first postoperative day. When the patient leaves intensive care, advance to transfers from bed to chair and ambulation. Chest and upper extremity mobilization exercises improve thoracic mobility. Use of a treadmill and ergometer can improve cardiovascular endurance and strength. Before discharge from the hospital, the patient should proceed to stair-climbing. This is the hallmark of recovery because many patients with advanced pulmonary disease find this task difficult if not impossible.

19. Name several postoperative complications of renal tranplantation.

Complications include bleeding, infection, and rejection. Exercise after transplantation increases exercise capacity and counteracts negative side effects of glucocorticoid therapy such as muscle wasting and weight gain. Muscle atrophy, anemia, cardiovascular deficiency, and fatigue are roadblocks to rehabilitation.

20. What is CGVHD and what does it have to do with bone marrow transplant?

CGVHD stands for **chronic graft-versus-host disease** and is an immune-mediated illness that strikes as many as 40% of patients who have survived 100 days following HLA-identical sibling bone marrow transplant. As the leading complication of allogenic bone marrow transplantation, CGVHD often leads to joint contractures and soft-tissue stiffness and induration. Severe musculoskeletal disability may follow when contractures set in.

21. What rehab procedures can be useful in patients with CGVHD?

Therapeutic Modalities and Techniques to Improve or Maintain ROM in Patients with GVHD

TYPE OF INTERVENTION	JOINT	THERAPY*
Preventive†	Hand	Resting hand splint
	Elbow	Air cast, molded splint made of aquaplast, fiberglass serial cast that can be bivalve and padded for skin protection
	Hip	Prone positioning
	Knee	Knee immobilizer
	Ankle	AFO, resting foot splint, high-top sneakers

Table continued on following page

Therapeutic Modalities and Techniques to Improve or Maintain ROM
in Patients with GVHD (Continued)

TYPE OF INTERVENTION	JOINT	THERAPY*
Restorative‡	Shoulders	Ultrasound and ROM, therapeutic excercise (AAROM), strengthening of antigravity muscles
	Elbow	Serial casting (bivalve and/or dynamic splints)
	Wrist/hand	Serial casting (bivalve and/or dynamic splints)
	Knee/ankle	Dynamic splint and/or serial cast

* Splints may be applied to restore and prevent complications with local changes and prevent further contractures. Application of splints is dependent on which joint is affected.
† Preventive therapy is joint focused, based on the location of sclerodermatous changes.
‡ Restorative therapy is applied if the loss of ROM is is progressing and/or potentially limiting the patient's functionally.
From Grant J, Young MA, Pidcock F, Christenson JR: Physical medicine and rehabilitation management of chronic graft versus host disease. Rehabil Oncol 15:13–15, 1997, with permission.

22. How does transplantation rehabilitation relate to the impairment, handicap, disability model?

Disablement terminology can be used to explain the impact of transplantation and rehabilitation interventions on persons with organ failure. The patient with end-organ failure experiences the effort of profound impairment (absence of an organ or organ functional deficit). The person may be limited in life roles, experience discrimination, and otherwise not achieve full participation in life activities (handicapped). Until transplantation, the medical and interdisciplinary rehab team teaches the patient disability-appropriate behaviors and equips the patient to maximize organ function, meet task demands, and achieve the fullest participation.

The transplant itself eliminates many impairments. Disabilities are eliminated with exercise targeted to task demands. Community reintegration and vocational rehabilitation helps in reaching full life participation.

BIBLIOGRAPHY

1. Grant J, Young MA, Pidcock F, Christenson JR: Physical medicine and rehabilitation management of chronic graft versus host disease. Rehabil Oncol 15:13–15, 1997.
2. Grant J, Young MA, Vogelsang G, et al: Chronic graft versus host disease after bone marrow transplant: A physiatric challenge. Presented at the annual meeting of the American Academy of Physical Medicine and Rehabilitation, Chicago, September 1996.
3. Latleif G, Young MA: Cardiac transplantation rehabilitation in a post-partum female. Presented at the Annual Assembly of the American Academy of Physical Medicine and Rehabilitation, Anaheim, CA, October 1994.
4. Young MA: Meeting the challenge: Rehabilitation and transplantation. Presented at the Annual Australasian Rehabilitation Medicine Faculty Meeting Symposium, Melbourne, Australia, August 23, 2000.
5. Young MA, McGuire MJ, Young MA: Optimizing rehabilitation and functional outcome in transplant survivors. Presented at the 3rd Mediterranean Congress of Physical Medicine and Rehabilitation, Athens, Greece, Sept 5, 2000.
6. Young MA, Stiens SA: Rehabilitation of the organ transplantation patient. In Braddom RL (ed): Physical Medicine and Rehabilitation, 2nd ed. Philadelphia, W.B. Saunders, 2000, pp 1385–1400.
7. Young MA, Stiens SA, McGill D, et al: Rehabilitation of the patient requiring transplantation. In Grabois MM, et al (eds): Physical Medicine and Rehabilitation: The Complete Approach. Cambridge, MA, Blackwell Science, 2000, pp 622–650.
8. Young MA, Tumanon R, O'Young BJ, et al: Vocational rehabilitation outcomes in solid organ transplant [abstract]. Arch Phys Med Rehabil 81:9, 2000.
9. Young MA, Young MM: Rehabilitation of the transplant patient: An international perspective. Presented at the Second Mediterranean Congress of Physical Medicine and Rehabilitation, Valencia, Spain, May 23, 1998.

10. Young MA, Young MM: Transplantation and rehabilitation: Enhancing functional outcome. Presented at the 11th European Congress of Physical Medicine and Rehabilitation, Goteburg, Sweden, May 26, 1999.
11. Young MA, Young M: Rehabilitation and transplantation: A new frontier. Presented at the Rehabilitation Medicine Society, Tel Aviv, Israel, 2001.

54. REHABILITATION IN CHRONIC RENAL FAILURE AND END-STAGE RENAL DISEASE

Sally Sizer Fitts, Ph.D., Christopher R. Blagg, M.D., and Diana D. Cardenas, M.D.

...the long-term risks of not exercising are greater than the risks of exercising.—Painter

1. What is renal failure?

Renal failure is the loss of the kidneys' ability to filter and eliminate metabolic waste products, to maintain normal fluid and solute homeostasis, to regulate blood pressure, and to produce hormones that prevent anemia and bone disease. The accumulation of metabolic waste products results in uremia. **Chronic renal failure** results from progressive, irreversible damage to the kidney. **End-stage renal disease** (ESRD) requires chronic dialysis or kidney transplantation to maintain life. The incidence and causes of ESRD vary from country to country and are changing as our population ages; but in 1998 in the U.S., diabetes mellitus accounted for 33.2% of patients, hypertension for 24.0%, glomerulonephritis for 17.2%, polycystic kidney disease for 4.6%, and other or unknown causes for 21.0% of patients alive on dialysis or with a functioning kidney transplant.

2. What is creatinine clearance?

Clearance (Cl) expresses the efficiency with which the kidney removes a substance from the plasma. The clearance is a measure of **glomerular filtration rate** (GFR) and is an assessment of renal function. **Creatinine** (Cr) is used to determine GFR because it is released from muscle at a constant rate, is stable in concentration in the plasma, and is freely filtered in the glomeruli.

The following equation calculates CrCl (in mL/min), which reflects renal plasma flow.

$$CrCl = \frac{U_{CR}}{P_{CR}} \times V$$

where U_{CR} = urine concentration of creatinine in mg/ml, P_{CR} = plasma concentration of creatinine in mg/ml, and V = urine flow in mL/min.

Normal creatinine clearance can be estimated with the following equation (the value is 15% less in women):

$$CrCl = \frac{(140 - Age\ [yr]) \times (lean\ body\ weight\ [in\ kg])}{P_{CR} \times 72}$$

3. How is renal failure treated?

Many patients with chronic renal failure are not referred to a nephrologist until they have developed severe uremia and its complications. However, current practice standards encourage beginning dialysis earlier, as this has been shown to result in better survival, less morbidity, and better rehabilitation.

The two types of dialysis are **hemodialysis** (HD) and **peritoneal dialysis** (PD). HD requires a permanent vascular access for external filtering of blood as it is pumped through a cellulose or synthetic filter to remove waste and water, either at an outpatient clinic or at home. The blood access for HD is usually in the forearm and may be either an arteriovenous fistula or a Gortex vascular graft. The typical HD regimen is 3–5 hours, three times weekly, and may result in an intermittent pattern of post-dialysis fatigue and fluid gain between dialysis sessions.

PD maintains a more steady state. PD requires a permanent intraperitoneal catheter for 4 to 5 daily manual exchanges of dialysate fluids to remove diffusible waste and excess water. PD is often supplemented by automated machine exchanges overnight at home. Both forms of dialysis require dietary management and some limitation of fluid intake.

Kidney transplantation is the optimal treatment for many ESRD patients. It requires immunosuppressive drugs, such as cyclosporine or prednisone, which have side effects such as weight gain, osteodystrophy, and mood swings.

4. What are the metabolic consequences of renal failure?

ESRD and its treatment affect every organ system. The metabolic consequences of renal failure include anemia (secondary to lack of erythropoietin normally produced by the kidneys), increased risk of heart and vascular disease, hypertension, secondary hyperparathyroidism, renal osteodystrophy, hyperuricemia, and episodes of hypotension. Related neuromuscular disturbances may include peripheral neuropathy, muscle wasting, sleep disorders, fatigue, restless legs, headache, and seizures. These problems continue and may progress, particularly if dialysis is inadequate, but are reversed with a successful kidney transplant or with more frequent and longer hemodialysis. Cardiovascular and cerebrovascular disease are the leading causes of death among ESRD patients.

5. Discuss the forms of renal bone disease seen with dialysis.

Secondary hyperparathyroidism is the most frequent cause of **renal osteodystrophy**, a generic term encompassing all skeletal disorders occurring in chronic renal failure and ESRD patients. High-turnover bone disease (**osteitis fibrosa**) is more common in hemodialysis (50–60%) than peritoneal dialysis patients, and low-turnover bone disease (**osteomalacia**) is more common in patients on peritoneal dialysis (60–70%). However, both can occur in some patients. Unmineralized adynamic (aplastic) bone lesions caused by aluminum deposition are seen less often since aluminum hydroxide phosphate binders have generally been replaced by calcium carbonate in recent years.

Secondary hyperparathyroidism causes increased bone resorption (osteopenia) and increased bone formation with unmineralized bone matrix (osteitis fibrosa). Three stages are recognized in the progression of secondary hyperparathyroidism in chronic renal failure:

(1) **Compensatory**—increased parathyroid hormone (PTH) levels with normal (or low) serum calcium levels and only subclinical skeletal changes

(2) **Hypercalcemic**—increased serum calcium levels secondary to hypersecretion of PTH

(3) **Osteitis fibrosa cystica**—severe symptomatic bone lesions (fractures and aching bones) that are preventable or treatable by parathyroidectomy. However, parathyroidectomy is rarely necessary today, with new vitamin D analogues and better management of serum calcium and phosphate levels.

PTH affects cortical bone more than trabecular bone, and lesions develop over many years. Most dialysis patients take calcium carbonate to bind phosphate, but excessive calcium supplementation may produce painful extraskeletal (soft-tissue) calcifications and possibly contribute to vascular calcification.

6. How do these metabolic changes and their secondary effects impact quality of life?

Uremia and its treatments affect every aspect of life—diet, work, recreation, sex, cognition, and sleep. Symptoms associated with uremia and dialysis include **fatigue, decreased exercise tolerance, sleep disorders, headache**, and **muscle cramps**, all of which can limit function and reduce quality of life. The **time required for dialysis** treatments and, for many patients, **post-dialysis fatigue** can limit the time and energy available for work and recreation. Recent work has shown that longer or more frequent dialysis can eliminate most of these symptoms.

Surveys show that dialysis patients, especially home hemodialysis patients, consider their subjective quality of life almost as good as that reported by the normal healthy population.

However, objective measures, including employment and exercise capacity, indicate substantial quality of life deficits among these patients. Clinical attention to dialysis adequacy Kt/v > 1.2 (where K = dialyzer clearance of urea per t = dialysis time per v = volume of distribution of urea in the body), nutrition, and treatment of anemia reduces mortality and morbidity and improves rehabilitation. Unfortunately, too many patients in the U.S. still receive inadequate dialysis.

7. How is exercise tolerance influenced by the metabolic effects of chronic renal failure and ESRD?

The exercise tolerance of persons on dialysis is only about 50% of normal. In dialysis patients over age 60, fatigue is the most frequent reason given for activity limitations, with dialysis patients being more limited in their ability to climb stairs, walk, and perform heavy work around the house than a control group matched for age, race, sex, and cardiac problems.

The low rate of employment, fatigue, and reduced exercise capacity in ESRD patients was long attributed to renal anemia. However, these explanations have been challenged recently, as correction of anemia does not restore normal exercise tolerance or physical activity. Exercise training also fails to increase the physical capacity of dialysis patients as much as predicted by their hematocrit increase, so other metabolic dysfunction(s) also must contribute. Early fatigue and build-up of lactic acid with mild exercise are consistent with reduced oxygen extraction, even in athletic dialysis patients, but the precise defect in muscle metabolism is not yet known. Decreased muscle mass, decreased capillary density in muscles, and lower proportion of type 2 muscle fibers are typical in dialysis patients. Extremely low oxygen extraction rates, even in exercise-trained and nonanemic renal patients, have been attributed to defective aerobic metabolism in the muscles. Recent experience with more frequent dialysis suggests that defective muscle metabolism may be related to chronic uremia resulting from inadequate dialysis. *Or* more simply stated, the physiologic mechanism is still unknown.

8. How is erythropoietin used in treating the anemia of renal failure?

Anemia was almost universal among dialysis patients until the availability of recombinant human erythropoietin (EPO) in the late 1980s. EPO treatment replaces the hormone normally produced by the kidneys that stimulates red blood cell production. Currently, most ESRD patients take EPO to maintain a hematocrit near the target value of 33–36%, although some nephrologists recommend a higher (normal) target hematocrit. Correction of anemia with EPO clearly improves strength, endurance, functional status, and subjective quality of life in patients with renal failure. Some athletic dialysis patients can maintain a normal hematocrit with EPO and aerobic exercise training.

9. How should patients with renal failure be evaluated for an exercise program?

Most patients can benefit from an exercise program at any time, but early intervention prior to initiation of dialysis is optimal to prevent disability and maintain employment, relationships, and physical activity. Physical therapy is not always required but can facilitate recovery from transplantation, hospitalization, or deconditioning for any reason.

Most guidelines for aerobic exercise recommend a training heart rate, which is not useful for people taking β-adrenergic blocking drugs to control hypertension. Perceived exertion is a better guide for exercise intensity, because β-adrenergic blocking drugs blunt the normal exercise-induced increase in heart rate. Each patient should be evaluated for the specific risk factors summarized by Harter and Moore before beginning any exercise program. Contraindications include medical instability or severe comorbidities, such as uncontrolled diabetes, cardiovascular disease, osteodystrophy, and arthritis. Painter summarized the issue simply: "Once specific risks have been ruled out, the risks of not exercising are even greater than the risks of exercising."

Almost every patient with chronic renal failure or ESRD can safely do mild stretching and strengthening exercises, and many are capable of meeting the new NIH recommendation to accumulate a daily total of 30 minutes of moderately intense physical activity. Patients should be selected more carefully for strenuous aerobic exercise. Painter's guidelines for exercise during hemodialysis include prolonged warm-up and cool-down, and limiting stationary cycling to the first 2 hours of he-modialysis. Protection of the dialysis access during exercise is important for all patients. Peritoneal dialysis patients must avoid abdominal pressure when full with dialysate, but may do abdominal strengthening and stretching exercises part way through an exchange when they are only half full.

Frequent monitoring by healthcare providers is important for the early identification of med-ically significant changes in exercise tolerance, minor injuries that can discourage the habit of regular exercise, or the need to advance individual goals. Patients should keep an exercise diary of activity, intensity, and duration.

10. What are the benefits of exercise for patients with chronic renal failure and ESRD?

The benefits of exercise include all the benefits for the general population, plus additional benefits related to the special challenges of renal failure and associated comorbidity. Regular phys-ical exercise can slow, stop, or reverse the progressive deconditioning that often characterizes the course of kidney disease, thus preventing progressive frailty, maintaining independence, reducing post-dialysis fatigue, and speeding patients' recovery from illness and surgery (including trans-plantation). Aerobic conditioning improves blood pressure control, often reducing medication re-quirements, and reduces cardiac risks—both of which are serious problems for many of these patients. Exercise training improves glucose tolerance and insulin sensitivity in diabetics, who make up about one-third of the dialysis population. Aerobic exercise during hemodialysis may in-crease the ease of fluid removal, and it clearly reduces hypotensive episodes and muscle cramping. Moore and colleagues showed normal, safe cardiovascular changes with stationary cycling during the first 2 hours of hemodialysis, but some increased risk during the third hour.

11. What are the difficulties or challenges of exercise for chronic renal patients?

Post-dialysis fatigue makes a person want to rest, but excessive rest leads to progressive de-conditioning, which then lengthens the time required to recover from post-dialysis fatigue. Regular exercise is the key to breaking out of this spiral of decline into disability. The time con-straints of dialysis mean less time is available to be physically active, so the habit of regular exer-cise becomes even more important to balance the forced inactivity required for dialysis treatments. Peritoneal dialysis patients often find exercise difficult because of their feeling of fullness, so some exercise part way through an exchange when less full of dialysate.

Dialysis is a life-saving treatment, but many patients also need rehabilitation services to resume living fully. Recent national legislation allows dialysis patients to work for pay without fear of losing Medicare coverage, but many need regular exercise and better dialysis more than employment to improve the quality of their lives.

BIBLIOGRAPHY

1. Fitts SS: Physical benefits and challenges of exercise for people with chronic renal disease. J Renal Nutr 7:123–128, 1997.
2. Fitts SS, Guthrie MR, Blagg CR: Exercise coaching and rehabilitation counseling improve quality of life for predialysis and dialysis patients. Nephron 82:115–121, 1999.
3. Kutner NG, Cardenas DD, Bower JD: Rehabilitation, aging, and chronic renal disease. Am J Phys Med Rehabil 71:97–101, 1992.
4. Life Options Rehabilitation Advisory Council: Exercise for the Dialysis Patient: A Comprehensive Program. Madison, WI, Medical Education Institute, 1995.
5. Moore GE: Selecting dialysis patients for an exercise program. Semin Dialysis 8:42–44, 1994.
6. Moore GE, Painter PL, Brinker KR, et al: Cardiovascular response to submaximal stationary cycling during hemodialysis. Am J Kidney Dis 31:631–637, 1998.
7. Painter P: The importance of exercise training in rehabilitation of patients with end-stage renal disease. Am J Kidney Dis 24(suppl 1):S2–S9, 1994.
8. Painter P, Carlson L, Carey S, et al: Physical functioning and health-related quality of life changes with exercise training in hemodialysis patients. Am J Kidney Dis 35:482–492, 2000.
9. Raj DS, Charra B, Pierratos A, Work J: In search of ideal hemodialysis: Is prolonged frequent dialysis the answer? Am J Kidney Dis 34:597–610, 1999.
10. Stefanovic V, Stojanovic M, Djordjevic V: Effect of adequacy of dialysis and nutrition on morbidity and work-ing rehabilitation of patients treated by maintenance hemodialysis. Int J Artif Organs 23:83–89, 2000.

55. CANCER REHABILITATION: GENERAL PRINCIPLES

Ki Y. Shin, M.D., Theresa A. Gillis, M.D., and Fae Garden, M.D.

1. Why is cancer rehabilitation necessary?

Advances in early detection and treatment allow more people with cancer to live longer. In the U.S., there are an estimated 8.4 million people alive today with cancer with 1.2 million new cases a year and a relative 5-year survival rate of 59%. These cancer survivors frequently are left with physical deficits and psychosocial problems that diminish their quality of life. Over 80% of persons with lung, colorectal, and prostate cancer report having **gait problems**. Significant problems in activities of daily living (**ADLs**) and **vocation** also exist. Up to 50% of persons with cancer may meet the diagnostic criteria for **clinical depression**. With early rehabilitation intervention, the disability caused by cancer and cancer therapy can be minimized.

Many physiatrists do not have significant experience rehabilitating cancer patients. This may be due to a lack of recognition of rehab needs, training biases, or physicians who are uncomfortable dealing with a patient population with a poorer prognosis. Cancer rehabilitation is medically, emotionally, and physically challenging. However, as in most rehabilitation patients, improvements in function and quality of life can be significant, and possibly even more meaningful among those patients anticipating a shortened life span.

2. Who are the members of the typical cancer rehab team?

Team members include the nurse, physical therapist, occupational therapist, social worker, speech and language pathologist, psychologist, primary oncologist, case manager, chaplain, and dietician. A physiatrist can evaluate medical rehabilitation issues and assist with diagnosis and management. Rehabilitation issues may include fatigue, nutrition, neurogenic bowel and bladder management, pain control, body image, lymphedema management, prosthetic and orthotic fitting, and management of spasticity, weakness, and imbalance.

3. Explain some of the nutritional concerns of the cancer patient.

Between 40% and 80% of all cancer patients develop clinical **malnutrition**. This is affected by tumor type, stage of disease, and mode of therapy used to treat disease. Clinical effects of malnutrition include poor wound healing, poor skin turgor (which can contribute to skin breakdown and decubiti), wound dehiscence, electrolyte and fluid imbalances, endocrine dysfunction, and compromised immune function. Decreased appetite from nausea and vomiting associated with chemotherapy, as well as endogenous cytokine release, can exacerbate the severity of malnutrition.

4. What are the potential adverse effects of cancer surgery on nutrition?

Surgical procedures such as **radical neck dissection** or **glossectomy** can impair mastication, swallowing, taste, and smell. Patients undergoing **gastrectomy** or **bowel resection** can develop gastric stasis, diarrhea, steatorrhea, megaloblastic anemia, malabsorption, and deficiency of vitamins B_{12}, D, and A.

5. What are the adverse effects of radiation therapy on nutrition?

Radiation treatment to the **head and neck area** can produce alterations in taste and saliva production. Food texture and sensation alterations can occur from irradiation of the oral mucosa. Ulcerations, stomatitis, or mucositis can also occur. Radiation to the **stomach and intestines** can cause acute nausea, cramps, and diarrhea. Patients with radiation damage to the intestines are usually started on lactose-free, low-residue oral diets. Small, frequent meals and increased fluids are also usually recommended.

6. What nutritional deficiencies can occur with chemotherapy?

Antimetabolite drugs, such as methotrexate, inhibit the metabolism of folic acid, which is necessary for the synthesis of DNA. The resultant **folic acid deficiency** can result in macrocytic anemia, leukopenia, and ulcerative stomatitis. The antimetabolites 5-fluorouracil and 6-mercaptopurine prevent nucleic acid synthesis by interfering with thiamine in DNA synthesis. Clinical **thiamine deficiency** is associated with paresthesias, neuropathy, and heart failure. **Vitamin K deficiency** results from long-term treatment with adjunctive antibiotics, such as moxalactam disodium, leading to a pronounced bleeding tendency.

7. How does cancer or cancer treatment affect female sexual function?

During or following cancer treatment, sexual dysfunction can occur. Changes in body image, stress and anxiety related to the diagnosis and treatment, and pain following a mastectomy can have a negative impact on sexual response. Fear of partner rejection can lead to the avoidance of sexual intercourse. Women who have undergone pelvic surgery or irradiation need to be counseled about the possible need for vaginal dilators to prevent stenosis as well as the possibility of bleeding with intercourse. Some women may need to use artificial vaginal lubrication and try changes from their customary sexual positions. Side effects of chemotherapy and radiation therapy, including nausea, fatigue, hair loss, and weight changes, can produce additional psychological and physical roadblocks to resuming sexual activity.

8. What are some sexual dysfunctions that occur in male patients undergoing cancer treatment?

Impotence, retrograde ejaculation, and infertility can result from damage to the vascular or nerve pathways following surgical treatment for prostate cancer. If permanent sterilization is anticipated, preoperative and pretreatment discussion of reproductive concerns, including sperm banking, should be undertaken. Sexual rehabilitation can include the use of oral medications such as Viagra, erectile assistive devices, and surgical reconstruction of the phallus. Performance anxiety, fear of rejection or failure, and treatment-induced symptoms described above can also inhibit sexual function and satisfaction.

9. What is paraneoplastic syndrome?

When tumors produce signs and symptoms at a distance from the tumor or its metastases, they are referred to as paraneoplastic syndrome, or remote effects of malignancy. By definition, these syndromes should not be produced as a direct effect of the tumor or its metastases. Paraneoplastic syndromes develop in a minority of cancer patients. Those caused by the production of polypeptide hormones are the most frequent and include:

1. ACTH/Cushing's syndrome
2. Syndrome of inappropriate secretion of antidiuretic hormone (SIADH)
3. Hypercalcemia
4. Hypocalcemia
5. Hypophosphatemia osteomalacia
6. Calcitonin production by tumors
7. Hypoglycemia
8. Lambert-Eaton syndrome

10. Discuss the manifestations of hypercalcemia in cancer patients.

Hypercalcemia is common in cancer patients, occurring in approximately 10% of patients. Not all cases are associated with bone metastases. Tumor types associated with hypercalcemia include breast, lung, renal cell, and multiple myeloma. Clinical manifestations of hypercalcemia include polyuria, nocturia, and polydipsia. Symptoms of anorexia, easy fatigability, and weakness also occur. Late symptoms of hypercalcemia include apathy, irritability, depression, mental obtundation, nausea, vomiting, vague abdominal pain, constipation, and pruritus.

11. What causes pain in cancer patients?

Cancer patients may experience a variety of painful conditions, related to both treatment and the tumor processes. The most common treatment-induced pains include **mucositis** from radiation or chemotherapy and **peripheral neuropathies** from chemotherapy, particularly taxanes, vinca alkaloids, and platinum. Both etiologies may produce such severe pains that narcotic analgesics are warranted. The most common malignant cause of pain is **tumor invasion of bone** from either a primary or metastatic lesion. **Compression** or **infiltration of peripheral nerves** by tumor is the second most frequent cause. Cancer pain occurs in 51% of all patients and 74% of those with advanced or terminal disease.

12. How can medications be used in managing cancer pain?

The World Health Organization recommends the stepwise use of non-opioid analgesics, adjuvant drugs, and opioids. **Aspirin** and **NSAIDs** are useful to control the pain of bone metastases because they are potent prostaglandin synthetase inhibitors. However, a therapeutic ceiling prevents significant dose-escalation of these medications. **Corticosteroids** produce analgesia by preventing the release of prostaglandin and are helpful in reducing pain from tumor infiltration of nerves and spinal cord. Adjuvant therapy includes **tricyclic antidepressants,** which block reuptake of serotonin in the CNS. **Carbamazepine, phenytoin, gabapentin**, and **methadone** can be effective in the treatment of neuropathic pain. Narcotic analgesics include (from weakest to strongest) **codeine, oxycodone**, and **morphine**. Transdermal preparations, sustained release formulations, and narcotics with longer half-lives than morphine are also available. There is no ceiling effect for these analgesics. Side effects may necessitate changes in route of delivery or rotation to another narcotic agent. Demerol (meperidine) is not recommended for the treatment of cancer pain due to its short duration of action and its potential for adverse CNS effects on repeated use. Narcotic analgesics are often *improperly underprescribed* in the treatment of severe cancer pain.

13. Describe some neurostimulatory and neuroablative procedures that are used in the treatment of cancer pain.

Neurostimulatory procedures include transcutaneous and percutaneous electrical nerve stimulation. This technique is indicated in the treatment of painful dysesthesias from tumor infiltration of a nerve. Dorsal column stimulation of the spinal cord has limited use in treatment of deafferentation pain in the chest, midline, and lower extremities. **Neuroablative procedures** include nerve root rhizotomy, which can be used to treat somatic and deafferentation pain from tumor infiltration of the cranial and intercostal nerves. Neuroablative procedures to the spinal cord include tractotomy of the dorsal root entry zone lesions, cordotomy, and myelotomy.

14. How can psychological interventions be used to manage cancer pain?

Psychological techniques may enable patients with cancer to regain a much-needed sense of personal control. Mental imagery, hypnosis, relaxation, biofeedback, music therapy, meditation, and other cognitive or behavioral methods can directly relieve pain as well as anxiety, which can enhance analgesia.

15. What is Pancoast's syndrome?

Pancoast's syndrome is caused by carcinomas in the superior pulmonary sulcus. The tumor produces pain in the distribution of C8 and T1–T2 nerves, as well as a Horner's syndrome. A shadow can sometimes be seen on chest films at the apex of the lung. Patients with Pancoast's syndrome usually complain of severe, unrelenting pain that often begins at the shoulder and vertebral border of the scapula. Radiation and surgery are recommended treatments.

16. What is the most common form of radiation-induced spinal cord damage?

Transient myelopathy or **Lhermitte's syndrome**, which may occur in patients being treated for head and neck tumors or lymphoma. The syndrome typically develops after a latent period of 1–30 months, with the peak incidence for onset of symptoms at 4–6 months after completion of treatment. Symptoms include electrical dysesthesias or paresthesias that radiate from the cervical spine to the extremities. These sensations usually occur in a symmetric fashion. Diagnostic imaging studies are typically normal. The syndrome usually resolves in 1–9 months after onset.

17. What is delayed myelopathy?

This irreversible condition typically occurs 9–18 months after completion of radiation treatment. The latent period for delayed myelopathy decreases with increased radiation dose and is also shortened in children. Functional deficits depend, for the most part, on the level of neurologic injury. Pain is not a prominent feature, in contrast to myelopathy related to metastatic spinal cord compression. Prompt initiation of steroid therapy with early symptoms may lessen the severity of the motor and sensory losses.

18. You are seeing a patient with suspected postradiation brachial plexopathy. How can this be distinguished from plexopathy due to tumor infiltration?

Plexopathy due to tumor invasion is up to 10 times more common than post-radiation plexopathy. Horner's syndrome (ptosis, enophthalmos), progressive pain, and lower trunk involvement are more common in neoplastic plexopathies. Upper trunk involvement is also more common in radiation plexopathy. Electrodiagnostic findings such as myokymic discharges and abnormal sensory conduction studies are more common in patients with radiation plexopathy.

19. Many patients undergoing cancer treatment have low platelet counts. Does the presence of thrombocytopenia affect the exercise prescription?

Vigorous exercise in the presence of thrombocytopenia may increase the risk of intra-articular bleeding. It is common practice to withhold resistive exercise therapy when platelet levels are < 10,000/mm^3. In early chemotherapy studies prior to the availability of platelet transfusions, the risk of intracerebral bleeding became more significant below this level.

20. How do cancer amputees differ from dysvascular or traumatic amputees?

Patients with cancer often face functional declines associated with chemotherapy or recurrent disease. Many sarcoma patients are treated with pre- and postoperative chemotherapy protocols, with the attendant risks of anemia, fatigue, anorexia and nutritional depletion, nausea, and cardiovascular toxicity while recovering from the amputation. Prosthesis fitting can also be complicated in patients who are receiving chemotherapy due to weight fluctuations caused by poor nutrition and/or edema. Irradiated skin is often less tolerant to prosthesis contact. All patients should be considered for prosthetic prescription, but special attention must be given to the cancer treatment protocol when planning fabrication, fitting, and training.

The energy costs of prosthetic gait may be particularly unrealistic in severely compromised patients; avoidance of immobility and deconditioning should be a primary concern for these patients *prior to* amputation. Cosmetic prosthesis should be offered to patients unable to use a functional limb.

21. What is meant by "limb salvage"? What procedures does this entail?

Limb salvage describes efforts toward maintaining a functional extremity and avoiding amputation in the treatment of sarcomas and bone metastases from other tumors. The plan may employ the use of reconstruction techniques with custom or modular segmental prostheses and/or allograft or autograft transfer of bony or muscular tissues. Limited resections of muscle groups, compartments, or partial bones may be necessary. Partial resections of the sacrum, pelvis, scapulae, and femur such as the Girdlestone procedure and internal hemipelvectomy are frequently seen. Cemented prosthetic hip and knee components and intramedullary rods of the humerus and femur are very common. Rehabilitation must be tailored to address intact and unstable structures.

22. What is the Van Nes procedure?

Tibial rotationplasty is used in the pediatric population to provide a functional "knee" joint after resection of tumors about the knee. The neurovascular structures about the knee must be free of tumor, and the popliteal vessels, sciatic nerve, and saphenous vein must be intact. The remaining distal tibia is rotated 180° and reattached to the femoral shaft, with the ankle serving as the knee joint. The quadriceps are joined to the gastrocsoleus complex, while the hamstrings are connected to the ankle dorsiflexors.

The advantages to the Van Nes procedure include preservation of femoral shaft length, particularly for very young children, as the rotated tibial growth plate is intact. At skeletal maturity, the patient has a substantial residual limb for prosthetic fitting. The skin of the foot tolerates prosthetic wear very well. The limb appearance is unusual but acceptable to the patients. A custom below-knee prosthesis is necessary.

As an alternative to rotationplasty, amputation and segmental endoprosthesis have advantages and disadvantages as well. Expandable endoprostheses must be used in children, with frequent lengthening at regular intervals, and these devices have a high rate of mechanical failure and loosening. Energy expenditure during gait following rotationplasty and above-knee amputation has been studied, but two separate studies were unable to show statistically significant differences in energy expenditure or cost between these two patient groups.

23. What is an internal forequarter amputation? Does it really exist?

No. Actually, the correct term is **en bloc upper humeral interscapulothoracic resection**, much more easily referred to as a Tikhoff-Lindberg resection.

24. How is the Tikhoff-Lindberg procedure done?

The procedure is appropriate for some tumors of the shoulder region which were previously subject to forequarter amputations. Resection of the proximal humerus, partial or total scapulectomy, and claviculotomy are required, with a humeral endoprosthesis implanted and fixed to the remaining clavicle or chest wall.

Early rehabilitation should avoid humeral motion, and after acute healing is complete, passive range beyond 90° abduction and adduction should not be attempted. Patients may choose to wear slings for additional support, particularly if the arm is large. Immediate postoperative compression with low stretch bandages may delay lymphedema development and permit early fitting with custom garments. Very limited passive shoulder motion remains, and the limb is essentially non-weight-bearing and nonlifting. Patients can retain active elbow motion and excellent hand and forearm function. A soft shoulder prosthesis allows a more cosmetic clothing fit.

25. What are the most common malignant bone tumors?

Carcinomas **metastatic to bone** account for > 40-fold more cases than all primary bone tumors combined. Breast cancer accounts for most bone metastases, with an incidence of bone metastases in this disease of 50–85%. Prostate carcinoma is the most common primary tumor for metastatic lesions in men, with bone metastases occurring in > 90% of patients with advanced disease. Lung, renal, bladder, thyroid, and bowel primaries each have an incidence of bone metastases of 20–40% at autopsy.

Myeloma is the most common primary malignant tumor of bone in adults, arising within the bone marrow from plasma cells. Osteosarcomas, Ewing's sarcomas, and chondrosarcoma are the most common tumors arising from bone tissue itself. In children, osteosarcoma, Ewing's sarcoma, and primitive neuroectodermal tumors (in descending order) are the most predominant primary malignant bone tumors.

26. When is a bone susceptible to pathologic fracture?

Pathologic fractures occur in 10–30% of patients with metastases and are seen most frequently in the long bones, particularly the femur and humerus. Bone strength is determined by the cortical and trabecular structure. Cortical destruction increases susceptibility of bone to torsional/rotational forces. The guidelines most frequently cited for increased risk of fracture are as follows:

1. Cortical bone destruction affecting ≥ 50% of the circumference as seen on anteroposterior and lateral radiographs or cross-sectional CT
2. Lytic lesions ≥ 2.5 cm in the proximal femur

3. Pathologic avulsion fracture of the lesser trochanter of the femur
4. Persisting or increasing pain with weight-bearing despite completion of radiotherapy
These estimates of fracture risk are used synonymously as indications for prophylactic fixation. An inherent limitation to this list is that tumor extent can be greatly underestimated by radiographs.

27. What rehabilitation methods may be used in managing bone metastases?

Some patients receive prophylactic fixation of metastatic lesions, employing internal fixation, methylmethacrylate and modular prosthesis, or other hardware. After operative management, restoration of mobility and self-care through a rehabilitation approach is essential.

The most painful bone metastases are treated with radiotherapy. During radiation, bone is placed at increased risk of fracture due to hyperemic softening of bone and necrosis of tumor cells, and complete reossification may not occur until 6 months or more after treatment. In theory, therefore, precautions and reduced load-bearing may be indicated for many months. During periods of greatest risk, and for nonsurgical candidates, unloading affected bones with assistive devices, braces, or immobilizers is recommended. Mobility issues with activity restrictions and adaptive equipment for ADLs should be addressed by physiatrists.

28. What are the most common initial symptoms caused by metastases to the spine?

Four symptoms characterize the clinical picture of spinal cord compression: pain, weakness, autonomic dysfunction, and sensory loss including ataxia. Pain is usually the initial symptom and can manifest as central back pain with or without radicular pain.

29. Does the pain of spinal cord tumor differ from the pain caused by a herniated intervertebral disc?

The pain caused by an epidural tumor is described as being worse when the patient is lying down. Patients may complain of being awakened from sleep several times during the night, and some may describe a need to sleep in a sitting position. Radiographs of the spine can reveal bony abnormalities at the painful site of suspected cord compression.

30. When should one consider epidural spinal cord compression in a cancer patient with back pain?

Always! The spine is the most common site for skeletal metastases, regardless of the primary tumor. Early diagnosis is essential, as the outcome is related to patient function at diagnosis— i.e., if a patient is paraplegic at diagnosis, he or she will remain so after treatment. Epidural spinal cord compression from metastasis occurs in 10–33% of cancer patients, and in 10% of these patients, cord compression is the presenting manifestation of malignancy.

31. When evaluating for spinal metastases, what radiologic studies are indicated?

In patients with cancer or high suspicion for malignancy or epidural spinal cord compression, MRI is often the first diagnostic test. Plain films and bone scan are of additional help in planning for surgical intervention and radiation therapy. In patients with back pain but without cancer or a high suspicion for malignancy, radiographs are often obtained when a patient does not respond to therapy. Although the vertebral body is usually the site first affected by metastases, 30–50% of cancellous bone here must be destroyed before change is seen on plain film. Therefore, destruction of the pedicle is usually discovered first on anteroposterior films. If back pain persists and radiographs are normal, bone scintigraphy or MRI is indicated. The sensitivity of bone scans for metastases is high. MRI clearly delineates epidural disease.

32. What interventions are most appropriate for metastatic spinal disease?

When epidural spinal cord compression is present, all patients require urgent intravenous steroid therapy. Studies show better functional outcomes and reduced pain with surgical resection and stabilization, followed by radiation. A posterolateral surgical approach allows access to the vertebral body, where most metastases occur. Laminectomies alone do not resect tumor and may further destabilize the spine. For patients who are not surgical candidates, radiation alone can be offered but it does not address concerns of spinal bony stability.

When tumor does not invade beyond the cortex, fluoroscopically guided injections of methylmethacrylate may be used to increase stability and reduce pain. Radiation therapy is the standard treatment for most bone-only spinal metastases.

33. What are some primary spinal cord tumors?

Ependymomas and astrocytomas are the usual intramedullary (located in the substance of the cord) tumors. Extramedullary tumors include neurofibromas and meningiomas. Most malignant lesions affecting the spinal cord are metastases from various primary tumors. Extradural spinal cord compression is a common neurologic complication of systemic malignancy.

34. What disability results after radical neck dissection? How is this best managed?

The spinal accessory nerve is usually sacrificed during radical neck dissection, causing loss of trapezius function. The scapula rotates upward and abduction is limited to only 60–70°. Shoulder pain frequently results, and lifting and overhead activities may become impossible.

Strengthening the levator scapulae, rhomboideus, and serratus anterior muscles may help stabilize the scapula, allow improved shoulder elevation, and reduce pain. Attempts to strengthen the deltoids, supraspinatus, or infraspinatus should be discouraged, as this only increases pain and further overworks the disadvantaged muscles. Pectoralis muscle contracture aggravates the protracted shoulder and results from lack of pull from the opposing trapezius. Therefore, pectoral stretches and maintenance of good scapular positioning is crucial. Some patients reduce their discomfort through use of a figure-of-eight orthosis, sling, or other orthoses to provide support against gravity, or by habitually hooking their hand on a pants pocket.

35. How do brain tumor patients differ from brain injury patients?

Most patients with primary brain tumors experience rapid improvement in function following tumor excision. Normal brain tissue has been compressed by tumor, so with pressure relief, recovery can be dramatic and the patient may return to normal function. However, many tumors recur, and with repeated excisions and invasion of normal tissue by tumor, further functions are lost. Radiation and chemotherapy can further limit recovery through lost plasticity and cognitive effects. Despite advances in treatment, most patients with glioblastoma multiforme or high-grade astrocytomas survive 2 years or less; therefore, rehabilitation goals should encompass this pattern of decline.

36. What is the most common primary brain tumor? Metastatic tumor?

Gliomas comprise about 60% of all primary CNS tumor. The most common tumors that metastasize to the brain are **carcinomas of the lung and breast**. Most brain metastases involve the cerebrum, with the frontal lobe being the most common site. Metastases to the cerebellum are less frequent, and those to the brainstem are the least frequent.

37. What rehabilitation needs are greatest among brain tumor patients?

Deficits experienced by brain tumor patients are clearly related to the involved structure. Cognitive deficits are quite prevalent and also related to the site of lesions. Neurobehavioral changes may be the most prominent problems faced by patients with tumors. Memory losses, reasoning and problem-solving skills, decreased energy or initiative, and inability to return to work are cited more frequently by family members as problems than difficulty with ambulation, bowel or bladder dysfunction, ADLs, or aphasia.

38. Describe the neuropsychological abnormalities found in patients with brain tumors.

The scope of cognitive effects ranges from subtle attention and motivational problems to frank delirium and clouding of consciousness. These deficits can be due to the primary effects of tumor or secondary effects of treatment. Patients with rapid-growing tumors, such as glioblastoma multiforme, exhibit behavioral and cognitive deficits secondary to rapid destruction of white matter tracts, increased intracranial pressure, and metabolic deficits. Patients with slow-growing tumors often do not demonstrate neuropsychological deficits, possibly due to a reorganization of cognitive functions to other brain regions.

Following radiotherapy to the brain, 14% of patients show subacute cognitive effects occurring 1–4 months after treatment; this effect is due to a reversible demyelination, and gradual improvement in functional status over the next 2–3 months distinguishes this condition from signs of early tumor recurrence. Up to 18% of neurologically normal cancer patients who receive chemotherapy have cognitive deficits after chemotherapy is discontinued. These deficits include impaired visual perception, verbal memory, and judgment.

39. Describe some available treatments of breast cancer.

Over the years, standard treatment of breast cancer has evolved from radical mastectomies to breast-conservation strategies. Modified radical mastectomies spare the pectoralis major muscle but include axillary dissection. Other surgical options include lumpectomy, segmental mastectomy, or total mastectomy with or without axillary dissection. Varying combinations of radiotherapy, hormonal therapy, and adjuvant chemotherapy have further reduced mortality. Sentinel node mapping, which traces the drainage pattern of the tumor site, can reduce the number of nodes resected.

40. Describe a postoperative rehabilitation program for women who have undergone mastectomy.

In general, postmastectomy patients without reconstruction are allowed to perform shoulder range of motion (ROM) to 40° of abduction and flexion immediately after surgery. Some physicians prefer the use of abduction slings or pillows immediately postoperatively with the goal of minimizing pain within this range. Immediately post-op, therapies consist of hand, wrist, and elbow ROM, positioning, and postural exercises. In addition, external rotation of the shoulder with the elbow maintained at the side and scapular retractions are indicated. After surgical drains are removed, active ROM can be increased. Supine abduction eliminates substitutions and compensatory bending, which patients may use during wall-climbing and overhead pulley exercises. When all sutures have been removed, facilitated and passive stretch may be pursued to the patient's limits of pain.

41. Define postmastectomy lymphedema.

Postmastectomy lymphedema is a collection of lymph in the interstitial tissues, resulting in a functional overload of the lymphatic system. The edema is usually confined to subcutaneous fat and skin. Lymphedema can follow lumpectomy, segmental resection, or radical mastectomy. Its etiology is likely multifactorial, caused by a combination of excision of lymph channels, inflammation of involved tissues, and coagulation of lymph. Fibrosis of breast tissue by radiation and local infection can also increase the risk of developing lymphedema. Some studies report that lymphedema affects between 25.5% and 38.3% of patients having axillary node dissection and radiation therapy.

42. Explain the conservative management techniques used for lymphedema.

Elevation, compression wrapping, manual lymph drainage massage techniques, and low resistance exercise of the distal musculature have been advocated. Compression of the affected extremity with low stretch bandages may be sufficient, but refractory edema may require a combination of compressive wrapping, manual lymph massage, and activity restrictions to control swelling. Some centers and therapists continue to use sequential compression pumps for lymphedema management with good results. There are few if any well-designed outcome studies comparing wrapping techniques and massage vs. compression pumps. Lymphedema treatments should be monitored closely for patient complaints of shortness of breath and significant pain. Ideally with either treatment, when limb circumference becomes stable without further improvements, the patient should be fitted for a custom support sleeve to be worn daily.

43. What concerns are raised when examining a patient with post-mastectomy lymphedema?

Recurrent disease, upper extremity deep venous thrombosis, and cellulitis can all exacerbate lymphedema. A proper evaluation and work-up should precede any conservative treatment program.

These same concerns should arise when patients with a history of pelvic, groin, or lower extremity tumors develop lower extremity edema.

44. What is a good website for cancer information?

www.cancernet.gov is a National Cancer Institute website affiliated with the NIH. It is updated regularly and has general as well as site-specific information including treatments, prognosis, and ongoing research.

BIBLIOGRAPHY

1. Bonica JJ: Treatment of cancer pain: Current status and future needs. Adv Pain Res Ther 9:589–616, 1985.
2. Byrd R: Late effects of treatment of cancer in children. Pediatr Clin North Am 32:835–851, 1985.
3. DeLisa JA, Miller RM, Melnick RR, et al: Rehabilitation of the cancer patient. In DeVita VT, Hellman S, Rosenberg SA (eds): Cancer: Principles and Practice of Oncology, 6th ed. Philadelphia, Lippincott Williams & Wilkins, 2001.
4. Dropcho EJ: Central nervous system injury by therapeutic irradiation. Neurol Clin North Am 9:969–988, 1991.
5. Fallowfield LJ, Baumm M, Maguire GP: Effects of breast conservation on psychological morbidity associated with diagnosis and treatment of early breast cancer. BMJ 293:1331, 1986.
6. Garden FH, Grabois M (eds): Cancer rehabilitation. Physical Medicine and Rehabilitation: State of the Art Reveiws, vol. 8, no. 2. Philadelphia, Hanley & Belfus, 1994.
7. Gerber L, Lampert M, Wood C, et al: Comparison of pain, motion, and edema after modified radical mastectomy vs local excision with axillary dissection and radiation. Breast Cancer Res Treat 21:139–145, 1992.
8. Harper CM, Thomas JE: Distinction between neoplastic and radiation-induced brachial plexopathy, with emphasis on the role of EMG. Neurology 39:502–506, 1989.
9. Kaplan HS: A neglected issue: The sexual side effects of current treatments for breast cancer. J Sex Mar Ther 18:3–19, 1992.
10. Lehmann JF, DeLisa JA, Warren CG, et al: Cancer rehabilitation: Assessment of need, development and evaluation of a model of care. Arch Phys Med Rehabil 59:410–419, 1978.
11. Mandi A, Szepesi K, Morocz I: Surgical treatment of pathologic fractures from metastatic tumors of long bones. Orthopedics 14:43–50, 1991.
12. Meyers CA, Abbruzzese JL: Cognitive functioning in cancer patients: Effect of previous treatment. Neurology 42:434–436, 1992.
13. Williams F, Maly B: Pain rehabilitation: 3. Cancer pain, pelvic pain and age-related considerations. Arch Phys Med Rehabil 75:S15–20, 1994.
14. Erickson VS, Pearson ML, Ganz PA, et al: Arm edema in breast cancer patients. J Natl Cancer Inst 93:96–111, 2001.

56. REHABILITATION OF THE INDIVIDUAL WITH HIV AND AIDS

Stephen F. Levinson, M.D., Ph.D., and Steven M. Fine, M.D., Ph.D.

1. Why have a chapter on AIDS in a book on rehabiltation?

For two major reasons—first, HIV/AIDS and its treatment can result in disability, and second, patients traditionally seen for rehabilitation may be infected with HIV.

2. What is the difference between HIV infection and AIDS?

Human immunodeficiency virus (HIV) infects and destroys CD4 lymphocytes, leaving patients susceptible to opportunistic infections. The Centers for Disease Control has defined AIDS as either a CD4 count < $200/mm^3$ (normal range, 400 to $1600/mm^3$) or HIV infection with a recognized opportunistic infection. Patients with high viral loads may progress from initial HIV infection to AIDS within a few years, whereas those with very low viral loads may remain free of symptoms for 15 years or longer.

3. Can I catch AIDS from my patients?

Transmission of HIV from patient to health care worker is rare and requires percutaneous or mucous membrane exposure to blood, bloody fluids, or other cell-containing body fluids. The risk of contracting HIV is *negligible if universal precautions are followed with every patient.* Even if exposed, postexposure prophylaxis with antiretroviral agents, started within an hour, can reduce the risk of contracting the virus.

4. When should a test for HIV be ordered?

HIV testing should be considered for anyone who requests it and for patients with symptoms of an opportunistic infection. HIV testing should be recommended to anyone with tuberculosis and considered for patients with risk factors such as IV drug use or in homosexual or bisexual men who develop zoster. Informed consent is required, as is follow-up counseling. Many states require reporting of positive results. Screening for antibodies to HIV is done with the enzyme-linked immunosorbent assay (ELISA), with the western blot used for confirmation. The HIV polymerase chain reaction (PCR) is used to measure viral load and should not be used for screening.

5. What should I know about the medications used to treat HIV?

Currently, three different classes of drugs are used in combination to treat HIV infection:

Nucleoside analogue reverse transcriptase inhibitors, including zidovudine, lamivudine, didanosine, zalcitabine, stavudine, and abacavir, are associated with bone marrow toxicity, peripheral neuropathy, pancreatitis, mitochondrial toxicities, and lipid abnormalities.

Non-nucleoside analogue reverse transcriptase inhibitors, such as efavirenz, nevirapine, and delavirdine, can cause neurologic side effects, rash, and hepatotoxicity.

Protease inhibitors, which include nelfinavir, indinavir, ritonavir, saquinavir, agenerase, and lopinavir, are associated with mitochondrial toxicity and lipid abnormalities.

HIV can rapidly develop resistance, and every effort should be made to ensure that patients do not miss even a single dose. If for some reason treatment with any agent needs to be interrupted, *all* antiretrovirals should be stopped to avoid the emergence of drug resistance.

6. What are the causes of disability in HIV infection?

General deconditioning often occurs in *Pneumocystis carinii* pneumonia, the most common opportunistic infection in AIDS. Kaposi's sarcoma presents as dark purple lesions that may be found anywhere on the skin, as well as in oral, lymphatic, and visceral sites. Dysphagia and edema are common, with pain being a particular problem when lesions involve the feet. HIV cardiomyopathy as well as cardiomyopathies associated with the treatment of associated malignancies should be kept in mind when planning a rehabilitation program. Other causes of disability include gastrointestinal (GI) and rheumatologic disorders and chronic fatigue. Neurologic disorders, however, are the most frequent cause of disability.

7. What GI disorders are seen in persons with HIV?

Diarrhea and **malabsorption** are commonly caused by HIV, opportunistic infections, and antiretroviral therapy. Good nutrition is important and supplementation may be required. **Swallowing disorders** may result from neurologic deficits, the sicca syndrome, or candidal and herpetic pharyngitis and esophagitis. A modified swallow or hyperalimentation may be instituted in patients who do not respond to treatment of the underlying cause.

8. What are the causes of chronic fatigue?

Fibromyalgia, pulmonary dysfunction, anemia, encephalopathy, endocrine dysfunction, myopathies, cardiomyopathy, psychiatric disorders, depression, and side effects of medications can contribute to fatigue. Although many patients complain that their medications cause fatigue, most gain energy when on effective antiretroviral therapy. As in any disease complicated by chronic fatigue, exercise, energy conservation, and pacing of activities can be helpful in building endurance.

9. What types of arthritis are seen in HIV?

Psoriatic arthritis, Reiter's syndrome, and reactive arthritis have all been described. An AIDS-associated arthritis may be chronic or transient, with a predominance of lower limb involvement. Treatment is with NSAIDs, physical therapy, and, if indicated, steroid injections. Avascular necrosis of the hip and other joints is common, painful, and difficult to recognize in HIV patients and may be related to weight-lifting, steroid use, and other poorly characterized factors. Diagnosis is based on MRI findings.

10. Discuss the myopathies seen in HIV.

Autoimmune polymyositis may occur at all stages of infection and is usually steroid-responsive. It is subacute and presents with proximal muscle weakness and thigh pain on exertion. Mitochondrial myopathy caused by nucleoside analogue therapy presents with the insidious onset of myalgias, tenderness, and weakness. HIV wasting syndrome gradually and symmetrically weakens the proximal muscles, predominantly in the lower extremities.

11. What neurologic complications are seen in HIV infection?

Cognitive dysfunction can result from HIV dementia, cryptococcal meningitis, iatrogenic encephalopathies, and from numerous encephalopathies listed in the table.

The **AIDS dementia complex** is a subcortical cognitive, behavioral, and motor impairment often seen during the late stages of AIDS. **Focal impairments** may include hemiparesis, ataxia, aphasia, dysarthria, swallowing disorders, and cranial nerve defects. **Movement disorders** such as hemichorea, ballismus, segmental myoclonus, parkinsonism, postural tremor, and dystonia are also seen. **Visual loss** from CMV retinitis can be particularly devastating.

Common Causes of Encephalopathy in HIV

Infection

Cerebral toxoplasmosis
- Most common cause of multifocal mass lesions
- Ring-enhancing on MRI
- Often rapid in onset, usually responsive to treatment
- May also cause encephalopathy and meningoencephalitis

Cytomegalovirus (CMV)
- Coinfection may play a role in subacute encephalitis
- May cause subacute progressive polyradiculopathy and myelitis
- Periventriculitis often involving cranial nerves
- Retinitis can cause blindness
- Often responds to treatment with ganciclovir and foscarnet

Progressive multifocal leukoencephalopathy (PML)
- Insidious onset, caused by JC virus
- May be halted or reversed with restoration of immune function

Herpes simplex virus (HSV)
- HSV-1 may cause acute encephalitis
- HSV-2 is usually more self-limited
- Both are associated with myelitis and autonomic dysfunction
- Responds to treatment with acyclovir

Varicella zoster virus
- Causes encephalitis, transverse and ascending myelitis, leukoencephalopathy
- Nerve palsies and painful zoster are common
- Responds to high-dose acyclovir instituted early in the course

Epstein-Barr virus (EBV)
- Causes encephalitis, acute cerebellar syndrome, acute psychosis, transverse or ascending myelitis
- May play a role in pathogenesis of primary CNS lymphoma

Bacterial or fungal brain abscesses

Neurosyphilis

Tuberculosis

Table continued on following page

Common Causes of Encephalopathy in HIV (Continued)

Malignant lesions
　　Lymphoma (second most common intracerebral mass lesion)
　　Metastatic Kaposi's sarcoma
　　Paraneoplastic syndromes
Cerebrovascular disorders
　　Thrombotic, embolic hemorrhagic, and vasculitic

---

12. What are some of the spinal cord dysfunctions seen in HIV infection?

Vacuolar myelopathy is a spinal cord disorder that is strongly associated with HIV encephalopathy and has a similar pathology. Patients present with progressive paraparesis, ataxia, posterior column loss, spasticity, and neurogenic bladder and bowel. Other causes of spinal cord dysfunction include aseptic, cryptococcal, and lymphomatous meningitis, spinal tuberculosis (Pott's disease), and viral myelitis from varicella-zoster, herpes simplex, cytomegalovirus, and HTLV-I-associated tropical spastic paraparesis. An association with multiple sclerosis has also been suggested.

13. Which neuropathies are seen in HIV infection?

Distal symmetrical polyneuropathy is seen in advanced disease, being present in virtually all cases at autopsy. Other causes of peripheral neuropathy include vitamin B_{12} deficiency, segmental herpes zoster, compression neuropathy and mononeuritis simplex and multiplex associated with vasculitis. Drug-induced neuropathies are also seen in association with treatment with dapsone, didanosine, ethambutol, isoniazid, rifabutin, rifampin, stavudine, vincristine, zalcitabine, and zidovudine.

Inflammatory demyelinating polyneuropathies, such as Guillain-Barré syndrome, are often seen early in HIV and may exhibit a relapsing and remitting course. These disorders must be distinguished from **progressive polyradiculopathy**, which occurs late in AIDS and is highly correlated with cytomegalovirus infection. Presenting as a subacute ascending flaccid paraparesis, progressive polyradiculopathy is rapidly fatal but may respond to ganciclovir if it is started within the first 24–48 hours.

14. How are focal deficits and spinal cord dysfunction managed?

The management of focal deficits requires an aggressive, comprehensive team approach specific to the particular deficits involved. The rehabilitation approach to myelopathy should take into account the prognosis and concomitant cognitive dysfunction. Over-rehabilitation (planning for expected further decline in function) is often indicated, provided the patient is emotionally ready. Gait disturbances may be managed with gait aids, wheelchairs, and orthotics. Home modifications and adaptive equipment should emphasize comfort and simplicity. Sphincter disturbances should be managed as in other neurologic disorders.

15. How can HIV-related neuropathies be managed?

Pain may be managed with first-generation tricyclic agents (e.g., amitriptyline), gabapentin (Neurontin), lamotrigine (Lamictal) and topical lidocaine (typically in a patch). Physical modalities, TENS, and footwear modifications may also be of use. Ambulatory aids, orthotics, and adaptive equipment may be helpful in the management of proprioceptive loss and symptomatic motor weakness. Light resistive exercise may be instituted if the lesions are incomplete and stable.

16. How does HIV present in children?

Children often exhibit a more rapid progression when infected *in utero* rather than perinatally. Common features include failure to thrive, diarrhea, and organomegaly. **HIV encephalopathy** is characterized by delayed developmental milestones, impaired cognition and expressive language, spastic diplegia and ataxia, and other cerebellar abnormalities. It often improves with antiretroviral treatment. The rehabilitation management is not unlike that in spastic diplegic cerebral palsy.

17. What about the psychosocial and vocational aspects of HIV?

Central to the rehabilitation of any individual is the relationship of the patient to his or her social support systems. In the person with HIV, the caregiver will play a crucial role in preventing the onset of AIDS and in the recovery of immune function. Treatment adherence is crucial and must be the central focus of any rehabilitation effort. Adherence to antiretroviral medications must be better than 95% to prevent the development of resistance. Adherence interventions can come in many forms and may include a counselor, medisets, various reminder systems, and frequent visits to health care providers. Even those who have progressed to AIDS often enjoy an astonishing recovery of function after effective treatment. People with HIV are often able to work for years without disability.

18. What is the future of HIV rehabilitation?

The future of HIV treatment is changing dramatically. The primary focus in recent years has shifted from the management of symptoms to the prevention of disease and debility. Persons who can achieve high levels of adherence to antiretroviral combinations may not progress at all, and those who have progressed may show dramatic improvement with treatment. Despite these tremendous advances, social and psychiatric issues, substance abuse, medication toxicities, and viral resistance prevent a large percentage of patients from benefiting fully. Many of these will experience disabilities amenable to rehabilitation. Fortunately, the principles of rehabilitation in HIV disease are similar to those in other disorders, and hence, rehabilitation professionals are well prepared to meet the challenge.

BIBLIOGRAPHY

1. Bartlett JG, Gallant JE (eds): Medical Management of HIV Infection 2000–2001. Baltimore, Johns Hopkins University School of Medicine, 2000.
2. Levinson SF, Fine SM: Rehabilitation of the individual with human immunodeficiency virus. In DeLisa JA, Gans BM et al (eds): Rehabilitation Medicine: Principles and Practice, 3rd ed. Philadelphia, J. B. Lippincott, 1998, pp 1319–1335.
3. Levinson SF, O'Connell PG: Rehabilitation dimensions of AIDS: A review. Arch Phys Med Rehabil 72:690–696, 1991.
4. Mukand J (ed): Rehabilitation for Patients with HIV Disease. New York, McGraw-Hill, 1991.
5. O'Dell MW, Levinson SF, Riggs RV: Focused review: Physiatric management of HIV-related disability. Arch Phys Med Rehabil 77:S66–S73, 1996.
6. O'Dell MW (ed): HIV-Related Disability: Assessment and Management. Physical Medicine and Rehabilitation: State of the Art Reviews, vol. 7. Philadelphia, Hanley & Belfus, 1993.

57. REHABILITATIVE MANAGEMENT OF RHEUMATIC DISEASES

Jeanne E. Hicks, M.D., Galen O. Joe, M.D., and Jay P. Shah, M.D.

GENERAL DIAGNOSIS, TREATMENT, AND REHAB

1. How do you distinguish between noninflammatory and inflammatory arthritis?

Noninflammatory arthritis is usually not associated with acute onset, fever, increased white blood cell (WBC) count and sedimentation rate (ESR), redness and heat in a joint; the joint fluid has < 2000 mm^3 WBCs; there is no extraarticular or systemic involvement; and x-rays are characteristic of a slow, progressive, degenerative process. The most common noninflammatory arthritis is **osteoarthritis. Inflammatory arthritis** is associated with an acute onset of redness, heat, swelling of joints, elevated ESR, joint fluid WBC count ≥ 50,000/mm^3, extra-articular and systemic involvement, and x-rays with soft-tissue swelling and sometimes erosions. **Rheumatoid arthritis** (RA) is the most common inflammatory arthritis.

2. Name the four distinct groups of inflammatory arthritis.

1. Inflammatory connective tissue disease (polyarteritis nodosa, juvenile rheumatoid arthritis, systemic lupus erythematous (SLE), dermatomyositis, polymyositis, mixed connective tissue disorders

2. Inflammatory crystal-induced disease (e.g., gout, pseudogout)

3. Inflammation induced by infectious agents (e.g., bacterial, viral, tuberculous, and fungal arthritis)

4. Seronegative spondyloarthropathies (e.g., anklyosing spondylitis (AS), psoriatic arthritis, Reiter's disease, inflammatory bowel disease)

These arthropathies may be either symmetrical or nonsymmetrical in relationship to the distribution of joint involvement.

3. What is the mechanism of action of aspirin?

Aspirin, or acetylsalicylic acid, has always been the foundation of management for rheumatic disorders with the attendant symptoms of pain, fever, and inflammation. It has been shown to block the synthesis of prostaglandins in the anterior hypothalamus, which is responsible for its **antipyretic effect**. It is a **prostaglandin synthesis inhibitor**, which is responsible for its anti-inflammatory effect.

4. What is the mechanism of action of NSAIDs? What are their common toxicities?

Nonsteroidal anti-inflammatory drugs (NSAIDs) suppress inflammation through the inhibition of prostaglandin synthesis and, in addition, inhibit leukocyte migration and the cyclooxygenase effect on platelets. The toxicities associated with chronic NSAID use include GI bleeding, pancreatitis, hepatotoxicity, decreased renal blood flow, and allergic interstitial nephritis.

5. What are the DMARDs? How has their use changed in recent years?

Disease-modifying antirheumatic drugs (DMARDs) are agents that have been shown to produce sustained improvement in the course of RA for at least 1 year. These improvements are supported by a reduction in synovitis, reduction of structural joint disease shown on x-rays, and enhanced physical function. The DMARDs vary greatly in their clinical structure, pharmacokinetics, modes of action, and profile toxicities. Many of these agents are used singly but more recently have been shown to be most effective when used in specific combinations.

6. What are SAARDs?

Slow-acting antirheumatic drugs (SAARDs), a subset of DMARDs, are classified according to their presumed mechanism of action (antimetabolite, cytotoxic, or immunosuppressor), alleged benefit, or observed onset of clinical effect. It usually takes several weeks or more of use to see clinical improvement. Examples include methotrexate, leflunomide, gold compounds, and cyclosporine.

7. What are the adverse effects associated with long-term methotrexate use?

Gastrointestinal toxicities such as stomatitis and dyspepsia are most common. Pulmonary and hepatic toxicity are the main concerns. Pulmonary hypersensitivity can occur in 2–6% and be life threatening but is usually reversible. Transaminitis occurs in 50%, but cirrhosis is rare. Teratogenicity is a known side effect. Pretreatment lever biopsy is recommended in patients with a history of alcohol abuse.

8. Do low-dose steroids cause muscle atrophy?

Muscle atrophy has been shown both in patients on high-dose steriods (prednisone > 15 mg/day) used in SLE and stable, active polymyositis, and on low doses (5–12.5 mg/day) used in these and RA. All of these diseases cause muscle atrophy from the systemic disease itself. Low patient activity levels can contribute as well.

9. Why is it important to measure function in arthritis patients?

Arthritis patients have physical impairments that affect their day-to-day ability to function, and treating the patient means addressing this function as well as controlling the pain and inflammation. Raising or maximizing the patient's functional level by appropriate rehabilitation strategies is an important component in the management of arthritis. Changes in their function during medication adjustment and rehabilitation reveal the patient's progress and help indicate, along with medical parameters of disease activity, when treatment regimens need adjustment.

10. How do you measure function in arthritis patients?

1. **Standard objective physical measures:** These consist of range of motion (ROM) testing, manual muscle testing, dynamometry strength and endurance testing, and timed functional tests.

2. **Functional assessments:** These comprise global and multidimensional self-report questionnaires of function in the physical, psychosocial, and vocational realm.

3. **Biomechanical:** Analysis of lower-extremity gait characteristics can be done via visual gait analysis and stride analyzers. Sophisticated motion analysis systems in laboratories can be used to determine upper- and lower-extremity function.

11. What is a global functional assessment? Which one is commonly used in RA?

A global assessment gives a general level of physical function without taking into consideration specific questions about multidimensional areas of function. The common one used for RA is the Steinbrocker Assessment devised in 1949 and revised by the American College of Rheumatology in 1993.

Revised Steinbrocker Global Assessment

1. No limitations

2. Adequate for normal activities despite joint discomfort or limitation of movement

3. Inadequate for most self-care and occupational activities

4. Largely or wholly unable to manage self-care; restricted to bed or chair

Adapted from Shumacher HR Jr (ed): Primer on the Rheumatic Diseases. Atlanta, Arthritis Foundation, 1993; Steinbrocker O, Traeger CH, Batterman RC: Therapeutic criteria in rheumatoid arthritis. JAMA 140:659–662, 1949.

12. What is a multidimensional functional assessment? What common ones are used to assess function in RA?

Multidimensional functional assessments measure function in a number of dimensions: physical, psychosocial, and vocational. Many self-report questionnaires now exist for use in the arthritis population.

Assessments Measuring Physical Health Parameters

	MOBILITY	SELF-CARE ROLES	COMMUNICATION	PAIN
American College of Rheumatology (ACR)	Global	Global	0	0
Stanford Health Assessment Questionnaire (HAQ)	++	+++	0	+
Arthritis Impact Measurement Scale (AIMS II)	+++	++	+	++
Sickness Impact Profile (SIP)	+++	+++	+	0
Short Form 36 ver. 2 (SF36)	++	+	0	+

0 = No questions in this area; + = few questions in this area; ++ = moderate number of questions in this area; +++ = many questions in this area.

Assessments Measuring Psychosocial Health Parameters

	SOCIAL INTERACTION	LEISURE/GROUP ACTIVITY	MENTAL
American College of Rheumatology (ACR)	0	0	0
Stanford Health Assessment Questionnaire (HAQ)	+	0	0
Arthritis Impact Measurement Scale (AIMS II)	++	++	++
Sickness Impact Profile (SIP)	++	++	+
Short Form 36 ver. 2 (SF36)	+	0	+

0 = No questions in this area; + = few questions in this area; ++ = moderate number of questions in this area; +++ = many questions in this area.

Most of these questionnaires have been validated in the RA population. However, there has been one recent questionnaire developed for children (Childhood Health Assessment Questionnaire, a modification of the HAQ) and a few exist for ankylosing spondylitis patients. Additional questionnaires are available to assess other specific areas as fatigue, depression, and altered sleep patterns in rheumatic disease patients. All these assessments are useful in evaluating function over time and can be used as outcome measures in medical trials assessing the effect of new drugs on disease control. In the latter case, they are usually used with other standard measures of disease activity (ESR and joint count) and function (50-ft walk time, manual muscle test, grip strength).

MODALITIES

13. Intra-articular temperature is normally lower than body temperature. What effect does application of superficial heat have on soft tissue and joint temperature in arthritis?

Superficial moist heat applied for 3 minutes causes elevation of the soft tissue temperature by 3°C to a depth of 1 cm and significantly increases the temperature of hand and knee joints. Superficial heat causes decreased soft-tissue pain by acting on pain receptors and by relieving muscle spasm. It also increases collagen extensibility, allowing for more effective stretching programs, but it is associated with increased collagenase enzyme in the rheumatoid joint, an enzyme which causes joint destruction. Therefore, it is best if cold is used on acutely inflamed joints, and heat reserved for subacute or chronic joints.

14. What are the benefits of deep heat?

Deep heat alone can penetrate deep capsular structures. In the presence of decreased motion of the shoulder and hip joints, in a subacute or chronic stage, deep heat is useful to increase tendon extensibility prior to a stretching exercise program.

15. What are the benefits of cold treatment on an acutely inflamed joint?

In treating the acutely inflamed or early subacute joint, the goal is pain relief. The use of cold seems most logical because it can increase the pain threshold, relax surrounding spastic muscles, and is associated with decreased indicators of inflammation (collagenase and WBC count) in the joint fluid. Strenuous exercise or stretching should be avoided immediately after use of cold modalities.

16. What are the contraindications of cold treatment?

Cold should not be used in patients with (1) cryopathies like Raynaud's phenomenon, cold hypersensitivity, cryoglobulinemia, or paroxysmal cold hemoglobinuria; (2) arterial insufficiency; (3) neuropraxia or other injury to superficial nerves; and (4) cognitive impairment or impaired sensation which would limit the ability to report pain or discomfort.

17. Discuss the detrimental effects of prolonged rest.

Rest is an accepted treatment for inflammatory rheumatic disease. However, prolonged rest can have detrimental effects. Decreased mobility may promote stiffening of periarticular structures, reduction of cartilage integrity, and decreased cardiovascular fitness, muscle mass and strength, bone density, and coordination.

18. List the factors to be considered in designing an exercise program for patients with inflammatory arthritis.

1. Assessment of local or systemic involvement
2. Stage of joint involvement
3. Type of pain
4. Age of patient
5. Comorbid medical conditions
6. Compliance
7. Preparation for exercise and exercise sequence

19. List the beneficial effects of exercise programs for patients with rheumatic diseases.

1. Increases and maintains joint motion
2. Re-educates and strengthens muscles
3. Increases static muscle endurance
4. Increases aerobic capacity
5. Decreases the number of swollen joints
6. Enables joints to function better biomechanically
7. Increases bone density
8. Increases overall patient function and well-being

20. What are the signs of excessive exercise in patients with rheumatic diseases?

1. Post-exercise pain of > 2 hours
2. Undue fatigue
3. Transient increased weakness
4. Increased joint swelling

If any or all of these problems occur, the program should be reassessed and appropriate adjustments made. The type of exercise, the duration, and its intensity need to be re-evaluated periodically in light of the disease stage and the particular condition of various joints.

21. Compare the indications and contraindications of passive exercise in patients with rheumatic disease?

The main purpose of passive exercise is to provide ROM. Passive exercise provides some stretch and compression to muscles and acts as a pump to enhance venous return. This form of exercise is beneficial for patients with severe weakness due to polymyositis or neuropathic disease, stroke, peripheral neuropathy, and vasculitis. Passive exercise is generally contraindicated in an acutely inflamed joint. Patients with acute joints may passively put their joints through an arc of motion once daily to prevent the development of joint contracture, but passive motion with many repetitions increases joint inflammation. This repetitive form of passive motion should be avoided in the presence of an acute joint.

22. When should forceful stretching of a tendon or joint be avoided?

Forceful **tendon stretching** should be avoided when it is inflamed, very tight, or lax. Forceful stretching of an inflamed tendon can increase inflammation and tendon sheath fluid accumulation. Forceful stretching of a very tight tendon can be very painful, and rupture might occur at the musculotendinous junction. Rupture can occur with quick forceful stretching of lax tendons as in SLE (particularly of the patellar and Achilles tendons). For a tight, noninflamed tendon, prolonged periods of stretch are more effective in lengthening the tendon without causing undue pain.

Forceful **joint stretching** should be avoided if there is a moderate or large effusion, joint inflammation, or joint laxity. Forceful stretching in the presence of joint effusion can cause a capsular rupture. Repetitive passive ROM with no stretching may increase joint inflammation. Forceful stretching of joints with much ligamentous and capsular laxity can cause joint subluxation (common in RA, juvenile RA, and SLE).

23. Which type of exercise is least likely to increase inflammation in an inflamed joint: isotonic, isokinetic, or isometric?

Isometric exercise is associated with the least joint inflammation and juxta-articular bone destruction.

24. What are the advantages of an isometric exercise strengthening program in patients with rheumatic disease?

Isometric exercise is ideally suited for restoring and maintaining strength in patients with decreased strength from rheumatic diseases, and for the recovery phase of dermatomyositis-polymyositis. An advantage of isometrics is that maximal muscle tension can be generated with minimal work, muscle fatigue, and joint stress.

25. Before prescribing isotonic exercise for a patient, what clinical criteria must be met?

Patients with inflammatory arthritis may begin isotonic exercise with low weights (1–2 lbs.) when they are *over the acute inflammatory period.*

26. What are some uses of water or pool-aquatic exercise in rheumatic disease patients?

Exercises in an aquatic setting decrease forces against joints by providing the buoyancy of water to support the painful joints and the warmth of the water to help decrease joint pain and muscle spasm. It is particularly useful in those patients with moderate to severe joint disease (e.g., RA, osteoarthritis) in which land exercise may be painful. It is also very useful to strengthen muscle in patients with polymyositis. Strengthening muscles 1 month prior to joint surgery often enhances the postoperative outcome. ROM, stretching, strengthening, and aerobic exercise can be done in the pool.

27. How do knee and hip effusions affect the surrounding muscle?

Hip effusions in RA patients have an inhibiting effect on contraction of the gluteus medius muscle. Likewise, knee effusions inhibit contraction of the quadriceps mechanism. This diminishes the effect of muscle-strengthening programs. It also allows for overpull by the stronger, less-atrophied hamstring muscles and makes the knee prone to flexion contracture.

It is recommended that moderate to large knee joint effusions, easily detected by clinical exam, be removed in rheumatic disease patients prior to initiating a quadriceps-strengthening program. It is harder to detect hip effusion clinically. However, if the patient is unable to strengthen the gluteus medius muscle and has pain with exercise, you may wish to check the hip by plain film or ultrasound to see if significant effusion is present. Removing a hip effusion is sometimes difficult and should be done by a professional skilled in this procedure.

28. What factors contribute to fatigue in patients with rheumatic disease?

Medication, chronic inflammation, anemia of chronic disease, abnormal posture and gait, decreased aerobic capacity, abnormalities of the sleep cycle, atrophy of muscle secondary to disease or chronic pain, and cardiovascular and pulmonary problems may contribute to fatigue. Fatigue is difficult to quantify because a decrease in overall stamina, true muscle fatigue, and lack of motivation all result in an inability to complete tasks.

29. You are asked to educate the rheumatic disease patient about energy conservation. What would your recommendations to the patient be?

1. Maximize biomechanical function of joints by using proper orthotics and assistive devices to maintain energy efficient ambulation and hand function.

2. Use appropriate clothing and adaptive devices; prepare proper environmental designs; maintain strength, ROM, and posture; take short rest periods during the day.

30. Name some appropriate techniques for joint protection.
   1. Avoid prolonged periods in the same position
   2. Minimize stress on particular joints by promoting good posture
   3. Maintain ROM
   4. Maintain strength
   5. Maintain good joint alignment
   6. Reduce joint pain
   7. Unload painful joint
   8. Avoid joint overuse during acute periods of pain
   9. Use appropriate adaptive equipment and splints when necessary
   10. Modify tasks to decrease joint stress

31. What is the purpose of prescribing orthotics for the rheumatic disease patient?
   To decrease pain and inflammation, and to improve joint alignment and function. Prevention of progression of joint deformity has not yet been clinically proven.

32. What are the most common areas in which braces are used in arthritis?
   Wrist-hand > foot-ankle > neck/back/knee.

33. Discuss the key reasons for referring rheumatoid patients for surgery.
   Pain due to joint destruction by inflammatory or degenerative arthritis is probably the commonest cause for surgical intervention. It is important to assess whether the patient with joint pain has had adequate medical and rehabilitative intervention before surgical referral. Pre- and postoperative muscle-strengthening exercises may help improve the surgical outcome of joint replacement. Synovectomy for pain is still done in RA. **Decreased function** due to pain and biomechanical inefficiency of joints is the second reason for surgery. Suspicion of a **pending extensor tendon rupture**, particularly in the RA hand, or actual **tendon rupture** is another valid reason for surgery. Elective tendon realignment and MCP replacement in RA should be carefully considered only if function will clearly be increased. **Deformity**, fixed or not, alone is usually not a reason for surgery, as significant deformity can be present and fairly good function maintained. Arthrodesis of unstable joints in a functional position, particularly the thumb or hind foot, is also useful.

34. What are the indications for joint replacement in the arthritic patient?
   Patients with RA, juvenile RA, osteoarthritis, and aseptic necrosis (AN) in SLE and polymyositis may require joint replacement. Common indications for replacement are persistent pain despite adequate medical and rehabilitative management, loss of critical motion in the involved joint, and significantly compromised functional status.

RHEUMATOID ARTHRITIS (RA)

35. Following total hip arthroplasty (THA), what hip movement restrictions and weight bearing precautions must be placed on a patient?
   Following THA, patients must avoid excessive flexion (> 90°), internal rotation, and abduction of the hip. They should avoid activities of hip bending > 90° for 6 weeks postoperatively. Ambulation training with a walker or crutches may start on postoperative day 2 or 3. Weight-bearing precautions depend on the type of prosthetic device used:
   Cemented THA—Weight-bearing as tolerated
   Bony-ingrowth THA—Toe-touch weight-bearing for 6 weeks, then advance to weight-bearing as tolerated.

36. Name the 7 criteria used to establish the diagnosis of RA.

1987 ACR Revised Criteria for the Classification of Rheumatoid Arthritis

CRITERION	DEFINITION
1. Morning stiffness	Morning stiffness in and around the joints, lasting at least 1 hour before maximal improvement
2. Arthritis of 3 or more joint areas	At least 3 joint areas simultaneously have had soft-tissue swelling or fluid (not bony overgrowth alone) observed by a physician. The 14 possible areas are right or left PIP, MCP, wrist, elbow knee, ankle, and MTP joints
3. Arthritis of hand joints	At least 1 area swollen (as defined above) in a wrist, MCP, or PIP joint
4. Symmetric arthritis	Simultaneous involvement of the same joint areas (as defined in criterion 2) on both sides of the body (bilateral involvement of PIPs, MCPs, or MTPs is acceptable without absolute symmetry)
5. Rheumatoid nodules	Subcutaneous nodules over bony prominences, or extensor surfaces, or in juxta-articular regions, observed by a physician
6. Serum rheumatoid factor	Abnormal amounts of serum RF demonstrated by any method for which the result has been positive in < 5% of normal control subjects
7. Radiographic changes	Radiographic changes typical of RA on posteroanterior hand and wrist radiographs, which must include erosions or unequivocal bony decalcification localized in or, most marked, adjacent to the involved joints (osteoarthritis changes alone do not qualify)

PIP = proximal interphalangeal joint; MCP = metacarpophalangeal joint; MTP = metatarsophalangeal joint. Adapted from Arnett FC, et al: The American Rheumatism Association 1987 revised criteria for the classification of rheumatoid arthritis. Arthritis Rheum 31:315, 1987.

For classification purposes, a patient is considered to have RA if he or she satisfies at least 4 of these 7 criteria. Criteria 1–4 must have been present for at least 6 weeks. Patients with 2 clinical diagnoses are not excluded. Designation as classic, definite, or probable rheumatoid arthritis is not to be made.

37. Describe the common articular distribution of RA.
RA causes a chronic, symmetric, erosive synovitis of the peripheral joints. It can involve all joints except the DIP joints of the hands. It can also affect the axial joints of the cervical spine.

38. What are the most common extraarticular manifestations of rheumatoid arthritis?
Skin—Rheumatoid nodules, vasculitic lesions
Neurologic—Entrapment neuropathies, myelopathies related to cervical spine instability
Cardiac—Inflammatory pericarditis, valvular dysfunction
Respiratory—Inflammation of the cricoarytenoid joint, interstitial lung disease
Hematologic—Hypochromic-microcytic anemia, Felty's syndrome
Systemic—Fatigue, malaise, fever

39. What is a rheumatoid factor? Is it pathognomonic for RA?
Rheumatoid factors (RF) are immunoglobulins (e.g., IgM) that react with the Fc portion of IgG molecules. They are found in the serum of 85% of patients with RA but are not pathognomonic of this disease. RFs are also found in some patients with Reiter's syndrome, psoriatic arthritis, sarcoidosis, the aged, bacterial endocarditis, and in 3% of apparently healthy people. RFs are of clinical value because their presence in high titer tends to correlate with severe and unremitting disease, RA nodules, and extra-articular manifestations of RA.

40. What are the x-ray hallmarks of RA?

The early x-ray abnormalities seen in RA are soft-tissue swelling and juxta-articular osteoporosis. Later changes include bilaterally symmetric joint-space narrowing and cartilage and boney erosions.

41. What are rheumatoid nodules and what is their clinical significance?

The rheumatoid nodule is characteristic of seropositive RA and is seen in up to 25% to 50% of patients. RF is found in virtually all patients with nodules. RA nodules are most commonly found over pressure points such as the olecranon prominence of the elbow, the extensor surface of the forearm, and the Achilles tendons.

42. How does a "swan neck" deformity develop?

The "swan-neck" deformity results from contracture of the interosseous and flexor muscles and tendons of the fingers, resulting in a flexion contracture of the MCP joint, hyperextension of the PIP joint, and flexion of the DIP joint. It commonly occurs in RA. However, it may be seen due to ligamentous laxity in SLE and polymyositis. This deformity, when reducible, can be corrected with a Silver Ring Splint.

43. What are boutonnière and mallet deformities?

The **boutonnière** deformity consists of hyperflexion of the DIP and hyperextension of the PIP joints. The **mallet** deformity is hyperflexion at the PIP. These are commonly seen in RA.

44. What joint contractures are most likely to be seen in a patient with long-standing RA?

Although the shoulder has several joints that make it highly mobile, it is most susceptible to joint contracture in a patient with long-standing RA. The capsule, bursae, and tendons may be inflamed and painful, leading to decreased use of the shoulder, which quickly results in loss of ROM and contracture.

45. A patient with a long history of RA presents to you with sudden onset of unsteady gait, paresthesias, and neck pain. A lateral x-ray of the cervical spine should be obtained to rule out what condition?

Atlantoaxial subluxation is common in RA. It may occur with up to 9–10 mm of subluxation with no neurologic findings. However, neurologic findings may occur early, and whenever they do occur, it is important to repeat the cervical spine x-ray and compare it to previous ones. High -resolution CT or MRI may show anatomical abnormalities in the presence of neurologic findings; surgery to reduce the deformity may be indicated. A neurologic consult is definitely indicated.

46. What are the most common foot abnormalities in patients with RA?

About 50% of patients with RA have forefoot problem, including widening of the metatarsal area, subluxed and prominent MTP joints, hammertoe, and hallux valgus deformities. Midfoot problems include decreased medial longitudinal arch, and hindfoot pronation with subtalar joint disease is common.

47. You are asked to prescribe proper footwear for a patient with RA. What shoe characteristics should your prescription contain?

In general, proper footwear for RA patients should include a shoe wide and deep enough to accommodate a soft insole or molded orthotic device without applying pressure over the toes. The upper part should be made of leather to allow proper ventilation and molding around the forefoot. The sole of the shoe should be either a crepe wedge or conventional heel-sole combination with a shank support system. If the sole-heel material is too soft, a flotation affect can occur at the ankle, which may cause hindfoot pain. Metatarsal relief, good arch support, and a firm heel counter to help control pronation at the hindfoot should be included.

48. Name some typical gait characteristics observed in patients with RA involvement of the feet.

Slow gait velocity
Decreased stride length
Prolonged heel contact
Short single-limb stance and longer double-limb support phase

49. What key muscles should be strengthened and stretched in RA?

STRENGTHENED	STRETCHED
Foot intrinsics	Toe extensors, peroneus, gastrocnemius
Quadriceps	Hamstrings, hip flexors, iliotibial band
Finger, wrist extensors	Hand intrinsics

Certain key muscles around joints affected by RA should be strengthened and stretched. Strengthening and stretching of these key muscles is particularly important to encourage muscle balance. Certain muscles become weaker than others, and an overpull of the stronger muscles around an RA joint may influence the creation of deformity or flexion contractures. For example, a weak atrophied quadriceps with overpull by the stronger hamstrings can create a flexion contracture of the knee.

50. What are the common indications for synovectomy in RA patients?

To relieve pain and inflammation associated with chronic swelling uncontrolled by medication, to retard the progression of joint destruction, and to prevent and retard tendon rupture.

SPONDYLITIS

51. Name the four disorders that make up the spondyloarthropathies.

Ankylosing spondylitis   Psoriatic arthropathy
Reiter's syndrome   Enteropathic arthropathy

52. What triad of disorders make up Reiter's syndrome?

Urethritis, conjunctivitis, arthritis. Reiter's syndrome, or reactive arthritis, typically follows a bout of urethritis or diarrhea 2–4 weeks previously (the urethritis may persist) and is presumed to involve the migration of bacterial antigens into these sites, where an inflammatory response ensues.

53. What is an enthesitis?

Inflammation at the site of a tendon or ligament attachment to bone. It is a pathologic hallmark of the spondyloarthropathies.

54. Which joint must be affected before establishing a diagnosis of one of the spondyloarthropathies?

The *sine qua non* of spondyloarthropathies is *sacroiliitis*. Early SI joint changes include superficial bony erosions and eburnation, which may enlarge, and are followed by progressive sclerosis and focal narrowing of the articular space. At more advanced stages, extensive sclerosis and focal ankylosis complete ankylosis of the synovial and ligamentous portions of the SI joint.

55. Which clinical test is used to measure the progression of spinal involvement in ankylosing spondylitis?

The **Wright-Schöber test** can be used to measure the progression of motion limitation in ankylosing spondylitis. This test measures the distraction on anterior spinal flexion measured vertically above the level of the posterior iliac spines. On anterior flexion, a reading < 10 cm is considered normal.

56. Describe an appropriate exercise program for a patient with ankylosing spondylitis.

The joint and spinal motion loss, muscle weakness, and decreased endurance seen in this disorder are less severe in patients who participate in an active and consistent ROM, stretching, strengthening, and aerobic exercise program, as well as maintain good posture. To be effective, the program must be done for the entire course of this chronic disease.

Posture advice includes sleeping on a firm mattress with no pillow or a very thin pillow; lying prone for 15–20 minutes twice a day; sitting upright in a chair that reaches to the thoracic level; having an eye-level computer; and placing reading materials on an eye-level stand. A twice-daily **ROM stretching program** should be done for the large peripheral joints most affected by ankylosing spondylitis (shoulder and hips), and **spinal extension exercises** should be done using the corner-pushup exercise. **Strengthening** of the shoulder, hip, and spinal extensor muscles should be done. **Aerobic exercise** in the pool (laps using a snorkel) encourages spinal extension. **Sports** or activities that involve heavy contact or encourage spinal flexion should be discouraged (golf, bicycling, bowling, crochet), and those encouraging spinal extension should be recommended (archery, table tennis, badminton).

OSTEOARTHRITIS

57. What is the pathophysiology of osteoarthritis (OA)?

The normal joint provides an extremely smooth bearing surface, permitting virtually frictionless movement of one bone over another within the joint; second; it distributes load, preventing concentration of stress within the joint. Although cartilage degeneration is the hallmark of OA, it does not represent the failure of a single tissue but of an organ—the diarthrodial joint. The primary abnormality in OA may reside in the articular cartilage, synovium, subchondral bone, ligaments, or neuromuscular apparatus. Nonetheless, the marked changes that occur in osteoarthritic cartilage and bone are cartilage wear and tear, decreased joint space, and osteophyte formation.

58. What types of sports activities typically increase the likelihood for OA?

High	Ballet (talus, ankle, MTP, hip)
	Soccer (ankle, talus, knee)
	Baseball (elbow, shoulder)
Low	Running (Hip)
Possible	Running (knee)
	Gymnastics (shoulder, elbow, wrist)

59. Which joints does OA typically involve? In which joints is it most likely to lead to disability?

In primary or idiopathic OA, the joints that develop OA (in order of decreasing frequency) are the knees, first MTP joints, DIP joints, carpometacarpal (CMC) joints, hips, cervical spine, and lumbar spine. It spares the elbows and shoulders, unless it is truly primary OA caused by an injury, fracture, or an occupation-related task.

Significant disability in OA is caused by involvement of the large weight-bearing joints of the hip and knee. CMC joint involvement in the hand causes pain and limitation in functional activities, particularly those of a repetitive nature. However, splinting of the CMC joint reduces pain and allows for a very functional thumb.

60. What are the most commonly encountered problems in a foot with OA?

Hallux valgus, with or without bunions; hallux rigidus with cocked toes, metatarsal head calluses, and abrasions on the dorsum of the toes.

61. What are the proven benefits of exercise in OA?

Patients can improve ROM, local muscle endurance, aerobic capacity, gait characteristics, balance, and overall function and decrease pain and disability.

POLYMYOSITIS

62. What are the five criteria for diagnosing polymyositis?
1. Symmetrical muscle weakness
2. EMG with myopathic pattern
3. Elevated CPK/aldose
4. Muscle biopsy with inflammation of muscle
5. Dermatologic features (dermatomyositis)

63. What are the types of polymyositis?
1. Idiopathic onset polymyositis
2. Adult dermatomyositis
3. Polymyositis-dermatomyositis associated with other connective tissue diseases (Sjögren's, RA, SLE, scleroderma, mixed connective tissue disease)
4. Polymyositis-dermatomyositis of childhood
5. Polymyositis-dermatomyositis with malignancy
6. Inclusion body myositis

Polymyositis and dermatomyositis are both seen in adults and children and can be associated with other connective tissue diseases or malignancy. Inclusion body myositis is a more recently recognized subtype associated with a slow progressive course generally unresponsive to treatment.

64. Describe an appropriate exercise program for polymyositis patients.
In the past, exercise for patients with polymyositis was not recommended because of fear that exercise would cause muscle inflammation. Currently, it has been shown that a 1-month isometric exercise program can increase strength in patients with inactive or stable active myositis without causing sustained CPK elevations. Patients with significant muscle atrophy and very weak muscles seem not to respond to a 1-month program.

It is reasonable to place polymyositis patients with chronic or stable active disease on a three-times-a-week or even daily **isometric program** consisting of 6–10 isometric contractions, each held for 6 sec, with a 20-sec recovery time between contractions. The main muscles to exercise are the deltoids, biceps, hip abductors, extensors, and quadriceps muscles. Those patients who also have distal weakness (20–40%) may wish to exercise wrist and hand muscles and ankle dorsiflexors/plantar flexors. A significant proportion of patients with inclusion body myositis have both proximal and distal weakness. A few studies support resistive exercise for myositis.

Adults and children with myositis also have decreased aerobic capacity. **Aerobic training** in adult myositis patients has revealed an increase in aerobic capacity without a disease flare. In chronic and stable active disease, isotonic exercise with 1-lb weights three times a week and low level aerobic programs on a cycle or in a pool can also be done. Exercise programs should be reassessed if there is increased muscle weakness and soreness along with significant CPK rises. For patients with very active or active unstable myositis, only a few isometric contractions three times a week should be done. If myositis patients have access to a pool, this is the best place for them to exercise.

Stretching exercises to maintain ROM should be done by all patients: chronic stable, active, and acute. Adult patients frequently lose significant shoulder motion, and children lose motion quickly in shoulders, elbows, hips, and knees, and sometimes wrist and ankles. Calcium deposits in the soft tissues around joints in childhood dermatomyositis make them particularly prone to loss of joint motion.

65. How can you stabilize the knee in the presence of a very weak quadriceps mechanism?
Patients with polymyositis often develop very weak quadriceps muscles and begin to fall when their strength is 3/5 or below. Although weakness is generally symmetrical in a proximal distribution in these patients, one quadriceps may be weaker than the opposite one. Bracing the limb with the weakest quadriceps will dramatically decrease the incidence of falling. The brace used is a short-leg Klenzack locked in 5° plantar flexion to create a stabilizing extension moment at the knee. This brace may also be used if there is concomitant plantar flexor weakness, as the locked position at 5° will prevent tripping on the toes.

Do not put a dorsiflexion assist on a brace when the quadriceps is weak. A flexion moment will be created at the knee and make it less stable. If the hip flexors are very weak this brace may be too heavy for the patient to clear the floor. A lighter plastic brace fixed in plantar flexion may be tried but is not as effective as the metal upright anchored with a metal plate into a firm heel-counter shoe. Braces which create a hyperextension moment at the knee should be used with caution in patients with joint involvement from arthritis as knee pain can be increased due to the hyperextension force.

SYSTEMIC LUPUS ERYTHEMATOSUS (SLE)

66. What are the criteria for the diagnosis of SLE?

1982 Revised Criteria for Classification of SLE

CRITERION	DEFINITION
1. Malar rash	Fixed erythema, flat or raised, over the malar eminences, tending to spare the nasolabial folds
2. Discoid rash	Erythematous raised patches with adherent keratotic scaling and follicular plugging; atrophic scarring may occur in older lesions
3. Photosensitivity	Skin rash as a result of unusual reaction to sunlight, by patient history or physician observation
4. Oral ulcers	Oral or nasopharyngeal ulceration, usually painless, observed by a physician
5. Arthritis	Nonerosive arthritis involving two or more peripheral joints, characterized by tenderness, swelling, or effusion
6. Serositis	Pleuritis—convincing history of pleuritic pain or rub heard by a physician or evidence of pleural effusion; *or* Pericarditis—documented by ECG or rub or evidence of pericardial effusion
7. Renal disorder	Persistent proteinuria > 0.5 gm/d or > 3+ if quantification not performed; *or* Cellular casts—may be red cell, hemoglobin, granular, tubular, or mixed
8. Neurologic disorder	Seizures—in the absence of offending drugs or known metabolic derangements; *or* Psychosis—in the absence of offending drugs or known metabolic derangements
9. Hematologic disorder	Hemolytic anemia—with reticulocytosis; *or* Leukopenia—< 4,000/mm^3 total on two or more occasions; *or* Lymphopenia—< 1,500/mm^3 on two or more occasions; *or* Thrombocytopenia—< 100,000/mm^3 in the absence of offending drugs
10. Immunologic disorder	Positive LE cell preparation; *or* Anti-DNA: antibody to native DNA in abnormal titer; *or* Anti-Sm: presence of antibody to Sm nuclear antigen; *or* False-positive serologic test for syphilis known to be positive for at least 6 months and confirmed by *Treponema pallidum* immobilization or fluorescent treponemal antibody absorption test
11. Antinuclear antibody	An abnormal titer of antinuclear antibody by immunofluorescence or an equivalent assay to any point in time and in the absence of drugs known to be associated with "drug-induced lupus" syndrome

Adapted from Tan EM, Cohen AS, Fries JF, et al: The 1982 revised criteria for the classification of systemic lupus erythematosus (SLE). Arthritis Rheum 25:1271–1277, 1982.

The proposed classification is based on 11 criteria. A person is said to have SLE if any 4 or more of the 11 criteria are present, serially or simultaneously, during any interval of observation.

67. Which sex is overwhelmingly affected by SLE?

SLE is primarily a disease of young women. Its peak incidence occurs between the ages of 15 and 40, with a female to male ratio of approximately 5:1.

68. What are the typical musculoskeletal and systemic manifestations of SLE?

Arthralgias are the most common presenting manifestations of SLE. These patients may develop arthritis with joint deformities (Jaccouds arthritis) and complain of muscle pain and weakness. They often have very significant **ligamentous** laxity, which can lead to dislocation of the shoulder, significant knee instability, and swan-neck deformities of the hands. The laxity makes them prone to tendon rupture during sports activities, particularly of the Achilles and patellar tendons. **Fatigue** and **psychological and neurologic disorders** may also be complications of SLE.

69. Describe an appropriate exercise program and its rationale for a patient with SLE.

Patients with SLE have prominent fatigue and significant decreased aerobic capacity has been shown in patients with mild SLE. These patients should be on an aerobic exercise program. Aseptic necrosis of the knee and hips often occurs due to the disease itself or steroids. An isometric and isotonic strengthening program for the quadriceps and hip musculature is important to help maintain biomechanical integrity.

FIBROMYALGIA

70. What are the common manifestations of fibromyalgia?

Fibromyalgia syndrome (FMS) is a myofascial pain syndrome characterized foremost by muscle point areas tender to pressure (**trigger points**). These areas are predominantly located in the neck, shoulder, and lower back, but also in the arms and legs. FMS is accompanied by **sleep disturbance** (decreased REM sleep time) and **fatigue**. It is also associated with decreased aerobic capacity by bicycle ergometry testing. In recent years, it has been noted that FMS can be seen in up to 70% of patients with chronic fatigue syndrome.

According to the 1990 criteria of the American College of Rheumatology, a patient is said to have fibromyalgia if both of the following criteria are satisfied. The presence of a second clinical disorder does not exclude the diagnosis of fibromyalgia.

1990 ACR Criteria for the Classification of Fibromyalgia

---

1. History of widespread pain (for at least 3 months)

   Pain is considered widespread when all of the following are present: pain in the left side of the body, pain in the right side of the body, pain above the wrist, pain below the wrist. In addition, axial skeletal pain (cervical spine or anterior chest, or thoracic spine or low back) must be present. In this definition, shoulder and buttock pain is considered as pain for each involved side. "Low back" pain is considered lower segment pain.

2. Pain in 11 of 18 tender point sites on digital palpation

   Occiput: bilateral, at the suboccipital muscle insertions

   Low cervical: bilateral, at the anterior aspects of the intertransverse spaces at C5–7

   Trapezius: bilateral, at the midpoint of the upper border

   Supraspinatus: bilateral, at origins, above the scapular spine near the medial border

   Second rib: bilateral, at the second costochondral junctions, just lateral to the junctions on upper surfaces

   Lateral epicondyle: bilateral, 2 cm distal to the epicondyles

   Gluteal: biltaeral, in upper outer quadrants of buttocks in anterior fold of muscle

   Greater trochanter: bilateral, posterior to the trochanteric prominence

   Knee: bilateral, at the medial fat pad proximal to the joint line.

Digital palpation should be performed with an approximate force of 4 kg. For a tender point to be considered "positive" the subject must state that the palpation was painful. "Tender" is not to be considered "painful."

Adapted from Wolf F, Smythe HA, Yunus MB, et al: The American College of Rheumatology 1990 criteria for the classification of fibromyalgia: Report of the multicenter criteria committee. Arthritis Rheum 33:160–172, 1990.

71. What treatments are used for fibromyalgia syndrome?

Fibromyalgia syndrome is managed by the use of **tricyclic antidepressants** such as amitriptyline. Because a decrease in aerobic capacity has been proven to exist in FMS patients, it is reasonable to place them on a **graded aerobic conditioning program**. Biopsy at the site of tender points has not shown any inflammatory reaction so the use of local steroid injection would seem not to be effective. **Local injections at trigger point sites** have been reported as helpful in relieving pain. The use of modalities of **heat/cold** and **TENS** deserve a trial, although there have been no definitive studies proving their benefit. Other treatments of unproven benefit but worth trying are **accupressure** and **massage** of tender areas.

JUVENILE RA (JRA)

72. What are the types of JRA and what are some common problems seen in these patients?

Common problems with JRA are decreased joint motion and strength, limb-length discrepancies, and gait abnormalities.

Types of JRA

Pauciarticular: involvement of 3 or less joints
Polyarticular: involvement of > 3 joints
Systemic: associated with a systemic onset of high fever, rash, and acute joint pain

73. You are asked to evaluate and recommend a treatment plan for a 5-year-old boy with pauciarticular JRA. Describe an appropriate exercise program and its rationale.

Children with JRA quickly lose strength around inflamed joints, and motion of the joint is compromised at an early stage. ROM and a few isometrics exercises are done even when the joint is acute. Incorporating exercise into play routines is important. Use of a tricycle can increase motion strength and conditioning. Pool programs are very helpful. The parent should be instructed in the importance of exercise and incorporate this into the child's daily routines.

ACKNOWLEDGMENT

Thanks is extended to Jessica Lipman, who was responsible for typing and organizing the tables for this manuscript.

BIBLIOGRAPHY

1. Hicks JE: Exercise in patients with inflammatory arthritis and connective tissue disease. Rheum Dis Clin North Am 16:845–870, 1990.
2. Hicks JE: Exercise in rheumatoid arthritis. Phys Med Rehabil Clin North Am 5(4):701–728, 1994.
3. Hicks JE: Modalities and devices for rheumatoid arthritis. J Musculoskel Med 17:385–398, 2000.
4. Hicks JE: Rehabilitation strategies for patients with rheumatoid arthritis. J Musculoskel Med 17:191–204, 2000.
5. Hicks JE, Gerber L: Rehabilitation of the patient with arthritis and connective tissue disorders. In DeLisa J (ed): Principles and Practice of Rehabilitation Medicine. Philadelphia, J.B. Lippincott, 1998, pp 1047–1081.
6. Hicks JE, Gerber L: Surgical and rehabilitation options in the treatment of the rheumatoid arthritis patient resistant to pharmacologic agents. Rheum Dis Clin North Am 21(1):19–39, 1995.
7. Hicks JE, Perry M, Gerber LH: Rehabilitation in the management of patients with osteoarthritis. In Moskowitz RW, Howell DS, Goldberg VM, Mankin HJ (eds): Osteoarthritis: Diagnosis and Medical/Surgical Management, 2nd ed, Philadelphia, W.B. Saunders, 2000, pp 413–446.
8. Hicks J, Nicholas J, Swezey R (eds): Handbook of Rehabilitative Rheumatology. Bayville, NY, Contact Associates, 1988.
9. Klippel JH, Dieppe PA (eds): Rheumatology. London, Mosby, 1998.
10. Munster T, Furst DE: Pharmacolotherapeutic strategies for disease modifying anti-rheumatic drug (DMARD) combinations to treat rheumatoid arthritis (RA). Exper Rheumatol 17(Suppl 18):S29–36, 1999.
11. Schumacher HR Jr: Primer on the Rheumatic Diseases, 12th ed. Atlanta, Arthritis Foundation, 2001.
12. Stitik TP (eds): Osteoarthritis. Physical Medicine and Rehabilitation: State of the Art Reviews, vol. 15, no 1. Philadelphia, Hanley & Belfus, 2001.

58. BURN REHABILITATION

W. Nicholas Sorensen, O.T.R., Steven V. Fisher, M.D., and Elizabeth A. Rivers, O.T.R., R.N.

1. Describe the type of injury occurring in a burn wound.

A burn is a permanent destruction of tissue proteins by an external agent. Jackson more precisely described this process by dividing the burn wound into three zones. The area of burn eschar—where protein destruction is most severe and cellular necrosis is complete—is called the **zone of coagulation**. Running deeper and peripheral to the eschar is the **zone of stasis**. Cells are less injured and the majority are initially intact. As circulation becomes increasingly impaired, however, blood flow to this region ceases (hence the name). Ischemia and necrosis follows. This happens, in severe burns, within an hour or two and lasts about 48 hours postburn. Sometimes, with swift and proper resuscitation, this condition of stasis is reversed and cellular recovery is seen within 7–10 days. The most peripheral is the **zone of hyperemia**. This area is marked by dramatically increased blood flow and negligible cellular injury. This area is not compromised unless infection of the burn wound occurs.

2. What different agents can cause a burn?

Thermal, electrical, chemical, and radiation. The first three are most commonly seen, while the latter is rare. Scalds are the most common overall cause, while flame remains the predominant one in patients requiring burn center admission.

3. How common are burns?

In the U.S., nearly 2 million estimated burn injuries occur each year. About 70,000 patients are admitted to a hospital, and about one-third of these patients require specialized burn center care.

4. How are burns classified?

First degree (superficial)	Involves only the epidermis. Skin is erythematous but not blistered.
Second degree	
Superifical partial thickness	Includes the epidermis and no more than the superficial one-third of dermis. Blistering is more prominent.
Deep partial thickness	Extends into middle two-thirds of dermis. Skin is angry, cherry red.
Third degree (full thickness)	Involves all of the epidermis and dermis. Eschar is prevalent.
Fourth degree	Deepest burns extending into muscle and bone

It is important to realize that most injuries are not of consistent depth, because of the variable skin thickness in different areas of the body, unless exposure to the agent is prolonged.

5. What factors can affect the severity or recovery from burns?

Burn depth, patient age, total body surface area (%TBSA), associated trauma, and premorbid health determine the severity of burn injury. The very young (< 5 years) and the very old (> 70 years) do not tolerate illness and trauma well, particularly burn trauma. Persons at the extremes of age are more fragile physiologically. They poorly tolerate massive fluid shifts and infectious complications associated with burn and its treatment. Patients in their 20s show the greatest survivability.

A very rough guideline to burn mortality is to add the percentage of body surface area burned to the patient's age. (Thus, a 20-year-old with a 75% TBSA burn injury and a 75-year-old with a 20% TBSA have roughly an equivalent mortality rate.)

6. Which is the worst kind of burn?

None of them are good; however, each has its unique problems. In general, **electrical burns** are deceptively deep, caused by serious damage relative to the relationship of resistance, electrical conductivity, and subsequent heat production. **Thermal burns** tend to cover a larger percentage of body surface area, which leads to a paucity of good donor sites. **Chemical burns** may appear deceptively superficial initially and have a higher incidence of paresthesias. **Radiation burns—** luckily we don't see them.

7. Outline the clinical findings and treatments for the various burn injury depths.

Assessment and Treatment of Burn Injury

DEPTH	HEALING TIME	PAIN	WOUND OUTCOME	TREATMENT MODALITIES
Superficial	1–5 days	Painful for 1–3 days Ibuprofen,* acetaminophen	No significant sequelae	Elevation decreases limb pain Keep wound clean Aloe or other moisturizer reduces dry skin and itching If needed (usually in electrical burns), therapy to prevent PTSD Sun protection
Superficial partial thickness	14 days	Painful for 5–14 days Acetaminophen with codeine or oxycodone gives adequate analgesia for wound care, exercise, and sleep	Possible pigment changes	Wound care Active exercise Protective prefabricated garments (e.g., Isotoners, Tubigrip) Sunscreen (PSF # > 15) Therapy to prevent PTSD
Deep partial thickness	21 days	Very painful until closure Methadone or morphine continuously for baseline pain control Parenteral or instant-release morphine and/or oxazepam and midazolam for dressing changes and stretching exerises	*If not grafted:* Probable pigment changes Reduced skin durability Severe scarring Sensory changes Apocrine changes Edema in dependent limbs *If grafted:* Reduced scarring	Wound care Analgesics, antipruritics, anti-inflammatories Active exercise Elevated positioning/orthotics External vascular support garments Moisturization and lubrication Daily living skills Psychological therapy Therapy to prevent PTSD Silicone inserts
Full thickness	> 21 days Graft needed	Nonpainful initially due to destruction of nerve endings Pain medication as above Carmamazepine, phenytoin, or amitriptyline	Same as above Additional sweating loss Possible loss of fingernails or toenails Possible additional sensory loss Alopecia over grafts	Same as above Postop positioning/immobilization Possible need for NSAIDs or etidronate disodium to prevent heterotopic ossification Very slow weaning from analgesics and anxiolytics Vibration for pruritus
Full thickness (4th degree)	Variable Graft needed Flaps may also be required	Nonpainful initially due to destruction of nerve endings Chronic pain treatment for neuromas and phantom limb pain and later bone spicules	Variable Possible amputations	Same as above Deep tendon massage Adapted equipment Prosthetic fitting if indicated Reconstructive surgery, including flaps

* Ibuprofen has the dual action of inflammation reduction at injury site and pain reception reduced at the CNS level. PTSD = post-traumatic stress disorder.

8. How do other types of thermal injuries differ from flame burns?

Conduction electrical injury is very different from thermal injury. Heat from conduction is produced in the body at areas of high resistance and does greater damage with duration of exposure. As cross-sectional area decreases, current density increases, thereby increasing resistance and heat. Unlike thermal burns, electrical injuries often cause severe damage to underlying bone and surrounding tissues. For these reasons, the location of the thermal injury will be very different in electrical injuries; the surface wound may initially look minor but the damage to deep structures can be devastating, resulting in limb loss. The incidence of neuropathies is higher, as is the incidence of post-traumatic stress disorder.

Although the wounds produced by **chemical burns** may appear similar to those produced by thermal insults, the extent and depth of burn may be initially underestimated. There may also be more tactile sensitivity and neuropathy. The healing burn may contract more than expected because of depth of injury.

Cold-induced injuries are classified as systemic (hypothermia) or local (frostbite). Frostbite occurs when the tissue reaches a temperature of $-4°$ C. Necrosis occurs with extra- and intracellular ice formation, cell dehydration and shrinkage, abnormal intracellular electrolyte concentrations, and denaturation of protein complexes. Several days are needed to determine the line of demarcation between necrotic and viable tissue. Hot-cold sensitivity and neuralgia frequently last for months or years postinjury. Early active ROM is vital as is edema control.

9. What is the "rule of nines"?

The rule of 9s is a convenient and fairly accurate way of estimating adult total body surface area (TBSA). The head and each upper limb are 9%. of TBSA. The anterior trunk, posterior trunk, and each lower limb are 18%, and the perineum is 1%. A child's body is different with the head as 18% of TBSA and the legs as 14% each. Burn centers document the extent of a burn by a detailed chart, such as the Lund-Bowder. As a rough estimate, the patient's hand is approximately 1% of TBSA.

10. When is it time to graft?

The best answer is that it varies. Skin grafting is a method of achieving wound coverage by transferring tissue from an uninjured source. A burn wound that will not heal within 21 days typically benefits from skin grafting, since the final functional and cosmetic result of a skin graft is superior to the poor-quality skin obtained by prolonged spontaneous wound healing. Early wound closure reduces pain, length of hospital stay, wound infection, risk of hypertrophic scarring, and additional medical complications. Presumed partial thickness burns are usually left to heal on their own. If the burn is clinically determined to be deep partial thickness and unlikely to heal within 3 weeks, grafting is recommended within this time frame. An obviously full thickness burn is grafted as soon as the patient is medically stable and a donor site is available. For a large burn (> 50% TBSA), the face and hands are almost always grafted first. Some very small deep partial thickness or full thickness burns are occasionally allowed to close spontaneously. Two examples are geriatric populations when donor skin is of very poor quality, and burns located in an area of the body where skin is particularly thick (e.g., palm or lower back).

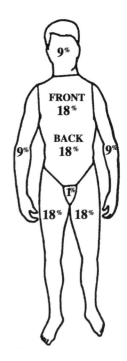

Rule of nines.

11. How can the rehabilitation team enhance the patient's success with graft healing?

The primary goal of inpatient burn care is wound closure. All efforts to optimize the "take" or adherence of the autograft are valuable. Some rehabilitation efforts are suspended while the graft site is immobilized postoperatively for a minimum of 3–5 days. For homografts (i.e., cadaver grafts), it is often useful to treat them similarly to autografts, especially in immunosuppressed patients who may "take" the graft for an extended period of time, which can be life-saving in large percentage burns.

Elevation of the affected limb prevents subgraft edema, optimizes graft take, and maximizes functional outcome. Grafted areas placed in a dependent position in the first few days can develop subgraft edema with consequent graft loss. For extremity grafts, immobilize the joint immediately proximal and distal to the graft.

Many factors contribute to the timing of ambulation after lower extremity grafting, including surgeon preference, previous cellulitis, complicating medical problems, age, and quality of skin graft take. In conclusion, the rule for post-operative movement from a rehabilitation perspective is "the earlier, the better"—without sacrificing the skin graft. The comprehensive rehabilitation process should continue concurrently even during the period of localized immobilization.

12. Do I need to look at the burn with the interdisciplinary team to determine and monitor the rehabilitation program?

Yes. Not only should you see the wounds with the dressings removed, but at least once a week you should see them with the surgical team while the wounds are exposed for care. This allows tight collaboration with the entire interdisciplinary team and facilitates a comprehensive review of the healing process, evaluation of range of motion (ROM), plans for therapy, and surgical procedures. All of this helps determine a coordinated and cohesive treatment plan and encourages the patient to become an active participant in his or her care.

13. What structures and functions are permanently altered in burned skin?

Consequences of Burn Injury by Depth of Injury

DEPTH OF BURN	ABSENT OR IMPAIRED MORPHOLOGY	WOUND CONSEQUENCES
Epidermis	Stratum basale	Damaged source for proliferating cells
	Stratum spinosum	Decreased protection against infection
	Stratum granulosum	Increased water loss
	Stratum corneum	Water loss, microorganism growth, entry of noxious agents
	Melanocytes	Repeated sunburn, pigmentation changes
Dermis	Altered collage	Decreased tensile strength
	Increased collagen	Hypertrophic scarring
	Aging collagen	Altered surgical response
Nerves	Affected	Pruritus/paresthesias
	Absent	Decreased sensation with future burn and trauma risk
Vascular system	Impaired autoregulation	Impaired venous and lymphatic return
	Absent	No healing (area dependent)
	Fragility	Reinjury risk
Basement membrane zone	Basal decidua and densa	Blisters
	Rete pegs and dermal papillae	Blisters, fragility
Epidermal appendages	Sweat ducts	Impaired thermoregulation
	Sebaceous glands	Loss of duct, sweat, and oil glands
	Hair follicle	Loss of hair root, resultant alopecia
Fingernail bed	Basal cells for proliferation absent	Malformed or absent nail

Adapted from Johnson CL: Wound healing and scar formation. In Campbell MK, Covey MH (eds): Topics in Acute Care and Rehabilitation. Frederick, MD, Aspen, 1987, pp 1–14.

14. When and why do I have to worry about heterotopic ossification?

Because it can lead to painful, frozen joints. Heterotopic ossification (HO) is the ectopic formation of bone usually observed around joints and tendons. The etiology is multifactorial, and its incidence in burns is rather difficult to quantify. In the general burn population, its incidence is reported to be between 1% and 3%. While HO is believed more common in larger-percentage burns, in patients whose wounds remain open for extended periods of time, and in joints with an overlying deep burn, it nonetheless remains difficult to predict. In fact, it may appear in joints with no overlying burn or in patients with a small (< 10% TBSA) percentage.

HO develops most often in elbows. Optimal treatment for burn-induced HO includes early recognition with modification of therapy to use only active ROM within the painfree arc.

15. Can neuropathies be prevented?

Only some. The incidence of peripheral neuropathy is estimated at 15–30% in burn patients; currently, it seems that only those caused by stretch and pressure from improper positioning or tight, bulky dressings are preventable.

The most commonly injured compressive sites are the peroneal nerve at the fibular head and the ulnar nerve at the elbow. Proper positioning to eliminate stretch and pressure on the brachial plexus will also reduce brachial plexopathies. The majority of neuropathies, however, are unavoidable. They are more commonly seen in patients with > 20% TBSA, with electrical burns exhibiting a higher incidence. The etiology may be infectious, metabolic, nutritional, toxicological, or drug-induced.

16. How is the decision to do an amputation made?

It often depends on where the amputation is needed. Most surgeons are initially conservative and attempt to salvage all possible length. However, definitive amputation should be planned with a physiatrist familiar with prosthetic fitting and function for limbs and with functional outcomes for digits. Longer is not necessarily better. The goals are always an optimal functional and cosmetic outcome. Excess fragile tissue may in fact be detrimental to properly fitting a prosthesis. A stiff phalangeal remnant that is tender, lacks subcutaneous padding, or is covered with thin epithelium can interfere with hand function much more than an amputated digit. In such cases, a ray amputation in which the corresponding metacarpal is removed along with the phalangeal remnant provides a more cosmetically appealing hand. Without a painful digital stump in the way, hand function is vastly improved.

17. Burn patients may take large amounts of narcotics for pain control. When should you suspect addiction?

Don't suspect it. Burn pain severity is extraordinarily complex. It cannot be predicted but is influenced by burn depth, location, patient age, gender, ethnicity, occupation, history of drug or alcohol abuse, and psychiatric illness. A burn medication protocol includes long-acting narcotics for background pain, short-acting opiates for procedural pain, as well as anxiolytics. Drug metabolism is markedly accelerated after a large burn. All medications including narcotics are quickly metabolized. It is very surprising to inexperienced physicians when, for example, a severely burned child needs 40 mg of morphine an hour for pain during the second month of hospital care, but large doses are appropriate.

Studies have shown that the patient's perception of pain is often greater than the burn staff believe it to be, suggesting that the patient has been undermedicated. New narcotic addiction does not occur in hospitalized burn patients despite the use of significant narcotic dosages. Premorbidly chemically dependent patients require increased doses of narcotic for adequate pain control. Chemical dependency treatment should not be initiated during the acute stage of wound healing.

18. Is patient-controlled analgesia (PCA) a reasonable choice for burn patients?

The answer is twofold. The first answer is "Yes, acutely." When an inpatient on the burn center controls the medication, the quality of supervised exercise often improves. PCA-administered morphine gives the patient a sense of recovered control. In many instances, the total dose of analgesic is actually reduced when a PCA pump is used.

The second answer is "No, not during the rehab phase." The IV should be removed as soon as possible. Oral morphine and its synthetic derivatives can be timed fairly precisely with scheduled therapy. The bottom line is to give the most appropriate analgesia for each stage of treatment.

19. Is pruritus in a burned patient a bad sign?

No. Itching is normal. Proper compression of healed burns and liberal use of antihistamines are the common methods for reducing itch to manageable levels. Long acting non-sedating antihistamines, such as loratadine (Claritin) or cetirizine (Zyrtec), have recently been used effectively, the latter in combination with cimetidine (Tagamet) especially to treat chronic urticaria. Frequent moisturization of burned tissue (at least qid), the use of vibration on troublesome spots (particularly at bedtime), and a controlled environment with good air conditioning, humidification, and circulation are all additional helpful modalities.

20. A burned child on the unit has become difficult to manage. What does this likely mean?

The cause of such behavior is multifactorial. Interdisciplinary reassessment with review of pain perception and treatment is a start. The goal is to manage pain and keep the child awake, participatory, and comfortable. Redirecting the child's attention by involving them in age-appropriate play with the use of imagery has been effective.

21. How can a child's pain be assessed?

Often, the best way is through the use of child-specific pain scales. The most widely used one is a visual analog scale that has several pictures of different faces representing variable levels of discomfort, ranging from none to extremely intense (corresponding to the 0 to 10 adult numerical scale). Ask the child to point to the pertinent one.

22. Can scar tissue that develops over burned areas be prevented?

No, but it may be minimized and partially controlled. A **hypertrophic scar** is a hard, red, collagenous bundle of connective tissue raised above the surface on the burn wound. Myofibroblasts remain continuously active in this hyperemic wound until some unknown factor causes their regression several months postburn. The patient, family, and burn team must accept the challenge of prolonged round-the-clock diligence to achieve flat, soft, mobile, supple, lightened, durable scars. Good outcomes happen when the people involved maintain an intensity, tenacity, and persistence greater than the scar tissue.

23. Why are burns disfiguring?

Typical patterns of facial burn disfigurement include lip and lid ectropion, loss of chin shelf and neck length, alopecia, canthal webbing, and microstomia. This can be minimized with continuous pressure garments and regular stretch for ROM. However, even after the burn wound is mature and scar tissue has receded, hypopigmentation, hyperpigmentation, wrinkling of thinned skin, puckering of the skin, shortened tissue length, and tethering of healed skin to underlying muscle, fascia, or tendon are noticeable sequelae. Pigmentation may be altered somewhat by reconstructive surgery, as can puckered skin or wrinkles. Surgical releases or Z-plasties add some lost tissue length. Nonetheless, plastic surgery is more the art of camouflage than the restoration of original skin qualities to burned tissue. There are no magic treatments, ointments, vitamins, or minerals that will eliminate disfigurement.

24. Can the whirlpool help burn healing?

No. Although whirlpools circulate water that can float dressings off, they may actually be deleterious. Problems include cross-contamination, skin maceration, edema, and rebound stiffness.

25. Whirlpools are still useful for burn wound debridement, right?

No. Spray is preferable to submersion. A mobile trolley used in tub rooms with installed overhead heat lamps facilitates this newer technique. The patient is kept warm, the debridement takes less time, and there is less chance of further increasing the hypermetabolic load.

26. Describe the process by which the patient's own skin will grow to cover a burn wound.

Appendages of epidermal cells that descend into the dermis at hair follicles and sebaceous glands are spared in **partial-thickness burns**. From these small projections, epithelial islands develop throughout the wound. Further epithelial cells proliferate from these islands ultimately to cover the entire surface. In **full-thickness injuries**, the epithelium must migrate exclusively from the periphery. Cellular migration and proliferation are most efficient in a moist environment free of microbial overgrowth. Healing is facilitated with moist, nonadherent dressings that are gently irrigated off the wound with removal of necrotic tissue.

27. Does eschar provide a protective covering for healing skin?

No. Dead dermis that remains attached to the wound bed is called **eschar** (pronounced *es-kar*). **Pseudoeschar** is dried serum and topical debris (it may be called a scab.) Since the wound cannot heal without a biologically friendly environment, it must be kept free of eschar. Open wounds should be covered with biological dressings to prevent pseudoeschar formation.

28. Do pressure garments prevent disfiguring scars?

No. They reduce and remodel tissue as healing occurs. Pressure garments are elastic vascular support apparel and custom contoured plates. They protect the fragile maturing burn wound from trauma and promote smooth remodeling if worn around the clock. They also help decrease itching, reduce edema, lessen hypertrophic scars, and speed wound healing. Pressure garments must retain their elasticity to be effective. They should be worn continuously, taken off only for wound care and bathing. Initially after wound closure, a soft, slightly compressive garment, such as an Isotoner glove or spandex athletic shorts, toughens the healing area and prepares the patient for tighter supports, such as Tubigrip or custom-measured garments.

All elastic support garments tent over concave body contours, allowing these valleys to fill in with scar tissue. Without diverse, interesting contours, the human body would look like a snowman and romance would be dead. Therefore, felt, elastomer, or silicone are frequently used as inserts in support garments or as an overlay to push the garment into the appropriate contours, thereby reducing scarring and contracture bands. This helps restore original flexibility and contour. Therefore, keeping the "kinks" is kinky.

29. How long do burn scars take to mature?

Patients always ask this question. The answer is: "6 months to 5 years, the median is about 18 months, and scarring gets worse before it gets better."

30. What about therapeutic positioning?

Proper positioning counteracts contracture by maintaining correct connective tissue length. Each patient requires an individual plan. Since edema is "glue," elevated, antigravity, antideformity positioning is essential. Alert patients accomplish this in planned activities, while sitting or walking. When patients are sedated, they do not move enough to prevent decubiti and contractures or to enhance venous and lymphatic return. Severely burned patients may be on bedrest for a prolonged time. Proper, varied bed positioning decreases edema; minimizes contracture development; prevents joint dislocations, neuropathies, and decubiti; and prevents complications of bedrest such as pneumonia or phlebitis.

The typical anticontracture positioning in bed consists of:
• Neck extension (no pillow)
• Shoulders abducted to 90° and flexed forward to 15°
• Elbows extended to > 15° and supinated
• Wrists and hands in the intrinsic plus position
• Hips extended and abducted 10° without external rotation
• Knees extended
• Ankles in neutral dorsiflexion

Consider all burned areas when planning positioning; no single one totally prevents all contractures. The patient and the burn team must communicate well to make time for medical treatments, occupational and physical therapy, and appropriate rest periods. Positioning, it must be remembered, never replaces active exercise.

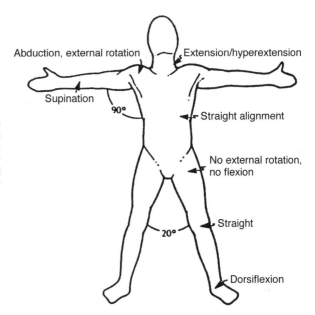

Anticontracture positioning. The patient is lying supine and is shown from a ventral view. (From Burn injury: Rehabilitation management in 1982. Arch Phys Med Rehabil 63:6–16, 1982, with permission.)

31. What is the best way to splint a typical burned hand?

In an intrinsic plus position. The usual clawed burn hand presents with hyperextension of the metacarpophalangeal (MCP) joints, flexion of the proximal and distal interphalangeal joints (PIP and DIP), thenar radial adduction and external rotation. The resting wrist-hand-finger orthosis should position the wrist in slight extension (~15°), the MCPs in 60–90° of flexion, the PIPs and DIPs in full extension, and the thumb in palmar abduction so thenar web space is maximized.

32. Are there any exceptions to this splinting program?

Yes, two. The first case is **PIP joints with tendon exposure**. Traditionally, PIP joints with open tendons have always been splinted in extension. This is perfectly appropriate if joint immobilization is not expected for an extended period of time (< 21 days). If the damage to the extensor mechanism is significant enough that return of normal function is unlikely, it often makes more sense to splint the joint into 25–30° of flexion. This may be done in conjunction with K-wire insertion by the surgical team. In the worst case, a PIP joint frozen into this position still remains partially functional. An alternative approach is to allow controlled collapse of the PIP joint so that a stable boutonnière deformity develops. The goal is to provide a functional sensate pinch.

The second case is in a hand with **extensive palmar burns**. In this case, the MCP, PIP, and DIP joints are extended, the digits abducted, the thumb in radial abduction, with the wrist slightly extended (~5°). If the hand is circumferentially burned, two splints should be fabricated—one intrinsic plus and one palmar extension—and their wear patterns modified according to need.

33. What about serial casts?

Serial casts are an extremely valuable way to reduce burn contractures. The scar will simply overpower any thermoplastic splint, no matter how good the fit or solid the construction. However, a well-made cast is stronger and provides firm total contact; it provides better contact to position the contracture on a stretch and allows remodeling of the scar in a lengthened state while minimizing skin breakdown. The first cast should be padded heavily at pressure points and bivalved to allow periodic examination of the skin for breakdown. The cast can kept on for 1–12 days. Most often it is worn for 2–3 days. A series of casts can be used to slowly lengthen serious burn scar contractures. It is important to vigorously exercise between casts to minimize loss of muscle strength.

34. How are CPMs used in burn rehab?

Continuous passive motion (CPM) machines, which passively move a joint through a controlled arc, are available for hands, elbows, shoulders, and knees. They may be used in individual special-need cases. If prolonged sedation is expected, if heterotopic ossification is suspected, or if there is complete temporary motor loss of an extremity (not uncommon in severe electrical injury), CPMs are useful. However, a CPM never replaces therapy. It is always true that an active patient and a passive therapist is better than a passive patient and an active therapist.

35. A face mask is used to cover the disfigurement, right?

No! Transparent face orthoses (TFOs) do not prevent infection either. However, these orthoses perform a valuable role by attempting to preserve normal facial contours, flattening hypertrophic scars, decreasing itching, providing UV protection, and, with adaptation, preserving corneal humidity via eye domes. A TFO worn 20 hours a day (with time off for hygiene, eating, and facial and neck exercise) is a very effective way to prevent distortion of facial contours and minimize hypertrophic scar formation during the maturation phase of wound healing. Fabricating, fitting, and revising these splints is a very therapist-intensive process and requires a significant commitment from the patient. It is essential that each TFO is continuously revised to keep up with the loss of facial edema and changes in scar tissue. However, in the hands of a skilled therapist, no other modality works as well. Once the patient sees the difference, noncompliance is no longer a serious issue.

36. Are transparent splints used elsewhere on the body?

Yes, most commonly on the neck. Often TFOs and TNOs (transparent neck orthoses) are used in combination.

37. Are there special considerations with microstomia?

As with all other contractures, prevention is better than cure. Microstomia splints can prevent horizontal lip contracture. Cheek pouches must be stretched with plastic syringe cases several times a day. These are also useful in obtaining a vertical circumoral stretch. These particular exercises are uncomfortable to do; however, given the prospect of not being able to eat one's favorite food or to easily perform some of the other more enjoyable oral activities (you are free to use your imagination) is usually motivation enough to do them.

38. Are silicone inserts effective at reducing hypertrophic scarring?

Sometimes. Some patients don't respond at all. A few develop contact dermatitis and cannot use them. However, those that do respond (typically between 50% and 60%) notice a difference. The hypertrophic scar feels softer, looks smoother, and may appear less erythematous. Best results are obtained when the patient wears them at night and does not exceed 12 hours of wearing time each day.

39. Do we know why silicone works? (Or why it sometimes doesn't?)

Nope. Research is ongoing.

40. No pain, no gain? Does this hold true for burn rehab, too?

Not necessarily. Burn rehabilitation does not have to be painful. Of course, there is unavoidable discomfort with treatment. After all, burn scar is very tough stuff. But there is a world of difference between tolerable discomfort and intolerable pain. The goal of rehabilitation professionals is to use medication and other pain reduction techniques to get gain without pain.

41. List the rehabilitation goals for outpatient burn care.

1. Facilitate wound closure
2. Prevent infection
3. Control edema
4. Regain joint and skin mobility
5. Regain strength and endurance
6. Resume independent self-care
7. Minimize hypertrophic scars
8. Teach skin protection techniques
9. Fit prostheses
10. Facilitate resumption of family roles
11. Develop a plan for return to part-time modified or full-time work, school, or play
12. Provide psychosocial support

42. Discuss the psychological effects seen in burn patients.

There are serious long-term psychological consequences from a burn. Normal responses to a major burn injury include fear, depression, grief, and despair. Concentration is impaired, sometimes for a long time. Distractibility, impatience, irritability, and frustration are typical. Returning to the site of the injury, especially if it is at work or home, often proves to be a formidable task. Sexuality is almost always impacted to some degree. Outpatient counseling, for the patient and family, can be required for an extended period. Premorbid drug and alcohol abuse may resurface postinjury and should be managed aggressively. Curiously, neither the degree of disfigurement nor the TBSA percentage correlate with psychological outcome.

43. Do children really return to school after being burned?

Yes. The sooner, the better. School and play are the work of children. After an injury, a child needs to go back to school as quickly as possible despite injuries, splints, scars, and ongoing therapies. Early reintegration promotes a positive body image and prevents disruptive, maladaptive, inappropriate behavior. Many burn centers have special school reentry programs specifically designed to help accomplish a smooth transition, most of which involve on-site visits to the school.

BIBLIOGRAPHY

1. Achauer BM: Reconstructing the burned face. Clin Plast Surg 19:623–636, 1992.
2. Campbell MK, Covey MH (eds): Topics in Acute Care and Trauma Rehabilitation: Burn Trauma. Frederick, MD, Aspen, 1987.
3. Elledge ES, Smith AA, McManus WF, Pruitt BA Jr: Heterotopic bone formation in burn patients. J Trauma 28: 684–687, 1988.
4. Fisher SV, Helm PA (eds): Comprehensive Rehabilitation of Burns. Baltimore, Wilkins & Williams, 1984.
5. Jordan CL, Allely R, Gallagher J: Self-care strategies following severe burns. In Christensen C (ed): Ways of Living. Bethesda, MD, AOTA, 1994.
6. Kloth LC, McCulloch JM, Feedar JA: Wound healing alternatives in management. In Wolf SL (ed): Contemporary Perspectives in Rehabilitation. Philadelphia, F.A. Davis, 1990.
7. Richard RL, Staley MJ: Burn Care and Rehabilitation: Principles and Practice. Philadelphia, F.A. Davis, 1994.
8. Ward RS: Pressure therapy for the control of hypertrophic scar formation after burn injury: A history and review. J Burn Care Rehabil 12:257–262, 1991.
9. Watkins PN, Cook E, May SR, Ehleben CM: Psychological stages in adaptation following burn injury: A method for facilitating psychological recovery of burn victims. J Burn Care Rehabil 9:376, 1988.
10. Williams WG, Phillips LG: Pathophysiology of the Burn Wound. In: Herndon DN (ed): Total Burn Care. London, W.B. Saunders, 1996.

VIII. Chronic Pain

59. PAIN MANAGEMENT

Jaywant J. P. Patil, MBBS, FRCPC, Anthony Guarino, M.D.,
and Peter Staats, M.D.

1. What is the internationally recognized definition of pain?

The International Association for the Study of Pain defines pain as "an unpleasant sensory and emotional experience associated with actual or potential tissue damage or described in terms of such damage." Pain is always a subjective experience. The application of the word is learned in childhood by experiences related to injury or trauma; how one reacts to pain may be influenced greatly by the individual's personality, mood, ethnic background, and past experiences of pain. Pain indeed is unpleasant and therefore frequently an emotional experience. Thus, the term pain has three important components:

1. A sensory component indicating biological underpinnings
2. An emotional component
3. As it is defined by the patient

There is no laboratory or imaging study that can show pain. This outlines the importance of believing our patients.

2. What are the dimensions of the pain experience?

Pain can be a multidimensional experience. Melzack and Casey suggest three distinct dimensions:

1. The **sensory-discriminative** dimension is the physical, sensory component of pain. Transmission of the sensory component of pain is well explained in basic neurophysiology. This dimension can be mapped in terms of time (e.g., intermittent vs. constant, acute vs. chronic) and space (location).

2. The **cognitive-evaluative** dimension is an on-going perception and appraisal of the meaning of the sensation. This dimension can be mapped in time (present, past, or future). This is the coping dimension of pain or "why should this happen to me, O Lord?" dimension of pain.

3. The **affective-motivational** dimension is the mood dimension of pain. It can be mapped in time within the social network.

All three dimensions can be seen in varying degrees in most pain experiences, be it acute or chronic pain. Remember the mnemonic **SAC**, which stands for **s**ensory, **a**ffective, and **c**ognitive dimensions of pain.

3. How do chronic pain and the so-called chronic pain syndrome differ?

Acute pain can persist and eventually become subacute and, with the passage of time, chronic in nature. **Chronic pain** is generally considered a pain that persists long after the expected healing time. Persons who suffer from pain make both physiologic and behavioral adaptations with time. Pain sufferers learn to cope and adapt to pain in different ways. Persons who suffer from **chronic pain syndrome** exhibit maladaptive patterns of behavior for dealing with persistent pain. Although there is no strict demarcation between acute and chronic pain, after the pain has been present for 3-6 months, it is termed chronic. Chronic pain syndrome refers to a constellation of biological as well as psychological changes that occur over time.

4. Name the five D's of the chronic pain syndrome.
   1. Drug abuse or misuse
   2. Dysfunction or decreased function in life
   3. Disuse resulting in loss of flexibility, strength, and endurance
   4. Depression or depressed mood
   5. Disability resulting in inability to perform activities of daily living (ADLs) or pursue gainful employment

   To these five D's previously described by Brena, one could add a sixth D—**disturbed sleep pattern**, where stage 4 sleep is significantly adversely affected.

5. What common pain behaviors are observed in clinical practice?
   In acute pain, one sees automatic-type behaviors that may or may not be helpful to the patient. **Respondent behaviors** are spontaneous responses to painful stimuli, such as holding one's foot after dropping a heavy object on it. With the passage of time, the pain does become subacute, and many **volitional behaviors**, such as walking slowly or using a cane, emerge in an attempt to decrease pain. **Chronic pain behaviors** are those behaviors that have been positively encouraged or enforced so that the frequency of that behavior is much greater than one would expect. For instance, rubbing a painful area of the body may be respondent behavior in the initial stages of pain, but if the pain sufferer gets the desired sympathy and TLC (tender loving care), the frequency of the behavior may increase, and then that behavior transforms itself into an **operant pain behavior**. This type of behavior may eventually control and limit the patient's mobility and function as the pain becomes chronic.

6. How does the DSM-IV 1994 classify chronic pain?
   The *Diagnostic and Statistical Manual of Mental Disorders, 4th edition* (DSM-IV) puts pain disorders under the general category of **somatoform disorders**. Pain disorders are further subclassified into:
   - Pain disorder associated with psychological factors (judged to have a major role in the onset, severity, exacerbation, and maintenance of pain)
   - Pain disorder associated with psychological factors and general medication conditions (judged to have an important role in the onset, severity, exacerbation, and maintenance of pain)
   - Pain disorder associated with general medical conditions

   Many patients who fall under the category of chronic pain syndrome could indeed come under the category of pain disorder associated with both psychological factors and general medical conditions according to the DSM-IV.

   Under the general category of somatoform disorder, in addition to pain disorder, there are also other psychiatric conditions, including somatization disorder, undifferentiated somatoform disorder, conversion disorder, hypochondriasis, body dysmorphic disorder, and somatoform disorder not otherwise specified. It appears that the DSM-IV has tried to define the processes that are involved in pain disorders in general. This approach seems to be a more practical and logical one. Why not call a spade a spade and not something else to confuse the issue? Other diagnostic labeling, such as fibromyalgia or myofascial pain syndrome, does not fully describe the pain process.

7. How is operant conditioning therapy used in a pain program?
   Behavioral and psychological therapy is a vital part of any good chronic pain program. It is assumed that the physiological disorder represents a combination of learned factors as well as biological determinants. The dysfunctional behavior in chronic pain is a product of faulty or inadequate learning to cope with the pain and may be alleviated by applying the techniques and principles of coping.

   The team treating the patient should have to reinforce positive behavior and discourage negative maladaptive behavior. The patient's family should become involved so that the family can also reinforce positive behaviors. In other words, operant conditioning or behavior modification programs reinforce positive behavior and ignore negative maladaptive behavior. Similar techniques of behavior modification are used to train children and pets with behavior problems. Strictly speaking, operant conditioning denies the importance of emotions, which are central in pain. Modern behavioral theories include concepts of emotions.

8. Outline a good 10-step approach to managing a patient with chronic benign pain.

1. **Accept that the patient's pain is real.** Find out why the patient experiences so much discomfort. Try and analyze to what degree the different dimensions of pain are contributing to the patient's total pain experience.

2. **Avoid excessive, unnecessary invasive procedures** and tests that do not help in the management of the patient's pain and only fuel the fires of the chronic pain process.

3. **Set realistic goals.** Make it clear to the patient that you are not trying to cure the pain, but rather to manage it and help the patient to be as functional as possible, despite the pain.

4. **Evaluate the patient's level of function.** Make realistic goals to increase function gradually in terms of different physical tolerances such as walking, sitting, standing, etc. The patient should be taught how to pace themselves and how to organize work activities so that he or she can carry out tasks despite the pain. In other words, the patient has to learn to work around the obstacle of pain, rather than letting pain restrict the quality of life.

5. **Prescribe pain medication on a time-contingency basis** rather than as-needed. Taking medication as needed may reinforce pain behavior and may not be the best way to approach chronic pain. Also, very gradually reduce the amount of narcotic pain killers taken.

6. **Prescribe an exercise program** for the patient, including a physical activity program, that should be very gradually increased over time. Many chronic pain patients have become deconditioned because of lack of activity due to the fear of pain. These patients need a reconditioning exercise program.

7. **Educate the patient and family** regarding the chronic pain process. If the patient and family understand the problem well, it then becomes easier to deal with it. The patient's focus should be directed not toward the pain but toward becoming more functional and active in society despite discomfort and pain.

8. **Help the patient get involved in recreational and pleasurable activities** to keep themselves physically as well as mentally busy. People who have something better to do don't hurt as much.

9. **If the patient has a nonrestorative sleep pattern, take action to restore a normal sleep pattern** so he or she gets adequate amounts of stage 4 sleep at night. Adequate sleep may help muscles relax completely, make patients psychologically less irritable during the day, and help them to cope better with pain.

10. **Treat depression.** If the patient suffers from some degree of depressed mood, a small dose of tricyclic antidepressants could help. It may also help stage 4 sleep.

9. What 10 factors may predispose a person with chronic pain to develop "chronic pain syndrome"?

1. A past history of anxiety, depression, panic attacks, or child abuse
2. Poor working conditions or no job to return to
3. Substance abuse
4. Multiple medical problems
5. Limited education with poor command of the local language (English)
6. Tendency to miss medical appointments
7. Inconsistent physical findings
8. Preexisting medical conditions
9. No response to different modalities of treatment
10. Previous injury claims with difficult rehabilitation

As a physician dealing with chronic benign musculoskeletal pain, one must be cognizant of these predisposing factors. In addition, your evaluation should consider other factors, such as stress, coping difficulties with the trials and tribulations of life (including pain), disturbed sleep pattern, depressed mood, and major psychosocial upheavals (such as marriage, separation, divorce, and ongoing litigation).

10. Describe the neurophysiologic process in the posterior horn of the spinal cord that contributes to chronic persistent pain.

Recent research has looked at the contribution of the dorsal horn cells in the production of chronic persistent pain. The **polymodal wide dynamic range neurons** (WDR) have many surface receptors, including the *N*-methyl D-aspartate (NMDA) receptors and neurokinin (NK) receptors. Excitatory amino acids released from sensory fibers, such as the A-delta fibers, act on the NMDA receptors, while **substance P**, which is released by the afferent C fibers, acts on both the NMDA and NK receptors. The action of substance P on the NK receptors results in decreased magnesium-dependent block on the NMDA receptors, which in turn results in influx of calcium ions into the WDR neurons. This results in increased depolarization of the NMDA receptors.

If painful sensations keep bombarding the WDR neurons with substance P transmitted via the C fibers, the WDR neurons undergo a **hyperpolarization state** or "wind-up." This wind-up phenomenon results in long-lasting cellular changes within the WDR neurons. There is loss of inhibitory mechanisms in the WDR neurons, which in turn results in continual pathologic persistent pain. One can prevent this pathologic state of hyperpolarization of WDR neurons by blocking the C fibers which release substance P with **opiates** or **nerve blocks**. It is now recognized that vigorous management of acute pain, postoperative pain, and preemptive analgesia (analgesia just prior to surgery) can prevent central sensitization and the process of "wind-up" that results in chronic persistent pain.

11. What is the role of tricyclic antidepressants (TCAs) in the management of noncancer chronic pain?

TCAs are used extensively in the management of chronic benign pain. In addition to having an analgesic effect on certain types of chronic pain, they also have a positive effect on the affective dimension of chronic pain. The normally used dosage of this medication is generally much smaller than that used in psychiatric practice. Often, 10–75 mg of amitriptyline or doxepin is effective in managing chronic pain. The medication can be given in one dose at nighttime, which also helps improve the quality of sleep. New TCAs that act on the serotonin pathway are available in the market, but their efficacy in the management of chronic pain is not yet well established. The efficacy of older TCAs, such as imipramine, amitriptyline, and doxepin, has been well established.

12. Is there a connection between fibromyalgia syndrome, myofascial pain syndrome, and chronic pain syndrome?

Fibromyalgia syndrome is a form of nonarticular rheumatism characterized by widespread musculoskeletal aching and stiffness associated with tenderness on palpation at characteristic sites called **tender points**.

Myofascial pain syndrome can present as localized muscle pain or a more generalized form of muscle pain. It is associated with stiffness, aching, gelling, tightness, numbness, tingling, weakness, or coolness in a localized area of the body, along with taut bands found in the involved muscles. There is tenderness in the muscle bands and **trigger points** that give rise to pain in sites remote from the trigger point. A localized muscle twitch response may be elicited by snapping or needling of the taut bands.

Both syndromes, when chronic, can be associated with deconditioning, psychosocial dysfunction, symptoms of depression, and disturbed stage 4 sleep or nonrestorative sleep pattern. It is possible that people who suffer from a generalized form of myofascial pain syndrome may fulfill the criteria for fibromyalgia. It is also possible that people who have tender points in fibromyalgia may also have trigger points in the same location.

In **chronic pain syndrome**, a patient suffers from chronic pain and has associated psychological abnormalities such as depression or anxiety. They also exhibit the typical five D's of the syndrome (see question 4). This patient may also present with tender points as found in fibromyalgia or trigger points as found in myofascial pain syndrome.

It is possible that a patient who starts with regional myofascial pain syndrome may eventually develop a spread of their pain over their body and fulfill the criteria for fibromyalgia syndrome. It is also possible that both groups of patients may later go on to fulfill the criteria for chronic pain syndrome. This makes one wonder whether we are looking at the same condition which tends to progress over time and which tends to get labeled by different physicians at different points in time. Unfortunately, this type of change in diagnostic labeling results in confusion for the patient and more anxiety, which in turns feeds into the chronic pain process or chronic pain syndrome.

13. Briefly describe the clinical guidelines for the use of opioids in chronic benign pain or chronic, noncancer pain.

1. Opioids should be considered only after all other conservative attempts at analgesia have failed.

2. A history of substance abuse, severe character pathology, or chaotic home environment should be viewed as relative contraindications.

3. A single practitioner should be primarily responsible for the treatment.

4. The patient should give informed consent before the start of therapy.

5. After drug selection, dosages should be given on a time-contingency or around-the-clock basis.

6. Failure to achieve at least partial analgesia with a relatively low dose in the nontolerant patient should raise the question about the potential treatability of pain syndrome with opioids.

7. Opioids should be considered complementary to other analgesics and rehabilitative approaches. Emphasis should be placed on improving the patient's physical and social functioning under the influence of analgesia provided by the opioids.

8. The patient should be permitted to escalate the dose of opioids transiently on days of increased pain.

9. The patient should be closely monitored initially and once stable on the opioids, monitored less frequently.

10. If an exacerbation of pain is not treated by transient small increased doses of opioids, the patient is best managed in a controlled environment in a hospital setting.

11. Evidence of drug hoarding, acquisition of drugs from other physicians, uncontrolled dosage escalation. and other forms of aberrant behavior must be carefully monitored and assessed. In some cases, gradual discontinuation of opioid therapy will be necessary.

12. At each visit, the physician must assess the degree of analgesia obtained by the patient, side effects of the opioids, physical and psychological functional status, and any drug-related aberrant behavior. All the observations should be well documented in the patient's medical record.

14. Do steroids have a role in patients with radiculopathies?

For patients with radiculopathies unresponsive to lesser conservative measures, and for whom surgery might be the only other option, transforaminal injection of steroids can be considered with the prospect of achieving substantial and lasting relief of the pain. If fluoroscopy is not available, patients might be offered temporizing, palliative therapy by means of an epidural.

15. What effect can facet blocks have in treating low back pain?

Facets can be the source of back pain with or without radiation. A facet injection is a diagnostic procedure that is therapeutic in many cases. It is best done under fluoroscopic guidance. Arthrography is performed to document needle position before injection of anesthesia. Findings on plain radiographs and arthrography may have little correlation with the patient's symptoms. With proper patient selection and technique, 55–65% of patients can gain immediate relief, and 20–30% can have long term relief (> 6 months). The therapeutic effect in some patients may be related rupture of the joint capsule and diffusion of the local anesthetic solution into the surrounding soft tissues.

16. When injections do not control facet disease, what nonsurgical intervention may provide long-term relief?

1. **Radiofrequency neuroablation** may quell lumbar and cervical facet disease.

2. **Lumbar medial branch neurotomy** may reduce pain in patients carefully selected on the basis of controlled diagnostic blocks. In a recent prospective study in appropriately chosen patients, 60% of patients obtained at least 90% relief of pain at 12 months, and 87% obtained at least 60% relief at 6 months.

3. **Percutaneous radiofrequency neurotomy** with multiple lesions of target nerves may provide lasting relief in patients with chronic cervical zygapophyseal joint pain confirmed with double-blind, placebo-controlled local anesthesia. In a recent study, the median time that elapsed before the pain returned to at least 50% of the preoperative level was 263 days in the active treatment group and 8 days in the control group.

17. What are some of the issues that can alter the interpretation of the result of diagnostic spinal blocks?

Injections can have false-positives and false-negatives, as caused by the following factors:

False-positives: placebo response, inadvertent spread of local anesthetics, systemic uptake of local anesthetics, injection of referred pain patterns, other effects of needle placement (inactivation of myofascial trigger points), and injection of an acupuncture site.

False-negatives: inability of the patient to determine pain relief, inability of the patient to differentiate procedural pain from ongoing pain, inaccurate needle placement, and inadequate volume or concentration of local anesthetic.

18. Does the sacroiliac joint contribute to low back pain?

Pain stemming from the sacroiliac joint accounts for some 1 in 6 patients with chronic low back pain. It cannot be evaluated by palpation alone. The most specific way to diagnose this problem is by differential blocks.

19. What are the indications for discography? What information can be obtained?

Discography is indicated in the evaluation of patients with unremitting spinal pain, with or without extremity pain, of > 4 months' duration, when the pain has been unresponsive to all appropriate methods of conservative therapy. Before discography, patients should have undergone investigation with other modalities (e.g., CT scanning, MRI scanning, myelography) that failed to explain the source of pain.

Important information should be gathered during the procedure. The volume of contrast injected and the pattern of the contrast distribution within the disc should be noted. The amount of resistance to the injection by the disc should be quantitated. The pain response is perhaps the most important part of the procedure and must be recorded exactly. Many physicians order CT scans afterwards.

20. When should a patient be considered for a spinal cord stimulator?

Spinal cord stimulation reduces neuropathic pain in a large number of patients. It should be considered when a patient fails physiotherapy, injection therapy, and medications. Patients should undergo a trial before permanent implantation and should undergo a psychological evaluation before the trial to rule out psychological impediments, if any, to a successful outcome.

21. What medications can be infused through an intrathecal pump?

Morphine and **baclofen** are the only two medications approved by the FDA for infusion through an implanted pump into the intrathecal space. The standard of care for medications placed into a pump has expanded and now other medications commonly used include hydromorphone, bupivacaine, clonidine, fentanyl and sufentanil. Rarely used drugs include the following: meperidine, methadone, ropivacaine, neostigmine, tetracaine, midazolam, and NMDA antagonists.

BIBLIOGRAPHY

1. American Psychiatric Association: Diagnostic and Statistical Manual of Mental Disorders. Washington, DC, American Psychiatric Association, 1994.
2. Bennett RM: Myofascial pain syndrome and fibromyalgia syndrome: A comparative analysis. Adv Pain Res Ther 17:43–65, 1990.
3. Bennett G, Burchiel K, Buchser E, et al: Clinical guidelines for intraspinal infusion: Report of an expert panel. J Pain Symptom Manage 20:S37–S43, 2000.
4. Bogduk N, Govind J: Epidural Steroids in Acute Lumbar Radicular Pain: An Evidence-based Approach. Newcastle, Australia, Newcastle Bone and Joint Institute, 1999.
5. Chaplin ER: Chronic pain: A sociobiological problem. Phys Med Rehabil State Art Rev 5:1–48, 1991.
6. Coderre TJ, Katz J, Vaccarino KL, Melzack R: Contributions of central neuroplasticity to pathologic pain: Review of clinical and experimental evidence. Pain 52:259–285, 1993.
7. Dreyfuss P, Halbrook B, Pauza K, et al: Efficacy and validity of radio frequency neurotomy for chronic lumbar zygapophyseal joint pain. Spine 25:1270–1277, 2000.
8. Executive Committee of the North American Spine Society: Position statement on discography. Spine 13:1343, 1988.
9. Guarino AH, Staats PS: Diagnostic neural blockade. Pain Digest 1997.
10. King JC, Kelleher WJ: The chronic pain syndrome: The inpatient interdisciplinary rehabilitative behavior modification approach. Phys Med Rehabil State Art Rev 5:165–175, 1991.
11. Krames E: A case for establishing hospital divisions of pain practice. Pain Med 3:212–216, 2000.
12. Lord SM, Barnsley L, Wallis BJ, et al: Percutaneous radio frequency neurotomy for chronic cervical zygapophyseal joint pain. N Engl J Med 335:1721–1726, 1996.
13. Maigne JY, Aivaliklis A, Pfefer F: Results of sacroiliac joint double block and value of sacroiliac pain provocation tests in 54 patients with low back pain. Spine 21:1889–1892, 1996.
14. Melzack R, Casey KL: Sensory motivational and central control determinants of pain: A new conceptual model. In Densholo D (ed): The Skin Senses. Springfield, IL, Charles C Thomas, 1968, p 427.
15. Patil JJP: Prevention and principles of treatment of chronic pain syndrome in soft tissue injury. Nova Scotia Med J 142:141–143, 1993.
16. Portenoy RK: Opioid therapy for chronic non-malignant pain: Current status. In Fields HL, Liebeskind JD (eds): Pharmacologic Approaches to the Treatment of Chronic Pain. Seattle, IASP Press, 1994, pp 247–287.
17. Raj PR, Neumann MM: Facet blocks. In Pain Medicine: A Comprehensive Review. St. Louis, Mosby, 1996, pp 266–270.
18. Wolfe F, Smythe HA, Yunus MB, et al: American College of Rheumatology 1990 criteria for classification of fibromyalgia: Report of Multicentre Criteria Committee. Arthritis Rheum 33:160–172, 1990.

60. MYOFASCIAL PAIN AND FIBROMYALGIA

Andrew A. Fischer M.D., Ph.D., David A. Cassius, M.D., and Marta Imamura, M.D., Ph.D.

1. Define the main components of myofascial pain: trigger points, tender spots, taut bands, and muscle spasm.

Trigger points are small exquisitely tender areas, which spontaneously, on compression, or with needle penetration cause pain in a distant region, called the referred pain zone. Treatment should be concentrated on the trigger point; therefore, it has to be identified from maps of referred pain zones.

Tender spots, in contrast to trigger points, induce pain locally. They are manifested by a point of maximum tenderness. When patients point with a finger to the area of most intense pain, the tender spot is located exactly underneath the pointing finger. Treatment should be concentrated upon this spot.

Taut bands consist of a group of muscle fibers that are tender and demonstrate hard consistency on palpation. The significance of taut bands is that they are an objective and very consistent palpatory finding associated with muscle pain. Trigger points and tender spots represent the most tender, pressure sensitive point within the taut bands. Physical findings over the tender spots and trigger points are therefore identical, and treatment of both is also the same.

Muscle spasm is also diagnosed by tenderness and hard consistency; however, the findings extend over the entire muscle and are not limited to selected fibers as in taut bands. Muscle spasm has been defined as an involuntary, usually painful muscle contraction that cannot be relieved completely by voluntary effort. EMG activity has been shown to be present during sleep in the spasmodic muscles, indicating that contractions are not voluntarily induced.

Tender points is an expression reserved for 18 spots the tenderness of which is specifically diagnostic of **fibromyalgia**. Therefore, it is important to distinguish these from tender spots and trigger points.

2. What are steps and criteria for diagnosis of trigger points and tender spots?

Tender spots and trigger points are small, exquisitely tender areas that cause pain spontaneously (referred to as active trigger points) or on their irritation or activation. The two most reliable criteria for diagnosis of trigger points, which showed highest kappa values, are **point (focal) tenderness** and **reproduction** (recognition) of symptoms on compression of the point of maximum tenderness.

In order to identify the immediate cause of pain:

a. Ask patient to point with one finger where the most intensive pain is.

b. Find the point of maximum tenderness or trigger point if the pain corresponds to a referred pain zone. Quantify the tenderness (degree of sensitization) by algometer.

c. Reproduction (recognition) of pain. Press over the maximum tender point and ask, is this the pain you are complaining about?

Pressure algometers are pocketsize force gauges fitted with a disc shaped plunger featuring a 1-cm^2 surface. Applied over the maximum tender spot, the pressure threshold (i.e., the minimum force that induces pain) is established. The critical value indicating abnormal degree of tenderness consists of a pressure threshold, which is lower by 2 kg/cm^2 relative to a normosensitive control point.

3. Describe an effective palpatory technique for diagnosis of point tenderness and spasm in muscles.

a. Position the patient in order to have access to the examined area.

b. While palpating the examined muscle, ask the patient to contract it so you can identify it.

c. Ask the patient to contract minimally the *antagonist* of the examined muscle. This maneuver instantaneously relaxes the examined muscle and makes it possible to "palpate through" it. Move your fingers *across the length of muscle fibers*. The taut bands, which are tender and of hard consistency as well as the most tender spots within them representing the tender spots or trigger points, can be easily palpated.

4. Describe the classification of trigger points according to location, chronicity, and latency.

Tender spots/trigger points can be classified according to **location**: muscle trigger points are referred to as **myofascial**. Trigger points can be located also in ligaments, pericapsular or other soft tissues, and periosteum. **Acute trigger points** are those of recent onset (hours or days), whereas they are **chronic** when long-standing (weeks, months, or years) but not necessarily incurable. An **active trigger point** is a focus of hyperirritability that is symptomatic, causing pain at rest. The pain can be local, over the maximum tender spot, or referred to an area specific for the muscle called a **reference pain zone**. A **latent trigger point** or tender spot is a focus of hyperirritability that is clinically quiescent with respect to spontaneous pain. Latent trigger points are also tender on compression and manifest all findings characteristic of active trigger points, including their location within the taut band, shortening and weakness of the muscle, proprioceptive dysfunction, and often production of specific referred autonomic phenomena in its pain reference zone. A local contraction of the taut band can be obtained by twitching across it. Latent trigger points or tender spots can be activated so that pain is produced by compression, overuse of the muscle, or on contrary prolonged rest in the same position. Further, psychological stress, changes in weather (barometric pressure), infections (particularly viral), metabolic changes, alterations in blood sugar level, or chilling of the muscle can activate these points.

5. Review the etiologic and perpetuating factors causing myofascial pain syndrome.

These factors include metabolic, nutritional, biomechanical, overuse, endocrine abnormalities, and psychological stress. Without removing the perpetuating factors, trigger points and tender spots have a tendency to recur. Therefore, for long-term results, eradication of trigger points/tender spots should always be combined with removal of the etiologic and perpetuating factors.

Mechanical stresses, nutritional inadequacies, metabolic and endocrine disorders, psychological factors, and chronic infection perpetuate trigger points. The most common sources of mechanical stresses are skeletal asymmetry and disproportion, poor posture, overuse of muscles, constricting pressure on muscles, and prolonged immobility. Nutritional inadequacies include low "normal" levels of vitamins B_1, B_6, B_{12}, and/or folic acid. Vitamin C deficiency causes postexercise stiffness and increases bleeding at injection sites. Adequate calcium, potassium, iron, and several trace minerals are also essential for normal muscle function. Borderline anemia is an important factor. Metabolic and endocrine disorders that commonly perpetuate trigger points are hypometabolism due to suboptimal thyroid function, hyperuricemia, and hypoglycemia. Psychological factors that inhibit rapid recovery include depression, tension caused by anxiety, and secondary gain or sick behavior. Chronic infection due to either viral or bacterial disease and some parasitic infestations can prevent recovery from myofascial pain syndromes. Other factors, such as allergy, impaired sleep, radiculopathy, and chronic visceral disease, may also have perpetuating roles.

6. List the diagnostic criteria for fibromyalgia.

  a. Widespread pain, defined as bilateral, extending above and below the waist

  b. Axial pain: over the cervical *or* thoracic spine area *or* lower back *or* anterior chest

  c. Tenderness over at least 11 of the following 18 specified tender points (all below are bilateral):

Occipital: at the suboccipital muscle insertions

Low cervical: at the anterior aspects of the intertransverse spaces at C5–7

Trapezius: at the midpoint of the upper border

Supraspinatus: at origins, above the scapula spine near the medial border

Second rib: at the second costochondral junctions, just lateral to the junctions on upper surfaces

Lateral epicondyle: 2 cm distal to the epicondyle of humerus

Gluteal: in upper outer quadrants of buttocks in anterior fold of muscle

Greater trochanter: posterior to the trochanteric prominence

Knee: at the medial fat pad proximal to the joint line

Quantification of pressure pain threshold over the tender points by algometric measurement makes the diagnosis reliable. The critical pressure pain threshold over the 11 tender points for diagnosis of fibromyalgia is 4 kg. The combination of criteria a+ b yields a sensitivity of 88.4% and a specificity of 81.1%.

7. What are the main differences between myofascial pain syndrome and fibromyalgia?

Fibromyalgia is a chronic musculoskeletal syndrome characterized by widespread pain and the presence of tender points, which are specifically diagnostic for the condition. **Myofascial pain syndrome** is considered a local or regional pain syndrome defined by the presence of trigger points or tender spots, which are localized areas of deep muscle tenderness within taut bands. Trigger points have a characteristic reference zone of perceived pain upon palpation.

Differentiation between Myofascial Pain and Fibromyalgia

	MYOFASCIAL PAIN SYNDROME	FIBROMYALGIA
Pain	Pain limited to taut band of muscle	Pain diffuse and not limited to taut band
	Pain caused by **trigger points**, which can be identified. Their activation by palpation reproduces patient's complaints.	Pain on compression of **tender points**. Pain is diffuse, not reproducible by activation of one tender spot.
Gender	Equal	Mostly female

Table continued on following page

Differentiation between Myofascial Pain and Fibromyalgia (Continued)

	MYOFASCIAL PAIN SYNDROME	FIBROMYALGIA
Critical level of tenderness	2 kg/cm^2 lower than normosensitive opposite side or surrounding area	4-kg pressure by fingertips, preferably by algometer
Symmetry	Asymmetric	Symmetric
Pain distribution	Limited to one region, not exceeding one quadrant of the body.	Involves at least three sites: right and left sides, plus above and below waist.
Tissues involved	Limited to muscle tissue only	Other than muscular tissues, such as medial knee fat-pad, humeral epicondyles, insertion of muscles in occiput, costochondral junction, greater trochanter. Muscular tender points are in upper trapezius, supraspinatus, and gluteus.
Tissues affected	Isolated or regional muscles (myotomes)	Generalized; involving most muscles and other tissues
Cause	Frequently acute muscle strain or chronic overuse of specific group muscles. (See Question 5.)	Insidious, beginning with generalized pain and often fatigue. Cause is not known.
Fatigue	No. Weakness and limitation of motion is confined to affected muscles.	Generalized involvement and fatigue.
Pathophysiologic basis	Local dysfunction in part of involved muscle. Point tenderness caused by focal sensitization of nerve fibers that becomes an irritative focus.	Decreased serotonin production causes lower general pain tolerance.
Diagnostic criteria	Local point tenderness. In case of trigger points, this is distant from referred pain. Pressure threshold is lower by 2 kg/cm^2 relative to normosensitive area. Reproduction of complaints by pressure over the trigger points. Relief of pain by needling of trigger points and/or infiltration by local ansesthetics.	Widespread pain for at least 3 months, affecting right and left sides, upper and lower body, as well as skeleton. Tenderness measured by pain on 4-kg pressure over 11 or more points out of 18 which are diagnostic of fibromyalgia (see question 6).
Reaction to treatment	Pressure pain threshold increases by 2 kg or more over the injected tender spot or trigger point. Corresponding pain is alleviated instantaneously. Spray and stretch or limbering exercises alleviate local trigger point pain.	Local injection of anesthetic does not relieve diffuse tenderness and pain. Trigger point therapy, however, is effective for relief of pain caused by tender spots or trigger points.

8. How do electrodiagnostic testing, imaging, and laboratory findings contribute to the diagnosis of myofscial pain syndrome and fibromyalgia?

Laboratory and radiologic investigations are largely unrevealing. They are usually useful for excluding other conditions that might be associated with or perpetuating both syndromes. At an initial evaluation, baseline blood tests include complete blood count, erythrocyte sedimentation rate, standard blood chemistry and thyroid function studies. If there is evidence of radiculopathy, EMG, CT, nuclear scans, or MRI may be useful. Some abnormal MRI findings in fibromyalgia patients are due to chronic deconditioning of the muscle. When there are clinical suspicions of systemic connective tissue disease or Lyme disease, serologic tests such as rheumatoid factor, antinuclear antibodies, and Lyme antibody assays may be of diagnostic value. Muscle biopsies should not be performed unless there is clinical evidence of inflammatory or metabolic myopathy.

9. What are peripheral and central sensitization?

Spinal segmental sensitization is a condition characterized by **hyperactivity, facilitation,** and **hyperexcitability** of a spinal segment that develops in reaction to an **irritative focus,** which constantly bombards the sensory ganglion by nociceptive stimuli. The irritative focus usually consists of a small area of damaged or dysfunctional tissue, where peripheral sensitization, or irritation of the nerve fibers, generates the continuous nociceptive stimuli causing sensitization of the CNS. The sensitization and hyperexcitability spread from sensory to motor components of the segment, inducing hypertonicity and tenderness (muscle spasm) and cause or activate tender spots/trigger points within the myotome. This **central sensitization** starts with the spinal segment. The most frequently affected segments are C5 and C6 as well as L5 and S1.

Peripheral sensitization is characterized by **hyperreactivity** of sensory nerve fibers to stimuli. The clinical manifestations of nerve fiber sensitization consist of **hyperalgesia** (increased reaction to painful stimuli such as scratching or pinprick) and **allodynia** (stimuli that normally fail to cause pain, such as pressure or compression, become painful). The usual mechanism of sensitization consists of local tissue damage, producing sensitizing, inflammatory, irritating substances, such as prostaglandins, bradykinin, etc. A vicious cycle develops between spinal segmental sensitization and irritative foci (tender spots/trigger points), each increasing the sensitization of the corresponding component.

10. How is spinal segmental sensitization diagnosed in clinical practice?

Spinal segmental sensitization is diagnosed by **hyperalgesia** and **pressure pain sensitivity** that extend over the sensory, motor, and skeletal areas supplied by the involved spinal segment, i.e., its dermatome, myotome and sclerotome.

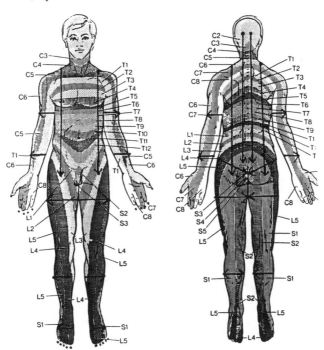

Dermatomes according to Keegan and Garret. These are the only correct dermatomes that correspond exactly to pain patterns (in the author's opinion). The arrows indicate sensory examination tracks, which allow very accurate and fast diagnosis.

Sensory testing for diagnosis of spinal segmental sensitization: Scratching the skin with the tip of an opened paper clip tests sensitivity to painful stimuli more precisely than a pinprick. The sharp object is slowly dragged across the dermatomal borders. Patients are asked to indicate if the sensation of the paper clip changed to sharper or duller. Use of **sensory testing tracks** allows more accurate diagnosis and requires only a fraction of the time as compared to the conventional pinprick method (see Figure).

Sensitivity of subcutaneous tissue is tested by the **pinch and roll method**. This test is performed by picking up the skin between the thumb and forefinger and rolling the tissue beneath. It is the most sensitive test for the diagnosis of sensitization. Electric skin conductance is an objective test of sympathetic dysfunction and can be measured by a microampere meter.

Motor testing for sensitization: Deep tissue (muscle) tenderness is assessed by digital pressure and quantified with a pressure algometer. Pressure pain threshold, which is the minimum pressure that induces pain, is considered abnormal if it is lower by 2 kg/cm^2 compared to a normosensitive control point.

Sclerotomal involvement consists of bursitis, tendinitis, and enthesopathy (attachment of taut band to bones). The table shows sensory and motor manifestations of spinal segmental sensitization at each individual spinal level.

Spinal Segmental Diagnosis

SEGMENT	MOTOR TESTING	REFLEX	DERMATOME
C1–2	Neck flexion		Skull
C3	Head lateral bend		Collar
C4	Shoulder shrug		Lower neck
C5	Shoulder abduction	Biceps, brachioradialis	Anterior shoulder, ventral arm + forearm
C6	Elbow flexion Wrist extension	Biceps, brachioradialis	Radial aspect of arm, forearm + thumb
C7	Elbow extension Wrist flexion	Triceps	Dorsal aspect of arm, forearm, digits 2–3
C8	Thumb abduction	Triceps	Ulnar aspect of arm + forearm + digits 5, 4
T1	Finger adduction		Ulnar aspect of arm + forearm; no digits; no hands
T2–L3			From spinous processes to ventral midline
T4			Nipples
T10			Umbilicus
T11 T12			End of rib cage
L1 L2	Hip flexion		Groin
L3	Knee extension	Patellar	Medial thigh, B/knee
L4	Ankle dorsiflexion	Posterior tibial	Medial thigh. B/knee, knee, big toe
L5	Toe extension	Posterior tibial	Lateral thigh > dorsum of foot > toes 2–4
S1	Hip extension		Lateral thigh, leg, foot, 5th toe
S2	Knee flexion		Medial thigh, leg
S3, 4, 5			Perianal

11. What is the relationship between spinal segmental sensitization (SSS) and musculoskeletal pain (particularly myofascial pain)?

Sensitization of the spinal segment corresponding to the tender spots/trigger points can be identified by proper examination techniques in the vast majority of musculoskeletal pain. Therefore, SSS should be identified or ruled out in musculoskeletal pain. If SSS is present, it should be treated and desensitized as a separate entity by paraspinous blocks, prior to therapy aimed at the peripheral cause of pain.

While tender spots/trigger points are irritative foci sending nociceptive signals to the spinal segment, the sensitized spinal segment induces sensitization in the periphery, causing tender spots/trigger points, muscle spasm, and tenderness. SSS may also activate or maintain the tender spots/trigger points. This vicious cycle in which the peripheral sensitized irritative focus causes SSS and the sensitized spinal segment mediates increased peripheral sensitization should be interrupted as soon as possible for effective pain relief. The clinical significance of SSS is that it is consistently associated with musculoskeletal pain, and desensitization of the involved segment alleviates the symptoms.

12. What is the specific treatment for spinal segmental sensitization (SSS)?

A special injection technique, the **paraspinous block**, effectively desensitizes the SSS and alleviates the pain in the segment. Parapsinous block consists of spreading local anesthetic (1% lidocaine) along the spinous processes and their connection in the form of the supra/interspinous ligaments. Paraspinous blocks are effective in specifically desensitizing (reversing to normal sensitivity) the sensitized segment and so relieving the segmental pain. This is manifested by normalization of the hyperalgesic dermatome on scratch, electric skin conductance, and pinch and roll; on motor testing, the tender spots/trigger points become less tender and the spasm within the corresponding myotome is relieved. Parapsinous block achieves this effect by blocking the nociceptive impulses from the sprained interspinous ligament(s), which acts as an irritative focus, mediating the SSS. This is a very simple procedure and no complications are encountered.

13. Describe injection techniques employed in treatment of these conditions.

Trigger point injections are special techniques to inactivate or eradicate tender spots/trigger points. **Injection** is the introduction of a foreign material into the body via a needle. The injected material is deposited in one location as a bulk. **Infiltration** in contrast spreads a material (usually anesthetic) over a larger area by depositing a small amount over multiple spots. **Needling** refers to repetitive insertion and withdrawal of a needle covering an area. The goal is to mechanically break up and distract the abnormal tissue, which causes pain usually because of inflammatory reaction.

Dry needling of tender spots/trigger points is effective in relieving pain and promoting healing. **Injection of medications** is also employed. Steroids are not necessary and may damage the muscle tissue. Anti-inflammatory injections (ketorolac) may be useful in acute widespread tender spots/trigger points. Use of botulinum toxin is limited by expense. **Needling and infiltration** combine both techniques, rendering improved results. Even adding saline to the needling improves the distraction and outcome. Using 1% lidocaine achieves the best effect. Infiltration with a small amount of anesthetic limited to the area of a tender spot/trigger point only inactivates the point, but there is no evidence of long-term results. The taut band usually remains intact and tender, possibly causing symptoms.

Needling and infiltration of the taut band aims to correct these deficiencies by extending the procedure over the entire taut band, using a thicker needle and more dense needling. This eradicates the entire treated part of the taut band and related tender spots/trigger points. Such outcomes were confirmed by improved pressure sensitivity quantified by algometry along with pain relief for up to 5 years follow up.

14. What is preinjection block and when is it used?

The idea of preinjection block is to interrupt the sensory impulses from the taut band and tender spot/trigger point so that needling and injection, which follow, can be carried out relatively painfree. Preinjection block consists of spreading 1% lidocaine on the side of nerve entry, along the taut band to be needled and infiltrated. Other advantages of preinjection block include prevention of central sensitization caused by needling or injecting a sensitized area. In addition, preinjection block relieves the neurogenic component of the taut band, shrinking it to about 20% of its original size. A "fibrotic core" located within the taut band is uncovered that is the sole target for the needling and infiltration. By shrinking the taut band, preinjection block allows one to concentrate the needling and infiltration on the fibrotic core, which makes the procedure more efficient and renders substantially better results.

15. Outline an algorithm for managing musculoskeletal pain with both short- and long term goals.

The **short-term goal** of treatment is to eradicate or at least inactivate the tender spots/trigger points in order to relieve the pain and restore function. This should be achieved before the patient leaves the office. The **long-term goal** is to remove the etiological-perpetuating factors causing the tender spots/trigger points in order to prevent their recurrence. For convenience, the management is broken down in four phases.

PHASE I: Identify the immediate cause of pain, which usually consists of tender spots/trigger points, muscle spasm, local injury, or inflammation, by using the following steps:

1. Ask the patient to point with one finger where the most intense pain is.

2. Identify the point of maximum tenderness by palpation and compress it while asking the patient, "Is this the pain you're complaining of?" This is called recognition of pain pattern.

3. Confirm that abnormal tenderness is present: measure the pressure pain threshold over the point of maximum tenderness using an algometer. Pressure threshold lower by 2 kg/cm^2 relative to a normally sensitive control point, which is usually on the opposite, nonpainful side, is considered abnormal tenderness.

Phase I has a short-term goal to relieve pain before the patient leaves the office. In the vast majority of cases, the immediate cause of pain lies exactly underneath the finger pointing to the area of most intense pain. When patients are unable to identify a specific point as the location of the most intense pain since the symptoms are diffuse, the cause may be a referred pain zone of a myofascial or ligamentous trigger point. The related trigger point should be diagnosed from maps and treated. The figure below shows referred pain zones of selected myofascial trigger points.

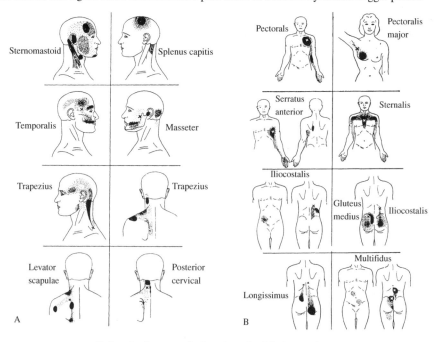

Referred pain zones of selected myofascial trigger points.

PHASE II: Diagnose the spinal segmental sensitization (SSS) and specify the segment corresponding to the trigger point/tender spot.

1. **Sensory: Diagnose the hyperalgesic dermatomes** (use sensory examination tracks) by:
   a. Scratching along the sensory diagnostic tracks
   b. Electric skin conductance, which objectively documents nerve fiber dysfunction
   c. Pinch & roll tests sensitization of subcutaneous tissue. (Most sensitive method!) Results can be quantified by pressure algometer.
2. **Motor: Diagnose the affected myotome**
   a. Trigger points/tender spots by palpation and algometry
   b. Taut bands by palpation (and objectively by tissue compliance meter)
   c. Muscle spasm by palpation (and objectively by tissue compliance meter)
3. **Sclerotome:** a. Enthesopathy; b. bursitis, tendinitis; c. epicondylitis

PHASE III: Treatment: Concentrate on the sensitized spinal segment corresponding to the immediate cause of pain (trigger points/tender spots, msucle spasm, neurogenic inflammation) or the associated supraspinous ligament sprain.

1. **Injections: for immediate and long-term relief of pain**
   a. Paraspinous block to desensitize the SSS.
   b. Preinjection block to anesthetize the painful sensitive area to be infiltrated.
   c. Needling and infiltration of the taut band to break up the entire underlying pathology around the trigger point/tender spot.
2. **Physical therapy:** to promote healing after injections, restore function, and prevent recurrence.
   a. **Modalities:** Heat or cold; electric stimulation (sinusoid surging and tetanizing currents), utrasound, TENS
   b. **Exercises:** Relaxation exercises and stretching—general and specific for the involved myotome, in which the pain generating points are located. Relaxation by activation of antagonist muscle(s).
   c. **Postural correction**

PHASE IV: Diagnosis and removal of perpetuating and etiologic factors:

1. **Mechanical:** Overuse, sport injuries, cumulative trauma disorder.
2. **Postural deficiencies, muscle deficiencies** (loss of strength or flexibility)
3. **Lab results:** Endocrine, metabolic, electrolyte, vitamin disorders

16. How would you treat a patient with fibromyalgia?

The rational basis for treatment of fibromyalgia includes enhancement of peripheral and central analgesia, improvement of sleep disturbances, diminishing mood disturbances, and increasing blood flow to muscle and superficial tissues. Analgesia can be obtained by central-acting analgesics such as amitriptyline and cyclobenzaprine. TENS, acupuncture, laser, injections of tender spots, and paraspinous blocks are other procedures less well documented. Individualized cardiovascular fitness programs allow increased blood flow to muscle and superficial tissues. Education programs include explaining that the illness is real regardless of unrevealing laboratory and imaging tests. Patients should be taught relaxation techniques.

17. Which medications are commonly used to treat fibromyalgia? Describe their mode of action and adverse effects.

CNS-active medications such as the tricyclic amitriptyline and cyclobenzaprine have been shown to be better than placebo in controlled trials. The doses of amitriptyline are 25–50 mg, usually given as a single dose at bedtime. This medication promotes stage 4 sleep and has a central analgesic effect due to potentiation of endogenous opioids as well as brain serotonin and other neurogenic amines. Potential adverse effects include the anticholinergic effects, which are important in patient compliance; even in low doses, dry mouth, constipation, fluid retention, weight gain, and difficulty concentrating are common. Atrioventricular blockade and closed angle glaucoma are contraindications. Cyclobenzaprine, 10 to 40 mg in divided doses, also improves pain, fatigue, sleep, and tender point count. Simple analgesics may be of limited help, and chronic use of opioids should be avoided due to tolerance and adverse affects.

18. What types of exercise are most beneficial in the treatment of myofascial pain syndrome and fibromyalgia?

Individualized exercise regimens and correction of postural deficiencies as well as lifestyle changes are usually recommended for these patients. For **myofascial pain**, the regimen consists of active limbering and relaxation exercises. Double-blind studies prove that such exercises are effective in the treatment of low back pain and its prevention, as long as the patient is doing them systematically. Postisometric relaxation has also been proven to be effective in a double-blind study; however, our experience demonstrates that the most effective treatment consists of inhibition of painful muscle spasm when a patient voluntarily contracts the antagonists. Spray of **vapocoolant** inactivates the trigger points/tender spots and makes relaxation exercises and passive stretching of the involved muscle more effective.

For **fibromyalgia** patients, cardiovascular fitness training of gradual increment is recommended. Low-impact aerobic activities, such as fast walking, biking, swimming, or water aerobics, for a minimum of 30 minutes three times a week in a range near target heart rate are recommended.

19. How do psychological factors affect treatment?

Many patients report depression, anxiety, and high level of stress. Most patients do not have an active psychiatric illness, and there is no evidence of specific personality type, such as obsessive-compulsive or somatoform disorders. Pain usually increases with stress and tension in these patients. As a perpetuating source of muscle spasm and chronic pain, psychological factors should be addressed in order to improve the final outcome.

20. What is the role of physiotherapy in management of trigger points and tender spots?

Physical therapy is an important component in treatment of any trigger point or tender spot in myosfacial pain syndrome and fibromyalgia. Physical therapy can be used independently or following injections of a trigger point. It promotes healing of the injected areas in the muscle and prevents recurrence of pain. Each injection should be followed by at least three sessions of physical therapy, consisting of moist heating pad for 20 minutes, followed by electrical stimulation using sinusoid surging current for 15 minutes over the injected areas. This induces strong periodic contractions and relaxation of the treated muscles. The contractions squeeze out the edema, which is formed at the injection site, and prevent inflammation caused by the injury. If a spasmodic component is present, tetanizing current is employed, followed by sinusoid surging current inducing periodic contractions for 10 minutes each. Usually three physical therapy sessions per week are required.

BIBLIOGRAPHY

1. Fischer AA, Imamura M: New concepts in the diagnosis and management of musculoskeletal pain. In Leonard TA (ed): Pain Procedures in Clinical Practice, 2nd ed. Philadelphia, Hanley & Belfus, 2000, pp 213–229.
2. Fischer AA (ed): Myofascial Pain: Update in Diagnosis and Treatment. Physical Medicine and Rehabilitation Clinics of North America, vol. 6, no. 1. Philadelphia, W.B. Saunders, 1997.
3. Fischer AA: Muscle Pain Syndromes and Fibromyalgia. New York, Haworth Medical Press, 1998.
4. Hackett GS: Ligament and Tendon Relaxation Treated by Prolotherapy, 3rd ed, Springfield, IL, Charles C Thomas, 1958, pp 27–36.
5. Keegan JJ, Garrett FD: The segmental distribution of the cutaneous nerves in the limbs of man. Anat Rec 102–409, 1948.
6. Mense S, Simons DG: Muscle Pain. Philadelphia, Lippincott Williams & Wilkins, 2000, pp 92–95.
7. Rachlin ES: Myofascial Pain and Fibromyalgia. St. Louis, Mosby, 1994.
8. Russell IJ: Fibromyalgia syndrome. In Loeser JD, Butler SH, Chapman CR, Turk DC (eds): Bonica's Management of Pain. Philadelphia, Lippincott Williams & Wilkins, 2001, pp 543–556.
9. Simons DG, Travell JG, Simons LS: Myofascial Pain and Dysfunction. The Trigger Point Manual, Vol. 1. Upper Half of Body, 2nd ed. Baltimore,Williams & Wilkins, 1999.
10. Travell JG, Simons DG: Myofascial Pain Dysfunction: The Trigger Point Manual: The Lower Extremities, vol. 1. Baltimore, Williams & Wilkins, 1983.

61. COMPLEX REGIONAL PAIN SYNDROME

Bryan O'Young, M.D., and Warren Slaten, M.D.

1. What is complex regional pain syndrome (CRPS)?
CRPS is a syndrome characterized by continuing pain, allodynia, or hyperalgesia, in which pain is out of proportion to the inciting event. The syndrome is associated with evidence of edema, changes in skin blood flow including color and temperature changes, or abnormal sweating activity in the region of pain at some time in the course of the condition. This diagnosis is excluded by the presence of conditions that would otherwise account for the degree of pain and dysfunction.

2. What is the difference between CRPS type I and CRPS type II?
In **type I**, there is a presence of an initiating noxious event or cause of immobilization *without presence of a known nerve injury*. In **type II**, there is *antecedent nerve injury*, though the signs and symptoms are not limited to the distribution of the injured nerve. Type I was previously known as reflex sympathetic dystrophy (RSD), and type II as causalgia.

3. Why were the names RSD and causalgia changed to CRPS?
The term CRPS has been used since 1993 because the International Association for the Study of Pain felt that the terms RSD and causalgia were inadequate to represent the full spectrum of signs and symptoms. The diagnostic criterion for CRPS is based on descriptive terms, rather than the poorly understood pathophysiology of the condition. The term "complex" was included to convey the reality that RSD and causalgia express varied signs and symptoms.

4. Besides RSD and causalgia, what were some of the other terms used to denote CRPS?
Sympathetically maintained pain syndrome
Algodystrophy
Shoulder hand syndrome
Sympathalgia
Sudek's atrophy
Post-traumatic osteoporosis
Traumatic vasospasm

5. What is sympathetically maintained pain (SMP)?
Pain maintained by sympathetic efferent innervation or by circulating catecholamines.

6. What is the difference between CRPS and SMP?
CRPS is a clinical diagnosis, whereas SMP is a pain mechanism. CRPS is characterized by components of both SMP and sympathetic independent pain. Therefore, a patient with CRPS may or may not have SMP. Besides CRPS, SMP is a pain mechanism for other pain syndromes, including peripheral neuropathies, post-herpetic neuralgia, and phantom pain.

7. Explain the known mechanisms of CRPS and SMP.
The precise mechanisms for the unique characteristics of CRPS are unknown. Many theories have been proposed explaining the mechanisms of SMP that may be involved in CRPS. These mechanisms are classified into central and peripheral processes:
Central Processes
• **Gate control theory**—Input from large-diameter fibers inhibits input from small, unmyelinated pain fibers, preventing central processing of the pain input. In SMP, it is believed that the large fibers are injured, with relative sparing of the small unmyelinated nociceptive fibers, so the pain input from the smaller fibers is unmodulated.

- **Turbulence theory**—Nerve injury causes formation of altered nerve input, creating "turbulence," which modifies the brain's perception of normal cutaneous afferent activity.
- **Wide dynamic range theory**—Large type-A myelinated afferent fibers are sensitized during trauma by type-C unmyelinated fibers. The afferent fibers are excited by sympathetic activity and then induce more pain.

Peripheral Processes

- **Artificial synapse theory**—At the site of nerve discontinuity, sympathetic efferent fibers propagate impulses to the somatic sensory afferents. This depolarization results in a perception of pain centrally and causes a release of pain-sensitizing substances peripherally.
- **Spontaneous discharge theory**—After nerve injury, regenerating axons result in excessive numbers of sodium and calcium channels and α-adrenergic receptors. These channels discharge spontaneously, and circulating catecholamines augment this activity, resulting in hyperalgesia and abnormal chemosensitivity.

8. Describe the traditional three stages for CRPS.

The staging of CRPS is a concept that is gradually growing out of favor. The course of the disease appears to be so unpredictable among various patients that staging is not helpful in the treatment of CRPS. The clinical features listed for each stage may not all be present. The rate of progression varies greatly from one individual to another. In addition, symptoms from stage I and II may fade as the disease progresses to stage III.

Stages of CRPS

Stage I (acute stage)
Onset of severe pain limited to the site of injury
Increased sensitivity of skin to touch and light pressure (hyperesthesia)
Localized swelling
Muscle cramps
Stiffness and limited mobility
At onset, skin is usually warm, red, and dry, and then it may change to a blue (cyanotic) appearance and become cold and sweaty.
Increased sweating (hyperhydrosis)
In mild cases, this stage lasts a few weeks, then subsides spontaneously or responds rapidly to treatment.

Stage II (dystrophic stage)
Pain becomes even more severe and more diffuse.
Swelling tends to spread and it may change from a soft to hard (brawny) type.
Hair may become coarse, then scant; nails may grow faster, then grow slower and become brittle, cracked, and heavily grooved.
Spotty wasting of bone (osteoporosis) occurs early but may become severe and diffuse.
Muscle wasting begins.

Stage III (atrophic stage)
Marked wasting of tissue (atrophic) eventually become irreversible.
For many patients the pain becomes intractable and may involve the entire limb.
A small percentage of patients develop generalized RSD affecting the entire body.

9. How is the pain described in CRPS?

The pain is best described as out of proportion to that expected from the initial injury. The initial and primary complaint in one or more extremities is described as severe, constant, burning, or deep aching pain. Any tactile stimuli of the skin may be perceived as painful (allodynia, pain to a benign stimulus). There may be prolonged sensation of pain (hyperpathia) after repetitive stimuli such as tapping. Although the pain may radiate in a dermatomal or nerve distribution, it is more often diffuse and nondermatomal. The pain is generally localized to the site of injury, and the pain and symptoms tend to become more diffuse with time. The pain usually starts in the extremity and with progression spreads proximally.

10. How does the clinical presentation and course of CRPS differ in children?

Frequently, there is no preceding neurologic or traumatic event, and the lower extremity is more often affected. Bone scan results are more variable and, when positive, show decreased rather than increased uptake. Osteoporosis is rare, and the prognosis is generally favorable.

11. Is there a gender difference in how men and women experience CRPS?

Like most forms of pain, CRPS affects men and women differently. Women exhibit greater coping skills, but they have a greater sensitivity to painful stimuli. Women over the age of 50 are likely to exhibit worse manifestations of the disease and progress more rapidly. Women with CRPS (in contrast to men) are more proactive about their disease and are more likely to seek early intervention when symptoms evolve. Allodynia is more flagrant in women than men.

12. Which diagnostic tests are helpful in the diagnosis of CRPS?

X-rays, triple-phase bone scan, sympathetic blockade, thermography.

13. What x-ray findings are typical in CRPS?

In the initial stages, x-rays may be normal. Periarticular osteoporosis may be found in later stages.

14. What are the findings in the triple-phase bone scan in patients with CRPS?

The blood flow and blood pool phases may show asymmetric uptake between limbs, whereas the static phase (most sensitive) shows increased periarticular uptake.

15. Are there abnormal laboratory findings in CRPS?

No. All are within normal limits (including calcium, phosphorus, and alkaline phosphatase).

16. Is there one or a combination of diagnostic tests that definitively establishes the diagnosis of CRPS?

No. Laboratory tests, x-rays, and triple-phase bone scan are helpful, but the diagnosis is established on clinical grounds.

17. What other diagnoses should be considered in the differential diagnosis of RSD?

Infectious arthritis	Scleroderma	Peripheral neuropathy
Systemic lupus erythematosus	Conversion reaction	Local trauma
Rheumatoid arthritis	Rotator cuff tear	Paraneoplastic syndrome

18. What are the principles for treating RSD?

1. Early recognition and diagnosis.
2. Early, aggressive treatment to break the cycle of sympathetic activity and pain.
3. Use of medications, including oral agents and sympathetic blocking injections.
4. Encourage normal use of the limb.
5. Symptomatic management, including pain management, avoiding contractures, and edema control.
6. Psychologic support, including patient education, relaxation training, and counseling.

19. Which drugs can be used to treat CRPS?

Medications commonly used to treat CRPS are based on the type of pain.

TYPE OF PAIN	MEDICATION
Constant pain associated with inflammation	NSAIDs (e.g., aspirin, ibuprofen, naproxen)
Constant pain not caused by inflammation	Agents targeting the CNS by an atypical mechanism (e.g., tramadol)

Table continued on following page

TYPE OF PAIN	MEDICATION
Constant pain or spontaneous (paroxysmal) jabs causing sleep disturbances	Antidepressants (amitriptyline, doxepin); oral lidocaine (mexiletene)
Spontaneous (paroxysmal) jabs and/or burning pain	Anticonvulsants (e.g., carbamazepine, gabapentin), lamotrigine
Localized nerve-related injury	Capsaicin cream and lidocaine patch
Sympathetically maintained pain	Clonidine patch, propanolol
Sympathetically maintained pain associated with vascular instability	Nifedipine
Muscle cramps (spasms and dystonia)	Clonopine, baclofen, tizanidine (can be difficult to treat)
Widespread, severe CRPS pain, refractory to less aggressive therapies	Oral opioids (use of opioids is debated due to their potential side effects. To obtain an appropriate informed consent, the patient should sign a physician-patient contract.)

20. Which physical modalities are used to treat RSD?

TENS to modulate inhibitory control of afferent input may provide some pain relief.

Contrast baths (alternating cold and hot water) for the affected extremity are believed to address the vasomotor component of the patient's symptoms.

Edema control measures, including elevation and gradient compression.

Desensitization techniques may increase the patient's tolerance of normal sensory input and decrease hyperesthesias.

Ultrasound provides pain relief with an inhibiting effect on the paracervical sympathetic ganglia.

21. What injection techniques are used to treat the patient with RSD?

Upper extremities—Bier block and stellate ganglion blocks.

Lower extremities—epidural block and lumbar sympathetic blocks.

22. What is a Bier block?

In this technique, guanethidine or reserpine is infused intravenously into the affected limb, followed by a pressure tourniquet around the affected limb at 100 mmHg above systolic blood pressure. These agents, which decrease sympathetic activity, are then allowed to circulate in a high concentration in the affected limb, until the tourniquet pressure is decreased.

23. How is a stellate ganglion block performed?

With the patient in the supine position and the neck extended, the needle is directed toward the tubercle of the C6 vertebral body (Chassaignac's tubercle). Once the needle comes into contact with the bone, the needle is withdrawn a few millimeters. The syringe is aspirated of either blood or cerebral fluid. Then, a 1-ml test dose is administered with the patient signaling a "thumb's up." The remainder of the solution is subsequently slowly administered with intermittent syringe aspirations.

24. What signs and symptoms suggest an effective stellate ganglion block?

Pain relief, Horner's syndrome (miosis, ptosis, nasal congestion, and anhidrosis), and an increase in skin temperature of the extremity. The patient needs to know that benefit from an injection is often short-lived (24–48 hours), and repeat injections may be required.

25. After comprehensive conservative care including medications and physical therapy and the use of sympathetic blocks, are there other treatment options for CRPS?

Yes. These include radiofrequency denervation, implantation of a spinal cord stimulator, and surgical paravertebral sympathectomy. These treatment options may work well in some patients with chronic intractable pain secondary to CRPS.

26. Which patients are good candidates for surgical paravertebral sympathectomy?

After 4–6 stellate ganglion injections, if the patient is still getting significant relief from injections but the relief is not lasting, then he or she may benefit from surgical sympathectomy. If injections have stopped having any effect, even temporary, then benefit from surgery is less likely. With surgery, risks to be considered include the possibility of sympathalgia, a painful condition of muscle fatigue and pain which is usually temporary, and Horner's syndrome, which may be permanent.

27. What is the prognosis for patients with CRPS?

Guarded. Early diagnosis and treatment improve the prognosis, but there is no definitive treatment at this time.

BIBLIOGRAPHY

1. Babur H: Reflex sympathetic dystrophy. J Neurol Orthop Med Surg 12:46–59, 1991.
2. Bonica J: Causalgia and other reflex sympathetic dystrophies. Postgrad Med 53:143–148, 1983.
3. Bonica J: The Management of Pain, 2nd ed. Philadelphia, Lea & Febiger, 1990.
4. Kirkpatrick A: Reflex Sympathetic Dystrophy/Complex Regional Pain Syndrome. Clinical Practice Guidelines, 2nd ed. Reflex Sympathetic Dystrophy Syndrome Association of America, 2000. Available on-line: www.rsds.org/cpgeng.htm.
5. Merskey H, Bodguk N (eds): Classification of Chronic Pain, Descriptions of Chronic Pain Syndromes, and Definition of Pain Terms, 2nd ed. Seattle, IASP Press, 1994.
6. Pittman D, Belgrade M: Complex regional pain syndrome. Am Fam Physician 56:2265-2275, 1997.
7. Raj P, Kelly J, Cannella S, McConn K: Multidisciplinary management of reflex sympathetic dystrophy. Pain Digest 2:267–273, 1992.
8. Schwartzman R, McLellan T: Reflex sympathetic dystrophy: A review. Arch Neurol 44:555–561, 1987.
9. Young MA, Baar K: Woman and Pain. New York, Hyperion Publishers, 2001.

IX. Rehabilitation in Sports and the Arts

62. SPORTS MEDICINE

Joel M. Press, M.D., and Jeffrey L. Young, M.D., M.A.

1. Can I skip this chapter if I am a general practicing physician?

A working knowledge of musculoskeletal anatomy and biomechanical principles is important no matter how specialized a physiatrist is. Most patients present with numerous musculoskeletal problems. Back, knee, and shoulder pain are common in patients hospitalized for stroke, traumatic brain injury, amputation, spinal cord injury, and arthritis rehabilitation. Sports medicine and sports technology also has led to many advances in care for the disabled. For example, adaptation of ski technology led to development of the "flex foot," and racing wheelchairs were precursors to lightweight chairs used today.

2. What is PASSOR?

The Physiatric Association for Spine, Sports, and Occupational Rehabilitation (PASSOR) is a section of the AAPM&R formed "to foster the growth of the specialty of physiatry in research, education, and the physiatric practice of musculoskeletal medicine with a special emphasis upon spine, sports, and occupational rehabilitation."

3. When discussing an injury with a patient, what important information do I need to find out?

1. *What was the mechanism of injury?* (What happened?)

2. *Is this a reinjury or was this an acute macrotraumatic event?* If the patient has been injured in the same area before, it implies either inadequate rehabilitation or the progression of chronic microtraumatic injury.

3. *Where else has the patient been injured?* A **kinetic chain analysis** of injuries often reveals events proximal or distal to the site of acute injury which haverendered the new site more vulnerable to overload.)

4. *What treatment did the patient receive?* An alarming number of musculoskeletal injuries do not receive adequate attention and proper rehabilitation.

5. *What other medical conditions does the patient have?* Do not assume that the patient is healthy just because they are an athlete. Many individuals with asthma, cardiac conditions, and metabolic and hormonal disorders are active participants in sports. Treatment regimens need to take this information into account.

4. What is involved in the preparticipation history and examination?

The history needs to include review of previous neurologic and musculoskeletal injuries and their rehabilitation, a thorough family and personal cardiovascular and respiratory disease inquiry, review of thermoregulatory and endocrine dysfunction, and evaluation for the presence or absence of unpaired organs.

The preparticipation history and examination is used to:

1. Detect conditions that will restrict athletic participation, predispose to injury, or limit the level of performance

2. Evaluate level of fitness and maturity

3. Determine general health

4. Establish an open physician-athlete relationship for maximal health education
5. Fulfill medical-legal requirements

5. What is a musculoskeletal examination?

In a complete musculoskeletal examination, the examiner notes inflexibilities and restrictions at the level of the joints, connective tissue, muscle, and fascia. Strength and dynamic and proprioceptive ability are also assessed. These findings, along with the neurologic exam, give a more complete diagnosis from an anatomic and functional standpoint. Biomechanical deficits and imbalances can be determined that may be important in prescribing a comprehensive rehabilitation program.

6. What are the most common sports injuries?

This depends on the sport. Athletes involved in high-impact sports that require jumping and landing on hard surfaces (e.g., basketball, volleyball) are at risk for injuries in the ankle and knee, such as anterior cruciate ligament tears, meniscal tears, and inversion sprains. Activities involving more upper-extremity movement (e.g., tennis, baseball, racquetball) may cause injury to the rotator cuff and elbow. Sports such as cheerleading, volleyball, gymnastics, and weight-lifting may predispose to back injuries due to hyperextension and repetitive extension.

Common Sports Injuries Due to Musculotendinous Overload

INJURIES	SPORT(S)
Acromioclavicular ligament sprain	Weight-lifting, gymnastics
Rotator cuff tendinitis	Baseball, tennis, swimming
Medial epicondylitis	Golf, baseball (pitching), tennis (forehand)
Lateral epidondylitis	Tennis (backhand)
deQuervain's tenosynovitis	Rowing, golf
Spondylolysis, lumbar spine	Gymnastics
Trochanteric bursitis	Running
Adductor tendinitis	Hockey
Iliotibial band friction syndrome	Running
Patellofemoral pain	Basketball, cycling, running, soccer, weight-lifting
Achilles tendinitis	Running, basketball
Ankle sprains	Baseball, basketball, soccer
Plantar fasciitis	Running, soccer, tennis
Flexor hallucis tendinitis	Dance

7. Why are inversion sprains so common in sports?

The ankle mortise is least stable, from an osteologic standpoint, when the foot is plantar-flexed. In this position, stability is conferred by the ligaments, particularly on the lateral side. Plantar flexion is accompanied by inversion, which further stresses the lateral structures, rendering them susceptible to injury. In sports such as basketball, soccer, football, tennis, and wrestling, which require explosive jumping, running, or lateral movement, the athlete is often on the ball of the foot with the foot in a plantar-flexed position. Eversion sprains are less common due to the greater strength of the medial ligaments and the obligatory coupling of eversion with dorsiflexion, which confers greatest osteologic stability.

8. Which entrapment neuropathies commonly occur in sports?

Entrapment (or compressive) neuropathies are an important cause of pain and limit the ability to participate in sports for many athletes. In the upper body, **thoracic outlet syndrome** can cause unilateral or bilateral dysesthesias in an ulnar and/or median nerve distribution. **Suprascapular nerve entrapment** induces weakness in the supraspinatus and infraspinatus or the infraspinatus alone. Long thoracic nerve compression results in shoulder dysfunction via reduced scapular control. **Musculocutaneous nerve entrapment** may result in biceps weakness or, more commonly, reduced sensation in the lateral forearm. Classic entrapment sites for the ulnar nerve are at the level of the cubital tunnel and Guyon's canal, while the level of the bicipital aponeurosis, pronator teres, and carpal tunnel are common sites for compression of the median nerve. In the lower body, important entrapment sites include the piriformis muscle which can compress the sciatic nerve, the fibular head where the common peroneal nerve is vulnerable, and the tarsal tunnel where the distal tibial nerve can be compressed.

9. What is a "stinger" or "burner"?

A traction or compression injury to the brachial plexus, probably at the rootlet level. These typically occur in the upper roots and are more common in contact sports, such as football, where head and neck contact result in extraforaminal root compression (college and professional) or increased acromiomastoid distance (high school) with upper plexus tension. Sharp, burning pain is experienced down the arm and generally lasts from seconds to minutes.

10. What injuries are associated with running?

Most running-related injuries occur in the lower extremities. Forces up to three times body weight are placed on the lower-extremity joints during running. In particular, injuries include plantar fasciitis, medial tibial stress syndrome, achilles tendinitis, patellofemoral pain syndrome, and iliotibial band friction syndrome. Stress fractures commonly occur in the tibia, metatarsals, and fibula and less commonly in the femur and pelvis.

11. What causes shin splints?

Shin splints, or medial stress syndrome, is due to overload of structures in the posteromedial or anterolateral leg. Enthesitis at the attachment of the soleus to the tibia may be the most common cause, but tibial stress fractures, posterior tibialis tendinitis/periostitis, flexor hallucis tendinitis, and tibialis anterior overload injuries may all contribute to the medial tibial stress syndrome.

12. Is surgery necessary for a meniscal tear of the knee?

No. Meniscal injuries associated with mechanical locking, loss of full ROM, and persistent pain that limits daily activity will probably require surgical treatment. However, due to the vascular supply to the peripheral 30% of the menisci, there is potential for healing. Many meniscal injuries that minimally affect daily activities during the first few weeks after injury can be cautiously watched for symptomatic improvement and possible resolution of symptoms. If symptoms persist after 6–8 weeks, definitive studies (MRI or arthrogram) and surgical consultation are typically indicated.

13. What is a hip pointer?

A contusion to the iliac crest with subperiosteal hematoma, usually the result of direct trauma. The injured athlete has difficulty walking and standing upright due to the pain and muscular tightening in that area. The true hip joint is unaffected.

14. How does the anterior cruciate ligament (ACL) become torn?

The ACL prevents anterior displacement of the tibia with respect to the femur and imparts control over knee rotation. There are a number of ways in which the ligament can be disrupted:

1. Deceleration of the leg via quadriceps contraction combined with valgus and external rotation forces upon a slightly flexed knee
2. Sudden internal rotation of a hyperflexed knee
3. Sudden hyperextension of the knee (landing from a jump)
4. Backward fall on a flexed knee accompanied by a forceful quadriceps contraction in an attempt to maintain an upright position
5. Direct blows to the knee (both laterally and medially directed blows will cause ACL disruption if of sufficient force)

15. Is it possible to participate in sports without surgical repair of the torn ACL?

Sometimes. The ACL provides the majority of rotatory stability at the knee. If it is torn, stability during lateral and twisting movements is lost. Most high-level athletes and young recreational athletes who wish to return to the same level of sports competition need surgical repair. Reconstructive surgery, typically done with a bone-tendon-bone graft harvested from the distal patella, middle one-third of the patella tendon, and the proximal tibia, reestablishes some of the restraint to rotatory instability. Following ACL reconstruction, an aggressive rehabilitation program is required. If the patient is incapable of adhering to or not motivated to follow a comprehensive program (typically 6–9 months), then surgery should be reconsidered. Some patients will do well without surgery and can return to sports activities. Keys to both nonoperative and postoperative treatment include aggressive hamstring strengthening and proprioceptive training.

16. What important considerations are involved in rehabilitation of patellofemoral pain syndrome?

Patellofemoral pain syndrome is often due to poor tracking of the patella into the trochlear groove throughout the full range of flexion and extension. Emphasis needs to be placed upon stretching posterior and lateral structures which may be tight (i.e., the iliotibial band, hamstrings, gastrocsoleus), strengthening structures that directly or indirectly move the patella medially (e.g, medial quads, hip external rotators), proprioceptive retraining of patellofemoral motion (e.g., taping), and strengthening exercises that do not increase patellofemoral joint reaction forces excessively.

17. How does the iliotibial band friction syndrome (ITB) occur?

ITB syndrome is a lateral knee pain syndrome due to overload of the ITB. Pain is produced as the ITB rubs over the lateral femoral condyle, typically between 20° and 30° of flexion. Pain may also occur over the lateral tibia at Gerdy's tubercle. Causes include running on uneven surfaces, sudden increases in running mileage, and incorrect footwear in either pronators or supinators.

18. What is "turf toe"?

A sprain injury of the plantar capsule of the MTP joint of the great toe. It is generally due to excessive forces placed on the MTP joint during push-off or running on hard surfaces (i.e., artificial turf in football and soccer). The athlete complains of pain and swelling of the first MTP joint which worsens with attempted push-off. Splinting for 7–10 days and/or taping to limit dorsiflexion are necessary to prevent further injury.

19. Describe the important aspects of rehabbing rotator cuff injuries.

Assessment of the entire kinetic chain (e.g., cervical, thoracic, and lumbar spine and upper and lower extremities) is especially important in the overhead athlete. Muscles should be strengthened both concentrically and eccentrically, individually and in groups. Progression should lead to activity/sports-specific conditions to maximize the chances for return to activity painfree. Rotator cuff rehabilitation must address:

1. Flexibility deficits, particularly in the external rotators and posterior capsule

2. Joint motion restriction within the sternoclavicular, acromioclavicular, scapulothoracic, and glenohumeral joints

3. Strength deficits, particularly in the scapular stabilizers (rhomboids, lower and middle trapezii, and serratus anterior) as well as the cuff muscles

20. What is a glenoid labral injury?

The glenoid labrum is a cartilaginous structure in the shoulder that helps deepen the glenuhumeral joint and articulates with the humeral head. The humeral head sits in the "shoulder joint" by its attachment to the glenoid labrum. Because the glenoid labrum is relatively small compared to the large surface area of the humeral head, the shoulder joint has a great deal of mobility at the price of stability. A glenoid labral lesion can occur when laxity in the shoulder capsule and/or weakness in the rotator cuff muscles occurs and small or large degrees of motion occur at the glenohumeral joint due to subluxation or dislocation of the shoulder, potentially tearing the cartilaginous glenoid labrum. Glenoid labral tears are more common in overhead athletes who do repetitive overhead motion due to the extraordinary forces across the shoulder joint.

21. How is tennis elbow treated?

Lateral epicondylitis is the result of repetitive eccentric overload of the extensors and supinators of the wrist. Rehabilitation focuses on stretching tight wrist extensors eccentrically, strengthening the wrist extensors, and avoiding aggravating factors. Limitations of motion at the shoulder, poor cervicothoracic posture, and poor "ergonomics" at the workplace must be corrected. Counterforce braces and, occasionally, corticosteroid injections can be helpful. (For more information on tennis elbow, see Chapters 41 and 42).

22. What is "little league elbow"?

Little league elbow is the consequence of repeated valgus overload in the skeletally immature elbow. During late cocking and acceleration, medial structures are stretched while lateral structures are compressed. The distraction forces on the medial side may cause enlargement or avulsion of the medial epicondyle and osteochondritis dissecans, while the compressive lateral forces may induce radial head and capitellar growth disturbance, fractures, and articular cartilage breakdown.

23. What is biker's palsy?

Entrapment of the ulnar nerve at the wrist at Guyon's canal. It occurs commonly in cyclists because of direct pressure on the ulnar side of the hand with standard handlebars. Sensory and motor symptoms are confined to the ulnar-innervated structures distal to this area, with sparing of the flexor carpi ulnaris muscle and the dorsal ulnar cutaneous sensory patch. Methods of prevention include wearing padded bicycle gloves and the use of "aero-bars" which allow weight-bearing through the forearm.

24. Which sports confer an increased risk of a herniated disk?

The usual mechanism of injury to the intervertebral disk is one of flexion combined with rotation. Sports that require these activities repetitively will cause damage to the peripheral annular fibers and ultimately disk herniation. In particular, baseball, golf, and bowling (the # 1sport in the U.S. from a participation standpoint!) have an increased risk of disk herniation.

25. Why do gymnasts get low back pain?

Gymnastics, like other sports that require a lot of hyperextension of the spine, can place excessive loads on the posterior structures of the spine. In particular, loads are placed on the pars interarticularis (the site of spondylolysis) and on the facet joints. Other sports with a high incidence of low back pain are cheerleading, weight-lifting, and football.

26. Why are passive modalities used so frequently in sports medicine?

Good question. There is no doubt that passive modalities are overused in general in musculoskeletal rehabilitation. Although they may have some benefit in the acute situation, long-term use has not been shown effective for any specific disorders.

27. What is functional musculoskeletal rehabilitation?

Functional rehabilitation implies that the exercises performed by the patient for a specific musculoskeletal disorder are done in the plane of motion, the type of contraction, and a coordinated fashion similar to the sport or activity that the patient performs. A functional rehabilitation program should "look like" the activity the patient performs on a daily basis with their specific sport. Straight-leg raises, for example, would be a means of strengthening lower-extremity musculature including the quadriceps muscle and hip flexors. However, there are very few "functional" activities that a person would do during the day that would simulate this motion. A more appropriate functional activity may be a partial squat or a step-up or step-down to activate the quadriceps and hip flexor musculature.

28. What are open and closed chain exercises and why are they used?

A closed kinematic chain (CKC) is operational when the distal segment is fixed and movement at one segment will move the other segments in a predictable pattern. An open kinematic chain (OKC) is operational when the distal segment moves freely. An example of a CKC movement is a simple squat, while an example of an OKC movement is throwing a baseball. Both types of exercises are used in sports injury rehabilitation depending on the type of motion that is being functionally addressed. Most running injuries involving the lower extremities will emphasize CKC activities, whereas upper-quarter shoulder and elbow injuries in tennis and throwing sports may emphasize OKC exercises.

29. What does "rehabilitation beyond the resolution of symptoms" mean?

Many musculoskeletal injuries appear to resolve despite whatever treatment patients are given. After treatment of the acute inflammation, symptoms from many ailments disappear, and athletes mistakenly assume it is safe to return to sport. However, stopping rehabilitation at this point is inadequate. Most musculoskeletal injuries in sports are the result of chronic overload, in which biomechanical alterations have occurred and microtraumatic tissue injury has occurred. These biomechanical changes, consisting of muscle imbalances, inflexibilities, and weaknesses, need to be addressed to prevent recurrence of injury.

30. When should you use the philosophy "no pain, no gain"?

In most cases of rehabilitation of musculoskeletal and sports injuries, the patient needs to be careful not to push beyond the limits of pain when significant muscle, tendon, bone, or ligament injury has occurred. Pain often will be a guideline that is approached but not forced past. On the other hand, the healthy patient who wants to "get stronger" is expected to experience some soreness of muscles after lifting the necessary weights to obtain strength gains. The assumption is that in the latter case, muscle has been subjected to systematically applied overload and that adequate recovery time has been given so that full recovery between exercise sessions has been achieved.

BIBLIOGRAPHY

1. Bruckner P, Khan K: Clinical Sports Medicine. Sydney, McGraw-Hill, 1993.
2. Cantu RC, Micheli LJ: ACSM's Guidelines for the Team Physician. Philadelphia, Lea & Febiger, 1991.
3. DeLee JC, Drez D: Orthopedic Sports Medicine: Principles and Practice. Philadelphia, W.B. Saunders, 1994.
4. Fu FH, Stone DA: Sports Injuries: Mechanisms, Prevention, Treatment. Baltimore, Williams & Wilkins, 1994.
5. Gray GW: Chain Reaction Festival. Adrian, MI, Wynn Marketing, Inc., 1999.
6. Griffin LY (ed): Sports Medicine: Orthopaedic Knowledge Update. Rosemont, IL, American Academy of Orthopaedic Surgeons, 1994.
7. Hamill J, Knutzen KM: Biomechanical Basis of Human Movement. Philadelphia, Lippincott, 1995.
8. Harvey JS (ed): Sports Medicine. Physical Medicine and Rehabilitation Clinics of North American, vol. 4, no. 3. Philadelphia, W.B. Saunders, 1994.
9. Kibler WB, Herring SA, Press JM: Functional Rehabilitation of Sports and Musculoskeletal Injuries. Gaithersburg, MD, Aspen Publications, 1998.
10. Nicholas JA, Hershman EB: The Lower Extremity and Spine in Sports Medicine. St. Louis, Mosby, 1986.
11. Nicholas JA, Hershman EB: The Upper Extremity in Sports Medicine. St. Louis, Mosby, 1986.
12. Press JM (ed): Sports Medicine. Physical Medicine and Rehabilition Clinics of North America, vol. 5, no. 1. Philadelphia, W.B. Saunders, 1994.
13. Saal JA (ed): Rehabilitation of Sports Injuries. Physical Medicine and Rehabilitation: State of the Art Reviews, vol. 1, no. 4. Philadelphia, Hanley & Belfus, 1987.
14. Simon SR: Orthopaedic Basic Science. Elk Park, IL, American Academy of Orthopedic Surgeons, 1994.
15. Weinstein SM, Herring SA: Nerve problems and compartment syndrome in the hand, wrist, and forearm. Clin Sports Med 11(1):161–188, 1992.
16. Young JL, Press JM: Rehabilitation of running injuries. In Buschbacher R, Braddom R (eds): Sports Medicine and Rehabilitation: A Sport-Specific Approach. Philadelphia, Hanley & Belfus, 1995.
17. Young JL, Casazza BA, Press JM: The physiatric approach to sports medicine. In DeLisa J, Gans BM (eds): Rehabilitation Medicine: Principles and Practice, 3rd ed. Philadelphia, Lippincott-Raven, Philadelphia, 1998, pp 1599–1625.

63. REHABILITATION OF THE PERFORMING ARTIST

Scott E. Brown, M.D.

You are an artist if you pay homage through one medium to all that you feel from an-
other. The scientific training permits of reliability and accuracy, not of adequacy. Thus,
from these it follows that medicine may be both a science and an art.—Alan Gregg
(1890–1957) (*Quoted by Wilder Penfield in* The Difficult Art of Giving.)

1. Who invented performing arts medicine?

Then—The first written reference to medical problems of musicians is found in *A Treatise
On The Diseases Of Tradesmen*, written by Bernardino Ramazzini in 1699. At the end of the 19th
century, a number of citations in the medical literature described a popular surgical procedure for
pianists at the time, wherein the extensor tendon slips between the third, fourth, and fifth digits
were cut to enhance isolated movement of the troublesome fourth finger. This procedure quickly
fell out of favor due both to complications and the finding of no further pianistic success for its
subjects. During the 1920s, Otto Ortmann published his experimental study of the physiological
mechanics of piano technique and Joseph Pilates invented his exercise equipment.

Now—In recent decades, the field has benefited from more rigorous scientific study. Alice
Brandfonbrener, initially with the Aspen Music School, and William Hamilton, Lyle Micheli, and
James Garrick, with Major Ballet companies in New York, Boston, and San Francisco, respec-
tively, have led the field with major research. The Performing Arts Medicine Association and the
International Association for Dance Medicine and Science were organized in the early 1990s.
Both organizations publish medically oriented journals.

2. How many artists are injured by performing their art?

In a survey of the members of the International Conference of Symphony and Opera
Musicians, 76% reported having had at least one medical problem severe enough to interfere
with performance, and 36% reported four severe problems. The annual incidence of injury in student musicians is 5.7/100 male conservatory students and 11.5/100 female conservatory students.
In dancers, injury has affected as many as 90% in some studies.

3. What are the special considerations in the physical examination of a musician?

Injured musicians expect a greater level of expertise from their doctors in specificity of diagnosis and treatment. It is no longer acceptable to prescribe simply absolute rest as the universal
solution to performance related problems.

If possible, a musician should be examined playing the instrument. Most will be able to
bring the instrument with them to the examination. Having a piano in the office is needed for
the keyboard players. Sometimes, a "house call" is required as for church organists. Problems
with embouchure (the position of the lips and mouth in playing a wind or brass instrument),
focal dystonia, ergonomic, and other technical problems will be missed if the musician is not
examined while playing. Videotaping in the office as well as during rehearsal and performance
can be a helpful adjunct.

A thorough but directed musculoskeletal and neurologic exam should be undertaken.
Underlying medical problems may present earlier in musicians who may be more sensitive to the
functional effects of minor impairment early in the course of disease. A careful search for tendon
anomalies should be done, especially in string and wind players. A common problem that can
cause difficulties in the left hand of violin players and the right hand of clarinet players is the
conjoined flexor sublimis tendons of digits four and five. Other specific problems to examine for

include hypermobility, hand span, dycoordination and uneven playing, muscle tension, and excessive gripping/pressure on the instrument.

4. For dancers, what areas should be included in the physical examination?

For dancers, a complete lower-extremity biomechanical evaluation must be done that includes:

Lumbar ROM
Pelvic tilt
Hip joint internal and external rotation with the hip in neutral (0° flexion or extension)
Femoral ante- or retroversion
Hamstring flexibility
Q angle
Tibial torsion
Toe out
Ankle ROM
Foot pronation
First MTP joint ROM

As with musicians, it may be helpful to see the performer dancing. The pointe position can only be assessed with the patient wearing toe shoes.

5. Is it better for a musician to have loose or tight joints?

While the legendary, virtuoso violin technique of Niccolo Paganini has usually been ascribed to his purported joint hypermobility, current research leans more toward the potential hazards of loose joints—34% of a large group of musicians with upper-extremity problems were found to be hyperextensible as compared to an incidence of approximately 6% in the general population. The inability to adequately stabilize a joint on a string or key leads to conscious or unconscious compensatory maladaptive ergonomic postures or excessive muscle tension. Applying further tension across an already hyperextended joint may further stretch the supporting ligaments and volar plates in the case of the digits. Splinting, proper muscle-strengthening exercises, and attention to technique are required. An extreme case in a violinist has been reported in whom each time the fifth digit was lifted off the string, the MCP joint dislocated, eventually leading to digital nerve compression.

6. What are the common nerve entrapments seen in musicians?

The most common symptom complex, that of numbness and tingling into the medial forearm and fourth and fifth digits, is usually attributed to thoracic outlet syndrome. As in the general population, the neurologic examination and electrodiagnostic studies are usually normal. Given the absence of objective findings, this has been called "**functional**" or "**symptomatic**" **thoracic outlet syndrome**. Most instruments are held or played in front of the body, potentially tightening the anterior chest and neck muscles. The resulting symptoms suggestive of **medial cord entrapment** may involve some nonaxonotmetic process or may be only a referred symptom. Management relies on stretching, posture, instrument modification, and proper pacing. **Carpal tunnel** and **cubital tunnel syndromes** are seen about equally frequently. If a focal dystonia is diagnosed, a thorough search for **entrapment neuropathy** should be undertaken.

7. What are the most and least dangerous instruments?

Highest injury rates in university-level student musicians are seen with piano, guitar, and harp. Intermediate risk includes the bowed strings, percussion, clarinet, saxophone, flute, and organ. Lower risk appears to include all brass instruments, oboe, and bassoon.

8. What is meant by "overuse" in performing artists?

In 1994, the Performing Arts Medicine Association formed a committee to clarify the term *overuse* among other confusing and ambiguous terms used routinely in the field. A thorough search and interpretation of medical and lay literature led to a description of the term overuse in two different contexts; the practice of overuse as a cause as distinct from the resulting syndrome effect. **Overuse practice** is an activity in which anatomically normal structures have been used in a so-called "normal" manner, but to a degree that has exceeded their biologic limits. The pathologic changes that may result from overuse practices (the overuse syndromes) depend on the tissues affected and the degree and type of damage (i.e., inflammation, fatigue, structural change, etc.). Many of the commonly used synonyms for overuse (i.e., repetitive stress injury) combine cause and effect into a single entity rather than considering them as separate events, reducing diagnostic precision.

9. Are performing arts injuries compensable under Workers' Compensation?

Most states recognize two general types of compensable adverse workplace events: accidental injury and occupational disease. The test for compensability relies on the demonstration by the claimant that the injury or disease arose out of the **activities required of the employment (AOE)** and that it occurred during the **course of employment (COE)**. Accidental injury is rare for musicians but common for dancers. An acute event will usually meet the AOE/COE standard. More problematic are the overuse syndromes, which are considered occupational diseases. Most performing artists play or dance outside their primary employment as teachers or sidemen with other groups or have a non-arts "day job" requiring hand use (computer keyboards). Causation in these cases is often disputed or may be apportioned among employers or nonemployee job positions. One must be an employee to be eligible for Workers' Compensation benefits. Most freelance work is done on an individual contractor basis and thus will not include Workers' Compensation benefits.

10. What are the goals of dance screening?

Dance screening is the preparticipation physical assessment of prospective dancers. The process has also been used for follow-up assessment after rehabilitation from an injury. The key objectives of a dance screening program are to:

Establish normative data

Uncover pathology

Quantify risk factors

Develop characteristics for a given level of performance

Establish baseline data to set educational, training, or rehabilitative goals

Determine if an individual dancer possesses attributes necessary for participation in that form of dance (controversial)

There is no universally agreed upon protocol for dance screening.

11. What is turnout?

Turnout refers to the total amount of external rotation of both lower extremities. Ideally, most of a dancer's turnout should come from true external rotation at the hip joint. The ideal classical ballet aesthetic has stressed 180° of turnout which would require the dancer to have 90° at each hip. This rarely occurs, requiring the dancer to cheat biomechanically to meet expectations of teachers and company directors in attaining the 180°.

12. How does a dancer cheat to increase turnout?

Lumbar hyperlordosis—This allows slight hip flexion, relaxing the Y ligaments and loosening the hip joint capsule, in turn allowing more external hip rotation.

Screwing the knee—While moving into a turned-out position, the knees are flexed which allows the hips to flex, thus increasing hip external rotation. Once in the turned out position, the knees are straightened with the hips following into extension. The hip capsule then tightens, forcing the femurs to internally rotate. With the knee already planted on the floor at maximal turnout, this internal hip rotation applies increased torsional stress to the knee, especially the medial collateral ligament and medial joint capsule.

Midfoot hyperpronation—A dancer forcing turnout below the knee will increase subtalar joint eversion and midtarsal abduction, which appears as excessive pronation. The foot rolls in, flattening the medial arch. The navicular bone will touch the floor.

Toe grab—In order to stabilize and hold a forced turnout, the great toe will flex, grabbing the floor.

Except for the contribution from tibial torsion, all turnout should come from external rotation at the hip. Many dancers do not adequately use the hip external rotator muscles to take full advantage of available motion.

13. How is the female athletic triad relevant to dancers?

The Task Force on Women's issues of the American College of Sports Medicine met in 1992 and outlined a position stand on the female athletic triad: **disordered eating, amenorrhea,** and **osteoporosis**. The Task Force found that the triad occurred not only in elite athletes but also in dancers. Disordered eating is a common obvious symptom of the pressure to adhere to an aesthetic of thinness. Exercise and anorexia produce a state of hypothalamic hypogonadism. Decreased ovarian hormone production and hypoestrogenemia result from hypothalamic amenorrhea, which ultimately produces osteoporosis. The Task Force found that the triad is often denied, a response common in the dance world. They encourage a high index of suspicion for osteoporosis and other less obvious medical sequelae such as arrhythmias, depression, and stress fracture if even one component of the triad is detected.

14. Who is Pilates?

Joseph Pilates was a German athlete who initially developed a philosophy of physical conditioning shortly after World War I as he helped to rehabilitate German soldiers. His approach incorporated not only physical exercise but stressed the mind-body interaction. Pilates felt that a lean body capable of fluid and effortless motion would engender similar functioning of the person as a whole. He stressed proper breathing and muscle stabilization during his exercise routines. As part of his approach, he designed a set of unique exercise equipment that he gave colorful names such as the reformer, trapeze table, and combination barrel. After coming to the U.S. in the 1920s, he opened a studio that quickly became popular with dancers. His reformer allowed various jumping and other analogous dance activities to be performed supine (gravity eliminated). This device continues to be popular in the dance world for cross-training and injury rehabilitation.

15. Should a pointe shoe be pointy?

The position of *en pointe* is one of the most basic dance positions. The foot must be supported with the ankle in 90° of plantar flexion. Weight-bearing forces are transmitted through the distal ends of the first three toes. The toe box or block of a pointe shoe usually tapers to support the toes and MTP joints but is not pointy. The box is usually made of glue-reinforced canvas, but modern plastics are beginning to be used. Pointe shoes are individually fitted onto the dancer's foot and further "broken in" by the dancer to get the right feel. There is no right or left as with conventional footwear. Proper fit must consider the fine line between avoiding compression problems and allowing sufficient medial-lateral stability. If there are no significant problems with corns or Morton's neuroma symptoms, fit can be assessed by holding the box over the foot while gently squeezing the metatarsals together. Length and depth must also be considered as well as whether the top of the box is longer than the plantar aspect. A longer plantar portion may lead to overpointing (> 90° of ankle plantarflexion), while a longer dorsal portion may lead to underpointing (< 90° of ankle plantarflexion).

16. What is the differential diagnosis of groin pain in a dancer?

A clunk or pop often described as a feeling of the hip joint coming out of place occurs when the **iliopsoas** snaps across the **iliopectineal** eminence, especially when the flexed, abducted externally rotated hip returns to the neutral position. Other causes of hip/groin pain include a torn acetabular labrum, femoral neck stress fracture, adductor sprain, and rectus femoris tendinitis and myofascial pain (especially in a poorly trained dancer who incorrectly uses this muscle to raise the leg forward).

17. A ballet dancer successfully rehabilitates a "groin pull" (adductor sprain) but continues to have difficulty with piroutte turns. Why might this be?

The pirouette turn is one of the fundamental movements in ballet. The process requires a series of rotational momentum transfers. For example, to turn to the right, the front-facing dancer extends one leg in front of the body, then rotates that leg in the horizontal plane around the side until it reaches its physiologic ROM limit. The momentum of the elevated leg is then transmitted back to the body to provide the angular force to complete the turn while the foot is brought back to the knee of the supporting left leg. The momentum transfer is accomplished by the adductor muscles of the right leg slowing its rotation by eccentric contraction as it reaches its ROM limit. The adductors may be stretched uncomfortably since the rotating right leg may continue to carry significant momentum as the end range is reached. Any reduction in allowing the rotating leg to its full range because of either conscious or subconscious protection of the adductor muscles shortens the time the rotating leg can build momentum. Less momentum will ultimately be transferred back to the body and the movement will have a jerky appearance or the turn will be incomplete.

Treatment must focus on fully rehabilitating the adductor muscles through their full length-tension curves for both concentric and eccentric contraction.

18. In dance, what harm can come from a bad attitude?

Attitude and arabesque are routine classical ballet positions wherein the gesture leg is held extended at the hip behind the body. The increased lumbar lordosis required for these maneuvers subsequently increases posterior element overuse stress. Facet pain and spondylolysis can result when additional biomechanical factors intensify the hyperlordosis such as femoral anteversion, psoas tightness, thoracolumbar fascia shortening, thoracic kyphosis, genu recurvatum, weak abdominal muscles, and volitional hyperlordosis while cheating turnout.

BIBLIOGRAPHY

1. Brandfonbrener AG: Joint laxity and arm pain in musicians. Med Probl Perform Art 15:72–74, 2000.
2. Brown SE: Workers' Compensation and performance injuries. Med Probl Perform Art 11:111–115, 1996.
3. Dawson WJ, Charness M, Goode DJ, et al: What's in a name? Terminologic issues in performing arts medicine. Med Probl Perform Art 13:45–50, 1998.
4. Laws K: Momentum transfers in dance movement. Med Probl Perform Art 13:136–145, 1998.
6. Novella TM: Pointe shoes: Fitting and selection criteria. J. Dance Med Sci 4:73–73, 2000.
5. Liederbach M: Screening for functional capacity in dancers: Designing standardized, dance-specific injury prevention screening tools. J Dance Med Sci 1:93–106, 1997.
7. Otis CL, Drinkwater B, Johnson M, et al: The female athletic triad. Med Sci Sports Exerc 29(5):i–ix, 1997.
8. Robson BE: The female athletic triad. J Dance Med Sci 2:42–44, 1998.
9. Ryan AJ, Stephens RE: Dance Medicine- A Comprehensive Guide, Pluribus Press, Chicago.1987.
10. Sataloff RT, Brandfonbrener AG, Lederman RJ (eds): Textbook of Performing Arts Medicine, 2nd ed. San Diego, Singular Publishing Group, 1997.
11. Teitz CC: Hip and knee injuries in dancers. J Dance Med Sci 4:23–29, 2000.
12. Winspur I, Wynn Parry CB: The Musician's Hand: A Clinical Guide. Martin Dunitz Ltd., London. 1998.
13. Winspur I, Wynn Parry CB: Musicians' hands: A surgeon's perspective. Med Probl Perform Art 15:31–34, 2000.

X. Rehabilitation and Industry

64. VOCATIONAL REHABILITATION COUNSELING

Ruth Torkelson Lynch, Ph.D., Rochelle Habeck, Ph.D., and Rhodora C. Tumanon, M.D.

The two essential tasks in life are to love and to work.—Sigmund Freud

1. What is a vocation? How does it relate to personhood and disability?

A vocation is a person's life work and financial means of self-sufficiency. In our culture, one's occupation typically plays a central role in personal and social identity and is viewed as a potential source of life meaning and satisfaction. From a psychological perspective, one's vocation is often an important medium for developing self-concept and self-esteem. From the social perspective, work determines much of one's social situation in the community, such as place of residence, social network, family well-being, income, insurance, and benefits. When disability interferes with one's vocational role, and that role has played a significant part in the person's identity and socioeconomic well-being, then the impact of disability has a far greater effect than on function alone.

2. What is a vocational rehabilitation?

It is a coordinated and systematic process of services provided by professionals to persons with disabilities, to enable the person with disabilities to sustain or gain employment, economic self-sufficiency, and independence.

3. Who is eligible for vocational rehabilitation services?

Persons with physical or mental impairment that constitutes or results in an impediment to employment

Persons who can benefit in terms of employment outcome from the provision of rehabilitation services

Persons requiring vocational rehabilitation services to prepare, secure, sustain, return, or regain employment consistent with the person's strength, resources, priorities, concerns, abilities, capabilities, interest, and informed choice

4. Who provides vocational rehabilitation services?

Comprehensive vocational rehabilitation to achieve work and independent living goals is a team effort that involves health care, psychosocial, educational, occupational, and technology and engineering service providers. They may include:

Rehabilitation counselors
Vocational evaluators
Career counselors and job-training instructors
Job developers and job-placement specialists
Case managers
Physicians and paramedical professionals (including rehab nurses, physical therapists, occupational therapists, speech therapists, audiologists, assistive technology specialists and engineers,

psychologists, neuropsychologists, social workers, orthotists and prosthetists, dietitians, and other related medical and surgical specialists)

Low-vision specialists and rehabilitation teachers for vision impairment

Sign-language interpreters

5. Name four roles that physiatry and other specialties play in vocational rehabilitation of persons with disabilities.

1. **Optimizing physical functioning**—assess medical or surgical stability and promote improvement in functional abilities; monitor treatment needs and options; assess and recommend physical demand characteristics for return to work (i.e., sedentary, sedentary light, moderate work, etc.); prescribe therapy and assistive devices including assistive technology and ergonomic adaptations that augment physical functioning for self-care and work.

2. **Promoting emotional and cognitive functioning**—assess the individual's cognitive, attitudinal, and behavioral status for work functions and for self-direction to accomplish competitive work performance; promote adaptation and adjustment to life changes and new levels and methods of functional ability.

3. **Promoting overall health and wellness** (e.g., nutrition, sleep, exercise) in addition to disability-specific health care (e.g., seizure or spasticity management) so individuals have the daily health and endurance to obtain and maintain employment.

4. **Enhancing social and community access**—be involved in disability prevention and advocacy for issues that enhance vocational rehabilitation efforts (e.g., access to education, employment, transportation, housing, and health care in the community).

6. Who are the qualified providers of vocational rehabilitation?

Providers of vocational rehabilitation have different levels of work classification and education. The work level is determined on the basis of the position description and the applicant's position and work experience. The minimum qualifications generally include a bachelor's degree or master's degree to as high as a doctorate. Most of the psychosocial, occupational, and job development providers are Certified Rehabilitation Counselors who are required to hold a master's degree with relevant supervised experience.

7. What does the rehabilitation counselor do?

They help determine the rehabilitation needs, identify resources and programs, and provide counseling and skill development for independent living and vocational functioning. Specifically, they:

1. Collect educational, medical, and psychological information to better understand the person's strength and limitations.

2. Help the person develop career and independent living goals and decisions.

3. Identify skills, knowledge, and training necessary to pursue a career consistent with the person's abilities and interests.

4. Provide and coordinate appropriate analyses (e.g., physical demands, reasonable accommodations) so the person can make an informed choice about their career options.

5. Develop an individualized plan for employment that lists the steps needed to reach the person's job goal.

6. Provide labor market information and other resources to obtain job leads.

7. Follow the person's progress at work to help in maintaining the job.

8. Who are case managers?

In a comprehensive rehabilitation setting, case managers may be rehabilitation counselors from an agency in the community or "in-house" rehabilitation counselors employed by the rehabilitation center. The case manager will:

1. Receive information about the person, including medical information, psychological, and educational and work history from rehabilitation counselors or referral sources.

2. Interview the person for goal-setting and decision-making.

3. Provide orientation to the program of services selected (i.e., vocational assessment, career development and job placement, retraining/educational services).

4. Provide information to the person regarding approved service and other rehabilitation professionals to facilitate services selected and received.

5. Possess sensitivity to different cultural beliefs and treatment practices.

6. Obtain informed consent and allow for informed client choice about services (including refusal of services).

7. Document the ability of persons served to make competent decisions.

8. Communicate to the person risks and possible consequences.

9. Manage crises.

10. Verify policies and procedures concerning intervention management for the benefit of the person served.

11. Assist in psychosocial needs and transitioning to the community.

9. What are the responsibilities of the medical core team?

The medical core team includes professionals in rehab nursing, PT, OT, speech and language pathology, and dietetics. This team provides restoration services which are directed to increase activity and functioning; to improve physical and mental capacities for work and mobility (e.g., balance, endurance for work, lifting abilities, proper body mechanics, transferable skills development); improve hand functions and coordination; and improve visual/perceptual function. Observation of attitudes, behavior, and functional difficulties is important. The medical core team should look for special needs of the persons served in the rehab setting (e.g., hearing and visual acuity difficulties; cognitive and memory skill deficiencies in both written and spoken communication; emotional status). Documentation of such observations from clinical and therapy settings will assist the vocational rehabilitation planning process.

10. What is "determination of severity" of disability and "order of selection" according to disability?

This is terminology used by the state and federal system of vocational rehabilitation services to clarify the level of physical and mental limitations and functional capacities that may impact employment outcomes (e.g., mobility, communication, self-care, self-direction, interpersonal skills, work tolerance, work behavior skills). **Order of selection** refers to the system that state/federal agencies use to prioritize individuals eligible for service. Individuals are deemed to automatically meet the criteria of **severity** when the person is a recipient of Social Security Disability Insurance (SSDI); a recipient of Supplemental Security Income (SSI) by reason of blindness or disability; or has major disabling conditions that preclude the person from obtaining and maintaining gainful employment without rehabilitation assistance.

11. What are alternatives for persons with severe disability when work capacities are very limited or when work tolerances are restricted?

- Supported employment (e.g., provide a job coach in a competitive work environment, place and train the individual directly in the workplace; build work supports and accommodations with the employer and coworkers, gradually modify the job coach intensity)
- Day programs (e.g., day centers with flexible hours)
- Home-based employment
- Sheltered work or enclave work (e.g., a group of workers with disabilities in competitive settings)
- Work-hardening programs (e.g., gradually increasing work hours and physical demands)

12. Who pays for vocational rehabilitation services?

The state or federal system of vocational rehabilitation provides state and federal funding through agencies within each state (e.g., Division of Vocational Rehabilitation, Department of

Rehabilitation Services). Other vocational rehab services are provided through funding from Workers' Compensation; Social Security Disability; private health, motor vehicle, or disability insurance; county or local social services; legal settlements; or nonprofit agencies serving persons with disabilities through donations and grant funding (e.g., Easter Seals, Goodwill Industries). Vocational rehabilitation services may also be provided by large employers (e.g., disability management, employee assistance programs) or by schools, colleges, and universities (e.g., high school to work transition services, university disabled student services).

13. How do environmental influences impact vocational rehab planning and service delivery?

An individual's characteristics and functional capacities are certainly not the only determinants of independent living and employment outcomes. Discriminatory policies and practices as well as environmental barriers (e.g., poor access to transportation, limited entrance into or movement within buildings, lack of modified tools and equipment) are also major handicapping factors. Vocational rehab services must address modifications in both the physical and interpersonal aspects of the worksite:

Physical structures (e.g., equipment or architecture)
• Modify the physical environment of the workplace
• Restructure job duties or processes so that essential functions can be performed
• Provide augmentative or assistive technology equipment, qualified readers, or interpreters
• Coordinate accessible transportation

Interpersonal elements (e.g., coworkers and supervisors)
• Teach direct supervisors how to facilitate accommodation needs with production and performance requirements
• Solicit supportive coworkers (**natural supports**) to provide accommodations or assistance
• Develop endorsement by management of the accommodation plan

Interventions will be most effective when the client, vocational rehab counselor, and individuals from the targeted environment are in close collaboration.

14. How are disability benefits affected by return to work?

Disability beneficiaries receiving Social Security Disability Insurance (SSDI) or Supplemental Security Income (SSI) can still receive benefits while they test their ability to work. The **SSDI** employment supports provide help over a long time (up to 9 years) of trial work. This support includes full cash payments for the first year, a 36-month extended eligibility period, and a 5-year period in which the individual can start their cash benefits again without a new application. Medicare coverage can be continued during this time or even longer, in some cases requiring a copayment as wages increase. The employment supports include consideration for the cost of impairment-related work expenses (e.g., attendant care services, transportation costs, work-related equipment). **SSI** employment supports offer ways to continue receiving SSI benefits and/or Medicaid coverage while working and in many cases the ability to receive checks again without filing a complete new application if the individual loses a job or is unable to continue working.

Many rehabilitation counselors and related professionals (e.g., social workers) have required additional training or specialization in benefits counseling to master the complexities of benefit systems. Details of SSA's program are availble at their web site: www.ssa.gov/work.

15. Define these work disability terms: SSDI, SSI, Ticket to Work, PASS, SGA.

SSDI—Social Security Disability Insurance provides benefits to individuals who are "insured" by workers' contributions to the Social Security trust fund through prior social security tax paid on their earnings or those of their spouses or parents.

SSI—Supplemental Security Income makes cash assistance payments to aged, blind, and disabled people (including children under age 18) who have limited income and resources. The federal government funds SSI from general tax revenues.

Ticket to Work program—This new program is being phased in nationally over a 3-year period with full implementation anticipated by January 1, 2004. The new law extends the years that an SSDI beneficiary can receive Medicare, allows more flexibility between employer-provided health plans and Medicare supplemental policies, expands state options and funding for Medicaid, and provides more funds to states in the form of grants to support working individuals with disabilities (details available at www.ssa.gov/work).

PASS—Under the **Plan for Achieving Self-Support**, an SSI disability benefits recipient may set aside income and/or resources over a reasonable time to enable them to reach a work goal and become financially self-supporting (e.g., use income set aside for occupational training, purchase of occupational equipment, establish a business). The PASS plan set-aside income and resources are not counted when determining SSI eligibility or payment amounts.

SGA—**Substantial Gainful Activity** refers to the earnings guidelines used to evaluate the work activity. This is only one of the tests to decide if an individual is considered disabled for SSDI or SSI.

16. Describe a possible vocational rehab plan for an individual with chronic low back pain who is returning to a preinjury job.

Vocational intervention at the **personal level**:
• Effective pain management and regular physician follow-up and use of support groups.
• Analysis of the person's functional capacities in relation to the demands of preinjury work.
• Counseling regarding the impact of the injury on the individual's career.
• Coordination of rehab efforts to maximize that individual's confidence, strength, endurance, and flexibility to perform the demands of the job.

Vocational intervention at the **environment level**:
• Detailed analysis of the work environment and job demands.
• Determine modifications to accommodate current functioning and reduce chances of further aggravation of the condition, consider ergonomic modifications.

Vocational plan—Develop and negotiate gradual return to work or temporary modified duty; plan with all parties to assist the individual in an early transition back to work.

17. Describe a plan for an individual with traumatic brain injury who was unemployed at the time of injury.

Vocational intervention at the **person level**—Assess residual skills and learning style; determine interests and aptitudes; develop a career plan.

Vocational intervention at the **environment level**—Consider requirements of suitable occupations and work environments and potential accommodation strategies (i.e., maximize residual functioning, reduce or modify tasks to require fewer of the individual's skill or knowledge deficits).

Vocational plan—Provide social skills training for use at the work environment; provide occupational retraining through continuing education or on-the-job training; use volunteer placement to develop general work behaviors or supported employment with a job coach to teach work skills at the job site; provide placement assistance or continue supported employment services depending on severity and capacities; provide adaptive technology for augmentation of work performance.

18. An individual with a spinal cord injury wishes to return to a former job, but has substantial limitations in performing essential duties of the job, even with accommodations. What are the options?

Same employer, same job—If the person can return to the prior job, then the counselor can prepare a list of proposed solutions to maximize access and job performance (e.g., modifications to enhance building access, streamline the work station, and accommodations for performance of job functions).

Same employer, different job—If return to the prior job is not feasible even with accommodations, alternative employment within the company could be pursued, including retraining for the new job duties and utilization of transferable skills from the preinjury job.

New employer, different job—If return to the same employer is not feasible, a new job with a different employer (e.g., a change in career) may be the next course of action. This choice often requires more time, training, and expense if the change is substantially different from the preinjury job. There are usually many skills, work behaviors, and knowledge that can be transferred from previous work experience even when a career change is made.

19. Where can vocational rehab services be obtained in the community?

1. **State-operated programs.** Each state has a public vocational rehab program that is funded through state and federal appropriations. Referrals can be made directly to the local officer of the state agency.

2. **Private sector providers.** This is the fastest-growing segment of vocational rehab service providers, due in part to privatization of service delivery. These providers may be found in independent practice, rehabilitation facilities, community agencies, linked regional networks, interstate corporations, and insurance companies. To make a referral to a private provider, the team should contact the payer to discuss the need for services and help determine who the appropriate provider will be.

3. **Employer-based programs.** Many employers, particularly large organizations that are self-insured, have some type of internal process for disability management, return to work, and employee assistance, especially since the advent of the ADA.

20. How is assistive technology used in vocational rehabilitation?

There are numerous technological advancements and devices to help people with disabilities augment and optimize their functional capacities for daily living and competitive employment. The vocational rehab counselor works closely with the patient, family, OT, employers, and educators to identify suitable and user-friendly accommodations. Development of an effective assistive technology plan requires careful attention to the functional demands of the job, school, and home environments as well as the tasks that the individual desires to participate in (including recreation and avocational pursuits). Even adaptations that improve the efficiency and reduce the energy demands of ADLs in the home can be identified as crucial to a vocational plan. ADL efficiency can help get the patient out of the home to work without expending excessive stamina just getting ready.

21. What is the role of career and training staff?

These groups of professionals generally are at the bachelor or masters level. They are often employed by job centers, vocational/technical schools, or college/university career or disability service centers. Individuals in these positions can be very helpful in providing information about the labor market, job vacancies, or educational requirements of various careers.

22. Who are the job development/job placement staff and what is their role?

These professionals assist persons with disabilities who are seeking competitive employment. They help identify potential employers, develop resumes and applications; prepare job search activities (e.g., identify potential employers, set up job trials); coach persons on effective interviewing techniques; provide practical job resources; and coordinate reasonable accommodations. Another viable option may be to set up internship training with the option to become a regular employee. Rehabilitation counselors and case managers may consult with a job placement specialist or provide job placement services themselves depending on the work setting.

23. What do vocational evaluators do?

Vocational evaluators assess the vocational options for individuals who experience barriers to employment due to physical, mental, and developmental disabilities. Behavior, emotional status, cognitive functioning, personality style, interest, academic achievement, vocational aptitudes, and work skills may be covered in a comprehensive, individualized vocational assessment. Communication skills, learning styles, and transferable skills analysis (including thorough job analysis) are also included. Work samples (e.g., situational and work site assessment) may be individually designed and developed with the active participation of the person with a disability. The vocational evaluator may be a professional with specific training in either vocational evaluation or rehab counseling.

BIBLIOGRAPHY

1. Bolton B (ed): Handbook of Measurement and Evaluation in Rehabilitation, 3rd ed. Gaithersburg, MD, Aspen, 2001.
2. Chan F, Leahy M (eds): Health Care and Disability Case Management. Lake Zurich, IL, Vocational Consultants Press, 1999.
3. Lynch RT, Leonard J, Powers JM: Vocational rehabilitation for injured workers. Phys Med Rehabil Clin North Am 8:297–310, 1997.
4. Maki D, Riggar T (eds): Rehabilitation Counseling: Profession and Practice. New York, Springer, 1997.
5. Parker R, Szymanski E (eds): Rehabilitation Counseling: Basics and Beyond. Austin, TX, Pro-Ed, 1998.
6. Power P: A Guide to Vocational Assessment, 3rd ed. Austin, TX, Pro-Ed, 2000.
7. Roessler RT, Rubin SE: Case Management and Rehabilitation Counseling: Procedures and Techniques, 3rd ed. Austin, TX, Pro-Ed, 1998.
8. Rubin S, Roessler R: Foundations of the Vocational Rehabilitation Process. Austin, TX, Pro-Ed, 2001.
9. Szymanski E, Parker R (eds): Work and Disability: Issues and Strategies in Career Development and Job Placement. Austin, TX, Pro-Ed, 1996.
10. Wolffe KE: Career Counseling for People with Disabilities: A Practical Guide to Finding Employment. Austin, TX, Pro-Ed, 1997.

65. OCCUPATIONAL MEDICINE AND REHABILITATION OF THE INJURED WORKER

Norman B. Rosen, M.D.

1. Why does the physiatrist play a unique role in occupational medicine?

Because of his or her **broad knowledge base** in such diverse fields as anatomy, kinesiology, neurology, physical and occupational therapy, injury assessment and management (with both acute and chronic disease management), and ergonomics and understanding of the multifactorial aspects of most occupational problems, the physiatrist plays a unique role. Because of **expertise in the conservative management** of both acute and chronic musculoskeletal conditions, he or she is well-suited to instruct workers, employers, and supervisors in aspects of injury prevention, disability management, and wellness recommendations.

By being available to **assess acute pain presentations**, the physiatrist can also give recommendations that are designed **to avoid long-term disability** and can more effectively triage complicated presentations. Based on a broad knowledge base and expertise in a variety of conservative management techniques, these recommendations can avoid unnecessary surgery and hasten recovery in those instances in which surgery has been recommended. The unique training of the physiatrist allows him or her to better **assess both premorbid and comorbid conditions** that may adversely impact on acute presentations. By being **outcome-oriented**, he or she must be aware of the importance of rapid return to work, work modification, and appropriate problem-solving to facilitate rapid return to function, including work.

2. What are the commonest musculoskeletal problems encountered in the workplace?

The common conditions encountered in the workplace are **low back pain** and **cumulative trauma (repetitive strain) syndromes**. Both of these conditions share in common acute or chronic *overload*, or more likely, symptoms are a result of a combination of both acute and chronic factors.

Low back pain affects 2–4% of the working population, and 80% of workers will experience an episode of low back pain sometime during their work careers. Although acute overload/overuse or acute trauma can precipitate the current dysfunction, often underlying pre-existing postural and mechanical factors are present that predispose the low back to trauma and prolong its treatment.

Cumulative trauma can involve any part of the body but commonly affects nerves, joints, ligaments, tendons, and muscles. The most common cumulative trauma syndrome other than low back pain includes carpal tunnel syndrome, ulnar nerve problems at the elbow, and lateral epicondylitis at the elbow.

3. Which groups of workers are most "at risk" for injury?

The youngest and oldest groups of workers are at greatest risk for injury—the youngest because of their lack of experience and the fact that they are untested and more prone to risk-taking, and the oldest because they may have allowed themselves to have become deconditioned and have developed other comorbid conditions making them more vulnerable to injury. Physiological changes associated with the normal aging process and psychological "burn-out" can contribute to injury.

4. Which factors most adversely impact on the development of low back pain?

Repetitive lifting, speed, load, stress, poor body mechanics, posture, deconditioning, weakness, vibration, cold temperature, and smoking. Obesity as a risk factor is more related to the associated deconditioning but must be vigorously treated in the treatment of low back pain, along with smoking cessation. Proper exercise should be prescribed.

5. What are NIOSH and OSHA?

NIOSH and OSHA are two government agencies dedicated to insure safety in the workplace. NIOSH, the National Institute of Occupational Safety and Health, establishes guidelines and standards for the work environment, individual job descriptions, and material handling. OSHA, the Occupational Safety and Health Administration, enforces these guidelines and standards in the workplace at the state and federal level.

6. To determine the maximum weight that is safe to lift, NIOSH has defined the "action limit" and the "maximal permissible lift." What are these?

The **action limit** is the weight that is safe for 99% of males and 75% of females to lift. The **maximal permissible limit** is the weight that 25% of males and 1% of females are able to lift.

7. Name eight job-related factors that the clinician should keep in mind when dealing with an injured worker, other than motivation and the issues pertaining to the physical impairment itself.

1. The age of the patient and the age that other workers in that same job generally "burn-out." Have other workers been injured in this job?

2. Level of conditioning, motivation to "wellness," adverse behaviors (smoking, alcohol, obesity, drugs).

3. Prior injuries, and recovery times, of other workers similarly injured.

4. Perception of the worker as to who was responsible for his or her getting hurt.

5. What is the nature of the job? Any sustained or unusual static postures? Repetitive stresses? Temperature?

6. Worker's sense of "being in control" of his work, job satisfaction.

7. How supportive have the supervisors and employers been of this patient's injury?

8. What are the *patient's* goals for embarking on a treatment program?

8. How should repetitive trauma and cumulative trauma syndromes be assessed?

Assessment of repetitive strain factors and cumulative trauma injuries includes:
- evaluating the job (job analysis)
- evaluating the worker (biomechanical, behavioral, cognitive-intellectual, and spiritual assessment)
- evaluating the work station (ergonomics)
- evaluating the technique used by the worker in performing his or her task

Questions to be asked should include: Any prior injuries? Recovery time? Are rest periods built into the work schedule? What is the nature of the repetitive injury? How much control does the worker perceive that he or she has over the work? Job satisfaction? What is his or her motivation to return to work with modifications? Does the worker blame anyone for the injury or condition?

The worker has to be assessed from a comprehensive standpoint, paying attention to physical, emotional, intellectual, ergonomic, and motivational factors. The work station should be evaluated from an ergonomic perspective. The technique used by the worker should be assessed from a biomechanical perspective.

9. What are the most common causes of recidivism among injured workers?

1. Incomplete healing of a prior event, including residual restrictions of ROM, strength, and balance.

2. Failure to comply with treatment recommendations, particularly a home exercise program.

3. Failure to take medications properly.

4. Failure to recognize and adequately treat underlying myofascial pain and dysfunction.

5. Failure to make the necessary behavioral changes (exercise, weight control, curtailing tobacco and alcohol use).

6. Failure of clinicians to address the psychosocial aspects of the presentation and deal with these effectively.

10. When dealing with resistant carpal tunnel obstruction, what other factors should the physician look for while pursuing conservative management?

1. Hand position while performing the task

2. Adequate strength and as normal an ROM as is possible in the proximal stabilizers, including the forearm, arm, and shoulder muscles and joints

3. Trunk stability while performing the activity

4. Posture

5. Vibration

6. Obesity

7. Pregnancy (in females) and systemic disease (thyroid, other endocrine and nutritional deficiency)

8. Presence of undetected and untreated areas of myofascial pain in muscles of forearm, hand, brachium, shoulder, and neck, which may mimic and potentiate carpal tunnel dysfunction.

11. In addition to median nerve compromise at the wrist, what other phenomena may complicate the picture?

Entrapment of the flexor tendons of the fingers

Cervical radiculopathy ("double crush" syndrome)

Undetected myofascial pain and dysfunction syndromes in proximal muscles (forearm and shoulders, in particular)

12. Name four strategies for rapidly and successfully returning an injured worker to work.

1. Validate the injured worker's complaints and explain the benign nature of the presentation, including options of treatment.

2. Encourage an immediate return to limited or light duty, using joint protection but encouraging the use of uninvolved parts of the body.

3. Deal with whatever work-related physical or emotional stresses are present. Utilize physical therapy to facilitate improved strength, flexibility, and work-tolerance.

4. Focus on "wellness" issues, as opposed to a limited focus on the impairment. See the "big picture."

13. How can one minimize a worker's dependency on a lumbosacral support?

Since abdominal muscles can become weaker if patients wear lumbosacral support, it is imperative that abdominal strengthening, adequate posture, and the frequent performance of pelvic tilts be taught. Patients should also be taught dynamic stabilization exercises, which are exercises designed to stabilize the spine while the patient performs a series of muscle-strengthening and stretching exercises. In addition, stretching of hip flexors, hamstrings, calves, and the low back should be performed, and in some instances, stretching of the rectus femoris may be necessary. The key muscle groups of the back include the quadratus lumborum, piriformis, gluteal muscles, and ileopsoas. Home exercise programs should be performed frequently and regularly.

14. What is the difference between symptom magnification disorders, somatization disorders, and malingering?

Exaggerated symptoms often complicate the clinical picture in these conditions. **Symptom magnification disorders** are behaviors that are out of proportion to the physical impairment that is present. They are usually a reflection of anxiety, depression, somatization, anger, and frustration. These syndromes have been referred to as somatopsychic dysfunction. **Somatization** is a true psychological preoccupation with bodily symptoms and is usually subconscious. This preoccupation with body symptoms can actually cause somatic symptoms and hormonal changes. Many cases labeled as psychosomatic are included in this category. **Malingering** is a conscious attempt to deceive and is marked by inconsistent behavior which is environmentally influenced.

15. What concurrent emotional factors should the clinician be aware of that may be contributing to "symptom magnification"?

The most important concurrent emotional symptoms that must be addressed by the clinician are anger, passivity, dependency, anxiety, depression, hopelessness, helplessness, and fear. Overt malingering is rare but, like the other conditions, should be countered with reassurance, rapid return to work or function in some capacity, exercise, wellness counseling, problem-solving, and close monitoring of function. Care should be taken not to "reward" the suspected malingerer with time off or with an unstructured program. In all instances, referral for appropriate mental health counseling is indicated, and counseling of spouses and significant others is also worthwhile.

16. What ergonomic modifications should be made to the work station of someone with back pain?

Sitting has been demonstrated by Nachmensen to increase intradiscal pressure more than standing or lying down. Chair modifications include a flexible, reclining backrest with high back, armrests, and the use of a lumbar support. Chair height should allow both feet to rest on the floor or on a footrest. Frequent changes in position and in routine are recommended. Workers should be allowed to take frequent stretch breaks, and a vigorous home exercise program should be encouraged. Computer monitors should be well positioned and keyboards angulated. Adequate light and ventilation should be assured.

17. What is a functional capacity evaluation (FCE)?

An FCE is set of supervised functional activities designed to objectively assess the ability of a worker to perform a set of tasks, including lifting, carrying, walking, handling of objects, sitting time, manual and gross dexterity, strength and endurance. In addition, some behavioral information can be obtained, and discrepancies between performance and complaints documented. This information is used to estimate the worker's abilities to return to work as well as to identify areas of deficiency that can be therapeutically addressed in a more focused fashion. Standardized measurements are used to direct injured workers to jobs more suited to their capabilities. Job modifications can be tested. Patients are generally subdivided into the following categories:

Sedentary: maximal lift and carry < 10 lbs; frequent lift < 5 lbs; able to sit 6 hr in an 8-hour workday

Light work: 10–20 lbs: maximal lift 20 lb; frequent lift around 10 lbs

Medium work: 20–50 lbs: maximal lift 50 lbs; frequent lift around 25 lbs

Heavy work: 50–100 lbs: maximal lift 100 lbs; frequent lift around 50 lbs

Very heavy work: > 100 lbs

Other factors affecting the FCE include ambulation, standing tolerance, manual dexterity, and cognitive-intellectual.

18. What are some ways of measuring pain?

Pain is a difficult symptom to measure. Some simple tools to measure pain include the pain drawing, visual analogue scale, happy face scale, observable behavior, and a variety of tests to assess anxiety state-trait, depression, functional capacity, and personal inventory. Most of these are self-reporting inventories and scales, and the clinician utilizes serial reports to ascertain improvement or worsening.

The Waddell signs were originally compiled to warn surgeons about operating on patients who scored high as having a poor surgical prognosis. These signs include:

1. Tenderness—diffuse and superficial, nonanatomic
2. Pain with axial loading or compression
3. Distraction—changes in straight leg raising
4. Regional weakness and sensory changes
5. Over-reaction

BIBLIOGRAPHY

1. Bonfiglio RF: LaBan MM, Taylor RS, et al: Industrial rehabilitation medicine management. In DeLisa JA, Gans BM (eds): Rehabilitation Medicine: Principles and Practice, 2nd ed. Philadelphia, J.B. Lippincott, 1993, pp 169–177.
2. Johnson EW (ed): Rehabilitation of the Injured Worker. Physical Medicine and Rehabilitation Clinics of North America, vol. 3, no. 3. Philadelphia, W.B. Saunders, 1992.
3. Moore JS, Garg A (eds): Ergonomics: Low-back pain, carpal tunnel syndrome, and upper extremity disorders in the workplace. Occup Med State Art Rev 7(4):593–790, 1992.
4. Rosen NB: The myofascial pain syndromes. Phys Med Rehabil Clin North Am 4:41–63, 1993.
5. Rosen NB: Physical medicine and rehabilitation approaches to the management of myofascial pain and fibromyalgia syndromes. Bailliere's Clin Rheumat 8:881–916, 1994.

XI. Pediatric Rehabilitation

66. GENERAL PEDIATRIC REHABILITATION

Frank S. Pidcock, M.D., and James R. Christensen, M.D.

1. What are the earliest signs of Duchenne muscular dystrophy?

Early diagnosis of Duchenne muscular dystrophy is desirable because its X-linked recessive mode of inheritance places the family at risk for giving birth to additional cases. The early developmental history is normal with age-appropriate achievement of milestones, such as raising head from prone and sitting independently. In retrospect, there is often a history of difficulty in arising from the floor, frequent falls, or an abnormally loud thud when walking. Neck flexor muscles are involved early, and these children have a characteristic difficulty in raising their heads when supine. These subtle deviations are regarded as permissible in the child who is just beginning to ambulate and go unnoticed or are attributed to clumsiness. Around age 3–6 years, the lag in motor development becomes inescapable. The child shows difficulty with climbing stairs, develops a waddling gait to compensate for proximal weakness with lordosis, and develops toe-walking to maintain the center of gravity over the feet and to prevent collapse at the knees.

2. Where is the genetic abnormality in Duchenne muscular dystrophy?

The Xp21 site on the short arm of the X chromosome. The surprise is the enormous size of the gene, which spans 2.3 million base pairs of DNA. It in turn codes for **dystrophin**, a muscle-specific protein of leviathan size. The specific function of this protein is still being determined, but it is believed to be a component of the muscle cell membrane. The protein participates in the stabilization of muscle cell membrane.

3. What is the most common peripheral neuromuscular disorder affecting infants? Is it really associated with all of the "fibs and positive sharp waves" you heard about in medical school?

Spinal muscular atrophy (SMA) type 1, which affects the anterior horn cell and is present in infancy (Werdnig-Hoffman disease), is the answer. Although electrodiagnostic evaluation of SMA demonstrates significant membrane instability with numerous fibrillations and positive sharp waves, clinical studies do not report an overabundance of these findings. In fact, if fibrillation potentials are profuse, think of other disorders, such as type I hypotrophy with central nuclei, mitochondrial myopathy, or storage diseases.

4. In children, when do motor nerve conduction velocities (MNCV) approach adult values?

MNCV parallel the development of myelination. Myelination begins at about the 15th week of conceptional age. After birth, there is a direct relationship between conceptional age (defined as gestational age plus age from birth) and MNCV, which is independent of birth weight. By 3–5 years, MNCV has reached adult values.

5. What musculoskeletal condition is common to preadolescent female gymnasts and professional football lineman?

Spondylolysis. It is the probable result of nonunion of a stress fracture of the posterior elements of the lumbar vertebrae brought on by repetitive high-stress hyperextension activities. The L5 vertebra is most commonly involved, but any spinal segment may be affected. Spondylolisthesis refs to slippage of one vertebra on the one below it and, if severe, may compress spinal nerve roots, causing an impingement syndrome. Just remember that *spondylo* means spine, *lysis* means a breakdown, and *listhesis* slips off your tongue.

6. When do you worry about idiopathic adolescent scoliosis?

Although idiopathic scoliosis is the most common form of childhood scoliosis, other causes must be considered before the diagnosis is made. These include relatively minor problems, such as a leg-length discrepancy or poor posture, as well as serious conditions such as vertebral and spinal cord tumors, osteoid osteomas, and spondylolisthesis. Muscle spasms and hysteria are other conditions that may present as a scoliosis.

Since idiopathic scoliosis is generally a painless condition, a report of **pain**, especially at the convexity of the scoliotic curve, must be taken seriously, and further evaluations to determine an etiology are mandatory. Other red flags which signal the need to evaluate a child in greater detail are **onset before puberty** and presentation in a **male**.

7. What degree of spinal curvature is of concern in cerebral palsy, muscular dystrophy, and idiopathic scoliosis?

The degree of curvature determines the recommended treatment. In muscular dystrophy, surgical stabilization should be done before the decline in vital capacity makes surgery risky. This occurs when the patient's vital capacity falls below 35% of expected, which equates to a curvature of 35° or more in muscular dystrophy patients. Surgery when vital capacity is < 25% of expected may lead to postoperative ventilator dependence. In patients with quadriplegic cerebral palsy, correction of scoliosis is usually indicated when the curvature exceeds 45°, but additional risk factors such as epilepsy, respiratory capacity, and overall general health make these children poor candidates for major surgery. These factors as well as alternative interventions such as the use of a spinal orthosis should be considered before surgery is undertaken.

8. Who was Gavriil Ilizarov and what was he doing in Siberia in the 1950s?

He was perfecting a technique for lengthening limbs. In 1951, Professor Ilizarov developed a surgical procedure for treating many pathological conditions of the musculoskeletal system. His method involves creation of an osteotomy followed by application of an external fixator to apply controlled distraction of the bone. The gap caused by slow separation of the ends of the bone is filled in with new bone tissue. The rate of lengthening is approximately 1mm/day. The amount of length achieved is related to the bone being treated and the etiology of the limb-length discrepancy. In general, the femur should not be lengthened more than 6 to 10 cm at one time. Upper limits for lengthening in other bones are: tibia, 10–15 cm; humerus, 10–15 cm; and forearm, 5–10 cm. Intensive therapy following the procedure for stretching soft tissue and muscle to accommodate the lengthening bone is essential to the success of the procedure. Therapy needs to continue throughout the entire lengthening phase of the procedure as well as during the period of bone consolidation that follows.

9. Should you be concerned if a newborn presents with an isolated Klumpke's palsy?

Yes! Dr. Eng teaches that she never observed an isolated Klumpke's palsy secondary to birth trauma. While the lower plexus may be involved, it is essentially always seen in conjunction with upper plexus injury. If a true isolated lower plexus injury is observed in a neonate, one must rule out other causes, such as spinal cord injury, outlet tumors (rare), and anomalous brachial plexus (very rare).

10. Should surgical exploration with microsurgical reconstruction be attempted for obstetrical brachial plexus injury?

The answer is not clear cut and a number of opinions exist. Proponents of surgery suggest that the absence of deltoid or biceps function at 3 months of age is the key clinical finding and that surgery is indicated. They believe that it should not delayed to more than 6 months of age if there is no evidence of further spontaneous recovery. A large study of 470 Swedish patients did not support this point of view. No difference in outcome was found in upper plexus palsies in those children in which surgery took place before or after 6 months of age.

11. Why are the neonatal reflexes an important part of the examination of infants suspected of having neurologic disorders?

The neonatal or primitive reflexes are part of the bundled software with which we are born. These provide a temporary set of automatic instructions for protecting the defenseless newborn in the hostile extrauterine world. These include the Moro reflex, asymmetric tonic neck reflex, tonic labyrinthine reflex, positive supporting, rooting, palmar grasp, plantar grasp, automatic neonatal walking, and placing. As the brain completes its myelination and the ability to control movements increases during the first year, the child needs to be able to control voluntary movements. If the neonatal reflexes persist beyond 4–6 months of age or manifest themselves in a mandatory fashion which "locks" the child in specific positions, they become chains that bind rather than rails to guide the child on the path to independent movement. Therefore, their presence in a persistent or obligatory fashion is one of the earliest clues of impairment to the motor control centers of the nervous system.

12. How do the asymmetric (ATNR) and symmetric (STNR) tonic neck reflexes differ?

The ATNR is one of the classic neonatal reflexes that gradually fades away by age 6 months to allow independent reaching and head-turning. It is a fencer's pose: head turned toward the opponent with rapier extended, and opposite arm flexed at the elbow with finger pointed toward the shoulder. In contrast, the STNR is the only reflex that is not present at birth and again absent at the first birthday. It provides postural stability as the child makes the precarious transition from crawling to standing. Think of it as the "Aesop's fables" reflex: when the child's neck is flexed, the arms flex and the hips extend, recalling the "dog and the bone." If the neck extends, the arms extend and the hips flex, a perfect position for steadying oneself before attempting to pull up to stand, reminiscent of the "fox and the grapes."

13. What is the earliest age at which a child can learn to operate an electric wheelchair safely?

Children attain the cognitive and perceptual skills required to safely drive a motorized wheelchair around 3 years of age. Because exploration of surroundings through movement is one of the chief means of learning in early life, introduction of an alternative to ambulation for children for whom mobility is severely limited is desirable as early as possible. Don't forget that a child in a wheelchair requires the same vigilant supervision as any other rambunctious preschooler.

14. Is cerebral palsy caused by obstetrical misadventure?

Unfortunately, the perception that cerebral palsy is caused by something that went wrong at birth has been a part of popular folklore since its initial description by William John Little in 1868. This issue has since been scrutinized carefully by many epidemiologists. An association between asphyxia at birth and the development of cerebral palsy was detected in only about 3% to 13% of cases. Furthermore, cerebral palsy rates have not shown a decrease despite major improvements in obstetrical and neonatal care between the 1950s and 1970s.

15. Do Apgar scores predict cerebral palsy or mental retardation?

The Apgar score was developed to quickly identify the newborn infant in need of resuscitation and has little predictive significance for the development of neurologic problems—unless it is depressed at 15–20 minutes after birth. In a large multicenter collaborative project, 4.8% of surviving infants had Apgar scores of < 3 out of 10 at 1 minute. In this group, the risk of cerebral palsy was only 1.7%. However, 15% of infants who had 5-minute Apgar scores of < 3 had cerebral palsy. A score of < 3 at 15 minutes was associated with mortality in about 53% of cases, with a risk for cerebral palsy of 36% in survivors.

16. How do brain MRI scans correlate with gestational age and type of cerebral palsy?

Most children with cerebral palsy who were born prematurely had periventricular leukomalacia (PVL) on brain MRI. The second but much less common finding was posthemorrhagic porencephaly. Abnormalities seen at term or near term in children with cerebral palsy were border zone infarcts, bilateral basal ganglia-thalamic lesions, subcortical leukomalacia, and multicystic encephalomalcia. Ninety percent of those with PVL were born prematurely.

In patients diagnosed with diplegia, most had PVL. In quadriplegic patients, term type brain injuries were seen in 22 of 45 patients and brain anomalies in 10 patients. In hemiplegics, 17 of 26 patients had unilateral lesions and 7 had bilateral lesions.

17. Are acquired spinal cord injuries (SCIs) more common in children than adults?

No. The incidence of all new SCIs is 10,000 per year in the U.S., but only 3–5% of those are in children under 15 years of age. However, if a child acquires an SCI, he or she is more likely to develop tetraplegia (56% of cases in children) than an adult. This increased susceptibility to cervical injuries can be explained in part by more ligamentous laxity, shallow angulation of the facet joints, incomplete ossification of vertebral bodies, and relative underdevelopment of neck muscles for a relatively large, heavy head. There are also pediatric disorders predisposing to SCI such as Down syndrome, juvenile rheumatoid arthritis, and skeletal dysplasias.

18. What is SCIWORA?

SCIWORA is a medical acronym that stands for "spinal cord injury without radiographic abnormality." About 20% of children under age 12 years having serious SCI do not have evidence of fracture or dislocation. The inherent elasticity of the fibrocartilaginous spine and its surrounding soft tissue in the growing child is believed to account for the phenomenon. Fifty percent of children with SCIWORA have delayed onset of paralysis up to 4 days following injury. Therefore, every effort should be made at the time of presentation to rule out potential spinal instability with CT and controlled flexion-extension radiographs.

19. Should every child born with myelomeningocele have it surgically repaired?

Advances in surgical care and antibiotics have taken away the need for haste in decisions regarding surgery. Charney et al. reported the relationship between time of surgery and eventual outcome in 110 newborns with myelomeningocele. They found no significant difference in mortality, development of ventriculitis, developmental delay, or worsening of paralysis among groups that were surgically repaired within 48 hours, 3–7 days, or 1 week to 10 months of life.

The fact is that currently most myelomeningoceles are surgically repaired shortly after birth and the children survive. Studies that look at functional outcome suggest that adults with myelomeningocele have difficulty achieving independence from parents, finding suitable living accommodations, and landing a reasonable job. The environmental support systems available to the child appear to be at least as important in determining life satisfaction as the severity of the medical condition.

20. Are there signs that help distinguish fractures resulting from child abuse versus accidental trauma?

Nonaccidental trauma to children unfortunately continues to be a serious health problem. A high index of suspicion, backed up by appropriate medical findings, is very important. Fractures suggestive of abuse include:

1. Multiple fractures in various stages of healing
2. Growth plate fracture
3. Transverse metaphyseal fracture ("bucket-handle" fracture) near the growth plate of femur, tibia, and humerus
4. Spiral fractures of long bones
5. Unusual locations of fracture (posterior rib, sternum, scapula)

The above fractures are helpful in establishing the diagnosis of child abuse. If abusive head trauma is being considered, important nonskeletal associated findings include retinal hemorrhages and subdural hemorrhages (especially when multiple and of different ages). It is extremely important to have a high index of suspicion when ruling out the possibility of a diagnosis of child abuse, because of the malignant nature of the syndrome and the significant risk of fatality following repeated episodes. Remember, we are all required by law to report any suspected abuse. If you're wrong, the result of the investigation is inconvenience and ruffled feathers. If you're right, the result may well be a saved life.

21. What is the Wee-FIM?

It's not just a small functional independence measure (FIM). Developed in 1987, the WeeFIM is a measure of functional abilities and need for assistance associated with disability in children age 6 months to 7 years. It can be used above the age of 7 as long as the child has delays in functional abilities. There are six subdomains which include items that are rated on a 7-point ordinal scale (from dependence to independence).

22. What is the COAT?

COAT stands for **Children's Orientation and Amnesia Test**. It is a 16-item test of orientation and memory designed for children recovering from traumatic head injury, which is easily administered at the bedside. It assesses three areas: general orientation, temporal orientation, and memory. Post-traumatic amnesia (PTA) is that period after the injury during which the brain is unable to store and recall new events or information. On the COAT, a score within 2 SD of the mean for age defines the end of PTA. The duration of PTA has been correlated with prognosis. In a controlled study by Rutter, children with PTA of < 1 week were doing well 27 months following injury. However, persistent psychiatric problems were noted in approximately 50% of children with PTA for > 1 week. PTA of > 3 weeks was associated with significant educational problems related to attention deficits and disinhibition.

23. Does outcome after traumatic brain injury (TBI) follow the general pediatric brain injury rule that "outcome is better with earlier insults" (due to plasticity of the developing CNS)?

Unfortunately, for younger children this is not the case. While some studies using narrower age ranges have shown no significant differences with age, others have shown that older children and adolescents do better than younger children.

Why does this not follow the general rule in pediatric brain injury? There are many possible explanations. Plasticity, which is so important in recovery from focal brain injuries (i.e., infantile strokes), may be at a disadvantage due to the diffuse nature of the injuries. The younger brain may be more susceptible to the effects of trauma due to its different physical (i.e., less myelinated) and neurochemical (i.e., increased excitatory amino acids) properties. Also, the mechanism of injury is different depending on age, which may result in differences in the primary injury. Also, if the injury results in deficits of new learning (which TBI does), the more one needs to learn in life, the more one is at a disadvantage.

24. Which groups are most at risk for injuries and therefore the focus of any injury prevention strategies in the rehab setting?

While the care and treatment of the patient with traumatic injuries are improving, prevention is the most effective intervention. Prevention should be given highest priority by any professional working with children.

Trauma is the major cause of childhood morbidity and mortality, and head trauma is the single most important determinant of the severity of injury and outcome. The incidence of TBI is highest in males aged 10–29 years, with the peak incidence between 15 and 19 years. A shocking statistic is that the estimated cumulative risk of brain injury for children through age 15 years is 4% in boys and 2.5% in girls.

Injury does not occur randomly across the population. **Race** and **socioeconomic status** are major determinants of risk. Death rates for unintentional injury among children < 15 years old vary with race: Native Americans > African-Americans > whites > Asian-Americans. For all races, injury death rates are inversely related to income level.

One of the most significant risk factors for a head injury is a **history of previous head injury.** This means that patients in a rehab setting are at higher risk for injury, which further highlights the importance of and need for injury prevention.

25. What injury prevention strategies are most effective?

The main principles of brain injury prevention include:

1. Anything that can decrease the amount and rate of energy transfer will decrease the severity of injury to the brain, if not prevent it entirely.

2. Strategies that rely as much as possible on "passive" or automatic strategies are likely to be more effective than those based solely on behavioral change, especially since behavior changes are most difficult to achieve in the population at most risk (e.g., adolescents, the poor, the intoxicated).

3. Strategies and recommendations should be focused and specific (e.g., don't say "be careful"—instead say "use a car seat, buy and use a bike helmet, and throw out the baby walker!").

Because of the limitations of education and other strategies in isolation, prevention will need to be approached from multiple simultaneous angles—passive strategies, education, financial incentives (e.g., bicycle helmet coupons/subsidies), and "mandatory use" legislation. However, the first step is for all professionals working with children to remember the need for and importance of prevention.

26. Is there such a thing as executive function in children?

The executive system describes those mental processes necessary for formulating goals, planning how to achieve them, and carrying out the plans effectively. Executive function can also be thought of as those processes that allow mental flexibility—the ability to mentally initiate and sustain thoughts and plans appropriately, inhibit unwanted thoughts and actions, and yet mentally "shift gears" when appropriate. Remember the mnemonic **ISIS**—initiate, sustain, inhibit, shift.

Executive dysfunction is commonly seen in children after closed head injury (as it is in adults). As with many other functions, it is developmental in nature and may become more obvious (and testable) with increasing age.

BIBLIOGRAPHY

1. Charney EB, Weller SC, Sutton LN, et al: Management of the newborn with myelomeningocele: Time for a decision-making process. Pediatrics 75:58–64, 1985.
2. Ewing-Cobbs, et al: The Children's Orientation and Amnesia Test: Relationship to severity of acute head injury and to recovery of memory. Neurosurgery 27:683–691, 1990.
3. Hresko MT: Thoracic and lumbosacral spine. In Steinberg GG, et al (eds): Ramamurti's Orthopaedics in Primary Care. Baltimore, Williams & Wilkins, 1992.
4. McDonald CM: Neuromuscular disease. In Molnar GE, Alexander MA (eds): Pediatric Rehabilitation, 3rd ed. Philadelphia, Hanley & Belfus, 1999, pp 289–330.
5. Okumura A, Hayakawa F, Kato T, et al: MRI findings in patients with spastic cerebral plasy. Dev Med Child Neurol 39:363–372, 1997.
6. Paley D, Kovelman HF, Herzenvberg JE: Ilizarov technology. Adv Oper Orthop 1:243–287, 1993
7. Rivara FP: Epidemiology and prevention of pediatric traumatic brain injury. Pediatr Ann 23:12–17, 1994.
8. Strombeck C, et al: Functional outcome at 5 years in children with obstetrical brachial plexus palsy with and without microsurgical reconstruction. Dev Med Child Neurol 42:148–-57, 2000.

67. DEVELOPMENTAL MILESTONES

Scott Benjamin, M.D., Melissa Trovato, M.D., Edward A. Hurvitz, M.D., Lisa Daley, M.D.,and Mark G. Greenbaum, M.D.

1. How can one understand developmental milestones and not just memorize the events and ages at which they take place?

It's actually a pretty logical progression. Think of development as a continuum, not single events, with one function building on top of another. Development proceeds in a head to toe direction. First developed is head control, then trunk control, then rolling which includes head, trunk, and some limb control. Sitting follows, then crawling, pulling to stand, cruising along furniture or with hand-held assistance. Then independent walking, running, etc.

In addition, think of mass activity replaced by individual, specific actions. Infants react to a stimulating toy with their whole body, while an older child will reach, crawl, or walk toward the toy.

2. How does muscle tone differ between premature and term infants?

The muscle tone of an infant born at 28 weeks gestation is completely hypotonic. Muscle tone increases first caudally, beginning with flexion of the thigh at the hip at about 30 weeks' gestation and progresses cephalad. Flexion of the four limbs appears at 36 weeks. In the full-term newborn, flexor tone predominates.

3. What are handy mobility milestones to remember?
- Rolling (first prone to supine, then reversed)—4–5 months
- Sitting independently—6–7 months
- Walking—1 year
- Runs—2 years
- Stairs (adult style)—4r years
- Skips—5 years (boys later than girls)

4. What are handy fine motor milestones to remember?
- Grasping items—4–5 months
- Hand-to-hand transfers—6 months
- Pincer—10–11 months
- Feed with spoon—18 months
- Scribble—18 months
- Copies circle—3 years
- Copies cross—4 years
- Copies triangle—5 years

5. What are handy language milestones to remember?
- Babbling—7–8 months
- Single words—1 year
- Body parts—18 months
- Short sentences—2 years
- Full sentences—3 years
- Paragraphs—4 years
- Knows colors—5 years

6. What are handy social skill milestones to remember?
- Interactive game (pat-a-cake) —9 months
- Takes off clothes (shoes)—15 months

- Copies housekeeping—18 months
- Parallel play—3 years
- Social interaction —4 years

7. What are some critical milestones to remember by age?

This table is a guideline. Use it for a rough estimate, not for diagnostic purposes (see question14). These are 50th percentiles.

AGE	GROSS MOTOR	FINE MOTOR	LANGUAGE	SOCIAL
6 month	Sitting	Hand to hand, palmar grasp	Makes sounds	
1 year	Cruising (walks holding on), early walking	Pincer grasp	"Mama," "Dada," one or two other words	Interactive game
18 months	Walks up stairs with help	Scribbling	10 words, body parts	Takes off clothes, feeds self, copies housekeeping
2 years	Running	Circular scribbling	Short sentences	
3 years	Stands on one foot, rides tricycle	Copies circle	Full sentences	Parallel play
4 years	Up stairs adult style	Copies cross	Speaks in paragraphs	Social interaction
5 years	Skips (boys later)	Copies triangle	Knows colors	

8. At what age do 50% of children walk independently?

12 months. Most children can walk with one hand held at 12 months. It may or may not be cause for concern and need for closer monitoring of skills if they have not attained this milestone.

9. At what ages does a child typically begin to go up and down stairs alternating their feet?

Children typically begin going *up* stairs alternating feet at **3 years** of age; they typically begin going *down* stairs alternating feet at **4 years** of age.

10. At what age is hand dominance usually established?

Usually by **2 years** of age. Early hand dominance may be a sign for a neurologic deficit, such as weakness due to hemiplegic cerebral palsy, with resultant decreased use of the affected side.

11. What do the words squeeze, palmar, scissor, chuck, and pincer all have in common?

They are different types of grasp that an infant progresses through beginning around 4 months of age. The squeeze grasp is first achieved with progression through the other grasp types until a fine pincer grasp is achieved at approximately 10–11 months of age.

12. What do I do if language development is delayed?

Order an **audiology evaluation** to check for hearing. Make sure the child is in an environment that stimulates language. Start speech and language intervention earlier rather than later.

13. Why have you not mentioned toilet training?

Toilet training varies by culture and by family. It generally starts at about 18 months and is usually completed by about 3 years. There is a wide variance, especially with overnight continence. Suffice it to say that children should be dry all day by age 3. Children with disabilities will often toilet train later, due to cognitive, mobility, sensory, or other problems relating to their diagnoses.

14. How do I use developmental milestones in practice?

One has to approach the disabled child with an understanding of normal development in order to use adaptive equipment to assistant the child in gaining increased interaction with the environment. For example, for a child with spina bifida, one might consider the following:

- **3–8 months**—use tumble form chair to allow the child to visually inspect the environment.
- **8–14 months**—place in 90° seat to allow bimanual interaction with the environment and sitting experience. Also, use sitting cart to allow exploration.
- **14–25 months**—place child in parapodium to provide standing experience and weight-bearing for developing bones and muscles.

15. How can development be assessed more formally?

The milestones presented above are only for very rough estimates of development. If you have any questions about the child, a standardized developmental assessment is indicated. The **Denver Development Screening Test** was the old standard in the clinic. Other scales have gained more favor over the past few years, but the Denver still allows a quick review of major developmental goals.

Several screening tools exist that are designed to be filled out by the caregiver in < 15 minutes. The **PEDS—Pediatric Evaluation of Development**—was developed by Francis Glascoe. It is an 8- to 10-question scale that can be completed in 2 minutes. The **Ages and Stages Questionnaire (ASQ)** and the **Child Development Inventory** are also popular.

Patients who need a full developmental evaluation should be seen by physical therapy, occupational therapy, speech and language pathology, and/or neuropsychology. Tests commonly administered include the following: The **Bayley Infant Neurodevelopmental Screen** is an assessment of developmental risk for infants aged 3 months to 24 months. The **Peabody Developmental Test of Motor Proficiency** is an assessment of gross and fine motor skills for ages birth through 83 months. The **Bruininks-Oseretsky** (B & O) is a scale of motor proficiency for children aged 4.5–14.5 years. There are many others, including those that address speech and language, and each institution will have its favorites.

16. What are the CAT/CLAM and Capute Scales?

CAT stands for **Clinical Adaptive Test**. CLAM stands for **Clinical Linguistic Auditory Milestones**. It is a tool developed by Dr. Arnold Capute at the Kennedy Krieger Institute to evaluate the development of language and visual motor problem-solving in children from 1 month to 3 years of age. The **Capute Scale** is the developmental quotient based on developmental age divided by actual age × 100.

17. What are the asymmetric tonic neck and Moro reflexes? What are their significance developmentally?

These are primitive reflexes. They should appear and disappear in sequence during certain stages in development, and their persistence may indicate CNS or other nervous system dysfunction. Both should disappear around 6–7 months, although they may be prolonged in the premature infant.

- **Asymmetric tonic neck reflex**—Turning the head to the side elicits ipsilateral arm extension and contralateral flexion and should dampen with repetition. (Fencer's posture as an obligatory response is abnormal at any age).
- **Moro reflex**—Placing the baby in a semi-upright posture, allowing initial neck extension and then release causes initial abduction and extension of arms, flexion of thumbs, followed by adduction and flexion of the upper extremities. Asymmetry is abnormal and may reflect brachial plexus, other limb injury, or CNS injury.

18. When does "stranger anxiety" appear?

Beginning at 5 months, the infant starts the process of operation and individuation—differentiating between his mother and himself. Eventually, the infant develops a sense of belonging to a central person, and by 7–8 months behavior towards strangers differs from that with familiar people. This behavior, termed "stranger anxiety," is manifested by crying or a look of wariness when handled by strangers.

19. What is the parachute response?

The infant is held in prone vertical suspension and then suddenly thrust downward by the examiner. The infant's upper and lower extremities extend and reach for support to protect from falling. These postural responses appear at 6–7 months. They are not suppressed; they persist for life. The postural responses, if delayed or absent, may indicate CNS dysfunction, immaturity, or motor neuron disease.

20. How is the hip examination important in the evaluation of children in a physiatry practice? What is Galeazzi's or Allis sign?

The hip examination is essential in the assessment of newborns, infants and children who are either nonambulatory or have abnormal muscle tone. As a physiatrist, one may encounter children with hip problems due to diagnoses such as cerebral palsy, spinal cord injury, or spina bifida. These conditions may carry an increased risk of hip subluxation or dislocation. Older infants and children with conditions such as these should have their hip ROM and knee height difference evaluated. Galeazzi's or Allis sign makes reference to the comparison of knee height, making note of a discrepancy. A discrepancy may be positive for hip subluxation.

BIBLIOGRAPHY

1. Amiel-Tison C. Neurological evaluation of the maturity of newborn infants. Arch Dis Child 43:89–93, 1968.
2. Behrman RE: Nelson's Pediatrics, 14th ed. Philadelphia, W.B. Saunders, 1992.
3. Carpenter DL, Batley RJ, Johnson EW: Developmental evaluation of infants and children. Phys Med Rehabil Clin North Am 7:561–582, 1996.
4. Glascoe FP: Early detection of developmental and behavioral problems. Pediatr Rev 21:272–279, 2000.
5. Illingworth RS: The Development of the Infant and Young Child, 9th ed. New York, Churchill Livingstone, 1989.
6. Molnar GE, Alexander MA (eds): Pediatric Rehabilitation, 3rd ed. Philadelphia, Hanley & Belfus, 1999.

68. CEREBRAL PALSY

Edward A. Hurvitz, M.D., and Rita N. Ayyangar, M.D.

1. What is cerebral palsy?

Cerebral palsy is a **static encephalopathy** caused by an **insult to the immature brain**, leading to a global dysfunction which always includes problems with **motor function** (i.e. tone, posture, movement). Although definitions vary, it is probably best to limit the onset of injury to the prenatal, perinatal, or immediate postnatal period. It is important to note that the lesion resulting in cerebral palsy is static; it does not progressively become worse. However, as children grow, their muscles may become tighter, and as they age, they may have increasing functional deficits, but neither of these problems are related to increasing loss of cerebral function. They are generally secondary effects of spasticity and other primary problems.

2. What causes cerebral palsy?

Cerebral palsy is often the result of an intraventricular hemorrhage in the premature infant or of episodes of anoxia. Usually, the cause is unknown. Recent literature suggests that infections during the prenatal period may play a significant role in its development. Congenital brain malformations and trauma can also be considered. **Risk factors** for cerebral palsy include prematurity, low birth weight, history of fetal deprivation, history of fetal wastage, abnormal presentation, and associated malformations, among others.

3. How is cerebral palsy diagnosed?

Clinical diagnosis based on the criteria mentioned in question 1 is the most common way. In less severe cases, developmental delays and the manifestations of spasticity may not be present for up to a year. Patients may, in fact, initially be floppy. The common complaints are developmental delay, trouble feeding, drooling, and the arms and/or legs feeling stiff with the legs often crossing over each other (scissoring). Sometimes, cerebral palsy can "go away," especially if the diagnosis is made in the first year of life. The most important thing to determine is that there is **no loss of milestones**, which would indicate a neurodegenerative disorder, hydrocephalus, or even a tumor. Metabolic testing to rule out other diagnoses is often indicated. An MRI or brain CT in a child whose development is delayed but progressing and who is known to have been premature, is of questionable value in most cases.

Part of the diagnosis is a description of the clinical manifestations; **spastic diplegics** have legs more involved than arms, **spastic quadriplegics** have total body involvement, and **spastic hemiplegics** have only one side involved with arm usually affected more than the leg. Some children may have dystonia, chorea, athetosis, or ataxia rather than spasticity, or they may have a combination of these symptoms. Pure ataxia is rare and is usually associated with a problem in the posterior fossa.

4. What are the most common questions parents have?

Will my child walk? Doesn't having cerebral palsy mean that you are retarded? What should I be doing now?

5. Well, will their child walk?

The best indicator of how they are going to do is how they are currently doing. Molnar used **sitting balance** at age 2 as an indicator of future walking; Badell described similar criteria for spastic diplegics. Bleck listed seven **primitive reflexes** and found that a child whose response was abnormal for two of these reflexes by age 12 months had a poor prognosis for walking. These were:

Should be Absent:	Should be Present:
Asymmetric tonic neck reflex	Parachute reaction
Symmetric tonic neck reflex	Foot placement
Moro response	
Neck righting reflex	
Extensor thrust	

Trahan and Marcoux identified topography of the impairments, presence of the Moro or asymmetric tonic neck reflex, presence of seizures, and ability to sit at 12 months as indicators of ambulation by age 6. Walking in these studies includes use of a walker or crutches.

6. What does the gait look like?

Children with hemiplegia will **toe walk** with plantar flexion and excess knee flexion on the involved side, and their involved arm held in flexion synergy. Diplegic children often have bilateral **equinovarus** deformity, **knees that are flexed and in valgus**, and "scissoring" (the feet crossing in front of each other with each step.) Rotational problems, including **femoral anteversion** and **tibial torsion**, will often cause internal rotation of the feet.

7. Is Cerebral palsy associated with mental impairment?

Not necessarily. Cerebral palsy covers a wide spectrum of clinical presentations. Many children have normal to above normal cognition, while others are severely impaired. Mental deficiency is noted in approximately 50–75% of children with cerebral palsy. Only about one third of diplegic children have some degree of mental impairment, but many have perceptual-motor deficits.

8. What should the parents be doing?

The parents should listen carefully to their medical professionals, remain calm, and obtain early intervention services for the child. The law requires that every state provide education for every child, with appropriate services for children with special needs. The parents should contact their local school district, inform them that they have a child with special needs, and have the child evaluated. The family will have an **IFSP** (Individual Family Service Plan) or, if the child is older than 3, an **IEPC** (Individual Education Planning Committee) with the school staff and determine the child's service eligibility. Children under 3 generally receive physical or occupational therapy once or twice a week.

9. Should you worry about seizures?

Many children with cerebral palsy have seizures. Children with spastic quadriplegia are most prone, followed by those with spastic hemiplegia. There is no need for a baseline EEG; evaluation and management can wait until there are symptoms.

10. What kinds of visual problems occur?

Strabismus is a common problem in cerebral palsy, due to an imbalance in the eye musculature. It is often treated with ophthalmologic surgery. **Hemianopsia** may be present with dense hemiplegia with a middle cerebral artery lesion.

11. What kind of problems does spasticity cause?

Spasticity is defined as a velocity dependent resistance to stretch. It is a common manifestation of the upper-motor-neuron syndrome (decreased dexterity, hyperreflexia, spasticity, paralysis). The most prominent finding is hypertonicity of the musculature and impaired motor control. (Reducing spasticity improves motor control, but of course does not normalize it—other aspects of the upper motor neuron syndrome are also playing a role.) Spasticity can cause **contractures** secondary to muscle tightness, especially in the gastrocnemius-soleus group, hamstrings, adductors, hip flexors, biceps, wrist flexors and opponens pollicus. **Hip dislocation** can occur due to tight adductors (see question 12). **Scoliosis** or **lordosis** from spasticity and weakness is another frequently noted problem that may worsen rapidly as the child grows through a growth spurt (see question 13). Spasticity can also cause difficulty with seating and interfere with caretakers ability perform transfers and other aspects of care.

12. What should be done about the hips?

In children with tight hip musculature, especially the adductors, the hips should be followed with plain x-rays on a regular basis (every year to year and a half). Hip dislocation is a common problem, occurring in 25–30% of the children. Orthopedic procedures such as **adductor tenotomies** or **derotational osteotomies** help prevent dislocation. Surgical reduction of a dislocated hip is indicated for ambulatory children or for nonambulatory children with pain or seating difficulties. In younger children, hip dislocation can lead to improper development of the hip joint and painful arthritis in young adulthood. In spastic quadriplegic children with very high tone, hip dislocation is very common. Unfortunately, results of surgical repair have been variable in this group, and surgery may not be indicated.

13. What should be done about the spine?

Children with cerebral palsy are at higher risk for scoliosis and lordosis. The incidence of scoliosis parallels that of neurologic involvement, with an incidence of 60% in children with spastic quadriplegia. Scoliosis in cerebral palsy progresses more rapidly and produces different curve patterns than idiopathic scoliosis. Hip dislocation and pelvic obliquity can contribute to worsening curves. Seating problems, pressure sores, and cardiopulmonary compromise are potential complications. Ambulatory children are managed with bracing and surgical techniques. Nonambulatory children are often best managed with molded seating but may need other interventions as well.

14. What should I do about the other limbs and joints?

Spasticity tends to lead to loss of range of motion (ROM) in a joint due to tight musculature, especially in muscles that cross two joints. In cerebral palsy, it is complicated by growth; bones grow faster than muscles, leading to greater loss of range. The main joints at risk are the ankles (plantarflexion) and flexion contractures at the knees, hips, elbows and wrists. The first line treatment is **stretching exercises**. **Serial casting** and **orthoses** are used, especially for the ankles, knees, and elbows. Casting can be combined with blocks (see question 15). If these methods fail, **orthopedic surgery** is indicated for muscle and tendon lengthening. Muscles that are lengthened will lose about a grade of strength. As children grow, the muscle continues to fail to keep up with bone growth, and all of the above interventions (including surgery) will need to be repeated.

15. When should antispasticity medications be used?

Spasticity medications (diazepam, baclofen, dantrolene, tizanidine, and others) are indicated for the treatment of **generalized spasticity**. They are useful in severely involved children to aid with hygiene and prevent mass extensor spasm. Their use to improve general mobility on a long-term basis is more controversial. They are occasionally used to see if the child might be a candidate for a rhizotomy or other more extensive interventions. Each drug has its own complications; diazepam and baclofen are sedating, baclofen and dantrolene sodium cause hepatic problems, and baclofen can lower the seizure threshold. Dantrium is a current favorite because of the seizure and sedation issue, but liver function tests must be monitored. The use of tizanidine in children is presently under investigation but has shown promise.

16. What are nerve/motor point blocks?

Motor point/nerve blocks are indicated for **spasticity affecting specific muscle groups**. They are commonly done to decrease scissoring due to adductor spasticity, equinovarus foot deformity during gait, and hamstring tightness.

Botulinum toxin injections lead to presynaptic inhibition of motor nerve function. It has become quite popular for treating focal spasticity in both the upper and lower extremities, as well as the neck and trunk. Tone reduction peaks at about 2–4 weeks after injection, and effects can last for 3–6 months. A variety of injection techniques are used, with some practitioners using EMG guidance and other visually locating motor points. The child's skin is commonly treated with EMLA cream or ethyl chloride spray for local anesthesia. Sedation or general anesthesia is used for younger children or more involved blocks.

Phenol and, less commonly, **alcohol** are neurolytic. They basically cause a chemical neurectomy that is effective for 3–6 months. An electrical stimulator is usually used to identify the proper location for injection. These agents can be used for motor point or nerve blocks, depending on the desired result. An aggressive stretching and motor re-education program is indicated after these procedures.

17. For whom is a rhizotomy indicated? What can it do?

The selective dorsal rootlet rhizotomy is a neurosurgical procedure designed to decrease the excitatory input to the motor neuron, thereby decreasing spasticity. It was popularized in the U.S. by Warwick Peacock in the early 1980s for children with cerebral palsy. The procedure consists of a laminectomy and exposure of the cauda equina. The dorsal roots are electrically stimulated, and various criteria are used for determining which parts of the root contain more fibers involved with abnormal reflexes. These rootlets are than severed. This technique allows for decreased tone without sacrificing significant sensation.

The ideal patient is a **young child (ages 3–8) with spastic diplegia who is quite ambulatory with a spastic gait**. Generally any child who could make significant functional gains if his or her spasticity was reduced could benefit, as well as children with significant seating problems. Children with poor head and trunk control, and children who use spasticity for functional purposes (e.g., extensor spasms to stand) are poor candidates for the procedure. After surgery, the children require an extensive physical and occupational therapy program to recover from postoperative weakness and to maximize functional gains.

18. What does an intrathecal baclofen pump do and for whom is it indicated?

The **intrathecal baclofen** (ITB) pump is an electronic programmable pump device that is implanted under the skin and connected to a catheter with its tip usually at about T12 so that it releases baclofen directly into the cerebrospinal fluid. As the drug is being delivered very close to its site of action (receptors are just 1 mm under the surface of the spinal cord), the dose required is often a 100 times less than the oral dose. The child initially receives an **intrathecal test dose** via a lumbar puncture to assess the effects of the medication over a period of 6–8 hours. The Ashworth or modified Ashworth scales are used to score spasticity. A child who is a **responder** (defined as a 1 point drop in the average lower extremity Ashworth scores) then goes on to get the pump implanted.

The pump is more effective for lower extremity spasticity, but improvements are noted in the uppers as well. The ITB pump allows flexibility of dosing, which can be a continuous infusion or may include intermittent boluses as well. Dose adjustments can be made by externally programming the pump using radiotelemetry. The pump must be refilled every 2–3 months via injection, and battery life currently necessitates replacement every 5–7 years. Patient acceptance has been high, despite the relatively high maintenance required for regular refills and management of complications. Common complications include infections such as meningitis, catheter kinks or breaks, pump malfunction, and overdosage which can cause hypotonia and respiratory problems requiring temporary ventilatory support. Acute withdrawal of the drug can be dangerous and high doses of oral baclofen or diazepam may be needed to avert a crisis.

ITB is used in both ambulatory and nonambulatory individuals. It is indicated for any child, weighing over 28 lbs with enough torso room for the pump, who would benefit from spasticity and/or dystonia reduction and can follow through with refill and maintenance needs.

19. When should I consult orthopedics? Neurosurgery?

The rhizotomy and baclofen pump **decrease spasticity** but have no effect on shortened, contracted muscles. Orthopedic surgery can **lengthen muscles** and change the biomechanics of gait through tendon transfers, but it does not change the basic neurology. A combination of techniques is often required to gain greatest improvement in gait. Gait laboratory analysis is useful in many cases for determining the appropriate interventions.

20. Who were Karel and Berta Bobath?

The Bobaths began treating children with cerebral palsy in the 1940s. He was a neurologist, and she was a physical therapist. The Bobath treatment program is based on normalizing movement patterns and inhibiting abnormal reflexes. Most therapists incorporate some of their techniques in treatment, along with a **neurodevelopmental therapy** (NDT) approach that encourages the child to sit correctly before they crawl, crawl correctly before they stand, etc.

21. What's new in physical therapy for cerebral palsy?

A common belief associated with neurodevelopmental therapy was that strengthening was bad for spastic musculature. It was thought that it would increase spasticity and abnormal reflexes. Recently, the benefits of strengthening have been reported. **Resistive exercises** have led to increased strength and improved gait pattern. Several new programs and treatment philosophies have emerged based on increased intensity of therapy. Some, like **conductive education**, require a short-term, but very intensive commitment by the family. The effectiveness of these programs is under investigation. **Hippotherapy** uses a horse as a tool in physical therapy; several beneficial effects have been suggested, and the programs are fun and motivating for the children.

22. What are AFOs?

Ankle foot-orthoses (AFOs) aid in gait by controlling the equinus or equinovarus deformity. The older type consisted of two metal sidebars going into the shoe. Most AFOs today are plastic, molded to the foot; they may be capable of dorsiflexion if constructed with an articulated ankle joint. Some braces, called **ground reaction AFOs**, are designed to prevent crouching by transferring force to the anterior shin during stance phase. They are effective only in the absence of significant knee or hip flexion contractures. For children with spasticity, AFOs are designed with features to decrease abnormal reflexes, including a foot plate that extends past the toe to discourage toe flexion and a metatarsal support to discourage stimulation to a particularly reflexogenic area of the foot. They are most effective during gait, but use during rest helps prevent contracture.

23. What are some of the seating issues in cerebral palsy?
The goals of seating are **proper postural alignment, comfort,** and **mobility**. Positioning should protect the joints and skin, support the trunk and pelvis to prevent deformity, and discourage abnormal reflexes. Extensor reflexes can be inhibited by keeping the hips, knees and ankles at **at least 90° angles**. Head support can discourage the asymmetric tonic neck reflex. Power chairs are important mobility devices for many children.

24. What kind of swallowing and nutritional problems are present?
Children with cerebral palsy may have difficulty with swallowing, speech, and drooling due to oral motor control problems. **Dysphagia** can lead to difficulty with adequate nutrition or aspiration. A dysphagia team, usually involving speech and language pathology, occupational therapy, and/or dietary specialists, evaluate the child clinically as well as with a videofluoroscopic swallow study using different consistency of food. **Fiberoptic endoscopic evaluation of swallowing** (FEES) is a direct visualization technique that gives a better view of the sequence and timing of swallowing, as well as the amount of residual food left with each swallow. Interventions include positioning and dietary changes, usually involving soft foods over liquids and full solids. Swallowing evaluations are helpful to resolve conflicts between families and the school about safety and appropriateness of oral feeding. With severe aspiration or caloric need problems, a gastrostomy tube is indicated. If the aspiration is asymptomatic, placement of a G-tube is somewhat controversial,and less of an absolute indication. Significant drooling problems are managed with glycopyrrolate, scopolamine patches, and surgery in most severe case.

25. How do I help kids who have communication problems?
Speech problems are often accompanied by spasticity, decreased coordination, and choreoathetosis. Augmentative communication devices must compensate for lack of speed and accuracy. Special switches have been developed to improve access to technology, as well as software that allows for greater options with fewer demands for accurate keyboard use.

26. What other equipment should I consider?
Various ADLs may require specialized seating. There are feeder seats, car seats, corner seats, and bath seats. Prone or supine standers are used to encourage weight bearing and standing activities. If children have difficulty sleeping at night, supine liers can position them more comfortably. Computers are important for school and recreation. An assisted technology assessment can aid with access problems. Specialty equipment may be commercially available or custom modified.

27. Describe some of the adapted recreational options for individuals with cerebral palsy.
Most recreational activities can be adapted, depending on the resources and willingness of the community. **Special Olympics** offers the child a chance to participate in peer level athletic competition. There are many adapted **horseback-riding programs**. Horseback riding can be recreational as well as therapeutic. **Computers** can open up many recreation opportunities. In today's world, a child who is severely impaired can interact on an even plane with others through the Internet.

28. What are some of the critical psychosocial issues to address?
Children with cerebral palsy are at high risk for development of psychological and behavioral problems. Like other children with disabilities, they often have difficulties with peer interaction and other issues of social competence. Higher functioning kids will have more awareness

of disability with resultant adjustment issues. Vocational issues, long-term care concerns, advocacy training, and access to proper resources are all factors to be considered when managing a family with a child who has cerebral palsy.

29. What is the best thing I can say to this family?
A family needs to hear that there will be support for them down the road, from their doctor and from their community. The physician should demonstrate this by listening to the family's concerns, providing medical information, and providing access to resources. They also need to know that cerebral palsy has a wide spectrum of clinical presentations and functional prognoses and that the effort they put in can make a positive difference in the final outcome.

BIBLIOGRAPHY

1. Bleck EE: Orthopedic Management of Cerebral Palsy. London, Mac Keith Press, 1987
2. Cornell MS: The hip in cerebral palsy. Dev Med Child Neurol 37:3–18, 1995.
3. Damiano DL, Abel MF: Functional outcomes of strength training in spastic cerebral palsy. Arch Phys Med Rehabil 79:199–125, 1998.
4. Deluca PA: The musculoskeletal management of cerebral palsy. Pediatr Clin North Am 43:1135–1150, 1996.
5. Gormley ME Jr: Management of spasticity in children (pt 1 & 2). J Head Trauma Rehabil 14:207–209, 1999.
6. Molnar GE: Cerebral palsy. In Molnar GE (ed.): Pediatric Rehabilitation. Baltimore, Williams & Wilkins, 1992, pp 481–533.
7. Sussman MD (ed): The Diplegic Child: Evaluation and Management. Rosemont, IL, American Academy of Orthopedic Surgeons, 1992.

69. NEURAL TUBE DEFECTS

Sam S.H. Wu, M.D., M.P.H., M.B.A., Jeffrey M. Cohen, M.D., and Steven A. Stiens, M.D., M.S.

1. What are neural tube defects (NTDs) and how are they categorized?
The neural tube closes between the 22nd and 29th day after conception, and neural tube defects (**myelodysplasia**) result from aberrations in neurolation.

Spina bifida is a general term used to describe a group of NTDs with failure of the vertebrae to fuse posteriorly. Spina bifida is further categorized into two subtypes:

(1) **Spina bifida occulta**: Although the overlying skin is intact, there is often skin pigmentation, hair tufts, or a dermal sinus with an associated underlying defect of the posterior bony elements of the vertebrae. This defect is usually demonstrable only on radiographic studies. There is no associated spinal cord malformation and the patient is generally asymptomatic.

(2) **Spina bifida aperta:** This defect has three variants. In myeloschisis, the neural tube defect is open and occurs prior to the 28th day after conception. It is most common at the thoracolumbar junction. In **meningocele**, the overlying skin is intact with presence of herniation of meningeal membranes. There is little or no defect of the underlying nervous system, and this defect produces little or no paralysis. In **meningomyelocele**, there is absence of overlying skin, with exposure of dysplastic spinal cord extruding posteriorly and often with leakage of CSF. This deficit produces lower extremity paralysis, sensory loss, and neurogenic bowel and bladder. It accounts for two-thirds of all NTDs.

2. What causes NTDs?
The etiology of NTDs is believed to be mutifactorial. Genetically, the recurrence rate is 2.4–5% after the birth of one child with spina bifida and doubles after two affected children. Most

NTDs occur as isolated defects with no other abnormalities. Trisomy 13 is associated with NTDs. Environmental factors include maternal hyperthermia in the first trimester, such as fever due to illness. Dietary factors include prenatal folic acid deficiency. Pharmacologic agents include aminopterin (a folate antagonist used as an abortion drug) and valproic acid (a widely used antiepileptic drug). Social factors include low economic status.

3. What is the incidence of NTDs?
There are geographic variations in the incidence:
Worldwide: 1/1000 live births
Wales and Ireland: 3–4/1000 live births
U.S. and Great Britain: 0.6/1000 live births

4. How do you detect and reduce the risk of NTDs prenatally?
1. NTDs allow for leakage of α-fetoprotein (AFP) and acetylcholinesterase isoenzymes into the amniotic fluid. Maternal serum AFP is tested at the 16th to 18th week postconception; however, it provides reliable detection in only 80% of cases. Elevated AFP can be seen in other defects beside NTDs, whereas elevated acetylcholinesterase isoenzymes are only seen in NTDs. Amniocentesis testing for elevated AFP and acetylcholinesterase isoenzymes, as a confirming test, is best performed by the 15th to 18th week postconception to minimize fetal risk.

2. Fetal ultrasound can screen for NTD by the 14th to 16th week postconception and has > 90% sensitivity. However, diagnosis should be confirmed by amniocentesis.

5. What are the leading factors affecting morbidity and mortality in individuals with meningomyelocele?
1. **Hydrocephalus** may occur in 95% of all children with meningomyelocele and requires shunt placement in up to 85% (see question 7).

2. **Renal failure** is a serious complication and may lead to death in patients with meningomyelocele. Reflux, hydronephrosis, and recurrent infection are the primary causes of renal failure.

3. **Pressure ulcers** are a major cause of morbidity in these adolescents and adults

4. **Tethered cord** is a defect in the normal ascension of the conus medullaris from its earlier distal position to the L1–2 vertebral level. This defect is due to the abnormal attachment of the spinal cord at its distal end (filum terminale). This defect can occur in 11–15% of children after meningomyelocele repair. The average age at diagnosis is 6 years. Signs and symptoms can include recent changes in lower-extremity motor strength or sensation; recent changes in functional mobility; and new onset of spasticity, back pain, scoliosis, or bowel or bladder incontinence.

5. **Hydromyelia** is a cavitation in the spinal canal and can present as neck rigidity, pain, weakness, or spasticity in the upper or lower extremities, rapidly progressive scoliosis, or worsening in bowel or bladder function.

6. **Obesity** is a frequent problem in individuals with meningomyelocele. Their reduced daily energy expenditure is due to paralysis, lack of muscle mass, and decreased physical activity.

7. **Latex hypersentivity** develops over time and can occur in up to 80% of patients with spina bifida. A negative diagnostic test does not rule out future sensitization. Therefore, these patients should avoid all exposure to latex containing material including catheters and other medical and nonmedical equipment.

6. Are there other CNS complications associated with myelodysplasia?
Congenital hydrocephalus, Arnold-Chiari malformation (herniation of cerebellar tonsil through the foramen magnum), Dandy-Walker complex (cystic dilatation of fourth ventricle), acquired hydrocephalus, tethered cord syndrome, and syringomyelia (up to 40% incidence).

7. What is hydrocephalus and how is it managed?
Hydrocephalus can be present in up to 95% of children with meningomyelocele. In the newborn, it may manifest as an increased rate of growth in head circumference, whereas in older children, it may manifest as signs and symptoms of increased intracranial pressure (ICP) such as

irritability, vomiting, and somnolence. It may also manifest insidiously with subtle changes in personality, a decline in school performance, or a decline in fine motor function. Arnold-Chiari type II malformation may also result from increased ICP as the cerebellum is displaced caudally with elongation and kinking of the fourth ventricle. Approximately 75–85% of children with meningomyelocele require the placement of a VP shunt to decrease ICP. Up to 50% of these children require shunt revision in the first year of shunting, with nearly all revised by 5 years of age.

8. What are the cognitive deficits in patients with MMC?

General intelligence: Low IQ scores are associated with higher level lesions. IQ scores are adversely affected by CNS infections and shunt malfunctions.

Higher-order cognitive functions: Regardless of IQ, many have significant impairments in problem-solving, conceptualization, efficiency of processing, and mental flexibility. Verbal performance is often better than quantitative. Therefore, neuropsychological testing is particularly valuable for quantification and remediation of these deficits.

Psychosocial involvement: Maladjustment to social roles is common and is prevented by mainstreaming in schools and provision of early intervention.

9. What are the bowel and bladder deficits associated with meningomyelocele?

Neurogenic bowel dysfunction can involve dyssynergy of intestinal peristalsis, total or partial absence of rectal fullness sensation, or a lack of anorectal sphincter control. More than 80% of children with meningomyelocele have neurogenic bowel dysfunction.

Neurogenic bladder dysfunction affects > 80 % of those with meningomyelocele. They may have partial or complete denervation of the bladder with poor compliance and poor contractility. In the vast majority (86%), the internal sphincter is incompetent. In a third, there is detrusor sphincter dyssynergia due to a partially functional external sphincter.

10. Describe the orthopedic deficits associated with meningomyelocele.

The level of spinal involvement dictates the types of musculoskeletal deficits and complications:

T6–12 Kyphosis, scoliosis, hip and knee flexion contractures and equinus foot

L1–3 Scoliosis, hip flexion and adduction contractures, hip dislocation, knee flexion contractures and equinus foot

L4–5 Scoliosis, lordosis, hip and knee flexion contractures, hip dislocation, knee extension contractures and calcaneovarus or calcaneus foot

S1–4 Cavus foot

11. What about surgery for meningomyelocele?

The goals of early surgery are prevention of infection and preservation of neurologic function. Adhesions between the arachnoid and dura are cut. Anomalous roots are identified and any ending blindly are excised. A water-tight closure of the dura is made, leaving maximal space for the enclosed spinal cord.

12. What are the major factors determining ambulation potential in individuals with meningomyelocele?

The degree of ambulation is dependent on multiple factors, including cognitive function, level of neurologic lesion, musculoskeletal complications, obesity, motivation, and age. Iliopsoas motor strength of 4/5 is associated with community ambulation, and 0/3 is associated with wheelchair use. In addition, gluteal and tibialis anterior motor strengths of 4/5 are strongly associated with ambulation without assistive devices.

13. What orthotic choices are available to improve ambulation in individuals with meningomyelocele?

Orthotics choices depend on the level of injury:

Mid thoracic: Patients generally are therapeutic ambulators in early age but later become wheelchair dependent. There is significant risk of fall.

1. **Parapodium:** provides structural support from the midthoracic level to the feet and allows for both standing and sitting. Children can ambulate therapeutically with a swing-through gait using a walker or crutches. However, as the child grows, the base plate of the parapodium needs to be enlarged to maintain stability; ambulation thus becomes more difficult in older children.
2. **Swivel walker:** a modification of the parapodium with a footplate attachment that translates lateral trunk movement to forward propulsion. It has increased ambulation efficiency over the parapodium.

Low thoracic/high lumbar: household level ambulation.

1. **Reciprocal gait orthosis:** comprised of bilateral hip-knee-ankle-foot orthoses with an elaborate cable system that links hip flexion in each hip with the contralateral hip extension. Energy expenditure for ambulation with this orthosis approaches that of wheelchair locomotion.

Mid lumbar: limited community ambulation.

1. **Hip-knee-ankle-foot orthosis:** may be needed for ambulation in presence of hip instability.
2. **Knee-ankle-foot orthosis:** to correct or prevent knee deformity.
3. **Ankle-foot orthosis:** may be adequate when knee extension strength is > 3/5.

Low lumbar/sacral: community ambulation.

1. **Floor reaction orthosis:** for non-fixed calcaneal foot deformity to increase knee extension moment.
2. **Ankle orthosis:** to stabilize ankle.
3. **Shoe modifications:** for foot deformities.

BIBLIOGRAPHY

1. Badell A: Myelodysplasia. In Molnar GE (ed): Pediatric Rehabilitation, 2nd ed. Baltimore, Williams & Wilkins, 1992.
2. Dise JE, Lohr ME: Examination of deficits in conceptual reasoning abilities associated with spina bifida. Am J Phys Med Rehabil 77:247–251, 1998.
3. Hays RM, Massagli TL: Rehabilitation concepts in myelomeningocele. In Braddom RL (ed): Physical Medicine and Rehabilitation. Philadelphia, W.B. Saunders, 1996.
4. Hobbins JC: Diagnosis and management of neural tube defects today. N Engl J Med 324:690–691, 1991.
5. La Marca F, Herman M, Grant JA, McLone DG: Presentation and management of hydromyelia in children with Chiari type-II malformation. Pediatr Neurosurg 26:57–67, 1997.
6. McDonald C, Jaffe K, Mosca V, Shurtleff D: Ambulatory outcome of children with myelomeningocele: Effect of lower extremity muscle strength. Dev Med Child Neurol 33:482–490, 1991.
7. Molnar GE, Murphy KP: Spina bifida. In Molnar GE, Alexander MA (eds): Pediatric Rehabilitation, 3rd ed. Philadelphia, Hanley & Belfus, 1999.
8. Shaw GM, Todoroff K, Velie EM, Lammer EJ: Maternal illness, including fever and medication use as risk factors for neural tube defects. Teratology 57:1–7, 1998.
9. Singhal B, Mathew KM: Factors affecting mortality and morbidity in adult spina bifida. Euro J Pediatr Surg 9:31–32, 1999.
10. Szepfalusi Z, Seidl R, Bernert G, et al: Latex sensitization in spina bifida appears disease-associated. J Pediatr 134:344–348, 1999.
11. Zurmohle UM, Homann T, Schroeter C, et al: Psychosocial adjustment of children with spina bifida. J Child Neurol 13:64–70, 1998.

XII. Medical Complications in Rehabilitation

70. COMMON MEDICAL PROBLEMS ON THE INPATIENT REHABILITATION UNIT

James K. Richardson, M.D., Paul T. Diamond, M.D., Steven A. Stiens, M.D., M.S., Isabel C. Borras, M.D., and Michael Freedman, M.D.

1. What is an emergency?

Stedman's Medical Dictionary defines an emergency as an "unlooked-for contingency or happening; a sudden demand for action." Prevention, minimization of the severity, and brisk effective response to these patient events are essential functions of the rehabilitation medicine team and allied health professions. Components of readiness include assessment of risk, preventive therapies, appropriate as-needed (PRN) medications, unit personal training, accessible energy equipment, and policies to address foreseeable situations. After events happen, it is useful to learn from them through review of the cases in a quality assurance committee. Recommendations from these reviews provide for more effective prevention and response in the future.

2. What habits should the clinician integrate and practice to recognize and prevent complications?

Open your eyes. Look at everything first. Look at all records quickly. Look at the patient's room, family, equipment, bed, patient head to toe, front and back, bedside vitals. Think up and down the **biopsychosocial hierarchy** of systems: **molecules** (metabolic), **cell (viability), tissues, organs** (ischemia, function, systems coordination, exercises), **person** (attitude, expectations), **two person** (involvement, expectations, awareness), **community** readiness. Then run the **problem list** mentally as you see patients or plan any change in care. Include practical problems that keep the team aware of risks the patient may have. Don't let bed rest cause problems. You must encourage your patients to **expectorate, animate, and be safe**.

FEVER

3. Does everyone with a fever have an infection?

No, especially on the inpatient rehab unit. An elevated temperature in a patient with C6 spinal cord injury who is situated on the south or west side of the unit in the late afternoon may simply reflect impaired autoregulation. Processes that are not infectious, such as connective tissue diseases, deep vein thrombosis (DVT), or pulmonary embolism (PE), may cause fever. An elderly diabetic patient who had a stroke may have overwhelming sepsis but not manifest an increased temperature.

4. A patient has a fever but doesn't have pneumonia or a urinary tract infection. What conditions should you consider?

On the inpatient rehab unit, the patient population has traits that predispose them to a number of difficult-to-diagnose fever etiologies:
- DVT or PE
- Sinus infection in patients with nasogastric tubes
- Osteomyeolitis underlying pressure sores
- Intra-abdominal, retroperitoneal, or paraspinal abscesses in trauma patients

- Blood-borne infection (after transfusions)
- Heterotopic ossification
- Infections related to "non-original" equipment, such as catheters, feeding tubes, orthopedic hardware, and ventricular shunts
- "Central fever" in patients with brain injury (cooling response to environment, good; to acetaminophen, poor)
- Drugs

5. List some drugs that commonly cause fever.

Penicillin derivatives	Nitrofurantion	Methyldopa	Procainamide
Sulfonamides	Isoniazid	Phenytoin	Amphotericin B
Thiazide diuretics	Hydralazine	Propranolol	Quinidine
Nitrofurantoin			

6. Some of my patients have fever now and then. When do I really need to worry?

Three common conditions that are associated with fever on a rehab unit and that can kill rapidly are DVT or PE, bacterial meningitis, and sepsis syndrome.

7. Is it always necessary to treat bacteriuria?

It is usually not necessary to treat asymptomatic bacteriuria. In patients with indwelling catheters, colonization frequently occurs within 2 weeks of catheter placement and alone is not an indication for antibiotic therapy. The diagnosis of UTI is made clinically. An appropriate course of antibiotics should be prescribed in patients presenting with pyuria, fever, or symptoms referable to the GU tract such as frequency, urgency, or dysuria. Clinical discretion is required, and in certain settings, such as in immunocompromised patients, the threshold to treat will be lower. For purposes of therapy, a distinction is made between acute "uncomplicated" and "complicated" UTIs. Uncomplicated UTIs typically result from *Escherichia coli* and, to a lesser extent, *Staphylococcus saprophyticus*, *Proteus mirabilis*, and *Klebsiella pneumoniae*. These infections typically respond to a short course of antibiotics. Most UTIs in the inpatient rehabilitation setting are classified as "complicated" because of the presence of comorbid illness, anatomic abnormality (e.g., neurogenic bladder), instrumentation, recent antibiotic use, or presence of resistant organisms. Infecting organisms vary and may include *Staphylococcus aureus*, *Pseudomonas aeruginosa*, *Enterobacter* species, *Citrobacter* species, *Proteus mirabilis*, enterococci, and B streptococci. Therefore, culture should be obtained in this setting along with sensitivities to confirm appropriate antibiotic selection. A course of ≥ 7 days may be indicated. Foley catheters should be changed after 24 hours of antibiotic therapy. In general, post-treatment surveillance cultures are not necessary unless clinically indicated.

8. Are drug-resistant organisms of concern on the rehabilitation unit?

Yes. The prevalence of colonization with vancomycin-resistant enterococcus (VRE) has increased significantly over the past decade. Patients with prolonged acute hospital stays and prior antibiotic therapy are at increased risk of VRE colonization. Recent data suggest that treatment with anti-anaerobic antibiotics promotes high-density colonization and may further increase the risk of spread. Transmission is through surface contact and is not airborne. Isolation procedures generally involve use of gown and gloves, private room isolation, and appropriate cleaning and disinfectant protocols. In patients who are colonized with VRE, clearing generally occurs within several months following discharge and may be documented by follow-up surveillance. Treatment options remain limited, and the associated mortality may exceed 35%. VRE colonization in the rehabilitation patient interferes with full participation in therapy programs and limits discharge options because many skilled nursing facilities do not accept patients who require isolation protocols. Methicillin-resistant *Staphylococcus aureus* (MRSA), another commonly encountered antibiotic-resistant bacterium, is transmitted through the air and requires droplet and contact isolation protocols. Unlike VRE, MRSA eradication protocols are available but generally take 2–3 weeks and are variably successful. Open wounds make successful eradiction of this organism less likely.

GASTROINTESTINAL DISORDERS

9. About 85% of my patients are intensely constipated, while the other 15% have diarrhea. Anything to worry about here?

Yes, in reality, the patients with diarrhea may be constipated and leaking liquid stool around a fecal mass. This is the ball-valve effect. Examine the belly, do a rectal examination, and check a flat plate if you are uncertain before treating the presumed "diarrhea" symptomatically, or you may contribute to the problem.

10. What about colitis due to *Clostridium difficile*?

Many patients on the rehab unit have had complications during their acute course that required antibiotics, and as a result, they are at risk for pseudomembranous colitis caused by *Clostridium difficile*. In diagnosing this condition, the presence of fecal leukocytes is a helpful, fast, and relatively sensitive finding but not very specific, as some patients with clearcut clinical *C. difficile*-associated diarrhea have minimal observable changes. The presence of *C. difficile* toxin in stool is the most reliable and specific diagnostic test. Stool culture for *C. difficile* is nonspecific and positive in 3% of the general population.

11. How do you treat pseudomembranous colitis?

For patients who are not seriously ill, **cholestyramine** to bind the toxin (a 4-g packet three times daily for 5–10 days) and **metronidazole** (500 mg orally three or four times daily for 10–14 days) to decrease *C. difficile* counts are effective treatments. For the seriously ill patient, oral **vancomycin** (125–250 mg orally four times daily) is recommended instead of metronidazole. Relapses are common on discontinuation of antibiotics, and retreatment may be necessary. At the end of antibiotic therapy, repopulating the gut with lactobacillus (using yogurt) is helpful.

12. Everybody who has had blood loss comes to the rehabilitation unit on tid iron. Does oral iron allow anemia to resolve more quickly?

If the patient is iron-deficient, yes; if the patient is not iron-deficient, no. However, it very effectively enhances anorexia in most patients when started immediately on a three-times-daily dose.

13. How do I evaluate the need for oral iron?

Check the iron indices. If the serum iron to iron-binding capacity ratio is < 0.15, give iron. If it is > 0.20, stop it. If it is in the "gray zone," then consider the situation. Previously well-nourished adult males usually have abundant iron stores. Regularly menstruating women and the poorly nourished usually have depleted iron stores. Remember, mild iron deficiency can occur with a normal mean cell volume, so err on the side of treating such patients. Serum ferritin reflects iron stores nicely if the patient does not have cancer, infection, inflammation, or liver disease, in which case the serum ferritin is falsely elevated.

If you decide to treat, give one dose of iron 30 minutes before a meal with orange juice or vitamin C in those with reflux esophagitis. Increase by one dose every 5 days until the patient is on a three-times-daily schedule; this should avoid problems with gastric irritation, nausea, and anorexia.

14. Everybody seems to come out of the intensive care unit on an H$_2$ antagonist. Do all patients need to stay on these medications?

Probably not. Three groups of rehabilitation patients would likely benefit from continued prophylaxis against GI bleeding:

1. Patients with complete T4 and higher spinal cord injuries seem especially prone to upper GI bleeds (possibly owing to unopposed parasympathetic stimulation to the stomach causing excessive release of acid).

2. Patients with a previous history of peptic ulcer disease or GI bleeding, especially if on anticoagulation.

3. Patients with an acute course complicated by multiple factors associated with GI bleeding, such as ventilator dependence, hemorrhage, shock from any cause, sepsis, multiple trauma, and steroid usage.

There is, however, a potential trade-off in terms of pneumonia risk. As a result, clinical judgment is needed to decide if the patient's risk for GI bleeding is offset by the possible increased risk of pneumonia with the use of H_2 antagonists.

15. Abdominal problems are difficult to diagnose in patients with SCI. Aside from GI bleeding, what else should I worry about?

- **Pancreatitis** also occurs with increasing frequency in the first 4–6 weeks after SCI; unlike GI bleeding, there is no change in risk depending on the level of injury.
- **Nephrolithiasis** may occur in young men with SCI in association with the hypercalciuria from bone demineralization. Such stones are radiopaque.
- These patients have slowed bile transit and are at increased risk for **cholelithiasis** and **cholecystitis**.

16. On a routine screening, renal ultrasound gallstones were identified in the gallbladder of 42-year-old man with C7 ASIA A SCI. Should an elective cholecystectomy be done?

Patients with SCI are at higher risk for gallstone formation due to autonomic dysregulation, rapid weight loss at time of injury, and poor gallbladder emptying. As a result, the prevalence of gallstones among persons with SCI is up to 30%.

Some symptoms of cholestasis and cholecystitis are translated through the sympathetic nerve branches from T6–10. Symptoms may be blunted in patients with lesions above T9. Sufficient clinical symptoms are experienced by those with lesions below T9 to allow presentation for cholecystectomy with similar morbidity and mortality as patients without SCI.

ELECTROLYTE DISORDERS

17. What is the most common electrolyte abnormality on the rehab unit?

Hyponatremia.

18. How do I tell if the hyponatremia is significant?

Serum sodium is a ratio of total body sodium to total body water—a low serum sodium by itself says nothing about whether total body sodium is too high, too low, or just right. Check the patient and assess his or her clinical volume status. Distended neck veins, presacral/pretibial edema, orthopnea, and rales all suggest hypervolemia or increased total body sodium. (It should be noted that patients with syndrome of inappropriate secretion of antidiuretic hormone [SIADH] and no other problem affecting their electrolytes have none of these signs and are clinically euvolemic, as they are able to excrete sodium normally.) Postural hypotension, decreased skin turgor, dry membranes, resting tachycardia, and increased blood urea nitrogen (BUN) to creatinine (Cr) ratio (> 20) all suggest hypovolemia and decreased total body sodium.

19. Which other labs should I look at?

Lab Values that Distinguish SIADH from Volume Depletion in Hyponatremia

	SIADH	VOLUME DEPLETION
BUN:Cr	< 20	> 20
Urine osmolality	> 200 mOsm/kg H_2O	> 400 mOsm/kg H_2O
Urine Na	> 40 mEq/hr	< 20 mEq/hr
Fractional excretion of Na*	> 2%	< 1%

* Fractional excretion of Na = [(urine Na/serum Na)/(urine Cr/serum Cr)] × 100.

20. After volume, and therefore total body sodium, status has been determined with laboratory and physical examination, what's next?

Decreased total body sodium. Consider giving volume with normal saline intravenously. Serum sodium will correct as the kidney senses adequate volume and stops reabsorbing water in the distal tubule.

Normal total body serum. The patient likely has SIADH, which is usually treated effectively with water restriction to approximately 1 L/day. A more humane alternative in patients with good left ventricular pump function is ad-lib water and high-salt diet combined with daily furosemide. Obviously, when drugs are contributing or causing SIADH, they should be discontinued or another drug substituted. Finally, if the SIADH is severe, then intravenous hypertonic saline and furosemide are likely required; at that point, call for medical consultation.

Elevated total body sodium. The patient likely has a concurrent pathologic process (e.g., congestive heart failure, cirrhosis) that is making the kidneys believe that the body is hypovolemic, and the lab values will usually reflect avid sodium and water conservation. Such situations suggest incomplete filling of the arterial tree, either due to deranged Starling forces (e.g., loss of intravascular colloidal osmotic pressure in cirrhosis) or pump dysfunction in heart failure. Fluid restriction is a mainstay of treatment. These situations can have an ominous prognosis—a patient trying very hard to remain a patient—and medical consultation is called for.

21. List some common causes of SIADH.

The major causes of SIADH are so ubiquitous on the inpatient rehab unit that it is almost surprising if some patients do not have it.

- CNS thrombotic or hemorrhagic event
- CNS infection or neoplasm
- Postoperative state
- Psychosis
- Prolonged nausea
- Lung disease
    Pneumonia
    Positive pressure ventilation
    Malignancy

- Drugs
    Carbamazepine
    Chlorpropamide
    Phenothiazines
    Cyclophosphamide
    Amitriptyline
    Other tricyclic antidepressants
    Morphine

22. How quickly should the sodium be corrected?

Correcting the sodium too fast places the patient at risk for acute cerebral shrinkage with mental status changes and possibly central pontine myelinolysis. It is prudent to correct the sodium by not faster than 10 mEq/L over 24 hours until the sodium reaches 125 mEq/L, and then more gradually, being careful to avoid overcorrection.

23. Do any other electrolyte problems occur on the inpatient rehab unit?

Yes, hypercalcemia can occur in young men with recent SCI. Such patients often have fatigue, apathy, and depression as the most prominent manifestations of hypercalcemia. Therefore, diagnosis in subjects with any kind of brain dysfunction requires a high index of suspicion. Other symptoms and signs include polydipsia, polyuria, nausea, and vomiting. The mnemonic is "**stones, bones, and abdominal groans**." Treatment includes mobilization of the patient to the degree possible, etidronate or pamidronate disodium, and a furosemide-induced saline diuresis.

24. Are there any special concerns for patients with diabetes mellitus on the inpatient rehabilitation unit?

Diabetes mellitus is always of concern, but it is particularly tricky to manage in rehabilitation inpatients. In that setting, the patient may go from completely inactive and relatively insulin-resistant to actively involved in an aerobic-conditioning program, which renders the patient more insulin-sensitive. The tapering of steroids may have the same effect. In general, it is probably better to be conservative during this time of change and tolerate a few episodes of hyperglycemia than to have recurrent hypoglycemia, especially in patients recovering from any kind of brain damage. Finally, fatal hyperkalemia has developed in patients with diabetes mellitus on NSAIDs; therefore, monitor serum K^+ in diabetic patients placed on these agents.

MENTAL STATUS CHANGES

25. The rehab team tells me that my profoundly brain injured patient has mental status changes, but he sure looks the same to me. What should I do?

Work it up. One of the real advantages of a team working with your patient for several hours per day is that they become very sensitive to the patient's cognitive and physical abilities. They can detect a drop-off in these abilities that is not evident with bedside examination. For example, loss of sitting balance in a low-level, incontinent patient might be hydrocephalus—which normally causes gait ataxia, incontinence, and cognitive dysfunction.

26. How do I work up acute or subacute mental status changes?

1. Think about structural or anatomic causes, metabolic causes, and drugs. A brain imaging study may be ordered to rule out hydrocephalus, edema, and thrombotic or hemorrhagic events.

2. Check the blood for white cell count, as sepsis can cause mental status change; also check the serum glucose, sodium, and calcium, and check the arterial blood gases for alterations in PO_2 and PCO_2. Cerebral hypoperfusion from myocardial infarction or arrhythmia can lead to mental status change. Emboli to the brain may occur, especially in those with atrial fibrillation, valvular abnormalities, myocardial infarction, or recent aortic or coronary catheterization.

3. Meningitis is common in patients who have had neurosurgical procedures, so check the CSF after ruling out hydrocephalus. If your clinical suspicion is high for meningitis, then antibiotics should be started immediately—even if that means that CSF has not yet been obtained.

4. If the patient is initially lethargic but recovers nicely within 24 hours, consider the possibility of an unwitnessed seizure.

5. Finally, and most importantly, look for drugs that might be diminishing cognitive function. Check anticonvulsant levels. Also consider the effect of drugs that might have been withdrawn recently, such as alcohol and benzodiazepines.

27. Which drugs might limit the recovery of a brain-injured patient or induce mental status change?

Benzodiazepines (short- and long-acting)

Phenothiazines (major tranquilizers)

Central sympathetic inhibitors (methyldopa, clonidine)

Anticonvulsants (phenobarbital/phenytoin)

DYSPNEA

28. What should I worry about when my patient gets short of breath?

Worry a lot about PE. In autopsy series of patients whose cause of death was unknown, PE still tops the list of causes. It is almost impossible to be too aggressive in working up and treating DVT or PE. Other considerations include hypoxygenation and hypoventilation or both. Start your evaluation with vital signs, heart and lung auscultation, and a transcutaneous O_2 saturation.

29. My patient with dyspnea has a low or intermediate probability ventilation-perfusion scan. What do I do?

Review your differential diagnosis. Check lower-extremity Doppler or ultrasound studies before subjecting your patient to a pulmonary angiogram or venogram, both of which have risks.

30. What if it is a weekend or night and I cannot get the studies done that I need?

If the patient has risk factors for DVT or PE and the most common symptoms and signs of PE (dyspnea, anxiety, tachycardia), or there is a respiratory alkalosis on arterial blood gas in a patient who cannot communicate symptoms, then the patient should be treated empirically with heparin until more definitive workup can be done. Heparin not only prevents further clot formation but has a relaxing effect on pulmonary endothelium after PE, which lessens the resultant perfusion defect and in turn lessens the patient's symptoms. If there is a contraindication to heparin, then transfer the patient to a monitored bed and place an inferior vena caval filter when and if the diagnosis is confirmed.

31. What other causes of acute dyspnea should be considered?

Dyspnea can be an anginal equivalent in any population, but given the percentage of patients with impaired sensation or ability to express themselves, **angina** as a cause of dyspnea is likely to be even more frequent on the rehabilitation unit. Patients with cervical SCI, diabetes, and cognitive dysfunctions or aphasia may all have difficulty reporting or sensing typical anginal symptoms. In addition, many patients on the inpatient rehab unit have abundant risk factors for coronary artery disease. Stroke patients have a greater mortality from coronary artery disease than stroke.

One bedside clue that suggests angina is the absence of a **tibial pulse**. If a patient is missing a tibial pulse, then that patient's risk of significant coronary artery disease is > 90%. Missing a leg due to vascular occlusive disease is another way not to have a tibial pulse, but the rule still applies—vascular amputees are at high risk for coronary artery disease and myocardial infarction.

32. Isn't there at least one relatively benign cause of sudden dyspnea in the inpatient rehab population?

Yes, a **mucous plug** can be a significant problem in rehab populations, who often have weakened expiratory force and cough. Aggressive pulmonary toilet with percussion/postural drainage, assisted cough, and suctioning are usually enough, but at times bronchoscopy and lavage are necessary.

33. Why do so many patients on the rehab service acquire pneumonia during their stay?

The risk factors for hospital-acquired pneumonia include impaired mentation, abnormal swallow, chronic debilitating illness, weak or absent cough, mechanical ventilation or tracheostomy, and possibly the use of H2 antagonists such as cimetidine. The endotracheal and tracheostomy tubes are particularly risky, as they allow microorganisms direct access to the bronchial tree, which quickly becomes colonized.

34. Are pneumonias more common on the right or left lungs after high cervical SCI?

The left. This may be due to the fact that the right mainstem bronchus is more directly aligned with the trachea, permitting greater success with suctioning and secretion clearance. Catheters introduced into the trachea during suctioning are more apt to enter and clear the right mainstem. As a result, postural drainage of the left lung by positioning the patient with the right side down may improve pulmonary toilet.

35. What is a good empiric therapy for hospital-acquired pneumonia while I await culture results?

Patients rapidly become colonized with gram-negative bacilli and *Staphylococcus aureus*, and thus those are the leading causes of hospital-acquired pneumonia. Reasonable empiric coverage includes a third-generation cephalosporin with good activity against *Pseudomonas* and an aminoglycoside.

Also, percussion, postural drainage, saline lavage, and suctioning are at least as important as antibiotics, and probably more important than antibiotics in typical rehab patients who have impaired cough. The antibiotics slow the rate of bacterial proliferation, but the pneumonia must be cleared by the rehabilitation team.

36. What can be done to prevent pneumonia?

- Incentive spirometry every 2 hours while awake.
- Intermittent high-pressure breathing, percussion, and drainage.
- Deep bagging to fully inflate the lungs twice per shift, assisted coughing, "quad coughing," nebulized bronchodilators.

- Mucus-thinning agents, as oral or nebulized medication.
- Preventive immunization with Pneumovax. Pneumococcal vaccine is indicated in adult patients over 50 and others with disability. Vaccination against influenza is available annually in the fall and is recommended for all people with disabilities that could put them at risk for pneumonia.

BLOOD PRESSURE ABNORMALITIES

37. Half of my patients have high blood pressure, and the other half have hypotension. What are common causes of hypotension on the inpatient rehab service?

Simple **bed rest** is a common cause of postural hypotension. Loss of postural reflexes is common after 3 weeks of bed rest in healthy people and after as little as several days to weeks in the elderly and those with major trauma or illness. **Disturbed autonomic function** is another cause and occurs in patients with autonomic neuropathy from Guillain-Barré, diabetes mellitus, certain antihypertensives, and other causes.

38. My patient is a little light-headed. Is that really anything to worry about?

Yes. Obviously, postural light-headedness can precipitate a fall, but it also can cause stroke and myocardial infarction in those with **systemic vascular disease**. Remember that the coronary arteries fill during diastole, so postural hypotension may be particularly concerning for patients with coronary artery disease.

Also, malignant arrhythmias due to autonomic dysfunction can occur in patients with **Guillain-Barré syndrome**. Any clinical evidence of tachy- or bradyarrhythmia or fluctuating blood pressure suggests that the Guillain-Barré patient deserves a monitored bed and close observation in an intensive care unit.

Finally, patients with **diabetes** who have significant autonomic dysfunction are felt to have an ominous prognosis, possibly due to erratic gastric motility, food absorption, and insulin timing.

39. How do I treat postural hypotension?

Mechanical efforts to enhance venous return, such as thigh-high compressive stockings, ace wraps, and abdominal binders, are recommended. Moving gradually and pumping the calves are recommended for those who are ambulatory. Graduated use of a tilt table may be necessary for those who are not.

Before starting new medications to improve the situation, look for medications that the patient is taking which may be worsening it. Diuretics, vasodilators, and anticholinergics such as tricyclic antidepressants should be stopped, and an adequate fluid and salt intake allowed. If further help is needed, sympathomimetic medication such as ephedrine or Midrin is helpful, particularly acutely, while fludrocortisone is helpful in more chronic situations. The latter medication may take several days to a few weeks to reach its maximal effect, which probably occurs through mechanism other than increasing plasma volume with salt retention (possibly improving "vascular tone" through an extrarenal mechanism).

40. A lot of my patients are on tricyclic antidepressants (TCAs). Except for anticholinergic side effects, they are safe, right?

The anticholinergic effects, such as dry mouth, constipation, urine retention, postural hypotension, and difficulty with visual accommodation, are usually tolerable, especially with time. More worrisome, however, is the use of TCAs in patients with cardiac conduction abnormalities. In older patients and those with cardiac risk factors, it is prudent to check an electrocardiogram prior to initiating the medication. Evidence of conduction problems, such as prolonged P-R interval or QRS complex widening, is a contraindication for the use of TCAs, which may result in complete heart block in such patients. There is little evidence to suggest that TCAs are negative inotropes, so they should be relatively safe in patients with impaired left ventricular function.

TCAs are actually antiarrhythmic for tachyarrhythmias, but the safety of using antiarrhythmic medication for tachyarrhythmias and TCAs together in this setting is uncertain.

41. What about the other half of my patients who seem to be hypertensive?

There are reasons why a high percentage of patients on the rehabilitation service may have hypertension. **Stroke patients** often have essential hypertension which underlies their disease. In general, blood pressure control goals of patients with recent stroke are modest. Most feel that maintenance of perfusion pressure in the post-stroke period is important, as the arteries in the injured region have lost their ability to autoregulate and, as a result, flow to the area that is markedly pressure-dependent. Therefore, in the hypertensive stroke patient, blood pressures should be lowered gradually during the weeks following the stroke.

Often, patients with closed **head injury** are hypertensive. These are often young patients, and since hypertension exerts its damaging effects over months and years, such patients can usually just be monitored. Should treatment be necessary, therapy that does not interfere with cognitive recovery or that helps the patient in some other way should be chosen. For example, clonidine should be avoided in general, and beta-blockers may be a good choice in brain-injured patients with rage reactions or headaches with vascular qualities.

42. Are there any hypertensive emergencies to worry about?

Yes. If your brain-injured patients have blood pressure increases, with any suggestion of change in neurologic status, they should be imaged with CT or MRI to rule out causes of increased intracranial pressure. Of course, malignant elevations of blood pressure can occur in patients with SCI.

43. Which patients are at risk for autonomic dysreflexia? What causes it?

Patients with spinal cord lesions above T6 are at risk for autonomic dysreflexia. It is caused by some noxious afferent input (usually a distended viscus, such as a full bladder or bowel) into the spinal cord below the level of the lesion, which in turn causes a large autonomic outflow. This outflow, which occurs below the level of the lesion, is unmonitored and therefore not modulated by higher centers in the brainstem and hypothalamus. Therefore, pronounced vasoconstriction occurs below the level of the lesion, as the vascular tree has sympathetic, but not parasympathetic, innervation. The high pressure is detected at vascular baroreceptors like those in the carotid bulb, and central modulation to lower pressure ensues. The vasculature above the level of the lesion has reduced sympathetic tone and dilates appropriately in an effort to decrease blood pressure. As a result, the patient often appears flushed above the level of the lesion and complains of a pounding headache characteristically behind the eyes, nasal congestion, and sweats. There may be a paradoxic bradycardia due to excessive centrally driven vagal tone to lower blood pressure.

44. How is autonomic dysreflexia treated?

Prompt treatment is important; blood pressure elevations can be malignant and cause intracranial hemorrhage. Sit the patient upright to reduce blood pressure. Check the bowel and bladder and evacuate these. (It is a good idea to use lidocaine gel during these procedures to minimize further noxious afferent input.) Usually, this is enough and the patient's pressure returns to baseline. If not, treat to control blood pressure while the search for the cause proceeds. Nitropaste is rapid in onset and easily removed should pressure go too low. If this is not effective, oral hydralazine, oral nifedipine, or intramuscular or intravenous morphine should be added to the regimen (the latter may be particularly helpful if the patient is in pain or anxious).

45. What are the potential causes of autonomic dysreflexia?

- **Gastrointestinal**—appendicitis, cholecystitis, diverticulitis, ischemic or perforated bowel
- **Genitourinary**—nephrolithiasis, endometriosis, epididymitis, testicular torsion
- **Dermatologic**—cellulitis, ingrown toenail, tight-fitting clothes, pressure sore, burn
- **Vascular**—aneurysm, deep vein thrombosis
- **Musculoskeletal**—heterotopic ossification, gout/pseudogout, joint infection

46. Is there any way to identify persons at greatest risk for developing a medical problem, requiring transfer off the inpatient unit and back onto an acute care floor?

Not without a crystal ball. However, some patient characteristics have been associated with an increased risk for transfer to an acute medical service: abnormal vital signs upon admission to the rehab unit, presence of a feeding or tracheostomy tube, impaired renal function, anemia, hypoalbuminemia, and history of DVT/PE.

BIBLIOGRAPHY

1. Bartlett JG: *Clostridium difficile*: Clinical considerations. Rev Infect Dis 12(suppl 1):S243, 1990.
2. Bone RC: The pathogenesis of sepsis. Ann Intern Med 115:457, 1991.
3. Criqui MHY, Langer RD, Frank A, Feigelson HS: Coronary artery disease and stroke in patients with large vessel peripheral arterial disease. Drugs 42(suppl 5):16–21, 1991.
4. Consortium for Spinal Cord Medicine, Clinical Practice Guideline: Acute Management of Autonomic Dysreflexia: Adults with Spinal Cord Injury. Paralyzed Veterans of America, 1997. [www.pva.org]
5. Dombovy ML, Vasford JR, Whisnant JP, Bergstralh EJ: Disability and use of rehabilitation services following stroke in Rochester, Minnesota, 1975–1979. Stroke 18:830–836, 1987.
6. Felsenthal G, Cohen S, Hilton B, et al: The physiatrist as primary physician for patients on an inpatient rehabilitation unit. Arch Phys Med Rehabil 65:375–378, 1984.
7. Goldstein LB, et al: Common drugs may influence motor recovery after stroke. Neurology 45:865–871, 1995.
8. Harkness GA: Risk factors for nosocomial pneumonia in the elderly. Am J Med 89:457, 1990.
9. Linstedt G: Serum ferritin and iron deficiency anemia in hospital patients. Lancet 1:205, 1980.
10. Massagli TL, Cardenas DD: Immobilization hypercalcemia treatment with pamidronate disodium after spinal cord injury. Arch Phys Med Rehabil 80:998–1000, 1999.
11. Robinson KM, Sigler EL, Streim JE: Medical emergencies in rehabilitation medicine. In DeLisa JA (ed): Rehabilitation Medicine: Principles and Practice, 2nd ed. Philadelphia, J.B. Lippincott, 1993, pp 792–795.
12. Rose BD: Renal function and disorders of water and sodium balance. In Rubenstein E, Federman DD (eds): Scientific American Medicine. New York, Scientific American, 1994.
13. Roth EJ, Wiesner S, Green D, Wu Y: Dysvascular amputee rehabilitation: The role of continuous noninvasive cardiovascular monitoring during physical therapy. Am J Phys Med Rehabil 69:16–22, 1987.
14. Stiens SA, Biener-Bergman S, Goetz LL: Neurogenic bowel dysfunction after spinal cord injury: Clinical evaluation and rehabilitation management. Arch Phys Med Rehabil 78:S86–S102, 1997.
15. Warkentin TI, et al: Heparin-induced thrombocytopenia in patients treated with low-molecular-weight heparin or unfractionated heparin. N Engl J Med 332:1330–1335, 1995.

71. HAZARDS OF IMMOBILIZATION: PREVENTING THE ADVERSE EFFECTS OF BED REST

Paul Corcoran, M.D., Eugen M. Halar, M.D., Kathleen R. Bell, M.D., and Steven A. Stiens, M.D., M.S.

1. Describe the adverse effects of bed rest on the various organ systems.

ORGAN SYSTEM	NEGATIVE EFFECTS OF BED REST
Muscles	Disuse atrophy, back pain
Joints	Contracture, loss of ROM
Bone	Osteoporosis
Urinary tract	Infection, calculi, incontinence

Table continued on following page

ORGAN SYSTEM	NEGATIVE EFFECTS OF BED REST
Heart	Deconditioning, diminished cardiac reserve, reduced stroke volume, resting and postexercise tachycardia
Circulation	Orthostatic hypotension, thrombophlebitis, pulmonary embolism
Lung	Atelectasis, aspiration, pneumonia
Gastrointestinal	Gastroesophageal reflux, anorexia, malnutrition, constipation, impaction, incontinence
Skin	Decubitus ulcer, maceration, monilial infection
Neurologic	Peripheral nerve compression
Psychological	Depression, disorientation, anxiety, hallucinations, sleep-wake cycle disturbance
Metabolism	Decreased metabolic rate, calcium loss, hypercalcemia, nitrogen loss, impaired glucose tolerance

2. What is a contracture?

Joint contracture is a limitation of passive joint range of motion (ROM) commonly resulting from a restriction (fibrosis) in connective tissue, tendons, ligaments, muscles, joint elements (capsule), and skin.

3. What four factors accelerate contracture formation in an immobilized limb?

The mnemonic **BITE** lists these nicely:

- **B** = **B**leeding
- **I** = **I**nfection, inactivity, and pain can contribute to development of contracture. Other factors include aging, systemic diseases (such as diabetes), and smoking.
- **T** = **T**issue **t**rauma
- **E** = **E**dema; **e**xternal factors (not in the joint capsule or muscle) such as spasticity, prolonged abnormal position

4. How long is a collagen fiber?

As long as it needs to be! This is why people instinctively stretch after awakening from sleep. We all know how good this morning ROM exercise feels, yet hospital routines may deny it to patients for days at a time. Coiled collagen fibers, not required to elongate regularly, become fixed in the shortened position. New cross-links form between fibers, making collagen fibers more packed and causing clinical contractures.

5. What are some ideas to prevent or treat contractures?

- Stretch, stretch, stretch, and **hold**—the longer the better
- Control spasticity—position to facilitate upper extremity and lower extremity extension
- Early functional activities
- Splints
- Heat the joints (ultrasound, paraffin dips for hands, warm hydrotherapy for comfort)
- Dynamic splints (spring-loaded assistance to push in direction of preferred range)
- Serial casting
- Surgical tendon release

6. Which organs and systems are helped by bed rest?

None, but some impaired body parts may receive short-term benefits from temporary rest: e.g., elevating the legs to treat shock or edema, maintaining basal metabolic levels during severe acute myocardial infarction, or briefly resting or splinting inflamed joints after trauma or surgery. The long-held notion that acutely inflamed rheumatoid joints should be strictly immobilized is being challenged by new studies comparing rest and activity.

7. How strong is a muscle?

It depends on the workload regularly imposed on it. Muscles must regularly exert 50% of their maximum strength in order to preserve that strength. If a muscle never exerts as much as 50% of its maximum strength, that maximum will diminish.

8. How fast does an inactivated muscle develop disuse atrophy?

Muscles lose about 15% of their baseline strength per week of total inactivity. Thus, 5 weeks of total inactivity costs 50% of the previous strength of the muscle. A plateau is reached at 25–40% of the original strength.

9. What two factors prevent osteoporosis by stimulating osteoblastic activity?

Muscle pull and weight-bearing, both of which are prevented by bed rest.

10. How quickly does osteoporosis begin?

Urinary calcium clearance increases four to sixfold within 3 weeks after total immobilization. High levels of calcium clearance persist until a new equilibrium is reached at a lower total calcium mass, a process that may take 6 months after complete quadriplegia.

11. Why do patients often complain of backache after bed confinement?

Their intervertebral joints are stiffer, their paraspinal muscles are weaker, and their vertebrae are more osteoporotic; hence, the futility of bed rest as therapy for back pain.

12. How does the gravity of bed rest affect urination and defecation?

A basic rule in the plumbing trade is, "S - - t doesn't run uphill." This rule also applies to the gastrointestinal and urinary tracts. It is no accident that the cloaca of all species is in their nether regions, while the mouth is on top. Every day in modern hospitals, attempts to swallow, urinate, or defecate in the horizontal position continually revalidate the law of gravity. The resulting dehydration, aspiration, constipation, and urinary stasis lead to the familiar UTIs and fecal impactions of bed-confined patients.

13. What fluid shifts occur with standing and lying down?

On standing up after remaining in the supine position for a sustained period, there is a 500–700 mL fall of intravascular fluid from the intrathoracic veins and capillaries to the lower-extremity veins, termed functional hemorrhage. Prolonged recumbence decreases the intravascular volume due to drops in aldosterone and antidiuretic hormone. Cardiovascular adaptation occurs with vasoconstriction, lower-extremity muscle contraction, and increased heart rate. The reverse occurs upon lying down. **Central fluid shift** is the mobilization of the blood into the chest, increasing venous return and cardiac preload.

14. What is the orthostatic reflex? Why is it lost during bed rest?

Falling blood pressure acts via the carotid baroreceptors to signal the medullary sympathetic center to trigger vasoconstriction in the muscular layers of the small arterioles. Like all muscles, these muscles atrophy from disuse when the body remains horizontal and/or weightless. The resulting orthostatic hypotension can cause syncope, with resulting falls and injuries in patients after prolonged bed rest, as well as in astronauts returning from space. The space program prevents this by carefully planned exercises during space missions; the terrestrial health care system has not yet adopted similar preventive exercises for bed-confined patients.

15. How fast can you recover from bed rest?

As a rule of thumb, it takes at least as long to recover cardiac conditioning from disuse as it took to deteriorate. It can take 2–3 times as long to recover muscle strength. So get off the couch and exercise.

16. What is the most common cause of sudden unexpected death in hospitalized patients?
Acute pulmonary embolism.

17. How does the internal pressure of skin capillaries compare with the external pressure on the skin?
Capillary filling pressures range from about 18 mmHg at the venous end to 35 mmHg at the arteriolar end, or about 0.5 psi. To maintain perfusion and avoid collapse of skin capillaries, the external pressure therefore must be kept below 0.5 psi. This means that a 150-lb patient in bed requires a minimum of 300 sq in of skin area for support. The good news is that this much area is in fact available on the dorsum of the head, trunk, and extremities of a recumbent person. The bad news is that firm V mattresses (e.g., hospital mattresses) prevent equal pressure distribution.

18. Can exercise prevent aging?
The depressing graphs of declining function with advancing age look suspiciously like the graphs of declining function with inactivity. Recent research in geriatrics and exercise physiology has demonstrated that, like the young, the elderly can improve strength and function through activity. Persons who choose a more active lifestyle can significantly retard much of what is erroneously called "the aging process." Maintenance of strength and flexibility can prevent falls. Continued regular sexual activity can diminish male impotence and female vaginal atrophy. Mental stimulation and involvement can retard the changes of Alzheimer's disease as well as those of "normal" aging. The maxim "use it or lose it" applies to all functions at all ages.

19. Name 10 strategies for minimizing the harmful effects of bed rest.
  1. Minimize duration of bed rest.
  2. Avoid strict bed rest unless absolutely necessary.
  3. Allow bathroom privileges or bedside commode.
  4. Stand the patient for 30–60 sec whenever transferring from bed to chair.
  5. Encourage the wearing of street clothes.
  6. Encourage taking meals at a table (not in bed).
  7. Encourage walking to hospital appointments.
  8. Encourage passes out of the hospital on evenings and weekends.
  9. Order physical therapy and occupational therapy as needed.
  10. Encourage daily ROM exercises as a basic part of good nursing care.

20. Imagine a patient with T3 ASIA A paraplegia on bed rest for healing a stage 3 ischial pressure ulcer. List all potential interventions that may prevent all the complications you might predict.
The patient's bed might be located near a window to allow light exposure. Otherwise, bright full-spectrum light should be available during daytime. Orders might include a prone gurney for ambulation; change position every 2 hours; alternating pressure air mattress "topper" for bed; emollients to skin; Theraband resistance exercise program emphasizing elbow extensors, shoulder depressors; hand exercises; side-lying bowel care ulcer side up; incentive spirometry every 2 hours and during the "commercials;" bedside computer access; and bedside "parties" with regular visits from friends and relatives. Activity prescriptions could include, for example, directed reading, on-line courses, assembling a photo album, writing a resume, writing Christmas cards, tying flies, mending clothes, or making models.

BIBLIOGRAPHY

  1. Asher RAJ: The dangers of going to bed. BMJ 2:967–968, 1947.
  2. Bailey DA, McCulloch RG: Bone tissue and physical activity. Can J Sport Sci 15:229–239, 1990.
  3. Berg HE, Dudley GA, Haggmark T, et al: Effects of lower limb unloading on skeletal muscle mass and function in humans. J Appl Physiol 70:1882–1885, 1991.
  4. Bortz WM: Disuse and aging. JAMA 248:1203–1208, 1982.

5. Browse NL: The Physiology and Pathology of Bedrest. Springfield, IL, Charles C Thomas, 1965.
6. Coyle EF, Hemmert MK, Coggan AR: Effects of detraining on cardiovascular responses to exercise: Role of blood volume. J Appl Physiol 60:95–99, 1986.
7. Deitrick JR, Whedon GD, Shorr E: Effects of immobilization on various metabolic and physiologic functions of normal men. Am J Med 4:3–6, 1948.
8. Fitts RH, McDonald KS, Schluter JM: The determinants of skeletal muscle force and power: Their adaptability with changes in activity pattern. J Biomech 24:111–122, 1991.
9. Greenleaf JE: Physiological responses to prolonged bed rest and fluid immersion in humans. J Appl Physiol 57:619–633, 1984.
10. Saltin B, Blomquist G, Mitchell JH, et al: Response to exercise after bed rest and after training: A longitudinal study of adaptive changes in oxygen transport and body composition. Circulation 38(suppl 7):VII-1–VII-78, 1968.
11. van den Ende CHM, Breedveld FC, le Cessie S, et al: Effect of intensive exercise on patients with active rheumatoid arthritis: A randomised clinical trial. Ann Rheum Dis 59:615–621, 2000.

72. SPASTICITY

Richard T. Katz, M.D.

1. What is spasticity?

Spasticity is "a motor disorder characterized by a velocity-dependent increase in tonic stretch reflexes (muscle tone) with exaggerated tendon jerks, resulting from hyperexcitability of the stretch reflex, as one component of the upper motor neuron syndrome." Tone is the sensation of resistance you feel as you range the patient at the bedside (while they are relaxed).

2. What causes spasticity?

The alpha motor neuron (the nerve cell that contols muscle contraction) is hyperexcitable. That is, less synaptic excitatory input is needed to cause the alpha motor neuron to fire or reach threshold. This is akin to a pot being "almost ready to boil."

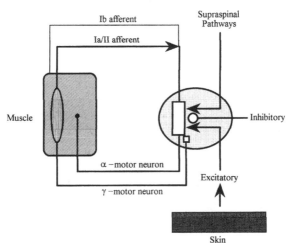

The basic neural circuitry is the segmental reflex arc, which consists of muscle receptors, their central connections with spinal cord neurons, and the motoneuronal output to muscle. This outflow is the summation of a host of different synaptic and modulatory influences, including: (1) excitatory postsynaptic potentials from group Ia and II muscle spindle afferents, (2) inhibitory postsynaptic potentials from interneuronal connections from antagonistic muscles and golgi tendon organs, and (3) presynaptic inhibition initiated by descending fiber input.

3. So are you telling me that if I could cure spasticity the patient would be cured? Are there other muscle or nerve defects involved?

Spasticity, unfortunately, is just one component of the **upper motor syndrome**, which has a whole host of features:

Abnormal behaviors (positive symptoms)
Reflex release phenomena: e.g., Babinski response
Hyperactive proprioceptive reflexes
Increased resistance to stretch
Relaxed cutaneous reflexes: e.g., loss of superficial abdominal reflex
Loss of precise autonomic control: e.g., autonomic dysreflexia

Performance deficits (negative symptoms)
Decreased dexterity
Paresis/weakness: changes in the way motor units fire
Fatiguability

4. I think I recognize spasticity when I see it, but how do I quantify it?

Now, here you have a problem. There is no uniform and practical way of quantifying the severity of spasticity. Most people use a crude scale developed by a clinician named Ashworth (the Ashworth Scale), which varies from 0 (none) to 4 (severe).

5. Should everyone with spasticity be treated?

A definite no. Patients should be treated when their spasticity interferes with present function, the potential for future function, or when the condition is painful. Ask yourself some simple questions. *Does it cause a gait disturbance?* Some people "walk on their tone" and if you decrease their extensor "synergy," they might be unable to ambulate successfully. Some people stand with their hypertonicity. In both cases the tone is serving a purpose for the patient. *Do spasms interfere with lifestyle?* Some spinal cord injured patients are literally thrown out of their chair by their flexor spasms; others may have adductor spasticity which causes a scissoring gait or precludes successful catheterization. Finally, spasticity is often very difficult to treat (such as in the severe stroke patient), and the clinician should be convinced the potential benefits of treatment clearly outweigh the possibility of side effects or drug toxicity. Functionally assessing the patients allows spasticity to be treated with a rational approach as outlined in the figure depicted at the bottom of the next page.

6. First things first—where do I start?

Start with two basic foundations. First, a daily stretching program is important and can have a significant effect that lasts for several hours after stretch due to synaptic changes that occur within the spinal cord circuitry. Second, avoid noxious stimuli. As seen in question 2, unwanted stimuli from overdistended bowel or bladder, pressure sores, or ingrown toenails play an important role in the local spinal circuitry of spasticity. Even an overly tightened leg bag may be a problem.

7. What is the role of drugs?

Drugs are most useful in the patient who has mild to moderate tone, and in all honesty, the drugs are only mildly to moderately effective. Don't fool yourself by starting drugs in a severely brain injured patient with drastic spasticity and marked dystonic posturing. The ideal patient for drugs is often the patient with less severe spasticity whether due to spinal cord dysfunction (e.g., spinal cord injury or transverse myelitis) or brain dysfunction (cerebral palsy, stroke, brain injury). Drugs and dosages for the treatment of spasticity which are available in the U.S are summarized in the table below.

Drug Treatment of Spastic Hypertonia

AGENT	DAILY DOSE	HALF-LIFE (HRS)	MECHANISM OF ACTION
Baclofen	10–80+ mg	3.5	Presynaptic inhibitor by activation of GABA B receptor
Diazepam	4–60+ mg	27–37*	Facilitates postsynaptic effects of GABA, resulting in increased presynaptic inhibition
Dantrolene	25–400 mg	8.7	Reduces calcium release, interfering with excitation-contraction coupling in skeletal muscle
Clonidine	0.1–0.4 mg (po) 0.1–0.3 mg (patch)†	12–16 (oral)	α_2-adrenergic agonist
Tizanidine	4–36 mg	8.4	α_2-adrenergic agonist

* Half-life of active primary metabolite is significantly longer.
† Patch is changed weekly.

8. Is baclofen the most effective drug?

It is surprising that baclofen (Lioresal) is used for as many indications as it is, as it is not a "wonder" drug. Baclofen is probably the drug of choice in spinal forms of spasticity and may help improve bladder control. There is a paucity of literature supporting its use in cerebral spasticity.

9. Diazepam is an antianxiety agent. Why use it for spasticity?

Available before baclofen was introduced, diazepam has proven to be a successful treatment for spastic hypertonia in spinal cord injury as well as other spinal forms of spasticity. It is generally

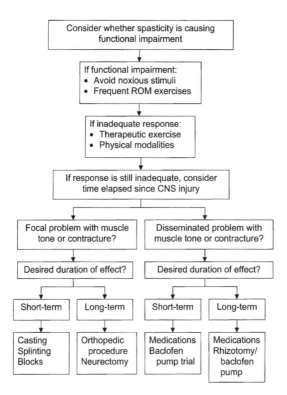

Treatment of spastic hypertonia.

unsuitable for patients with brain injury (traumatic or vascular) due to its ability to cause very significant cognitive impairment.

10. Doesn't dantrolene sodium have the ideal mode of action for spasticity?

In a word, yes. Dantrolene sodium (Dantrium) reduces muscle action potential-induced release of calcium into the sarcoplasmic reticulum, decreasing the force produced by excitation-contraction coupling. Thus, it is the only action that acts right where we want it—at the spastic muscle. Dantrolene sodium was initially embraced with a tremendous amount of excitement, which was dampened when a small number of patients developed severe hepatic insult and died. Nonetheless, there do not seem to be many new cases of this irreversible liver damage, which is puzzling. It is the preferred agent for cerebral forms of spasticity such as hemiplegia or cerebral palsy, but may be a useful adjunct to the treatment of spinal forms of spasticity.

11. Is tizanidine available in the United States?

Yes, for approximately 5 years. Tizanidine is an imidazoline derivative (like clonidine) and has an agonistic action at central α_2-adrenergic receptor sites. Unlike clonidine, it is much less potent in lowering blood pressure. It has been shown to be effective in patients with spinal and supraspinal injury. It is better tolerated than diazepam in hemiplegics and has been beneficial to patients with multiple sclerosis.

12. How effective is clonidine as a spasticity drug in spinal cord-injured patients?

Fairly effective, but it is not highly dramatic. Clonidine (Minipress), a traditional antihypertensive agent which has been largely supplanted by newer antihypertensives, has been shown to be fairly effective in controlling spasticity for patients with spinal cord injury. An adhesive patch (Catapres-TTs) is available for week-long transdermal delivery.

13. Is gabapentin as good for spasticity as it is for seizures?

Gabapentin is an analog of GABA and has been shown to be effective in spasticity management of patients with spinal cord injury and multiple sclerosis. It frequently causes somnolence as well as dizziness, ataxia, fatigue, and nystagmus. Anti-seizure dosages are generally required.

14. What is the most significant advance in the treatment of spasticity in recent years?

Hands-down winner is **intrathecal baclofen** delivered via a subdermal pump. A pump can be implanted subcutaneously in the abdominal wall, with a catheter surgically placed into the subarachnoid space. In this manner, higher dosages of these medications can be placed near the spinal cord—the desired site for action of the drug—while largely avoiding the CNS side effects associated with increased oral intake. The pump may be refilled on a monthly basis by transcutaneous injection. Eligible patients should be those who are significantly disabled by their spasticity and have failed more conservative measures.

15. Drugs act in a general manner, but what if the effect of spasticity is more focal?

If the problem is focal, there are short- and long-term solutions that may be considered. Chemical neurolysis or **phenol block** uses 2–6% aqueous phenol solutions to chemically disrupt nerves within a trunk or at the motor point where it attaches to muscle. The phenol causes protein coagulation and necrosis which may last 3–6 months.

Musculocutaneous blocks may be useful in the hemiplegic with upper-extremity elbow flexion synergy, or the C5 quadriplegic who has elbow flexion unopposed by a paretic triceps. **Median nerve blocks** may help the hemiparetic patient with a flexed wrist or fingers curled within the palm. **Obturator blocks** have been used in the patient with scissor gait, a frequent concomitant of cerebral palsy. Hip flexor spasms or flexor contractures may be improved by performing **paravertebral lumbar spinal nerve block** (although these require quite a high level of skill). **Tibial nerve block** can help the patient with an equinovarus posture (pointed foot turned inward) during gait.

More recently, **botulinum toxin** has been used in the spastic patient to weaken dystonic muscles in an analogous manner to its use in blepharospasm, strabismus, cervical dystonia, and focal dystonia. Commercially available preparations are botulinum toxin A, and more recently type B. It works at the neuromuscular junction by inhibiting the release of acetylcholine. The effect of the injection in a muscle lasts about 3 months, and as many as 3% of patients develop significant neutralizing antibodies with chronic treatment. The injection does not need to be as precise as with a phenol block, as the toxin diffuses through muscle membranes.

16. Are there any nonpharmacologic alternatives to nerve blocks for patients with focal spasticity?

Casting is another technique that can be done frequently in a patient with focal contracture due to spasticity. Limbs can be stretched and then casted in a lengthened position. Casts can be changed every few days or weeks to gradually stretch contracted structures. Casting is limited, however, in that it can only achieve mild increases in joint range. To achieve more dramatic increases, one must incorporate a surgical procedure.

17. What does the orthopedic surgeon offer the spastic patient?

There are a long list of orthopedic surgical procedures that have been proposed for spastic patients. The **SPLATT** procedure deserves mention as an especially effective treatment for the equinovarus foot. An acronym for **S**plit **A**nterior **T**ibial **T**ransfer, it involves splitting the tibialis anterior tendon distally. Half is left attached to its site of origin, while the distal end of the lateral half of the tendon is tunneled into the third cuneiform and cuboid bones. This provides an eversion force which balances the spastic inturning at the ankle, giving the patient a solid platform on which to place weight during gait. **Achilles tendon lengthening** is often performed in conjunction with the SPLATT to decrease the toe-pointing equinus posture. These procedures can dramatically improve the gait pattern of a hemiplegic patient.

18. Are dorsal rhizotomies effective for children with cerebral palsy?

Although there was a wave of initial enthusiasm, careful scrutiny of the dorsal rhizotomy literature begs caution. **Rhizotomy** refers to the surgical section of nerve roots, and this has been carried out for a long time. Cutting the anterior (motor) nerve root is undersirable, as it causes denervation atrophy which predisposes to pressure sores. Cutting the posterior (sensory) nerve root seems preferable, as it decreases the sensory input to the spinal cord circuitry. By selectively sectioning nerve rootlets rather than entire dorsal roots, the neurosurgeon can decrease the amount of spastic tone while minimizing sensory loss necessary for skin protection and motor control.

BIBLIOGRAPHY

1. Katz RT: Spastic hypertonia. In Braddom R (ed): Physical Medicine and Rehabilitation, 2nd ed. Philadelphia, W.B. Saunders, 2000.
2. Keenan MA, Kozin S, Berlet J: Manual of Orthopaedic Surgery for Spasticity. New York, Raven Press, 1993.
3. Smyth MD, Peacock WJ: Surgical treatment of spasticity. Muscle Nerve 23:153–163, 2000.

73. METABOLIC BONE DISEASE

Charles E. Levy, M.D., Jeffrey Rosenbuth, M.D., Valery F. Lanyi, M.D., and Bryan O'Young, M.D.

Our greatest glory is not in never falling, but in rising every time we fall.
—Confucius

1. Which disorders are considered metabolic bone diseases?

Metabolic bone diseases are disorders of the skeletal system due to an alteration in bone cell function causing loss of skeletal integrity and strength. The major metabolic bone disease seen by physiatrists is osteoporosis, but this category also includes Paget's disease, osteomalacia, renal osteodystrophy, hyperparathyroidism, osteogenesis imperfecta, and osteopetrosis.

2. What is peak bone mass? When is it achieved?

Peak bone mass (PBM), the highest level of bone mass achieved as a result of normal growth, generally occurs at age 30–35 for cortical bone and likely earlier for trabecular bone, with variation at specific skeletal sites. For example, PBM of the femoral neck is achieved in the 17th year, whereas the lumbar vertebrae usually reach their maximum between ages 18 and 24 years. Bone mass of the other regions of interest either shows no difference in women between age 18 and menopause or is maximal in 50-year-old women, indicating slow but permanent bone accumulation continuing at some sites up to the time of menopause. Bone mineral density (BMD) is generally accumulated through adolescence, after which it declines at variable rates depending on anatomic location.

3. What happens to PBM at menopause?

Starting around the fourth or fifth decade of life, bone mass declines at a rate of 0.3–0.5% per year. This is actually true in men and women, but after menopause in women, bone mass loss accelerates up to 10 times the initial rate for a period of 5–7 years. The cumulative losses of bone mass range from 20% to 30% in men and 40% to 50% in women.

4. What is osteoporosis?

Osteoporosis is a disease of bone characterized by a reduction in bone mass that is caused by an imbalance between bone formation and bone resorption. In osteoporosis, normally mineralized bone is present in decreased density, resulting in skeletal fragility and an increased risk of fracture. In contrast, the amount of bone tissue in **osteomalacia** is normal (or increased), but there is reduced mineral content to the organic component ratio, leading to a "softening" of bone. The World Health Organization defines osteoporosis as BMD > 2.5 standard deviations (SD) below the young adult mean. **Osteopenia**, likewise, is defined when BMD falls between 1 and 2.5 SD below the mean. Normal values for BMD are based on nomograms including age and sex correction factors.

5. Is osteoporosis only a significant problem in women?

No. Although 1 in 3 women will have sustained a hip fracture by the age of 80, 1 in 6 men will have suffered the same complication. In fact, the lifetime risk of hip, wrist, or vertebral fracture is approximately 40% for white women and 13% for white men. Men have a greater lifetime risk for hip fractures than for prostate cancer. After the age of 75, half of the population and an equal number of men and women are affected by osteoporosis.

6. What are the symptoms of osteoporosis?

Like many diseases associated with aging (e.g., hypertension), osteoporosis is largely asymptomatic until the occurrence of a catastrophic event, which will likely be the fracture of a wrist, tibia, humerus, hip, or vertebra. Fractures are often preceded by movements that seem trivial and, when affecting the spine, usually occur more commonly in the low thoracic or lumbar vertebrae. The initial pain of the typical compression fracture resolves in 4–6 weeks. An accumulation of compression fractures can lead to postural deformity, which can include the dorsal kyphosis and exaggerated cervical lordosis known as the "dowager's hump," with accompanying chronic thoracic or low back pain, nuchal myalgia, and abdominal protrusion and gastrointestinal discomfort. In severe cases, restricted excursion of the thoracic cage predisposes to pulmonary insufficiency and pneumonia. Radiation of pain down one leg is uncommon, and patients are mostly free of pain between fractures.

7. Is all osteoporosis the same?

No. It is important to break down osteoporosis into subcategories. First, one should distinguish localized versus generalized disease. **Localized osteoporosis** includes primary disorders, such as reflex sympathetic dystrophy and transient regional osteoporosis. Secondary causes of localized osteoporosis include immobilization, inflammation, tumor, and necrosis.

Generalized osteoporosis includes primary and secondary forms. By far, the most common type of primary generalized osteoporosis is involutional osteoporosis, which can be further broken down into postmenopausal osteoporosis (type I) and age-associated osteoporosis (type II). Type I generally affects women between the ages of 50 and 65 years, whereas type II affects those over age 70. Finally, there is general osteoporosis that results from a secondary disease process (type III).

Classification of Osteoporosis

CLASSIFICATION	CLINICAL COURSE	REMARKS
Primary		
Involutional		
Type I (postmenopausal)	Affects women only within menopause, lasting 15–20 yrs	Predominantly trabecular bone loss in axial skeleton
Type II (age-associated)	Men or women over age 70	Proportional loss of trabecular and cortical bone
Idiopathic juvenile	Age 8–14, self-limited (2–4 yrs)	Normal growth; consider secondary forms
Idiopathic young adult	Mild to severe, self-limited (5–10 yrs)	
Secondary (type III)	Dependent on underlying cause	Usually reversible to some extent after treatment of the primary disease
Endocrine		
Gastrointestinal		
Bone marrow disorders		
Connective tissue disorders		
Malnutrition		
Lymphoproliferative diseases		
Medications		
Cadmium poisoning		
Others		
Regional		
Reflex sympathetic dystrophy	Three overlapping clinical stages: typical course lasts 6–9 mos, followed by spontaneous or assisted resolution	Radiographic changes may occur in first 3–4 wks, showing patchy demineralization of affected area; triple-phase bone scan shows increased uptake in involved extremity before radiographic changes; brief tapering dose of corticosteroids often warranted.

Table continued on following page

Classification of Osteoporosis (cont.)

CLASSIFICATION	CLINICAL COURSE	REMARKS
Transient regional osteoporosis	Localized, migratory, predominantly involves hip, usually self-limited (6–9 mos)	Rare; diagnosis by clinical suspicion, radiograph, and bone scan; treatment similar to that for reflex sympathetic dystrophy

8. Describe the history and physical examination for osteoporosis.

History and physical examination should focus on assessing risk factors, such as nutritional insufficiencies, endocrine or gastrointestinal disease, alcoholism, medications known to affect bone (e.g., corticosteroids, certain anticonvulsants), and secondary amenorrhea (anorexia and extreme exercise). One should examine the body habitus for signs of anorexia, cushingoid appearance, hypogonadism, goiter, gynecomastia, and barrel chest in patients with chronic obstructive pulmonary disease (COPD); perform lung auscultation for the distant breath sounds and wheezes of COPD; and observe for signs of inflammatory disease.

9. What laboratory tests are warranted?

The medical work-up is aimed at determining the cause and extent of osteoporosis.
- Serum chemistries, including calcium, phosphorus, protein, cholesterol, alkaline phosphatase, hepatic enzymes, renal function tests, and thyroid function tests
- Complete blood count and erythrocyte sedimentation rate (ESR), to rule out inflammatory processes and anemias associated with malignancies
- Serum testosterone (in men) to rule out hypogonadism
- Urinalysis screens for proteinuria due to nephrotic syndrome and for low pH due to renal tubular acidosis
- 24-hour urine
- Serum parathyroid level and vitamin D levels
- Multiple myeloma is unlikely with normal serum protein electrophoresis, ESR, and hematocrit
- Serum and urine markers of bone resorption such as urinary pyridinolines, telopeptides, serum bone specific alkaline phosphatase, and osteocalcin
- Iliac crest bone biopsy/marrow aspiration

10. What are the different methods of assessing bone mass?

Radiographs can be confirmatory but are not a reliable screen for osteopenia.

Single photon absorptiometry (1960s) requires water or gel immersion. It typically measures density at the radius and the calcaneus.

Dual photon absorptiometry (1970s) is used to study the spine, hip, and whole body without immersion.

Dual energy x-ray absorptiometry (DEXA) (1980s) has improved resolution, with shorter time of study and lower levels of radiation than dual photon absorptiometry. This is the preferred measure by most researchers and practitioners studying osteoporosis. It should be performed on both vertebrae and femoral neck areas. BMD > 2.5 SD below the mean correlates well with osteoporotic fractures.

Quantitative computed tomography (CT) (1980s) separately measures cortical and cancellous bone on existing CT instruments and measures true bone mineral density. However, radiation exposure is hundreds of times greater than for DEXA. This method is expensive.

Broadband ultrasound (1990s) may be as useful as densitometry without radiation.

11. What are some indications for bone mass measurement?

In general, bone mass measurement is indicated if the results would influence the patient and physician to use pharmacologic, dietary, and lifestyle interventions to prevent osteoporosis. Some examples include:

1. **Menopause**. Hormone therapy is often guided by BMD measurement.

2. To **confirm the radiologic diagnosis** of osteopenia. Even seemingly obvious vertebral compression fractures may actually represent old juvenile epiphysitis, positioning problems of the radiograph, or normal variations in vertebral body shape.

3. **Long-term glucocorticoid steroids**. Findings of significantly reduced bone mass may lead to reduction in dose.

4. **Primary hyperparathyroidism**. BMD measurement may help identify candidates for parathyroid surgery among those at risk for severe skeletal disease with asymptomatic primary hyperparathyroidism.

5. **Amenorrhea in a younger woman** for any reason (anorexia, hyperprolactinemia, excessive exercise).

6. **Strong family history** of osteoporosis or presence of other risk factors.

7. To determine if osteoporosis **therapy has been effective**.

12. Who was Julius Wolff? What is Wolff's law?

Wolff, a professor of surgery at the University of Berlin, published his famous monograph, *The Law of Bone Remodeling*, in 1892. The essential tenet of this work was that static stress to a bone—whether it be compression, tension, or shear—would cause bone to remodel along mathematically predictable lines. Wolff collaborated with Professor Culman, a mathematician from Zurich who developed a method of analyzing the structural stresses in various components of bridges, building frames, and cranes. To test Wolff's supposition, Culman assigned his students the task of drawing the stresses on a particular hypothetical crane, which, unbeknownst to the students, was shaped to resemble the human femur. The students' vectors closely resembled the trabeculae of the actual femur, thus confirming what was later called Wolff's law. In essence, this law states mechanical use (weight-bearing) results in increased cortical bone mass and strength, whereas disuse leads to bone atrophy.

13. What is the evidence for the use of exercise as a preventative measure in osteoporosis?

1. Wolff's law describes how applied load can cause changes in body weight and bone size and affect architecture of bone.

2. A study of flaccid and spastic paraplegics by Abramson in 1961 demonstrated that involuntary motion from spasticity may delay development of osteoporosis in spinal cord–injured persons.

14. What is the relationship between immobilization and osteoporosis?

Following extended immobilization (either external such as for fractures or self-imposed because of pain), evidence of osteoporosis can be noted on x-rays within 2–3 months.

15. Is there a relationship between muscle strength and osteoporosis?

Sinaki has demonstrated that extensor strength of the back muscles and BMD have a positive correlation.

16. What are the effects of weightlessness on bone mineral density and what strategies can be applied?

Data supplied from NASA suggest that astronauts develop acute osteoporosis once deprived of gravitational forces. Resistive exercises within gravity-deprived space improve BMD. It also suggests that walking may be one of the prime methods of intervention.

17. Describe the physical therapy and exercise considerations for osteoporosis.

Several studies confirm the fact that weight-bearing exercise improves bone mineral density. Aerobic low-impact exercises, such as walking and bicycling, are generally recommended. The height of the bicycle seat, saddle style, and handle bar height and style should be adjusted for an upright spinal alignment. Research also supports the contention that high-intensity strength training offers the multiple benefits of preservation of bone mineral density, improvement of muscle mass and strength, maintenance of balance, and decrease in hip and vertebral fractures. In fact, even a decrease in the number of hours sitting per day has been shown to be protective against hip fractures.

The National Osteoporosis Foundation Scientific Advisory Board Position Paper on Exercise and Osteoporosis (1991) describes five important principles of therapeutic exercise for osteoporosis:

1. Principle of specificity. Activities should stress sites most at risk for fracture, and skeletal protection should be provided for those areas with severe loss of bone mass.

2. Principle of progression. A progressive increase in intensity is required for continued. improvement.

3. Principle of reversibility. The positive effects of an exercise program will be lost if stopped.

4. Principal of initial values. Those with an initial low capacity will have the greatest functional improvement.

5. Principle of diminishing returns. There is a limit to improvements in function, and as the limit is approached, greater effort is needed for increasingly smaller gains.

Although swimming is unlikely to improve bone mineral density, it provides chest expansion, spinal extension, and low-impact cardiopulmonary fitness, and therefore it has a place in an osteoporosis regimen. A home program of physical therapy should include deep breathing, back-extension exercises, pectoral stretching, isometric exercises to strengthen the abdomen, and avoidance of kyphosis.

18. Which back exercises should be avoided for those with postmenopausal spinal osteoporosis?

Spinal flexion exercises predispose osteoporotic women to vertebral compression fractures.

19. Why is bracing used for vertebral compression fractures?

For the **acute treatment of back pain** due to a compression fracture, an orthosis can provide enough immobility to allow a patient to lessen the duration of bed rest. Bracing decreases spinal motion, allowing paraspinal muscles to cease painful guarding, and also provides a physical barrier to reinjury.

For **chronic back pain**, bracing substitutes for weak muscles, reduces ligamentous strain, and offers some protection against the occurrence of new fracture. Patients are able to endure greater activity and achieve fuller independence.

Occasionally, **certain sports or recreational activities** demand application of a brace, which is then removed when normal activity is resumed.

20. What bracing options are available?

1. The simplest brace is the **elastic binder**, which functions as a reminder to restrict motion and also increases intra-abdominal pressure.

2. The heat-moldable plastic **thoracolumbar orthosis** (TLO) is shaped to the patient's contours and then applied in an elastic support, often fabricated by a physical therapist. This usually takes only minutes to fabricate and is generally a less-expensive option.

3. For greater control, an orthotist can fit a hyperextension **thoracolumbosacral orthosis** (TLSO), such as the Jewett and CASH (cruciform anterior sternal hyperextension) braces.

4. Further restriction may be obtained with a custom-molded **plastic body jacket**.

5. **Posture-training supports** consist of small pouches containing weights up to 2 lbs. The pouch, suspended by loops from the shoulders, is positioned just below the inferior angle of the scapula to counteract the tendency to bend forward and may be worn for 1 hour twice a day.

Continued use of spinal orthotics is generally discouraged because of the increased likelihood of weakening and atrophy of trunk muscles and decreased spinal mobility.

21. What other therapeutic options should be considered?

Home modifications can reduce the risk of falling. Elimination of throw rugs and application of nonskid tape on the outer edges of steps (of different colors if possible to aid those with poor visual acuity) can improve safety. Lighting dark hallways and rails at stairwells and in the bathrooms can blunt common household perils. Ramps can replace stairs. A transfer tub bench that straddles the bathtub with two legs in the tub and the remaining two legs positioned on the dry bathroom floor eliminates the need to step over the edge of the tub. An additional benefit is that the user can wash his or her lower limbs with less bending.

Work simplification is aimed at reduction of vertebral compressive forces. Proper body mechanics demand that heavy items are carried at waist height and close to the body. Repositioning desks, files, and telephones can spare trunk flexion. Pacing helps defer fatigue, as does alternating tasks that demand sitting with those that require standing. Wheeled carts of the proper height and backpacks can decrease vertebral strain of carrying. Rotating platforms (e.g., lazy Susans) can decrease the need to reach, and a swiveling, wheeled office chair with a lumbar support can be adjusted to support and position the spine. Electric can openers, knives, and mixers, lightweight cups and bowls, and levered door closures ease kitchen tasks. Long-handled reachers, shoehorns, sock aids, and sponges facilitate dressing and grooming.

22. What are the pharmacologic considerations in osteoporosis?

Drugs are used to achieve two goals: (1) pain control or (2) slowing or reversal of the underlying disease process.

23. Discuss the options for pain control for vertebral compression fractures.

Back pain due to a vertebral compression fracture usually resolves in 4–6 weeks. **Bed rest** may be helpful initially, but it should be of limited duration. Beyond 1 week, cardiovascular deconditioning, loss of strength, and further loss of bone density usually outweigh the benefit of pain avoidance. Modalities such as **moist heat** and **massage** may alleviate symptoms.

Nonsteroidal anti-inflammatory drugs (NSAIDs) are often helpful, although the physician must screen and monitor against the occurrence of peptic ulcer and renal diseases. Smaller doses are often appropriate for the elderly. Although **opioids** may offer meaningful relief from pain, they often slow gastrointestinal motility, causing constipation, particularly in the elderly. Furthermore, there is some risk of drug dependence.

24. What role does calcitonin play in the treatment of osteoporosis?

Calcitonin directly inhibits osteoclastic activity, reducing bone resorption so that vertebral bone mass is increased. Some reports even show decreased fracture incidence. It may be administered subcutaneously, intramuscularly, or nasally. A high incidence of nausea, transient facial flushing, and inflammatory reaction is associated with injected calcitonin; the incidence of these side effects drops dramatically with nasal administration. Calcitonin exerts an analgesic effect and is often prescribed in the acute postfracture period. Concurrent adequate intake of vitamin D and calcium is essential.

25. What advantages does alendronate offer in comparison with the other bisphosphonates?

Bisphosphonates (etidronate, pamidronate, and alendronate) are phosphatase-resistant analogues of pyrophosphates, which are naturally occurring inhibitors of bone resorption. The bisphosphonates bind to hydroxyapatite, preventing its dissolution and impairing osteoclast function. As a result, there is a reduction in the frequency of osteoclast activation. The dosage of **etidronate** (Didronel) necessary to inhibit bone resorption unfortunately also impairs mineralization of newly synthesized bone matrix. To avoid this unwanted effect, it is typically dosed for 14 days every 3 months. **Alendronate** (Fosamax) has a much more favorable ratio of osteoclast suppression to bone mineralization inhibition. It is about 1000 times more potent than etidronate in terms of inhibiting bone resorption and therefore can be dosed daily. As is the case for calcitonin, calcium and vitamin D intake should be supplemented. Postmenopausal women with osteoporosis taking alendronate have shown increases in bone mineral density of the lumbar spine, femoral head, and greater trochanter as well as a reduction in vertebral fractures.

26. Calcitonin and the bisphosphonates produce their effects by inhibiting osteoclasts, thus impairing bone resorption. Are there any agents that stimulate new bone formation?

Sodium fluoride stimulates osteoblast proliferation and increases bone formation. Various formulations of fluoride have been available in Europe for many years. Unfortunately, too much fluoride can increase bone fragility. A slow-release form of sodium fluoride embedded in wax has been effective in decreasing the incidence of vertebral fractures and increasing spinal bone mass in severely osteoporotic women. At the time of this printing, an advisory committee of the U.S. Food and Drug Administration has recommended approval of slow-release sodium fluoride for the treatment of osteoporosis, but this treatment still awaits official sanction.

Anabolic steroids have been shown to increase bone mass but are also associated with liver toxicity, masculinization, and hypercholesterolemia.

Testosterone has been demonstrated to increase bone mass in elderly men with hypogonadism.

Parathyroid hormone (PTH) may be of benefit when administered parenterally.

27. What are SERMs?

Selective **e**strogen **r**eceptor **m**odulators. **Raloxifen** has an agonist effect on bone and probably vascular endothelium and lipids. It does not cause endometrial hyperplasia. **Tamoxifen** is a mixed estrogen agonist-antagonist that increases BMD as much as calcium supplementation but not as much as estrogen. Its advantage is that it appears safe for use in women with a history of breast cancer.

28. What are codfish vertebrae?

Codfish vertebrae refer to a radiographic finding in osteoporosis. This deformity occurs when there is expansion of the intervertebral disks into the superior and inferior vertebral endplates, causing an exaggerated bioconcavity. Fuller Albright, a pioneer in metabolic bone disease, noted in 1948 that this bioconcavity resembled the vertebrae of codfish, which are naturally bioconcave. In order to remember this term, a codfish in profile can be imagined in the interspace between the vertebrae (see Figure).

Radiographic findings in osteoporosis are nonspecific. Anterior vertebral compression fractures are common. Often, the external architecture of bone will be preserved, but mineral density is diminished. Loss of striations and a decrease in cortical thickness of the proximal femur are classic findings. Fractures of isolated vertebral bodies at T4 or higher is unusual and suggests malignancy.

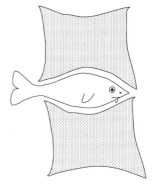

Codfish vertebrae. A representation of a lateral radiographic view of two vertebrae displaying an exaggerated bioconcavity. (Codfish is shown for illustrative purposes only. This is not ordinarily seen.)

29. What are the origins of the osteoblast and osteoclast?

The progenitors of both types of cells are located in bone marrow. **Osteoblasts** are members of a cell line derived from pluripotent mesenchymal stem cells called fibroblast colony-forming units (CFU-F). **Osteoclasts** arise from the hematopoietic granulocyte-macrophage colony-forming unit (CFU-GM).

30. What cytokines and colony-stimulating factors activate the development of osteoblasts and osteoclasts?

   Osteoblasts
      Interleukin-1
      Tumor necrosis factor
      Parathyroid hormone
      1,25-dihydroxyvitamin D_3
   Osteoclasts
      Interleukins-1, -3, -6, and -11
      Granulocyte-macrophage colony-stimulating factor
      Macrophage colony-stimulating factor
      Tumor necrosis factor
      Leukemia inhibiting factor
      Stem cell factor

31. How are estrogens and interleukin-6 connected in the pathophysiology of postmenopausal osteoporosis?

Estrogens inhibit the genetic transcription of interleukin-6. Therefore, loss of estrogens leads to greater amounts of interleukin-6, leading to increased numbers of osteoclasts. Ultimately, the homeostasis of bone formation and resorption is disrupted, favoring bone loss.

32. How does this apply to hypogonadal men?

Androgens exert a similar influence on interleukin-6 as estrogens.

33. What is coherence therapy? What does ADFR stand for?

Coherence therapy attempts to coordinate the normal sequence of bone remodeling throughout the body to allow strategic pharmacologic intervention. This intervention is aimed at limiting the resorption stage, which is broken down into four phases that can be remembered with the acronym ADFR:

   A—The **activation** stage is initiated with an agent such as phosphate, parathyroid hormone, thyroid hormone, 1,25-dihydroxyvitamin D_3, or growth hormone, which increases the number of remodeling units and coordinates their cycles (coherence).

   D—**Depression** follows this stage wherein an agent such as etidronate, calcitonin, estrogen, or calcium is applied to reduce the amount of bone removed by osteoclasts.

   F—Next comes the **free** stage, during which osteoblasts are left unimpeded to complete bone formation, usually for 2–3 months.

   R—**Repetition** is the final stage, wherein the cycle is repeated. Typical durations range from 3–6 months, with the hope and expectation that a little more bone will be added with each cycle.

34. What are the typical dosages used in estrogen replacement?

Estrogen therapy in postmenopausal women leads to reduced rates of bone loss and fracture and a reduced incidence of cardiovascular disease. Disadvantages are an increased risk of endometrial cancer (although this risk can be reduced when progesterone is added), small increased risk of breast cancer, and the resumption of menses. Bone mass measurement may be used to stratify risk: women whose bone mass is ≥ 1 SD above the young adult mean are relatively free from risk of fracture, although repeat measurement in 5 years may be warranted. Of course, reduction of cardiac risk by itself may be justification to start estrogen replacement.

Two types of 30-day regimens are commonly used in estrogen replacement: cyclic and continuous. The **cyclic** regimens include a resumption of menses. Estrogen, at 0.625 mg, is given daily for 25 days. This is combined with progesterone on days 12–25. Alternatively, estrogen can be taken for all 30 days with 5–10 mg of progesterone given daily for the first 14 days.

Likewise, there are two common **continuous** doses. For women without a uterus (i.e., hysterectomy), estrogen alone at 0.625 mg/day can be given, because there is no fear of endometrial carcinoma. A daily dose of 2.5 mg of progesterone can be added to the above schedule to provide protection against endometrial hyperplasia, while still avoiding the return of menses. The long-term safety and benefit of this schedule are still being evaluated.

35. How much calcium should be consumed daily by different age groups?

Optimal Calcium Requirements Recommended by the National Institutes of Health Consensus Panel

AGE GROUP	OPTIMAL DAILY INTAKE OF CALCIUM (MG)
Birth–6 mos	400
6 mos–1 yr	600
1–5 yrs	800
6–10 yrs	800–1200
11–24 yrs	1200–1500
Men: 25–65 yrs	1000
Women: 25–50 yrs	1000
Postmenopausal women on estrogens: 50–65 yrs	1000
Postmenopausal women not on estrogens: 50–65 yrs	1500
Men and women > 65 yrs	1500
Pregnant and nursing women	1200–1500

Dietary recommendations should be tailored to individual preferences. For example, 1 oz of Swiss cheese = 1 cup of milk = 1 cup of yogurt = 1 oz of calcium-enriched orange juice = approx. 300 mg of calcium. For individual patients, a consultation with a dietitian may be helpful. Others may be adequately served with educational pamphlets and charts. Calcium intake < 2000 mg/day is unlikely to be harmful.

36. How serious is the problem of hip fracture?

Hip fracture is a significant cause of morbidity and mortality in caucasian women ≥ 50 years and, to a lesser extent, caucasian men of similar age. Ninety percent of osteoporotic hip fractures are intertrochanteric and femoral neck. Some 17.5% of these women will ultimately sustain a hip fracture (compared to 6% of men) and will account for a large percentage of the anticipated $45 billion in direct medical costs attributable to osteoporosis in the next 10 years. Most hip fractures in osteoporotic individuals require operative management with a resulting 1-year morbidity rate of 14–36%. Perioperative risk factors are significant, and many patients also have poorly controlled systemic diseases.

37. Can any factors help predict who will sustain a hip fracture?

Caucasian postmenopausal women are at greatest risk. Furthermore, those with lower bone density are more likely to sustain a hip fracture. Poor self-rated health, a history of hyperthyroidism or maternal hip fracture, treatment with anticonvulsants, barbiturates, or long-acting benzodiazepines (half-life ≥ 24 hours), caffeine intake, and inactivity (< 4 hours on one's feet) raise the risk of hip fracture independent of bone mass. Findings on physical exam that are associated with fracture include inability to rise from a chair without using one's arms, resting tachycardia, poor depth perception, and poor perception of visual contrast. Taller, thinner women are also at increased peril.

38. How significant is osteoporosis in individuals with spinal cord injury (SCI)?

Fractures are common in individuals with SCI and occur at rates double that of controls, with up to one third of patients with long-term SCI reporting fractures. Complication rates are as high as 40%. Internal fixation can be unstable, and delayed fracture healing is often seen. In paraplegia, up to half of the lower extremity bone mass is lost, although the lumbar spine often has normal bone density.

BIBLIOGRAPHY

1. Cooper C, Barker DJ: Risk factors for hip fracture. N Engl J Med 332:814–815, 1995.
2. Cummings SR, Nevitt MC, Browner WS, et al: Risk factors for hip fracture in white women. N Engl J Med 332:814–815, 1995.
3. DeLisa JA (ed): Rehabilitation Medicine: Principles and Practice, 3rd ed. Philadelphia, J.B. Lippincott, 1998.
4. Downey JA, Myers SJ, Gonzalez EG, Lieberman JS (eds): The Physiological Basis of Rehabilitation Medicine, 2nd ed. Stoneham, MA, Butterworth-Heinemann, 1994.
5. Favus MJ (ed): Primer on the Metabolic Bone Diseases and Disorders of Mineral Metabolism, 2nd ed. New York, Raven Press, 1993.
6. Gregg EW, et al: Physical activity and osteoporotic fracture risk in older women. Ann Intern Med 129:81–88, 1998.
7. Grisso JA, Kelsey JL, Strom BL, et al: Risk factors for falls as a cause of hip fracture in women. N Engl J Med 324:1326, 1991.
8. Harris ST, Watts NB, et al: Four-year study of intermittent cycle etidronate treatment of postmenopausal osteoporosis: Three years of blinded therapy followed by one year of open therapy. Am J Med 95:557–567, 1993.
9. Kattke FJ, Lehrmann JF (eds): Krusen's Handbook of Physical Medicine and Rehabilitation, 4th ed. Philadelphia, W.B. Saunders, 1990.
10. Manolagas SC, Jilka RL: Mechanisms of disease: Bone marrow, cytokines, and bone remodeling: Emerging insights into the pathophysiology of osteoporosis. N Engl J Med 332:305–311, 1995.
11. Matkovic V (ed): Osteoporosis. Physical Medicine and Rehabilitation Clinics of North America, vol. 6, no. 2. Philadelphia, W.B. Saunders, 1995.
12. Matkovic V, Heany RP: Calcium balance during human growth: Evidence for threshold behavior. Am J Clin Nutr 55:992–996, 1992.
13. Ott SM: Osteoporosis in women with spinal cord injury. Phys Med Rehabil Clin North Am 12:111–131, 2001.
14. Sturtridge W, Lentle B, Hanley DA: The use of bone density measurements in the diagnosis and management of osteoporosis. Can Med Assoc J 155:924–929, 1996.
15. Wahner HW: Diagnostic procedures and new techniques [course handouts]. Presented at the 55th Annual Assembly of the American Academy of Physical Medicine & Rehabilitation, 1993.
16. Watts NB: Osteoporosis: Methods to prevent fractures in patients at high risk. Postgrad Med 95:72–86, 1994.
17. Watts NB, Harris ST, et al: Intermittent cyclical etidronate treatment of postmenopausal osteoporosis. N Engl J Med 323:73–79, 1990.

74. HETEROTOPIC OSSIFICATION

Jay V. Subbarao, M.D., M.S.

1. What is heterotopic ossification?

Heterotopic ossification (HO) is the formation of bone in abnormal locations caused by metaplasia of the mesenchymal cells into osteoblasts. It is classified as progressive or nonprogressive and is commonly periarticular. HO may be difficult to distinguish from a callus in a healing fracture and should be differentiated from periosteal reaction, which occurs due to irritation or inflammation close to the long bones.

2. What are some other names used for this condition?

1. Myositis ossificans
2. Para-osteoarthropathy
3. Ectopic ossification
4. Osteosis neuratica
5. Para-articular bone formation
6. Neurogenic ossifying fibromyopathy

3. How often does HO occur?

The incidence of HO depends on diagnostic measures, type of institution (acute or rehabilitation hospital), study design, and length of follow-up on patients. Clinically significant HO occurs in 20% of patients following head injury and in 20–30% after spinal cord injury (SCI). Ten percent of all cases cause severe restriction in joint motion or ankylosis.

4. What causes HO?

The exact etiology is unknown. However, genetic predisposition is suspected. Initial studies suggest an association with human leukocyte antigens (HLA). There are no tests for predicting susceptibility to HO, but warning signs include spasticity, pressure ulcers near joints, and proliferative osteoarthritis in multiple joints (males).

5. How do exercise and physical therapy affect HO formation?

Some experimental studies noted that bleeding and hematoma precede HO formation, leading to the implication that aggressive physical therapy may cause HO. However, this is not supported by the clinical experience. For example, an SCI patient who undergoes stretching of the hamstrings with similar force on both sides rarely shows clinical evidence of hematoma or other soft-tissue hemorrhage, and even if HO were to form, it usually involves only one joint. Also, HO occurs in only 20% of SCI patients, while all SCI patients undergo similar rehabilitative exercise programs. It is also reasonable to believe that HO is less likely to occur in a mobilized joint than one that is immobilized.

6. There is soft tissue all over the body, so can bone form anywhere?

HO is always periarticular and occurs in an area with neurologic deficit (i.e., below the level of lesion). Common sites include the hip, knee, shoulder, and elbow. HO may not affect the entire extremity, and bilateral involvement may occur. In neurologically compromised patients, HO is often found around proximal joints. Upper-extremity involvement is more common in patients with brain injury than with SCI. Interestingly, just because HO occurs at the hip or knee does not necessarily mean that HO formation will occur all along that extremity.

7. How can I tell if HO exists when I make daily rounds?

This is not easy. While the joint involved may initially present with eythema, swelling, and intense pain, the most pathognomonic finding is the gradual loss of ROM in the involved joint. To determine if stiffness, e.g., in the knees, is due to bed rest, check the ankle and hip on the same side. Generally, they are not as limited as the knee, or for that matter, the opposite knee is also not as stiff as the one that is red and swollen. Patients with HO rarely have accompanying systemic findings such as fever or leukocytosis.

8. Should any redness around the joint make me think of HO then?

Watch out! Other conditions may resemble HO, including cellulitis, deep vein thrombosis, hematoma, abscess, septic arthritis, and all other acute inflammatory processes. To complicate things, there are reports that deep vein thrombosis may coexist with HO. Also, check for edema distal and proximal to the joint and for spasticity in that extremity, as these may influence the diagnosis and future management. Often, the existence of HO is suggested by the therapist who notes decreasing ROM of the involved joint.

9. Can I rely on any laboratory tests to detect HO?

An elevated serum alkaline phosphatase (SAP) is common with HO. However, an elevated SAP also occurs in healing fractures and surgical procedures. If HO is suspected, the SAP may be helpful in diagnosis, but elevation does not correlate with severity of HO.

10. What about x-rays?

Roentgenograms can show the presence of bone formation. However, they are always negative in the first 2 weeks, and they do not help in assessing loss of function. Orthopedic surgeons can use x-rays to grade HO.

11. Are any imaging procedures helpful?

Radionuclide bone imaging can provide evidence of hyperemia, shown by pooling of contrast around the suspected joint. This technique involves injecting ^{99cr}Tc-methylene diphosphonate followed by imaging in **three phases**: pictures taken immediately after injection, within 2 minutes, and then at 2 hours. Phases 1 and 2 are very sensitive and often positive in early stages of HO and therefore effective for early detection. In fact, phase 3 images may be positive for up to 4 weeks prior to seeing any noticeable changes in plain x-rays. CT and MRI are not useful unless there is need to study the effect of HO on soft tissues.

12. Once HO is suspected, what are the treatment options?

Active and passive ROM
Positioning joint in optimal functional position
Medications to arrest calcification (etidronate disodium, EHDP)
Anti-inflammatory drugs
Radiation to the involved joint
Manipulation of involved joint
Surgical resection

13. Is joint rest helpful or not? What about physical therapy?

In its acute phase, short-term rest of the involved joint for up to 2 weeks is acceptable. Rest is essential to reduce inflammatory changes and microscopic hemorrhages which may lead to HO formation.

The patient must participate in general conditioning and ROM exercises to the uninvolved joints to prevent loss of function. Gentle active or assisted movement through painless ROM of the affected joint is recommended. Passive ROM can be performed on patients without voluntary movement. More aggressive movement is initiated after the inflammatory response subsides (approx. 2 weeks). If there is any increase in redness and swelling, joint motion should be discontinued. If ROM continues to decrease, immobilize the extremity in a functional position so that if ankylosis occurs it is still functional.

14. How does EHDP work?

Ethilidene hydroxydiphosphonate (EHDP) is commonly used to control new bone formation. Studies suggest that it inhibits growth of hydroxyapatite crystals by preventing the precipitation of soluble amorphous calcium phosphate. EHDP also slows the rate of osteoblastic and osteoclastic activity. Unfortunately, there are no conclusive studies on humans that show EHDP controls HO formation. Since HO is a self-arresting process, it is difficult to determine if treatments are helpful or if progression has stopped on its own.

15. Does EHDP dissolve any of the bone already formed by HO?

No.

16. Since we cannot do anything once HO forms, can we prevent it?

Some medications such as ibuprofen, aspirin, and indomethacin are used as preventative therapy. However, their effectiveness is unproven. Indomethacin is postulated to inhibit prostaglandin synthesis and is commonly prescribed at 25 mg three times a day for 2 weeks. The use of EHDP preoperatively before surgical resection is recommended.

17. What is the role of radiation?

Prophylactic radiation has been used in patients with nonneurologic disorders. However, it has not been studied extensively, and there is a theoretical risk of skin breakdown. Single low-dose gamma radiation postoperatively is being used in " high-risk patients" following total hip arthroplasty revision or excision of HO in SCI patients.

18. Can we crack it?

There are studies that recommend manipulation of ankylosed joints under anesthesia. Manipulation is commonly done in cases involving burns, post-traumatic myositis ossificans, and joint replacement, which are nonneurologic. Manipulation following a neurologic injury may be justified when a patient has a residual functional extremity, but there are risks. It is also important to keep in mind that HO is stronger than osteoporotic bone. Forcible manipulation may result in fracture of bone.

19. When is surgical resection indicated?

Surgical resection is not intended to excise the HO entirely, prevent recurrence, achieve complete ROM in that joint, or arrest progression. The main indication should be a very clearly defined **functional limitation** which can be corrected by surgery. It is recommended to wait 1 year after onset of HO. There should also be evidence of arrest as evidenced by normal or decreasing serum alkaline phosphatase, lack of increased uptake in the triple-phase bone scan, and an x-ray showing evidence of "mature bone." Also, prior to surgery, the patient should not have any evidence of inflammatory signs or joint pain or infection in the skin or urine. To promote a quick recovery, a general conditioning and stretching program should be started prior to surgery.

20. What two types of surgical procedures are used?

Wedge resection and excision. Wedge resection is the most commonly used. Excision is less commonly used and does not remove all the new bone.

21. Describe the postoperative course.

Postoperatively, gentle mobilization should occur within 48 hours after surgery to facilitate effective drainage of the hematoma. Positioning of the joint depends on the type of function desired, e.g., increase in flexion or extension. Superficial infection often occurs in these patients, and therefore it is essential that the patient be involved in functional activities as soon as possible to prevent complications, such as urinary tract infection, pressure ulcers, and deconditioning from immobilization. Postoperative x-rays may show new bone formation, but keep in mind that the goal of surgery is functional gain, and improvement in function is how one should measure the surgical outcome.

BIBLIOGRAPHY

1. Chantraine A, Minaire P: Para-osteo-arthopathies: A new theory and mode of treatment. Scand J Rehabil Med 13:31–37, 1981.
2. Citta-Pietrulungo T, Alexander M, Steg N: Early detection of heterotopic ossification in young patients with traumatic brain injury. Arch Phys Med Rehabil 73:258–262, 1992.
3. Ebraheim N, Kim K, Jackson WT, Kane JT: Heterotopic ossification and pseudoarthrosis in the shoulder following encephalitis: A case report and review of the literature. Clin Orthop 219:291–298, 1987.
4. Freed JH, Hahn H, Menter R, Dillion T: The use of the three phase bone scan in the early diagnosis of heterotopic ossification. Paraplegia 20:208–216, 1982.
5. Garland DE, Razza BE, Water SRL: Forceful joint manipulation in head injured adults with heterotopic ossification. Clin Orthop 169:133–138, 1982.
6. Garrison SJ: Update on heterotopic ossification in spinal cord injury. Curr Concepts Rehabil Med 5:1–35, 1989.
7. Lal S, Hamilton B, Heinemann A, Berts HB: Risk factors for heterotopic ossification in spinal cord injury. Arch Med Rehabil 70:387, 1989.
8. Michelsson JE, Ravschning W: Pathogenesis of experimental heterotopic bone formation following temporary forcible exercising of immobilized limbs. Clin Orthop 178:265–272, 1983.
9. Orzel JA, Rudd TG: Heterotopic bone formation: Clinical, laboratory, and imaging correlation. Clin Sci 26:125–132, 1985.
10. Stover SL: Heterotopic ossification after spinal cord injury. In Bloch RF, Basbaum M (eds): Management of Spinal Cord Injuries. Baltimore, Williams & Wilkins, 1986, pp 284–301.

11. Stover SL, Garland DE, Nilsson OS: Heterotopic ossification. Clin Orthop 263:1–120, 1991.
12. Stover SL, Niemann KMW, Miller JM: Disodium cidronate in the prevention of postoperative recurrence of heterotopic ossification in the spinal cord injured patient. J Bone Joint Surg 58:683–687, 1976.
13. Subbarao JV: Heterotopic ossification. In Grabois M, Garrison SJ (eds): Physical Medicine and Rehabilitation: The Complete Approach. Malden, MA, Blackwell Science, 2000.
14. Subbarao JV: Pseudoarthrosis in heterotopic ossification in spinal cord injured patients. Am J Phys Med Rehabil 13:88–90, 1990.
15. Subbarao JV, Nemchausky BA, Gratzer M: Resection of heterotopic ossification and didronel therapy— regaining wheelchair independence in the spinal cord injury. J Am Paraplegia Soc 10:3–7, 1987.
16. Varghese G, Williams K, Desmer A, Redford J: Nonarticular complication of heterotopic ossification: A clinical review. Arch Phys Med Rehabil 72:1009–1013, 1991.

75. PRESSURE ULCERS

Michael M. Priebe, M.D.

1. The axiom goes, "where there is no pressure, there is no ulcer." Why does pressure causes ulceration?

Tissue ischemia. When tissues are compressed between a bony prominence and an external surface, capillaries are compressed and blood flow is obstructed, leading to ischemia. However, pressure is not the only contributor to ischemia.

2. How much pressure is too much?

Kosiak, in his classic 1961 study of the etiology of pressure ulcers, found a clear relationship between pressure and time in producing tissue changes in rat muscle. Constant pressure of 35 mmHg applied for up to 4 hours did not cause microscopic changes in the muscle fiber of neurologically intact and paraplegic rats, but 70 mmHg applied for 2 hours did produce moderate microscopic changes. *In general, the more pressure applied, the shorter the duration needed to produce tissue changes.* He also found that alternating pressure, in which the tissue was relieved of pressure for 5-minute intervals every 5 minutes, showed consistently less ulcer potential or no change compared to tissue subjected to an equivalent amount of constant pressure.

While Kosiak's experiment is very important in understanding the pathophysiology of pressure ulcers, it still does not answer the question of how much pressure is too much. Theoretically, if we keep the pressure below the mean arteriolar perfusion pressure of 32 mmHg, we should be safe. However, there is a continuum of pressure across the microvascular bed, dropping to 20 mmHg in capillary loops and 12 mmHg in venules. How much pressure is too much? We don't really know.

3. What are the three primary objectives of pressure management?
1. Even distribution of pressure
2. Minimize shear forces
3. Frequent pressure relief

4. Which tissues are most sensitive to pressure?

Tissues vary in their sensitivity to pressure. Interestingly enough, muscle is the most sensitive and skin is most resistant to pressure-induced ischemia. This explains, in part, the natural history of many deep pressure ulcers: a single insult, usually sustained high pressure over a bony prominence, leads to tissue ischemia and necrosis, which is worse at the muscle-bone interface. The affected area appears clinically as an area of induration, erythema, and warmth, but with intact skin. Within a few days to a week, even with complete pressure relief, the wound opens, revealing a deep crater filled with necrotic tissue.

5. If muscle is the most sensitive tissue to pressure, why do surgeons use muscle flaps (myocutaneous flaps) to close large pressure ulcers?

Myocutaneous flap procedures are based on the basic surgical principle of minimizing deadspace. Myocutaneous flaps do not provide a "cushion" as mistakenly assumed. They provide well-vascularized tissue to fill the large deadspace left after resection of a pressure ulcer. In fact, within a year or less, the bulk of the muscle in a myocutaneous flap has often atrophied due to chronic pressure. However, the blood supply is still intact, and the wound remains healed.

Another benefit is that the surgeon is often able to move the suture line—a very vulnerable region due to the formation of scar tissue, which has very poor tensile strength initially—away from the site of maximum pressure.

6. Name some other factors leading to pressure ulcers.

Shear forces: The pressure capable of disrupting blood flow can be reduced by half in the presence of significant shear forces.

Elevated tissue temperature: Increased temperature leads to higher metabolic demands in tissue, including muscle. This increases the likelihood that a pressure event will lead to tissue damage.

Malnutrition and anemia: Serum albumin positively correlates with pressure ulcer stage and negatively correlates with pressure ulcer risk. Hemoglobin < 10 mg/dL delays wound healing.

Peripheral vascular disease and smoking: Adequate oxygen in the wound bed increases local resistance to infection and enhances collagen formation. A good blood supply is necessary to provide nutrients and oxygen to the wound and remove toxins and waste products.

Altered sensation, mobility, and mental status: These result in decreased recognition of impending tissue damage or decreased ability to shift weight from pressure areas.

Maceration: This decreases the skin's tolerance to mechanical stress.

7. At what anatomic sites are pressure ulcers most likely to develop?

They develop most commonly over areas of bony prominence:

Sacrum (most common)	Ischium	Malleolus
Coccyx	Trochanter	Heel

8. What does pressure ulcer location tell us?

The location tells us what caused the pressure ulcer. Location is often predictable and depends on the individual's activity level. Persons who spend much or all of the day lying in bed most often develop pressure ulcers over the sacrum, trochanters, and heels. Persons who are sitting develop pressure ulcers over the ischii, coccyx, and trochanters. The location of a pressure ulcer often suggests its origin, thereby allowing for focused interventions for treatment and prevention.

9. How does sitting put pressure on the trochanters?

The trochanters do bear weight during sitting. If there is a pelvic obliquity present, whether due to decreased flexibility of the hips, contractures, or scoliosis, excessive pressures will occur at the trochanter (and ischium) on the low side. These trochanteric ulcers tend to form posterior to the greater trochanter rather than directly lateral to it (which is seen in side-lying ulcers). Use of a wheelchair with a sling seat that is over stretched may also contribute to trochanteric pressure ulcers.

10. What are four critical elements of assessment of a pressure ulcer?

1. Location
2. Stage
3. Dimensions
4. Tissue quality (wound bed, exudate, surrounding tissue)

11. How are pressure ulcers staged?

The National Pressure Ulcer Advisory Panel has defined four stages for pressure ulcers:

Stage I: Nonblanchable erythema of intact skin, the heralding lesions of skin ulceration. Note that reactive hyperemia can normally be expected to be present for one-half to three-fourths as long as the pressure occluded blood flow to the area. Hyperemia should not be confused with a Stage I pressure ulcer.

Stage II: Partial-thickness skin loss involving the epidermis and/or dermis. The ulcer is superficial and presents clinically as an abrasion, blister, or shallow crater.

Stage III: Full-thickness skin loss involving damage or necrosis of subcutaneous tissue that may extend down to, but not through, underlying fascia. The ulcer presents clinically as a deep crater with or without undermining of adjacent tissue.

Stage IV: Full-thickness skin loss with extensive destruction, tissue necrosis, or damage to muscle, bone, or supporting structures (e.g., tendon or joint capsule). Note that undermining and sinus tracts may also be associated with Stage IV pressure ulcers.

12. What is the best treatment for a pressure ulcer?

There is no single right answer. Every patient is different, and every wound unique. There are, however, a few principles to guide the treatment approach.

1. **Prevention is paramount.** As with most things in life, an ounce of prevention is worth a pound of cure. In the case of pressure ulcers, an ounce of prevention may be worth a pound of flesh. Careful attention to risk factors allows early detection of persons at risk for developing a pressure ulcer so that preventive efforts can be made.

2. **The underlying systemic and systematic problems that initially led to the development of the ulcer must be corrected.** This principle is the one most often ignored. Biologic, psychosocial, and environmental problems must be addressed to maximize the rate of healing and minimize the risk of recurrence.

3. **Wounds must be adequately cleansed and debrided before healing can occur.** Eschar, the tough, leathery, or dry matter covering a wound, is not a beneficial natural dressing that can be left in place. Not only does the eschar prevent proper staging of the wound, but it also harbors bacteria and prevents the formation of granulation tissue and epithelialization of the wound. Chronic, nonhealing pressure ulcers without eschars may also benefit from debridement to stimulate the acute wound-healing cascade.

4. **Maintain a moist wound environment.** A moist environment provides the optimal conditions for cell migration and mitosis. A dry wound impedes the healing process. Many products are available to assist in maintaining a moist wound environment (see question 16).

13. Which is the best way to debride a pressure ulcer?

The fastest and often most effective is **surgical**, or "**sharp**," **debridement**. Small wounds may be debrided at the bedside, but extensive wounds should be debrided in the operating room. This is often necessary early in the management in Stage III and IV pressure ulcers and is urgent in the face of advancing cellulitis or sepsis.

Mechanical debridement, primarily using wet-to-dry gauze dressings, can be effective to further remove necrotic tissue. Hydrotherapy and wound irrigation can assist in debridement and soften the eschar, making mechanical debridement easier.

Both sharp and mechanical debridement are nonselective, and healthy tissue can be damaged while attempting to remove necrotic tissue. Moistening dressings prior to their removal decreases the damage to healthy cells but is also less effective in debriding necrotic tissue. Wet-to-dry dressings should only be used for debridement and discontinued once the wound bed is clean.

Enzymatic debridement uses commercially available ointments containing enzymes to degrade the devitalized tissue in the wound bed. It is selective and generally does not damage healthy tissue. However, it is slow and cannot degrade large volumes of dead tissue.

Autolytic debridement, essentially using the body's own enzymes to degrade dead tissue, can be very effective in noninfected wounds. This is accomplished by placing an occlusive dressing over the wound and allowing the wound fluid to collect under the dressing. Be very careful, though, because if the wound is infected, you have just created an abscess. The wound fluid helps to soften the eschar and begin the separation of healthy from nonviable tissue, making sharp debridement easier.

14. The saying is, "You can put anything on a pressure ulcer, except the patient, and it will heal." True?

Yes and no. The human body is amazing in its ability to heal itself, often in the face of continued injury or insult. However, scientific evidence demonstrates that many agents used historically in wound care actually delay healing and epithelialization. Povidone-iodine, hydrogen peroxide, acetic acid, and sodium hypochlorite, commonly used in the past to cleanse wounds, are cytotoxic to human fibroblasts and delay wound healing. The cellular toxicity of these agents exceeds their antibacterial potency.

15. What is the difference between the tried-and-true normal saline wet-to-dry dressings and the myriad of new-fangled wound dressings?

It is important to first differentiate between "wet-to-dry" dressings and "wet-to-moist" dressings. Many times, physicians order wet-to-dry dressings when they mean wet-to-moist. Normal saline wet-to-dry dressings are used for debridement of necrotic wounds. However, wet-to-moist dressings, in which the dressing is changed before it dries out, can be used to maintain a clean, moist wound bed and have been used for years to heal pressure ulcers. It is hard to argue with success.

The real difference between wet-to-moist saline and gauze dressings and the newer dressings is essentially ease of care. Because wet-to-moist dressings need to be changed every 6–8 hours to maintain moisture, nursing care costs and "burden of care" are very high. Newer dressings can often be changed once a day or less, depending on the type of dressing chosen and the degree of wound exudate. However, regardless of the dressing chosen, the same principles apply—correction of underlying factors, adequate debridement of the wound, and a moist wound environment.

16. How does one know which type of dressing to choose?

Dressings differ in their properties, such as absorptive ability, oxygen permeability, adherence to the wound bed, patient comfort, ease of use, and need for a secondary dressing. These characteristics distinguish one from the other and help determine which would be the best alternative for a particular wound. Dressings such as transparent membranes, hydrocolloids, hydrogels, alginate products, and foam dressings are each suited to maintaining a moist wound environment in different wounds. It is important to match the dressing to the wound.

Properties and Common Uses of Five Major Classes of Wound Care Products

	PROPERTIES	USES
Transparent membranes	Moist healing principle Semi-permeable Allows O_2 exchange Prevents bacterial entry Promotes epithelial migration	Prevents shear and friction Stage 1, 2 and shallow 3 ulcers Clean, granulating, nondraining Autolysis Secondary dressing Change when leaks or excess fluid
Hydrocolloids	Occlusive barrier Forms gel with wound exudate Creates moist wound environment Prevents bacterial contamination Available in wafers, paste, powder, or granules	Stage 1, 2, 3, and some 4 ulcers Minimal to moderate exudating wounds Prevents shear and friction Secondary dressing Aids in liquefaction, nonsurgical debridement Change when leaks (if < 24 hr try another dressing)

Table continued on following page

Properties and Common Uses of Five Major Classes of Wound Care Products (cont.)

	PROPERTIES	USES
Hydrogels	Water, polyethylene oxide with other compounds Primary wound covering Provides moist wound environment Various absorption abilities Good for patient comfort Nonadherent to wound bed	Stage 2, 3, some 4 pressure ulcers Burns Autolysis—softens eschar Granulating or necrotic wounds
Alginate dressings	Hydrophilic, nonwoven fiber Converts to gel with wound exudate Calcium and sodium exchange Creates moist environment Nonadherent to wound Available in packing or sheets	Light to heavily draining wounds Stage 2, 3, and 4 pressure ulcers Burns, vascular ulcers, graft sites May be used with infected wounds Can pack deep wounds to fill deadspace
Foam dressings	Semipermeable, absorptive, non-woven, polyurethane dressing Combines moist healing and absorbency No dressing residue in wound Nonadherent to wound Thermal insulation Comfortable, trauma-free removal Can be used with topicals	Minimal to heavily draining wounds Donor sites Burns (1st and 2nd degree) Shallow pressure ulcers Skin tears

Adapted from Cuttino C: Dermal Wound Management in Long Term Care Settings Conference, Houston, TX, February 1994. King of Prussia, PA, Heath Management Publications, 1994.

17. When are antibiotics indicated in the management of pressure ulcers?

When there is evidence of infection associated with the pressure ulcer. The problem is defining what constitutes an infection. Clearly, when there is evidence of sepsis or cellulitis, urgent care, including debridement and systemic antibiotics, is needed. However, in the absence of overwhelming infection, what is the best way to determine the need for antibiotics? Wound cultures are generally useless because all pressure ulcers are colonized with bacteria. The Agency for Health Care Policy and Research suggests that wound cleansing and debridement will, in most cases, control colonization, purulent drainage, foul odor, and local inflammation. If a pressure ulcer is not healing after 2–4 weeks of optimal treatment, a 2-week trial of a broad-spectrum topical antibiotic may be helpful, e.g., silver sulfadiazine or triple antibiotic ointment. Systemic antibiotics are reserved for cases with evidence of osteomyelitis, cellulitis, or signs of systemic infection.

18. How is osteomyelitis underlying a pressure ulcer diagnosed?

Osteomyelitis underlying a pressure ulcer will impede wound healing and necessitate a very different approach to wound management. However, overdiagnosis of osteomyelitis may subject a patient to unnecessary treatments.

The gold standard for diagnosis of osteomyelitis is pathologic examination of a **bone biopsy**. Plain radiographs can be helpful, but changes on x-ray develop late in the course of osteomyelitis. Bone scans are rarely useful because of the high false-positive rate in the presence of a pressure ulcer. MRI has been shown to be sensitive and specific for osteomyelitis underlying a pressure ulcer.

19. Is electrical stimulation or other adjuvant therapy useful in the management of pressure ulcers?

The role of adjuvant therapies in pressure ulcer care has a long and controversial history. The problem is lack of controlled trials using these forms of therapy. Clinical trials using **electrical**

stimulation have demonstrated an enhanced rate of pressure ulcer healing in chronic stage III and IV pressure ulcers unresponsive to conventional treatment. It may also be useful for recalcitrant stage II ulcers. Its therapeutic benefit is hypothesized to be due to increasing circulation as a result of electrical stimulation. Use of this form of therapy has been limited to a small number of research centers and is not widely accepted.

Small clinical trials using **growth factors** have demonstrated an increased rate of pressure ulcer healing in persons with spinal cord injury. Future research is necessary to appropriately evaluate new and potentially beneficial therapies.

BIBLIOGRAPHY

1. Bergstrom N, Bennett MA, Carlson CE, et al: Treatment of Pressure Ulcers: Clinical Practice Guideline no 15. Rockville, MD, Agency for Health Care Policy and Research, 1994, AHCPR publication no. 95-0652.
2. Consortium for Spinal Cord Medicine. Pressure Ulcer Prevention and Treatment following Spinal Cord Injury: A Clinical Practice Guideline for Health-Care Professionals. Washington, DC, Paralyzed Veterans of America, 2000.
3. Cuddigan J, Frantz RA: Pressure ulcer research: Pressure ulcer treatment. Adv Wound Care 11:294–300, 1998.
4. Darouiche RO, Landon GC, Klima M, et al: Osteomyelitis associated with pressure sores. Arch Intern Med 154:753–758, 1994.
5. Dinsdale SN: Decubitus ulcers: Role of pressure and friction in causation. Arch Phys Med Rehabil 55:147–154, 1974.
6. Hess CT: Wound care products: A directory. Ostomy/Wound Manag 40(3):70–94, 1994.
7. Kosiak M: Etiology of decubitus ulcers. Arch Phys Med Rehabil 42:19–29, 1961.
8. Linder RM, Morris D: The surgical management of pressure ulcers: A systematic approach based on staging. Decubitus 3:32–38, 1990.
9. National Pressure Ulcer Advisory Panel: Pressure ulcers prevalence, cost and risk assessment: Consensus development conference statement. Decubitus 2:24–28, 1989.
10. Panel for the Prediction and Prevention of Pressure Ulcers in Adults: Prediction and Prevention: Clinical Practice Guideline no. 3. Rockville, MD, Agency for Health Care Policy and Research, 1992, AHCPR publication no. 92-0047.
11. Rees RS, Robson MC, et al: Becaplermin gel in the treatment of pressure ulcers: A phase II randomized, double-blind, placebo-controlled study. Wound Rep Reg 7:141–147, 1999.
12. Robson MC: The role of growth factors in the healing of chronic wounds. Wound Rep Reg 5:12–17, 1997.

76. NEUROGENIC BOWEL DYSFUNCTION: EVALUATION AND ADAPTIVE MANAGEMENT

Steven A. Stiens, M.D., M.S., and Lance L. Goetz, M.D.

This is a fundamental principle of medicine, that whenever the stool is withheld or is extruded with difficulty, grave illnesses result.
—Maimonides (1135–1204)

1. How are the large intestine and pelvic floor innervated?

Colonic peristalsis is orchestrated by a series of nerve cells linking the brain to the colonic mucosa. The **vagus** (vagabond) nerve wanders from the brainstem and innervates the gut all the way to the splenic flexure of the colon. The **nervi erigentes** (inferior splanchnic nerve) carries pelvic parasympathetic fibers from the S2–4 conal spinal cord levels to the descending colon and rectum. The descending colon receives sympathetic innervation from the **hypogastric nerve** (L1, 2, 3). The intrinsic nervous system of the intestine includes unmyelinated fibers from postganglionic parasympathetic ganglia and interneurons that coordinate peristalsis. **Auerbach's (intramuscular, or myenteric) plexus** is located between the circular and longitudinal muscle layers. **Meissner's (submucosal or under the mucosa) plexus** relays sensory and local motor responses. The external anal sphincter is supplied by the somatic **pudendal nerve (S2–4)**, which innervates the pelvic floor.

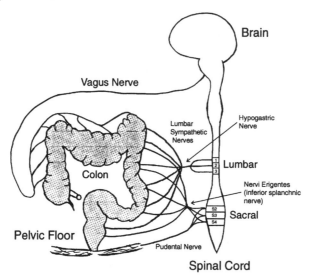

Nerve connections to the colon.

2. What is the "law of the intestine"?

In 1899, two English physiologists, W.M. Bayliss and E.H. Starling, reported that the intestines, even when removed from the body, have an inherent tendency to produce peristalsis toward the anus. This has become known as the "the law of the intestine." Whenever the intestinal wall is stretched or dilated, the nerves in the myenteric plexus cause the muscles above the dilation to constrict and those below the dilation to relax, propelling the contents toward the anus.

3. What is the normal physiologic sequence of steps that lead to defecation?
Reflex activity

1. Giant migratory contractions start at the cecum and advance stool through the colon to the rectum.

2. Stool distends the rectum as the internal sphincter relaxes (rectal inhibitory or sampling reflex), triggering a conscious "urge."

3. External anal sphincter and puborectalis muscle contraction retains stool (holding reflex).

Voluntary activity

1. Relaxation of the external anal sphincter and puborectalis releases stool.

2. Contraction of the levator ani, external abdominals, and diaphragm combined with glottic closure elevates intra-abdominal pressure and propels stool out.

4. How are the types of neurogenic bowel dysfunction defined and classified?

Neurogenic bowel is a term that relates colon dysfunction (constipation, incontinence, and discoordination of defecation) to lack of nervous control. The **upper motor neuron (UMN) bowel** results from a spinal cord lesion above the conus medullaris and typically manifests as fecal distention of the colon, overactive segmental peristalsis, underactive propulsive peristalsis, and a hyperactive holding reflex with spastic external anal sphincter constriction and the requirement for mechanical or chemical stimulus to trigger reflex defecation. The **lower motor neuron**

(LMN) bowel results from a lesion that affects the parasympathetic and somatic pudendal cell bodies on axons at the conus, cauda equina, or inferior splanchnic nerve and the pudendal nerve.

5. What patterns of colonic and pelvic floor dysfunction are observed with UMN and LMN lesions?

The UMN bowel has been described as "spastic" due to the excessive colonic wall activity observed. Surface EMG studies have demonstrated increased muscular activity in the colon after spinal cord injury. Colonic transit is normal until the descending colon is reached. There, movement is characterized by excessive segmentation waves and less frequent propulsive mass action. The striated muscle of the external anal sphincter, normally under voluntary control, remains tight due to spasticity of the pelvic floor.

The LMN bowel findings include low descending colonic wall tone and a flaccid pelvic floor and anal sphincter. No spinal-cord-mediated reflex peristalsis occurs. Slow stool propulsion is coordinated by the myenteric plexus alone, and incontinence is common with movement. The denervated colon produces a drier, rounder (scybalous) stool because the prolonged transit time results in increased absorption of moisture from the stool.

6. What is the internal anal sphincter?

The internal anal sphincter is the thick layer of colonic smooth muscle that surrounds the anal canal at the distal rectum. It is the major contributor to the resting pressure of the closed anal canal. Closure is maintained by tonic excitatory sympathetic (L1, 2) discharges. Internal sphincter tone is inhibited by anal dilatation by stool (**rectoanal inhibitory reflex**) or digital stimulation. Those experienced in bowel care are frequently able to palpate an increase in internal sphincter tone after defecation, which is a clinical sign that defecation is over and bowel care should be completed.

7. What is the difference between a bowel program and bowel care?

Although the terms are frequently interchanged, the most correct usage is as follows. A **bowel program** is the individualized comprehensive management plan for prevention of the problems that come with neurogenic bowel dysfunction. A bowel program has a variety of components, which include diet, fluid intake, physical activity, medications, and consistent scheduled bowel care. **Bowel care** is the individualized procedure for initiating and completing a bowel movement. It is the process for assisted defecation. Bowel care may include any or all of the following steps: preparation, positioning, checking for stool, inserting rectal stimulant medications, digital rectal stimulation, manual evacuation, recognizing completion, and clean up.

8. How is digital stimulation done?

Digital rectal stimulation is a technique for inducing reflex peristaltic waves of the colon to evacuate stool. It is done by gently introducing the entire gloved and lubricated finger into the rectum. This and moving the finger in a circular pattern opens the external anal sphincter by providing a stretch stimulus that reduces spastic tone and outflow resistance. Stimulation is produced by rotation of the gloved finger in a firm circular manner, maintaining contact with the rectal mucosae and dilating the proximal rectum. It is important to continually maintain contact with the mucosae. Rotation is continued until relaxation of the bowel wall is felt, flatus passes, stool comes down, or the internal sphincter constricts. This maneuver activates peristalsis locally (coordinated by the myenteric plexus) and stimulates conal-mediated reflex peristalsis. Digital stimulation ideally should require no more than 1 minute to generate peristalsis, but can be repeated every few minutes as needed to aid in stool evacuation.

9. Describe the bowel care used to facilitate reflex defecation for a person with an UMN bowel.

Persons with UMN injuries need a scheduled trigger of defecation every 1–3 days. Without the ability to feel the stool in the rectum or to easily initiate reflex defecation, a person with spinal cord injury must regularly assume the need for bowel movements to predictably eliminate stool and avoid colonic overdistention. The defecation reflex is stimulated digitally with a finger (or assistive device) inserted in the rectum (digital stimulation) and/or with appropriate stimulant medication.

The initial stimulant medication trigger is typically a suppository, enema, or minienema, which produces a mucosal contact stimulus that initiates conus-mediated reflex peristalsis. The stimulant medication is placed against the mucosa in the upper rectum. After the active ingredients have had time to dissolve and disperse, stool flow begins and is augmented as necessary with digital stimulations. Digital stimulations are repeated every 5–10 minutes if no stool passes. The end of the bowel care is signaled by cessation of gas and stool flow, palpable internal sphincter closure, or the absence of stool from the last two digital stimulations. Patients frequently "sense" the end of defecation. This sensation signaling the end of bowel care is possibly mediated by visceral afferents or partial sacral sparing of anal afferents.

10. What events and intervals mark the progress of the bowel care?

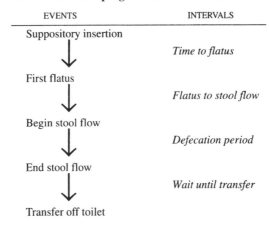

EVENTS	INTERVALS
Suppository insertion	
↓	*Time to flatus*
First flatus	
↓	*Flatus to stool flow*
Begin stool flow	
↓	*Defecation period*
End stool flow	
↓	*Wait until transfer*
Transfer off toilet	

11. What is the gastrocolic response?

Feeding induces increased propulsive colonic motility mediated by cholinergic motor neurons. Some have referred to this increase in gut motility as the **gastrocolic reflex**, but the mechanism may not be exclusively neural. The mechanism of this cholinergic stimulation is yet to be conclusively defined. Proposals include central vagal mediation, intrinsic colon pathways, and humoral mediation via cholecystokinin or gastrin. This increase in peristasis is facilitated by a fatty or proteinaceous meal and blunted by atropine. Some investigators have reported that the gastrocolic response is less robust after spinal cord injury.

12. Describe the techniques to produce defecation and maintain continence in persons with LMN bowel dysfunction.

Persons with LMN injuries often have more difficulty with their bowel care due to the absence of spinal reflex peristalsis and low anal sphincter tone. The rectum must be cleared of stool more frequently, usually one or more times per day, to prevent leakage of stool that cannot be retained by the patulous external sphincter. Rectal stimulant medications are not generally recommended for patients with LMN bowel because the absence of a spinal cord-mediated reflex peristalsis limits their effectiveness. Some patients wear tight underwear or bicycle pants to support the pelvic floor and help retain stool.

The LMN bowel care procedure usually consists of removing stool with the finger (manual evacuation) and using digital stimulation to increase peristalsis. Continence is improved by modulation of stool consistency with a high-fiber diet. Plant fibers such as psyllium hydromucilloid "regularize" stool by absorbing excess water and retaining it to prevent dry hard stool.

13. What if the bowel care routine becomes excessively long, dependent, or complicated by autonomic dysreflexia or intractable bleeding hemorrhoids?

Some persons with long histories of spinal cord injury (SCI) may have limited ability to independently manage their own bowel care, develop difficulty maintaining continence, or evolve excessively long ineffective bowel routines with insufficient results. A **colostomy** will offer independent bowel management, less incontinence, and reduced bowel care time, with a resultant improvement in quality of life. A colostomy is generally an elective procedure and is usually reversible, although people with SCI who elect for colostomy seldom have it reversed. Colostomies are often considered if severe bilateral grade 3 decubiti are present. Fecal diversion reduces wound contamination and simplifies care.

14. How can complications related to the neurogenic bowel be prevented?

Complications include hemorrhoids, impaction, colonic diverticuli, rectal prolapse, perirectal abscess, megacolon, and colonic cancer. Current prevention strategies include a high-fiber diet to maintain a soft stool. Supporting the pelvic floor with a gel or air cushion to distribute pressure over the entire perineal surface prevents the enlargement of hemorrhoids and maintains closure of the anal sphincter.

Following a regular schedule of bowel care sessions is important, even if stool elimination does not occur each time. Missed bowel care can contribute to excessive stool buildup, making the stool drier and more difficult to eliminate. Retained stool can overstretch the colon wall, reducing the effectiveness of peristalsis and resulting in longer bowel programs with poor results. Hemorrhoids can be prevented through frequent digital stimulations (to minimize the time necessary for the bowel program) and by avoiding constipation.

15. What laxative preparations should be avoided as chronic medication? Which are preferred?

Stimulant laxatives that are **anthraquinone derivatives**, such as senna, aloe, and cascara preparations, should be avoided because they can cause neuropathic damage to the myenteric plexus. Pigments from such laxatives also can stain the colonic mucosa (melanosis coli). **Stool softeners**, such as docusate sodium and mineral oil, are preferred for ongoing use because neither organ damage nor tolerance develops. **Daily fiber supplements** containing cellulose, polysaccharide, or psyllium can improve stool consistency if adequate fluid intake is maintained. **Chronic suppository use** is not known to cause colonic complications. Attempts to wean from suppositories and rely solely on reflex emptying from digital stimulation can be made over time.

16. What medications are used to augment the bowel program?

Oral

Psyllium hydromucilloid, calcium polycarbophil—maintains stool moisture and bulk.

Docusate sodium—a surface-acting emulsifying agent that lubricates and maintains stool moisture.

Suppositories to trigger defecation

Glycerine—mild stimulus, lubricating.

Bisacodyl (phenolphthalein derivative)—a polyphenolic molecule that produces colonic mass action on contact. Provides a stronger chemical stimulus. Bisacodyl may be compounded with a vegetable oil or a potentially faster-acting polyethylene base.

CO_2-generating suppositories—produce reflex defecation in response to colon dilatation. Not uniformly reliable in persons with SCI.

Enemas to trigger defecation

Theravac minienemas (rapid acting)—contain docusate sodium, polyethylene glycol, and glycerine with or without benzocaine (which can reduce the incidence of autonomic dysreflexia by locally anesthetizing the rectal wall).

Bisacodyl enema with a water base

Large-volume enemas should be reserved for patients that are refractory to other medications

17. How can diarrhea in patients with neurogenic bowel be managed?

Diarrhea can be related to GI infection, food intolerance, or use of antibiotics (most common treatment for a urinary tract infection). Treatment in these patients is similar to that for patients without a neurogenic bowel: antidiarrheal agents, laboratory evaluation for infectious causes (including *Clostridium difficile*, when indicated), and discontinuation of offending agents. Commonly, diarrhea alternating with constipation is related to partial bowel obstruction with flow of diarrhea around an impaction. A rectal exam is essential in evaluating these patients and may relieve the obstruction. Higher impactions are revealed by stool-filled loops of bowel on plain radiographs and require complete evacuation of the bowel, usually with oral magnesium citrate preparations.

18. What is a continent appendicocecostomy stoma? And what good is it for bowel care?

The Malone procedure surgically produces a catheterizable stoma that enters the cecum for self-administration of antegrade enemas to initiate bowel care. Through an 8-cm incision in the right lower quadrant, the appendix is localized and brought to the surface of the abdomen to form a stoma by amputating the tip to expose the lumen. The appendix is sewn into place and stoma can be covered with a bandaid. Bowel care is done by catheterizing the cecum through the appendix, then infusing 100–400 cc of saline to trigger defecation. Bowel care is completed in the classic manner with repeated digital rectal stimulation to promote peristasis and liberate stool and enema liquid. The Malone procedure has been done on many patients with spina bifida and a few with SCI with good success.

BIBLIOGRAPHY

1. Connell AM, Frankel H, Guttmann L: The motility of the pelvic colon following complete lesions of the spinal cord. Paraplegia 1:98–115, 1963.
2. Glick ME, Meshinpour H, Haldeman S, et al: Colonic dysfunction in patients with thoracic spinal cord injury. Gastroenterology 86:287–294, 1984.
3. Gore RM, Mintzer RA, Calenoff L: Gastrointestinal complications of spinal cord injury. Spine 6:536–544, 1981.
4. House JG, Stiens SA: Pharmacologically initiated defecation for persons with spinal cord injury: Effectiveness of three agents. Arch Phys Med Rehabil 78:1062–1065, 1997.
5. King J, Stiens SA: Neurogenic bowel management in physical medicine and rehabilitation. In Braddom R (ed): Physical Medicine and Rehabilitation, 2nd ed. Philadelphia, W.B. Saunders, 2000.
6. King R, Biddle A, Braunschweig C, et al: Clinical practice guidelines: Neurogenic bowel management in adults with spinal cord injury: Guideline group, consortium for spinal cord medicine. Washington, DC, Paralyzed Veterans of America, 1998.
7. Stiens SA, Biener-Bergman S, Goetz LL: Neurogenic bowel dysfunction after spinal cord injury: Clinical evaluation and rehabilitation management. Arch Phys Med Rehabil 78:S86–S102, 1997.
8. Stiens SA, Braunschweig C, Cowel JF, et al: Clinical practice consumer guideline: Neurogenic bowel: What you should know—a guide for people with spinal cord injury: Consortium for spinal cord medicine. Washington, DC, Paralyzed Veterans of America, 1999.
9. Stiens SA: Reduction in bowel program duration with polyethylene glycol based bisacodyl suppositories. Arch Phys Med Rehabil 76:674–677, 1995.
10. Stiens SA, Pidde T, Veland B, David M: Accidents Stink: Bowel Care 202 [video]. PVA Education and Training Foundation, 2001. [1-800-424-8200.]
11. Sun EA, Snape WJ, Cohen S, et al: The role of opiate receptors and cholinergic neurons in the gastrocolonic response. Gastroenterology 82:689–693, 1982.
12. Yang CC, Stiens SA: Antegrade continence enema for the treatment of neurogenic constipation and fecal incontinence after spinal cord injury; Arch Phys Med Rehabil 81: 683–685, 2000.

77. UROLOGIC DISORDERS IN REHABILITATION

Inder Perkash, M.D.

1. What is meant by a neurogenic urologic disorder? What are some common conditions leading to this disorder?

A neurourologic disorder is defined as a loss of voluntary control on initiation of micturition and/or an inhibition of micturition. This loss of control leads to either **retention** or **incontinence** of urine. Neurourologic disorders usually result from CNS lesions (e.g., cerebrovascular accident, head injury, intracranial tumors, spinal cord injuries [SCI], multiple sclerosis, and myelodysplasia) but may result from peripheral nerve injury as well (e.g., diabetic neuropathy). After a complete SCI lesion, there is usually a total lack of voluntary control on voiding, and as a result, there is usually retention or inadequate voiding.

2. What are the neural pathways linking the bladder to the CNS?

The human bladder is supplied by both the parasympathetic (motor and sensory) and sympathetic nervous systems. The bladder outlet at the pelvic floor is innervated by the somatic nervous system through the **pudendal nerves**.

The micturition center in the spinal cord is localized primarily in the interomediolateral region of **spinal cord segments** S2–4, with S3 being the most important root for bladder innervation. The pelvic parasympathetic nerves (S2–4) innervate the detrusor muscle and carry both motor and sensory fibers. However, the cell bodies of the parasympathetic fibers are located in the bladder wall. In other words, preganglionic fibers originate in the spinal cord, and postganglionic fibers originate in the bladder wall and innervate the bladder through short loops.

The innervation to most striated muscles of the pelvic floor, including those of the periurethral and anal sphincter, is through the pudendal nerve arising from S1–4.

There is ample evidence that the actual organizational center for micturition is localized in the **pontine-mesencephalic reticular formation**. Lesions above this level (suprapontine) are usually associated with detrusor hyper-reflexia, whereas infrapontine supraconal lesions are always associated with detrusor sphincter dyssynergia.

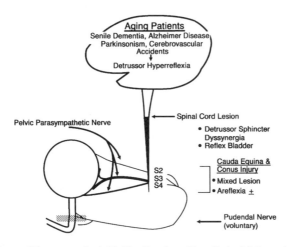

CNS lesions leading to different neurologic bladder disorders. (From Perkash I: Incontinence in patients with spinal cord injuries. In O'Donnell P (ed): Geriatric Urology. Boston, Little, Brown, & Co., 1994, pp 321–325; with permission.)

3. Describe the physiology of micturition.

When the bladder fills to about 100 mL, there is a minimum sensation of filling, but when it fills to about 300–400 mL, there is usually a feeling of fullness sensed by the brain (frontoparietal cortex). This sensation can be depressed and therefore micturition is inhibited. However, one can instantly initiate voiding when desired. Therefore, both initiation and inhibition are under voluntary control of the cerebral cortex, and continence is maintained. During sudden vigorous activities, such as jumping, coughing, or dancing, continence is maintained reflexively through the spinal cord, the **holding reflex**.

The bladder's response during filling is to accommodate and not lead to an increase in intravesical pressure. This very high compliance is due to passive viscoelastic properties of the bladder wall and possibly to intact β-adrenergic sympathetic innervation. Any fibrotic changes due to chronic infection and/or a neurologic lesion can reduce compliance and lead to much higher pressures during bladder filling.

4. What happens after spinal cord injury (SCI)?

Below the level of injury, there is complete loss of voluntary control; therefore, initially, there is retention of urine. However, later there is a tendency to develop a hyper-reflexic bladder with spontaneous voiding.

The basic function of local spinal cord reflexes is to hold urine. Normally, any sudden impact in the lower abdomen or strenuous activity, such as dancing or coughing, will lead to an instant reflex contraction of the external urinary sphincter and thus prevent leakage of urine. In spinal cord lesions, however, this **holding reflex** manifests with increased EMG activity of the external urethral sphincter during filling of the bladder or at attempted voiding and thus prevents leakage of urine. In people with SCI, this pathologic reflex is demonstrated by simultaneous cystometrographic and EMG studies of the external urethral sphincter during gradual bladder filling. When detrusor contraction attempts to empty the bladder, there is a reflex external sphincter contraction. This is referred to as **detrusor-sphincter dyssynergia** and is responsible for inadequate reflex voiding in SCI patients.

5. What is the role of sympathetic innervation of the bladder and bladder neck?

Efferent sympathetic nerves to the bladder and urethra originate in the intermediolateral nuclei of spinal cord segments T11–L2 and promote urine storage and continence. These nerves traverse the paravertebral ganglia to the hypogastric plexus to the bladder wall, bladder neck, and posterior urethra. They carry both motor and sensory fibers.

The bladder wall (fundus or body) primarily exhibits β-adrenergic receptors and responds to norepinephrine by relaxing. There is also an abundance of β-adrenergic receptors at the bladder base, which includes the upper trigone vesicoureteral junction. This helps bladder storage by relaxing the bladder muscle.

The bladder neck (vesicoureteral junction) is predominantly supplied with α-adrenergic fibers. There is a high density of α-adrenergic receptors along the bladder neck, particularly in males. This helps to prevent retrograde ejaculation and also helps close the bladder neck during bladder filling. Since α-adrenergic activity leads to closure of the bladder neck, α-adrenergic blockers (α-antagonists) have therefore usually been used to improve voiding by relaxing the bladder neck.

6. What basic bedside neurologic assessments provide initial clinical data for urologic management?

A basic neurourologic clinical exam should include a clear history for difficulty or inability to void. It should also include a quick, general neurologic exam to document any neurologic deficit. The exam should include **perianal sensation** (touch, pinprick), anal tone and voluntary contraction of the **anal sphincter** with digital examination, and **bulbocavernous reflex** (anal contraction with squeeze of the head of the penis). Rectal examination is also important to evaluate possible obstruction due to benign or malignant enlargement of the prostate. Because toe plantar flexors and hip external rotators are innervated by the S1 and S2 segments, their examination provides information on the integrity of sacral motor branches supplying the external urethral sphincter (S2) muscle.

An abdominal examination is important to feel for a distended bladder, as well as palpation before and after attempted voiding. In SCI patients, attempted voiding can be evaluated by **suprapubic tapping** over the bladder, **Valsalva maneuver**, and **credé** (suprapubic pressure). However, objective evaluation of micturition problems can only be accomplished by urodynamic testing.

Postvoid residual (PVR) measurements are made by allowing the patient's bladder to fill naturally to capacity and then having the patient attempt voiding voluntarily in a natural position (standing or sitting). Measurement of the voided volume is compared with the residual volume obtained by catheterization or ultrasound. A PVR > 100 mL or more than about 20% of the total voided urine is considered abnormal.

7. How is a routine urodynamic evaluation done?

Because flow rates are difficult to determine in completely paralyzed patients, other objective urodynamic parameters must be used, including cystometry and urethral pressure profiles. The term **video urodynamics** refers to the simultaneous pressure flow studies with fluoroscopic visualization of the lower urinary tract. Similar studies can also be done using transrectal ultrasonography to simultaneously visualize the lower urinary tract.

Cystometry is the recording of intravesical pressures during bladder filling. It requires introduction of a catheter through the urethra and slow filling of 24–40 mL/min of fluid at body temperature. During bladder filling, intravesical pressure usually does not rise above 20 cm H_2O prior to bladder contraction. In patients with bladder wall fibrosis due to repeated infections, the bladder filling pressure rises more suddenly, and it rises above 20 cm H_2O and at lower volume. Such a situation is noticed because of reduced compliance. Normal persons have a feeling of fullness at around 400 mL, when they feel a desire to void.

It is difficult to study flow rates in patients with SCI, and therefore pressure/flow studies cannot be accomplished. Some information can be obtained by gently tapping the suprapubic area over the bladder, which can lead to voiding. Post-void residuals can then be determined either with ultrasound or by catheterizing the bladder.

8. What is a urethral pressure profile? How is it useful?

A urethral pressure profile (UPP) is the pressure curve provided by the measurement of intraurethral pressure during withdrawal of a pressure sensor along the bladder neck, prostatic urethra, and the rest of the urethra. Profilometry can be performed on an empty or full bladder. Maximal urethral pressure is usually noticed close to the bulbous urethra. The UPP has limited value in patients with neurogenic bladders. In the presence of obstruction, the fall in UPP is more marked just beyond the site of obstruction.

9. What is detrusor compliance?

Compliance is defined as the increase in bladder pressure per unit of volume and is calculated by the change in volume divided by the change in pressure ($\Delta V/\Delta P$). The detrusor wall is composed of roughly equal amounts of muscle and collagen. When the collagen is more abundant, the elasticity decreases, the detrusor becomes stiffer, and the pressure rises faster during filling. Hypertrophic, spastic (neurogenic) detrusor muscle can also have a varying degree of reduced compliance.

10. What is detrusor sphincter dyssynergia?

The normal process of voiding includes a balanced synergy of simultaneous bladder wall contraction and sphincter relaxation. **Detrusor sphincter dyssynergia** is a pathologic hyperactive holding reflex characterized by the presence of involuntary pelvic floor (urinary sphincter) EMG activity during detrusor (bladder wall) contraction. This is observed in patients with spinal cord lesions below the pons and is absent in those with intracranial lesions. In normal persons, it is sometimes difficult to differentiate involuntary sphincteric activity such as dyssynergia from voluntary contractions to inhibit micturition. A careful evaluation is therefore required to diagnose detrusor sphincter dyssynergia in a patient with a normal neurologic examination.

11. How are the bulbocavernous reflex and sacral evoked potential tested? Why?

Bulbocavernous reflex is a polysynaptic (S2–4) crossed sacral withdrawal reflex and a nociceptive reflex of very constant latency. Clinically, it can be tested by squeezing the glans or clitoris and feeling the contraction of anal sphincter muscle. This reflex is present in all normal persons and in those SCI patients with lesions above the conus. The bulbocavernous reflex can also be recorded objectively by stimulating the dorsal nerve of the penis and picking up the EMG response (50–200 µV) in the anal sphincter muscle or from the perineal striated muscle.

The **sacral-evoked response** can be obtained either by stimulating the dorsal nerve of the penis with a ring electrode or by placing a stimulating needle on the left or right side of the bulbocavernosus muscle in the perineum to define a unilateral lesion. The first latency (about 12 msec) can be recorded over T4–L1 on the back, which represents the sensory peripheral conduction time. The central conduction time can be recorded at the scalp, which is usually 50 msec. Patients with previously diagnosed neurologic disease or those found to have subtle abnormalities on neurologic screening are candidates for this type of evaluation. The sacral-evoked potential testing and somatosensory-evoked potential testing should not be used as screening tests but rather as objective measurements of the location, presence, and nature of afferent penile sensory dysfunction. The findings of this testing can aid in anatomic localization of the lesion as peripheral, sacral, or suprasacral.

12. Which type of neurourologic dysfunction is typically seen with upper motor neuron lesions in SCI patients?

Vesicoureteral dysfunction depends on the site of lesion and any preexisting or associated disease, such as diabetes mellitus, radiculopathy, enlarged prostate, urethral stricture, or even ethanol abuse. Initially after an acute spinal injury, there is widespread autonomic paralysis (spinal shock phase); this often recovers by 3–6 weeks but can take longer. The reappearance of reflexes below the level of injury heralds the end of the spinal shock. The bladder can easily become overdistended due to neglect during this period. As a result, reflex voiding may not immediately ensue. Later, the appearance of detrusor sphincter dyssynergia leads to intermittent voiding (squirting of urine alternating with retention of urine). Bladder emptying can then be accomplished with intermittent catheterization. Baseline urodynamic testing is usually performed 6–8 weeks after acute injury.

13. What is the best way to provide bladder drainage in patients with acute SCI?

During the first 7–14 days, an indwelling catheter may be left in the urethra for continuous bladder drainage to prevent inadvertent bladder overdistension. A small catheter (F14 or 16) is recommended, which prevents urethral irritation and allows periurethral secretions to drain easily around it. Most patients who have severe injuries require fluid intake/output monitoring since they are on intravenous fluids.

Intermittent catheterization can be started as early as 7–15 days after injury. Fluid intake may need to be restricted to < 1500 mL/day. The bladder is drained with a straight catheter (F14) every 4 hours with a goal bladder volume of no more than 500 mL. After the establishment of reflex bladder, the patient is evaluated objectively with urodynamic monitoring of intravesical voiding pressures (leak pressure). A cystometrogram (CMG) may need to be repeated to evaluate voiding pressures following the use of anticholinergics to reduce detrusor contractions. Persistently high voiding pressures > 40–50 cm H_2O with sustained rise during CMG may necessitate a further increase in the dosage of anticholinergics. To start, patients are given oxybutynin (Ditropan, anticholinergic), 2.5–5 mg two or three times a day, to lower intravesicle pressure to < 40–50 cm H_2O. Patients who do not tolerate regular oxybutynin, particularly because of dryness of the mouth, can be given either longer-acting oxybutynin or tolterodine. There is some evidence that tolterodine may have less effect on muscarinic receptors in the salivary glands. There is also some evidence that oxybutynin is more lipid-soluble and thus may have higher concentration in the brain. This might influence reversible short-term memory problems. This helps to achieve continence between catheterizations, and therefore patients do not have to wear external drainage and leg bags.

14. Which method provides optimal long-term drainage of the neurogenic bladder?

Patients who have a reflex bladder, particularly tetraplegics, cannot catheterize themselves but can wear an external drainage condom, and they should considered for surgical reduction of outflow obstruction. To reduce outflow resistance and to have them void at low pressure, transurethral sphincterotomy or stenting of the urethral sphincter is considered. This also helps to reduce the autonomic dysreflexia triggered by detrusor sphincter dyssynergia.

A patient with a small retractile phallus with reflex bladder may be considered for a penile implant. Other patients who cannot self-catheterize and have a small retractile phallus may need an indwelling catheter or suprapubic cystostomy.

In female patients who cannot self-catheterize and are incontinent, vesical or supravesical diversion, such as a suprapubic cystostomy or bowel pouch, may be considered. Continent reservoirs that can be catheterized through sites on the abdomen area also available. Recently, such patients are also being considered for sacral nerve root implants to accomplish an electrically controlled bladder.

15. What is autonomic dysreflexia? How is this condition treated?

A sudden paroxysmal rise both in systolic and diastolic blood pressures with compensatory slowing of the pulse rate is observed clinically in dysreflexia. It usually happens in patients with spinal cord lesions above T5–6. Symptoms may include a pounding headache and sweating.

Autonomic dysreflexia is commonly precipitated by a full bladder and/or rectum or by other painful stimuli. To relieve the condition, the bladder is emptied by suprapubic tapping and/or immediate catheterization. Immediate blood pressure reduction can also be achieved with nitropaste, nifedipine, 10 mg sublingually, or by chewing the caplets and swallowing them for rapid absorption. Long-term management includes prevention of the triggering mechanism and may require the chronic use of α-adrenergic blockers, such as prazosin, terazosin, or a ganglionic blocker. Permanent resolution of dysreflexia (caused by voiding dysfunction) can sometimes be accomplished by transurethral sphincterotomy or following placement of a metallic stent in the posterior urethra.

16. Describe the usual protocol for urologic follow-up of these patients.

Patients with SCI are monitored with **radionuclide renal perfusion imaging** to evaluate glomerular filtration and renal plasma flow and with annual **ultrasound** of kidney to detect renal parenchymal loss, hydronephrosis, and stones. If hydronephrosis of the kidneys or ureters is noticed or deterioration of the renal function is found, a full work-up including **intravenous urogram** and **voiding cystourethrogram** is done. **Cystoscopic examination** is also done to evaluate outflow obstruction or to rule out other bladder problems such as bladder tumors. A yearly cystoscopic examination is recommended for patients who are heavy smokers or use chronic indwelling catheters.

17. What bladder problems are seen in patients with brain injury?

Following head injury or other intracranial lesions, the bladder is hyper-reflexic, but there is no dyssynergia. Initially, there may be retention of urine, and patients can be managed with an indwelling catheter followed by intermittent catheterization every 4–6 hours. Some patients may have an enlarged prostate which may require treatment later. Involuntary leakage of urine can be controlled with a small dosage of oxybutynin or tolterodine. Inadequate voiding due to internal sphincter resistance can be improved with the use of terazosin, an α-receptor antagonist, starting with a dose of 1 mg at night. Effectiveness of this therapy on voiding needs to be assessed with postvoid residual measurements, then gradually increasing the dose as needed over several days. All autonomic drugs are GI irritants and therefore should be given with meals. Initially, patients may not tolerate the hypotensive effect, and so they are given a low dose until they get used to the drug.

In patients with intracranial lesions such as parkinsonism, the bladder also is hyper-reflexic. The use of drugs (anticholinergics) to manage tremors may lead to retention of urine. In all such patients with detrusor hyper-reflexia, a transurethral resection of the prostate can sometimes result in permanent incontinence.

18. What are the common urinary tract complications of neurogenic bladder? How can they be prevented?

- The earliest changes are noticed as trabeculations seen inside an irregular, thickened bladder wall and even small diverticuli seen on voiding cystographic studies.
- Vesicoureteral reflux has been recorded in 10–30% of poorly managed patients. The presence of reflux is a serious complication since it leads to pyelonephritis and renal stone disease.
- Severe bladder outflow obstruction can result in bilateral hydronephrosis and hydroureters and even an overdistended areflexic bladder.
- Repeated bladder infections can lead to bladder wall changes and marked reduction in the compliance of the bladder.

All of these bladder wall changes can be prevented to some extent by adequately draining the bladder at a pressure below 40 cm H_2O, either by intermittent catheterization along with the use of anticholingergic drugs or by timely surgical relief of the outflow obstruction.

19. How common are urinary tract infections (UTIs) in SCI patients?

UTIs and their sequelae are the most frequent medical complications experienced by SCI patients. In persons who have long-term indwelling catheters or suprapubic catheters, the presence of bacteriuria is almost universal. The incidence of bacteriuria is reduced significantly in patients who can perform intermittent self-catheterization.

20. What is a significant UTI?

A UTI accompanied by a 1.5°F rise in body temperature with positive urine microbial culture and a large number of pus cells. Ordinary spun urine showing > 5–10 pus cells/high-power microscopic field is considered significant to indicate tissue infection. If this is noticed in patients on intermittent catherization, it may require treatment. In the absence of fever, an asymptomatic infection may not be treated in patients with Foley indwelling or suprapubic catheters.

21. What preventive measures can be taken to reduce the risk of UTIs?

Patients wearing external condom drainage with voiding pressures < 50 cm H_2O are relatively safe, but they need to clean their external drainage bag and tubing with 6% bleach. A thorough washing will clean the appliances. Personal hygiene with shower and adequate cleaning of the perineum and a daily cleaning of the cushion cover may reduce pelvic floor colonization and subsequent anterior urethral heavy colonization.

22. List the drugs used in the management of bladder problems and their desired effects.

Pharmacologic manipulation of bladder function is shown in the table. Tolterodine and oxybutynin as anticholinergics are available to manage detrusor hyperreflexia. Most of the autonomic drugs that change arteriolar tone also seem to have effect on the bladder neck, e.g., α-agonists constrict the bladder neck and α-blockers relax the bladder neck.

Pharmacologic Manipulation of Bladder Function

DESIRED FUNCTIONAL CHANGE	DRUGS	MODE OF ACTION
Improve bladder emptying		
Facilitate bladder contraction (muscarinic action)	Acetylcholine (clinically not used)	Normal neurotransmitter of the cholinergic receptors. It cannot be used for therapeutic purposes.
	Bethanechol (clinically used)	Limited indications. It should not be used with outlet obstruction or in suspected coronary disease. It could be used in selected patients along with α-sympathetic blockers and in patients with atonic or hypotonic bladder.
Decrease outlet resistance	Prazosin, terazosin, doxazosin (clinically used) Phenoxybenzamine (mutogenic in laboratory animals) Tamsulosin (newer selective blocker)	α-Adrenoceptor blockers improve voiding by opening bladder neck.
Improve bladder storage		
Reduce bladder contraction	Atropine, propantheline, oxybutynin, tolterodine, trospium chloride	Anticholinergic action (antimuscarinic action).
Increase outlet resistance	Phenylephrine, ephedrine	Sympathetic agonist response on α-adrenergic receptors.
Improve bladder storage and increase outlet resistance	Tricyclic antidepressants	Central and peripheral anticholinergic effects and also enhances α-adrenergic effect on bladder base and proximal urethra.

BIBLIOGRAPHY

1. Cardenas DD, Hooton TM: Urinary tract infection in persons with spinal cord injury. Arch Phys Med Rehabil 76:272, 1995.
2. Perkash I: Intermittent catheterization failure and an approach to bladder rehabilitation in spinal cord injury patients. Arch Phys Med Rehabil 59:9, 1978.
3. Perkash I: Management of neurogenic dysfunction of the bladder and bowel. In Kottke FJ, Stillwell GK, Lehmann JF (eds): Krusen's Handbook of Physical Medicine and Rehabilitation, 3rd ed. Philadelphia, W.B. Saunders, 1982, p 724.
4. Perkash I: Long-term urologic management of the patient with spinal cord injury. Urol Clin North Am 20:423, 1993.
5. Perkash I: Urologic diagnostic testing. In Lennard TA (ed): Pain Procedures in Clinical Practice, 2nd ed. Philadelphia, Hanley & Belfus, 2000, pp 66–74.
6. Perkash I: Contact laser sphincterotomy: Further experience and longer follow-up. Spinal Cord 34:227, 1996.
7. Perkash I: Controlling UTIs in patients with spinal cord injuries: Maintaining low intravesical voiding pressures is crucial. J Crit Illness 11(Suppl):11, 1996.
8. Reid G, Kang YS, Lacerte M, et al: Bacterial biofilm formation on the bladder epithelium of spinal cord injured patients: II. Toxic outcome on cell viability. Paraplegia 31:494, 1993.
9. Rutkowski SB, Middleton JW, Truman G, et al: The influence of bladder management on fertility in spinal cord injured males. Paraplegia 33:263, 1995.
10. Schwantes U, Topfmeier P: Importance of pharmacological and physicochemical properties for tolerance of antimuscarinic drugs in the treatment of detrusor instability and detrusor hyperreflexia—chances for improvement of therapy. Int J Clin Pharmacol Ther 37:209–218, 1999.
11. Sugiyama T, Park YC, Jurita T: Oxybutynin disrupts learning and memory in the rat passive avoidance response. Urol Res 27:393–395, 1999.
12. Silver JR, Doggart JR, Burr RG: The reduced urinary output after spinal cord injury: A review. Paraplegia 33:721, 1995.

13. Thyberg M, Ertzgaard P, Gylling M, Granerus G: Effect of nifedipine on cystometry-induced elevation of blood pressure in patients with a reflex urinary bladder after a high level spinal cord injury. Paraplegia 32:308, 1994.
14. Van Kerrebroeck PE, Amarenco G, Thuroff JW, et al: Dose-ranging study of tolterodine in patients with detrusor hyperreflexia. Neurourol Urodyn 17:499–512, 1998.

78. COMMUNICATION AND SWALLOWING IMPAIRMENTS

Donna C. Tippett, M.P.H., M.A., CCC-SLP

1. Who should be referred for a speech-language pathology evaluation?

Anyone with a suspected communication or swallowing impairment should be referred for a speech-language pathology evaluation. The effects of communication and swallowing problems can be minimized, and sometimes eliminated, with proper evaluation and treatment. If there is a question regarding the appropriateness of a referral, speech-language pathologists can perform a screening before giving a lengthy assessment. It is appropriate to obtain a speech-language pathology consultation within 24–48 hours after an individual is admitted to the hospital for an acute event, especially if dysphagia is suspected. Indications of dysphagia include drooling, "squirreling" of food in the mouth, gurgly voice after swallowing, and coughing after swallowing. Orders for speech-language pathology consultations are increasingly part of the admitting orders and are included on stroke pathways.

2. Discuss some of the causes of communication disorders and dysphagia.

Speech-language disorders are serious, treatable conditions that affect 16–18 million Americans, and swallowing disorders affect between 6 and 10 million Americans. The etiologies of these disorders may be **developmental** (e.g., language delay secondary to mental retardation, dysarthria secondary to cerebral palsy) or **acquired** (e.g., aphasia following left hemisphere stroke, cognitive/communicative impairment following traumatic brain injury, dysarthria associated with multiple sclerosis, alaryngeal speech following laryngectomy, dysphagia secondary to brainstem stroke). The personal cost of communication and swallowing disorders is high, affecting people's lives at home, school, and work. These disorders exact a price from society, too, involving losses in productivity, special education costs, and medical expenses.

3. What influences prognosis and candidacy for speech-language intervention?

It is difficult to make a definitive statement regarding candidacy for speech-language treatment given the diversity of patient populations and disorders seen by speech-language pathologists. However, it is usually true that treatment should be deferred for patients who are obtunded, sedated, or very ill. Variables that may be of prognostic value include:

Age at onset of disorder: The older the patient, the poorer the prognosis.

General health: The healthier the patient, the better the prognosis.

Motivation and cooperation: High degrees of motivation and cooperation are favorable prognostic signs.

Environmental factors: Family support can facilitate carryover of treatment objectives.

Etiology: Progressive diseases are associated with poorer outcomes, but treatment may still be indicated to facilitate communication and swallowing via compensatory strategies.

Initial speech-language pathology evaluation: Responsiveness to diagnostic treatment is a favorable outcome variable.

Rao states that individuals who are *not* candidates for aphasia treatment are those who demonstrate perseveration, severe auditory comprehension deficit, inability to match objects, unreliable yes/no responses, jargon, and empty speech without self-correction.

4. How are the aphasias classified?

There is no universally accepted nomenclature, and several schemes use different names for the same combination of symptoms (e.g., Wernicke's aphasia = receptive aphasia = syntactic aphasia). The advantages and disadvantages of aphasia classification continue to be debated in the literature, although one clear benefit is efficient communication among clinicians. Rao identifies six classification systems:

Aphasia Classification Systems and Examples

SYSTEMS	EXAMPLES
1. Severity	Mild, moderate, severe
2. Modality	Receptive vs. Expressive
3. Behavioral	Simple aphasia, aphasia with visual involvement
4. Statistical	40th percentile on the Porch Index of Communicative Ability
5. Linguistic	Semantic aphasia, syntactic aphasia
6. Syndrome	Broca's aphasia, global aphasia

The syndrome classification system, associated with the **Boston school of aphasia**, relies on an examination of fluency, comprehension, repetition, and word finding to make the diagnosis.

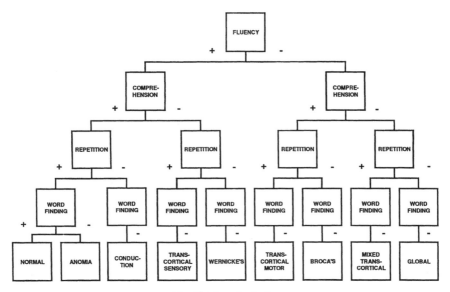

Classification of aphasias.

5. How can the clinician distinguish between fluent and nonfluent aphasias?

Aphasias are often difficult to classify in practice. It is most important for a physician to recognize that a language problem is present and to initiate a referral to speech-language pathology. It is also important to distinguish **fluent aphasias** from language of confusion or psychotic speech. Fluent aphasias localize to the temporal area of the brain and may not be associated with a hemiparesis, making some people think that the individual is just bananas. However, these patients often have a hemianopsia or other subtle neurologic deficit. **Dysfluent aphasias** are associated with more anterior lesions, near the motor strip, and are usually associated with a right hemiparesis, so the diagnosis of a left hemisphere lesion (e.g., CVA, tumor, abscess) is readily apparent.

6. What are language of confusion and language of generalized intellectual impairment? How are these different from aphasia?

Neuropathologies of Language

	ETIOLOGIES	FEATURES	DISTINGUISHING CHARACTERISTICS
Language of confusion	Diffuse, bilateral cerebral hemisphere damage, often traumatic	Difficulty in attention, concentration, and endurance Faulty memory Disorientation Impaired integrative language abilities Irrelevant and confabulatory conversational language	Intact vocabulary, syntax, and naming abilities Performance can be improved if structure is provided
Language of generalized intellectual impairment	Diffuse, bilateral cerebral hemisphere damage (e.g., dementia)	Disorientation Memory deficits Impaired judgment Impaired affect Perseveration Anomia Circumlocution Jargon	Language impairment is roughly proportional to impairment in other cognitive functions Evidences a lack of information rather than irrelevance
Aphasia	Commonly left unilateral cerebral hemisphere damage	Impaired ability to understand and/or express language (i.e., listening, reading, speaking, writing)	Language impairment is disproportionate to impairment of other intellectual functions No gross disorientation

7. Describe the typical communication deficits seen in patients with right cerebral hemisphere damage.

These patients demonstrate relatively **intact language** but **impaired communication abilities**. Key features are insensitivity to context (i.e., missing nuances and subtleties), difficulty organizing information in a meaningful way (e.g., answering questions with tangential, unnecessary information), difficulty "reading" facial expressions and gestures, inability to understand figurative language, lack of affect, caustic sense of humor, impulsivity, left neglect, denial of deficits, better performance on structured than open-ended tasks, and writing errors (e.g., omission of strokes, letters, or words; perseveration of strokes, letters, and words; failure to dot *i*'s and cross *t*'s; extra capitalization). Some have noted that these kinds of communication deficits have been demonstrated by individuals without documented right strokes (overworked residents)!

8. Define apraxia.

Apraxia is a **disorder of the execution of learned movement** that cannot be explained by weakness, incoordination, sensory loss, or lack of attention to commands. **Cortical lesions** are considered the neuroanatomic basis for apraxia in general. Two anatomic explanations for apraxias have been advanced. In the **disconnection theory**, apraxia results because motor areas are isolated from cortical areas subserving language comprehension and visual abilities.

For example, the motor ability to whistle may be intact and an individual may whistle spontaneously, but when asked to whistle, the individual cannot perform this action on command. In the second theory, apraxia is thought to result from lesions occurring in cortical centers, which store **movement patterns**. This theory does not explain why these movements can be performed adequately at times.

Apraxias include those of **construction, dressing, gait**, and **speech**. Apraxia of speech is characterized by highly variable and unpredictable substitutions of sounds (often unrelated to intended sounds), blockages and repetitions similar to stuttering, and slow effortful output secondary to reduced capacity to program the positioning of speech muscles and the sequencing of muscle movements for the volitional production of sounds. There is no significant weakness, slowness, or incoordination of speech muscles in reflexive or automatic acts.

9. What is agnosia?

Agnosia is a **disorder of recognition** that may occur in any of the major sense modalities despite adequate perception in these modalities (e.g., audition, vision, tactile sensation). An **auditory agnosia** is an inability to match an environmental noise with its sound source. For example, a patient may not be able to recognize a watch from its ticking but can identify a watch placed in his hand. A **visual agnosia** is an inability to identify an object on visual confrontation. For example, a patient may not be able to identify his wife when shown a picture but can describe her appearance (e.g., blonde hair, blue eyes).

10. How are the dysarthrias classified?

Dysarthria is a **speech impairment**, not a language impairment like aphasia. Individuals with dysarthria are often difficult to understand and may have "slurred speech." They do not have problems with listening, reading, writing, or spoken language (e.g, vocabulary, grammar).

As with the aphasias, the dysarthrias can be classified in a variety of ways—by age at onset, etiology, cranial nerve involvement, or speech component involvement. A well-known classification system is the Mayo Clinic approach, which reflects neuroanatomic and neurophysiologic bases for dysarthrias. Six types of dysarthrias are described based on perceptual features:

Flaccid (in bulbar palsy)
Spastic (in pseudobulbar palsy)
Ataxic (in cerebellar disorders)
Hypokinetic (in parkinsonism)
Hyperkinetic (in dystonia and chorea)
Mixed (in disorders of multiple motor systems, such as multiple sclerosis)

11. Explain some of the terminology associated with aphasia.

Neologism: substitutions of entirely invented words for correct ones (e.g., *poofle* for *doctor*)

Semantic paraphasia: word substitutions belonging to the same semantic class (e.g., *chair* for *table*)

Phonemic paraphasias: substitutions of one sound for another (e.g., *fable* for *table*)

Telegraphic speech: speech output includes substantive words (e.g., nouns, verbs) and omits grammatical modifiers (e.g., articles, conjunctions, pronouns; "girl eat cake")

Agrammatism: sparse, hesitant groping speech limited to the most essential content words

Logorrhea: "press of speech;" fluent speech with unnecessary words and neologisms; speech is more abundant than normal speech

Echolalia: meaningless repetition of other's utterances, meaningless repetition of other's utterances

Palilalia: pathologic repetition of syllables or sounds; associated with degenerative brain diseases

Affluent aphasia: aphasic syndrome occurring in the wealthy

12. Name some common evaluation tools used to assess language disorders in adults.

Tests of Language Disorders in Adults

TESTS	PURPOSES	AREAS ASSESSED
Boston Diagnostic Aphasia Examination	Generate test scores for diagnosis of classic anatomically based aphasias	Conversational and expository speech Auditory comprehension Oral expression Understanding written language Writing Supplementary language and nonlanguage tests
Western Aphasia Battery	Classify various aphasic syndromes and evaluate severity of impairment	Spontaneous speech Comprehension Repetition Naming Reading Writing Praxis Construction
Brief Test of Head Injury	Quickly identify and measure cognitive and language abilities typically impaired in individuals with TBI	Orientation/attention Following commands Linguistic organization Reading comprehension Naming Memory Visual-spatial skills
Ross Information Processing Assessment	Quantify and qualify cognitive/linguistic deficits commonly associated with TBI	Memory Temporal and spatial orientation Organization Knowledge of general information Problem solving and abstract reasoning Auditory processing
Dementia Rating Scale	Briefly and easily measure lower level cognitive abilities in individuals with cortical impairment, particularly of the degenerative type	Attention Conceptualization Initiation/perseveration Construction

13. How is speech production assessed?

Speech production can be assessed by examining nonspeech and speech aspects of each component of oral motor function in a systematic fashion. The functional component approach by Netsell and Daniel includes the respiratory mechanism, larynx, velum/pharynx, tongue, lips/face/teeth, and jaw. Examples of nonspeech and speech tasks to assess each component are:

Nonspeech and Speech Tests of Oral Motor Function

COMPONENTS	NONSPEECH TASKS	SPEECH TASKS
Respiratory mechanism	Breathing rate at rest	Maximum sustained phonation
Larynx	Elevation with swallow	Ability to change pitch
Velum/pharynx	Velar position at rest	Maintenance of oral/nasal contrasts
Tongue	Lingual range of movement	Lingual articulation
Lips/face/teeth	Facial symmetry	Labial articulation
Jaw	Mandibular strength against resistance	Mandibular assist for articulation

Speech production can also be assessed by using tests such as the Frenchay Dysarthria Assessment. Finally, speech intelligibility is rated at single word and connected speech levels. Physicians can assess speech production briefly by asking patients to repeat words and phrases, rapidly produce words such as *Topeka* or *buttercup* to test speech diadochokinesis and by rating the intelligibility of conversational speech.

14. What are VAT, VIC, MIT and PACE therapy?

These represent treatments designed to address specific problems.

VAT—Using **Visual Action Therapy**, global aphasic patients learn to associate objects and their functions with action pictures and drawings of objects and later to produce gestures to indicate objects.

VIC—Using **Visual Communication Therapy**, global aphasic patients learn to use a system of arbitrary symbols to respond to commands, answer yes/no questions, and express needs and feelings.

MIT—**Melodic Intonation Therapy**, used with Broca's aphasics, capitalizes on preserved melodic production in the right hemisphere to facilitate speech production. Patients are taught to intone phrases, initially in unison with the speech-language pathologist and later independently.

PACE—**Promoting Aphasics' Communicative Competence** emphasizes a functional rather than a question/answer approach. The patient and clinician convey information in conversation using whatever means is necessary—speech, gesture, drawing, writing, mime.

15. What are some communication alternatives to natural speech?

Alternatives can be divided into oral and nonoral options. A familiar **oral option** is the use of an electrolarynx by a laryngectomy. Electrolarynges are also useful short-term communication options for individuals who have tracheostomy tubes with inflated cuffs. **Nonoral options** include handwriting, gesture, and augmentative communication systems, which range from simple alphabet and picture boards to sophisticated computer systems. Amer-Ind is a gestural communication system based on American Indian hand signals, which can be used with stroke patients. Augmentative communication systems can facilitate communication between caregivers, family members, and intubated or tracheostomized patients in intensive care settings.

16. Describe the three stages of swallowing.

It is customary to divide the process of swallowing into three stages, although these divisions are arbitrary.

1. The **oral stage** includes manipulation of food in the mouth, creation of a "bolus," and propulsion of the bolus into the pharynx by the tongue.

2. The **pharyngeal stage** includes initiation of the swallow response, velopharyngeal apposition, elevation and anterior movement of the larynx, epiglottic tilt, closure of the larynx, pharyngeal constriction, and opening of the cricopharyngeus.

3. In the **esophageal stage**, boluses are moved through the esophagus into the stomach by peristalsis.

17. Does the presence of a gag reflex indicate that swallowing function is preserved?

No. There is a widespread misperception that the presence or absence of the gag reflex can predict swallowing function. The gag reflex is commonly tested as an indicator of swallowing function, and individuals without gag reflexes are often referred for swallowing evaluations. However, the gag reflex is a protective reflex to keep foreign material from entering the foodway and airway. It is *not* related to swallowing function. Leder showed that the gag reflex can be absent in individuals who swallow normally and intact in individuals with dysphagia. Presence or absence of the gag reflex is difficult to assess because the response can be diminished with repeated attempts at elicitation.

18. How useful is the bedside swallowing study?

The bedside swallowing study provides useful information about speech/oral motor status, oral stage of swallow, level of alertness, appropriate position for feeding, and ability to self-feed.

There are limitations, however, particularly regarding pharyngeal events. Logemann et al. showed that experienced dysphagia clinicians missed aspiration 40% of the time at the bedside in individuals who were subsequently shown to aspirate on videofluoroscopy. This is because aspiration can be "silent"—i.e., without any outward indication such as coughing or throat clearing. The bedside evaluation is not adequate for determining the physiological basis for dysphagia or for planning treatment, and the videofluoroscopic swallowing study remains the "gold standard" for evaluation of swallowing. More recently, Logemann et al. studied the sensitivity and specificity of a 28-item screening test. They identified variables that could classify whether or not patients aspirated 71% of the time, have an oral stage dysphagia 69% of the time, pharyngeal delay 72% of the time, or a pharyngeal stage swallowing problem 70% of the time.

19. What are instrumental swallowing evaluations?

A **videofluoroscopic swallowing study** is a radiographic evaluation conducted by a speech-language pathologist and radiologist. Patients are given liquid and solid foods impregnated with barium. Various maneuvers may be tried to facilitate safe, effective swallowing. Logemann developed the "modified barium swallow study" in which specific food types and amounts are used.

A **fiberoptic endoscopic evaluation of swallowing** (FEES) involves passing an endoscope transnasally into the hypopharynx so that the foodway and airway can be observed before and after (but not during) the moment of swallowing. The image is blocked or "whited out" at the moment of swallow by the pharynx closing around the endoscopic tube. Solids and liquids are dyed green to improve visualization. FEES was first described by Langmore et al. and can be performed at the bedside by a speech-language pathologist. A modification of the FEES is the FEESST, which includes laryngopharyngeal sensory testing.

Less commonly used instrumental assessments are electromyography, manometry, scintigraphy, and ultrasound.

20. How much aspiration is too much?

The relationship between dysphagia, aspiration, and aspiration pneumonia is complex. Langmore et al. showed that the presence of dysphagia and aspiration are necessary but not sufficient conditions for the development of aspiration pneumonia. Important risk factors are dependency for oral feeding, dependency for oral care, number of decayed teeth, tube feeding, more than one medical diagnosis, number of medications, and smoking. Aspiration of refluxed gastric contents is particularly injurious to the lung, as pH ≤ 2.4 destroys lung tissue.

21. What are some common compensations and exercises for dysphagia?

Recommendations for swallowing compensations and exercises are made by speech-language pathologists based on the results of bedside and instrumental swallowing evaluations.

Swallowing Compensations	Purposes
Neck flexion	Increase airway protection by putting the epiglottis in a more overhanging position.
Head/neck rotation	Decrease retention of boluses by turning head/neck to the weaker side, closing off that side and directing boluses to the stronger side.
Mendelsohn maneuver	Sustain laryngeal elevation during swallow to increase airway protection.
Supraglottic swallow	Adduct vocal folds to achieve improved airway protection.
Masako maneuver	Protrude tongue through central incisors to increase pharyngeal constriction.

Swallowing Exercises	Purposes
Shaker exercises	Head raising exercises to augment opening at the cricopharyngeus.
Lingual range of movement and strength against resistance exercises	Improve oral manipulation and control of boluses.
Yawning exercises	Increase movement of the back wall of the throat.
Falsetto exercises	Increase laryngeal elevation.
Thermal/tactile stimulation	Improve initiation and timing of swallow response

22. How does a unidirectional speaking valve facilitate safe swallowing in a patient with a tracheostomy?

A unidirectional speaking valve allows inhalation to occur at the level of the tracheostomy and exhalation through the larynx, mouth, and nose. Valve candidates must have generally intact laryngeal structure and function (valves cannot be used with individuals who have had laryngectomy). This unidirectional flow of air can sweep penetrated material out of the airway. Valves also restore cough and throat clear which can facilitate airway clearance. Commercially available valves are the Passy-Muir, Montgomery, and Shikani-French.

BIBLIOGRAPHY

1. Duffy JR: Motor Speech Disorders: Substrates, Differential Diagnosis, and Management. Baltimore, Mosby, 1995.
2. Fujiu M, Logemann JA: Effect of a tongue-holding maneuver on posterior pharyngeal wall movement during deglutition. Am J Speech-Lang Path 5:23–30, 1996.
3. Goodglass H, Kaplan E: Assessment of Aphasia and Related Disorders. Philadelphia, Lea & Febiger, 1972.
4. Langmore SE, Terpenning MS, Schork A, et al: Predictors of aspiration pneumonia: How important is dysphagia? Dysphagia 13:69–81, 1998.
5. Langmore SE, Schatz K, Olsen N: Fiberoptic endoscopic examination of swallowing safety: A new procedure. Dysphagia 2:216–219, 1988.
6. Leder SB: Videofluoroscopic evaluation of aspiration with visual examination of the gag reflex and velar movement. Dysphagia 12:21–23, 1997.
7. Logemann JA: Evaluation and Treatment of Swallowing Disorders. Austin, TX, PRO-ED, Inc., 1998.
8. Logemann JA, Lazarus C, Jenkins P: The relationship between clinical judgment and radiographic assessment of aspiration. Presented at the American Speech-Language-Hearing Association Annual Meeting, Toronto, November 1982.
9. Logemann JA, Veis S, Colangelo L: A screening procedure for oropharyngeal dysphagia. Dysphagia 14:44–51, 1999.
10. Netsell R, Daniel B: Dysarthria in adults: Physiologic approach to rehabilitation. Arch Phys Med Rehabil 60:502–508, 1979.
11. Rao PR: The aphasia syndromes: Localization and classification. Top Stroke Rehabil 1(2):1–13, 1994.
12. Rao PR: Adult communication disorders. In Braddon P (ed): Physical Medicine and Rehabilitation. Philadelphia, W.B. Saunders, 2000.
13. Shaker R, Kern M, Bardan E, et al: Augmentation of deglutitive upper esophageal sphincter opening in the elderly by exercise. Am J Physiol 272(6 Pt 1):G1518–1522, 1997.
14. Tippett DC: Tracheostomy and Ventilator Dependency: Management of Breathing, Speaking and Swallowing. New York, Thieme, 2000.
15. Tippett DC, Sugarman J: Discussing advance directives under the Patient Self-Determination Act: A unique opportunity for speech-language pathologists to help persons with aphasia. Am J Speech-Lang Pathol 5(2):31–34, 1996.
16. Wertz RT: Neuropathologies of speech and language: An introduction to patient management. In Johns DF (ed): Clinical Management of Neurogenic Communicative Disorders. Boston, Little, Brown, 1985.

XIII. General Therapeutics

79. THERAPEUTIC EXERCISE

Ralph M. Buschbacher, M.D., and Mark Randall, Psy.D., Dr.P.H., M.A.

1. What are the three types of muscle fibers?

Type I—slow twitch oxidative
Type IIa—fast twitch oxidative
Type IIb—fast twitch glycolytic

Muscle Fiber Types

Slow twitch fibers: Type I
  a. Low activity level of myosin ATPase
  b. Slow speed of contraction
  c. Less developed glycolytic capacity than fast twitch fibers
  d. Contain numerous mitochondria and mitochondrial enzymes to sustain aerobic metabolism
  e. Fatigue-resistant and suited for prolonged aerobic exercise
  f. Labeled SO (slow oxidative)
• Type I fibers are used for activities that require endurance, in postural muscles, and in low-intensity activity. These types of fibers generate energy primarily through the use of oxidation, which provides great endurance

Fast twitch fibers: Type II
  a. High capability for electrochemical transmission of action potentials
  b. High activity of myosin ATPase
  c. Rapid level calcium release and uptake by sarcoplasmic reticulum
  d. High rate of cross-bridge turnover
• All of this relates to the ability to transfer energy rapidly for quick force contractions.
  Type IIa: Considered intermediate because fast contraction speed is combined with a fairly well-developed capacity for both aerobic and anaerobic energy transfer. Are referred to as FOG (fast oxidative glycolytic) fibers.
  Type IIb: Greatest anaerobic potential; true fast glycolytic fibers

2. What determines the fiber type of a given muscle cell?

The fiber type is determined by the nerve fiber that innervates it. All fibers innervated by a given motor neuron have the same physiologic and histochemical properties. The type of motor neuron and pattern of nerve impulses transmitted play the main role in determining the mechanical and histochemical properties of the muscle fibers. After denervation, if nerve regrowth and sprouting occur, the muscle fiber will take on the characteristics determined by the new nerve fiber.

3. What is the Henneman size principle?

Motor units are recruited in order of increasing size, increasing contraction strength, and diminishing fatigue resistance. Therefore the smaller, less powerful, fatigue-resistant fibers are almost always recruited before the larger, more powerful, fatigable fibers regardless of speed of contraction. This makes sense, as these fibers are weaker. When first moving a muscle not much strength is needed, and activating the weaker fibers (motor units) gives more fine motor control. When more strength is needed, larger and larger fibers are recruited to give larger gross muscle strength.

4. What are the determinants of muscle strength?

Muscle size: Per unit of muscle tissue, muscle strength is determined by the cross-sectional area of the fibers. This generates a force of $3.6 \, kg/cm^2$.

Muscle shape: Differently shaped muscles have different functional cross-sectional areas. (see Question 5).

Insertion site: Insertion sites farther from the axis of rotation give greater strength but over a smaller arc, while insertion closer to the axis of rotation gives a greater range of motion (ROM) with less strength.

Torque curve: Muscles may have different torque curves. This means that muscles are not equally strong throughout their entire ROM or range of contraction. This depends, again, on the shape, size, and insertion sites of the muscles as well as the specific biomechanics of the body part in question. Exercise equipment is sometimes designed to match the torque curve of the specific muscle groups (see below).

Neural factors: Neural factors include synchronization of muscle firing, how quickly the fibers are recruited, and how many fibers can be recruited simultaneously.

5. Describe the different types of muscle shapes.

There are two main types of muscle shapes, parallel and pennate. There also exist various combinations and variants of these.

Parallel muscle fibers travel the entire length of the muscle. A muscle fiber ordinarily contracts by about 50% of its resting length (length if removed from the body). Thus, parallel muscle fibers can generate a large amount of shortening (but have lesser strength).

Pennate muscles have fibers that insert onto the muscle tendon at an angle, which allows a greater number of muscle fibers. While the total size of the muscle may be the same as in a parallel arrangement, the total effective cross-sectional area is greater and thus provides greater strength. Since the muscle fibers shorten by about 50% of its resting length and the fibers attach at an angle onto the tendon, the total movement is less than in parallel muscle fibers.

6. What did Moritani and deVries show in regard to the relationship between strength and hypertrophy?

Moritani and deVries showed that in the first few weeks of a training program, there is an increase in strength not related to hypertrophy. An increase in integrated EMG activity during this time period implies that there are neural factors leading to increased strength. This may be due to increased synchronization and coordination of muscle firing. Only later does hypertrophy take effect. They also showed that neural training effects are transferred to some extent to the opposite (untrained) limb. Moritani and deVries also found that elderly subjects had a strength increase with weight training primarily due to neural learning, not hypertrophy.

7. Describe the different types of muscle contraction.

Isometric: Isometric means "equal distance." This refers to a contraction that does not result in movement about a joint. In a living person, however, there are no true isometric contractions, since there is some internal shortening within the muscle and connective tissues. Examples of isometric exercise include pushing on a wall, holding a briefcase, or lifting a very heavy weight. Heavy weight lifting is considered "isometric-like."

Isotonic: Isotonic refers to an equivalent force being exerted or weight being lifted throughout the entire ROM of contraction of the muscle. Traditionally, this has referred to lifting free weights. However, when lifting free weights, the force is not constant. When the arm is by the side (for instance, in lifting a weight through elbow flexion), the first few degrees of ROM do not result in much vertical lift and do not require much force. When the arm is at about 90°, the torque required is greatest and then it drops again as the elbow is flexed further. Thus, the person can only lift a weight equivalent to that which can be lifted at the weakest part of this ROM. Exercise equipment has been developed that attempts to match the force exerted by the muscles so that the resistance approximates the **torque curve** of the muscle. This is commonly known as

cam varied resistance and was popularized by the Nautilus Company. In these exercises, a "cam" (a pulley that is spiral-shaped or shaped like the nautilus seashell) varies the effective resistance of the weight. The goal is that the muscle can be trained maximally at all parts of its ROM.

Isokinetic: Isokinetic means "equal speed." No matter how hard the subject pushes against the machine, the speed of movement remains constant. This allows the person exercising to exert maximal force at all parts of the ROM. However, this is not a natural type of motion and requires great motivation. Speeds generated by isokinetic machines may not match physiologic speeds seen in functional daily and athletic activities. Isokinetic equipment was developed so that maximum muscle tension can be applied throughout the whole ROM.

8. What are the different types of muscle movement?

Concentric: This is a shortening contraction—basically, what we would see when picking up a weight.

Eccentric: This is a lengthening contraction—i.e., what we would see when lowering a weight. Eccentric contractions have potential for developing greater muscle tension. This makes sense, since you can lower a heavier weight than you can lift. With greater tension, there is a higher potential of causing injury. Lengthening contractions are probably responsible for delayed-onset muscle soreness and are probably better at generating muscle hypertrophy than concentric contractions. Eccentric contractions occur commonly in daily life, although they are somewhat counterintuitive when planning a resistance exercise-training program. For instance, when walking, a good bit of the energy expenditure and work occurs during slowing down of the limb and controlling the "heelstrike" to "footflat" part of the gait cycle.

9. What is plyometric exercise?

Plyometric exercises are functional types of exercise, which apply the principle of a brief stretch followed by contraction. A brief stretch (such as during a muscle stretch reflex) will elicit a contraction, and by briefly preloading (stretching) the muscle, this is felt to facilitate the subsequent contraction. Exercises utilizing this principle include jumping up and down or jumping over boxes. Pylometric exercise is useful because many sports involve plyometric-type maneuvers. However, it is also more likely to cause injury.

10. What is endurance exercise? Endurance fitness?

Endurance exercise is the prolonged reciprocal use of large muscle groups. It is differentiated from **muscle endurance**, which refers to the length of time that a muscle can contract at a given tension.

The terms **stamina**, **endurance fitness**, **cardiovascular fitness**, and **aerobic fitness** refer to the body's ability to generate ATP aerobically. Aerobic energy, or the long-term energy system, is primarily measured by an individual's $\dot{V}o_2$max. $\dot{V}o_2$max is considered the fundamental measurement in exercise physiology, but it is not the only determinant of aerobic/endurance exercise capacity. Other factors, such as the number of capillaries, enzymes, and fiber type, exert a strong influence on one's capacity to sustain a high level of aerobic/endurance exercise.

11. What are the different types of flexibility exercises?

Static stretching: Static stretches involve stretching the muscle and staying in that position for some time period. Generally, at least 15–20 sec is required to provide any benefit. Static stretching is relatively safe.

Ballistic stretching: Ballistic stretching involves bouncing-type maneuvers. This exercise was popular several decades ago, but it is now out of favor because the muscle stretch reflex is activated in a manner similar to plyometric exercise and will actually hinder the stretching.

Proprioceptive neuromuscular facilitation: For this type of stretching, the muscle is stretched to its fullest extent, and then the person contracts that muscle against the direction of the stretch. While joint position does not change, this is felt to cause internal shortening of the connective tissues of the muscle, and after a few seconds of contraction, the muscle is relaxed and again stretched a bit more. This is generally done three times in any given position and can sometimes be done with a partner.

Passive stretching: Also known as relaxed stretching or static-passive stretching, in this form of stretching exercise the person stretching assumes a position and holds it with another part of the body or with assistance from a partner or some apparatus such as a machine. Ways to accomplish a passive stretch might be to use body weight or free weights to stretch certain muscles. For example, when standing with the ball of the foot on a step and the heels hanging down, body weight will stretch the gastrocsoleus complex.

Dynamic stretching: Dynamic stretching is different from ballistic stretching in that ballistic stretching forces a limb or part of the body beyond its usual ROM. Dynamic stretching involves moving parts of the body in a controlled manner (e.g., dance or martial arts) and gradually increasing the reach and speed of movement.

12. What is the Delorme technique? The Delorme axiom?

Delorme developed a technique that he called **progressive resistance exercise** to strengthen muscles. In progressive resistance exercise, the subject is tested to determine the maximum weight that he/she can lift 10 times using good form and technique—this is called the "10 repetition max," or 10 RM. Delorme would have the person lift at various percentages of the 10 RM starting at 10%, 20%, 30%, etc., up to 100% (later he modified this to 50%, 75%, and 100% of 10 RM). Subjects exercise daily and then retest to determine a new 10 RM each week. The progressive part refers to the progression from week to week, not from 50%, to 75%, to 100%.

The **Delorme axiom** states that high-intensity, low-repetition exercise builds strength, and low-intensity, high-repetition exercise builds endurance, and that each of these two types of exercise is incapable of producing the results obtained by the other type. This is an oversimplification, and deLateur has shown that as long as exercise is carried out to fatigue, there is transfer from high-intensity to low-intensity exercise and vice versa.

13. What is the Oxford technique?

The Oxford technique basically turned the Delorme method on its head by doing the exercises at 100% 10 RM, then 75% 10 RM, then 50% 10 RM. This was felt to keep the muscle more fatigued. The Oxford technique was developed by Zinovieff.

14. What is the Hellebrand technique?

Hellebrand used a similar principle as deLateur, but used a metronome. When a given target speed for lifting repetitions is reached, the weight is increased to lower the speed. It is difficult to remain motivated doing this protocol, and listening to the metronome can be annoying.

15. How do the effects of free weights, pulleys, and cam varied resistance differ during ROM?

Free weights are simple. Any type of weight that is lifted can be used as an approximation of isotonic exercise. The actual muscle tension is not equal throughout the ROM, which is a limitation of using free weights. Body builders use various body positions to get around this limitation.

Pulleys even out the tension throughout the entire ROM of the muscle. The pulley creates the same amount of resistance throughout the entire ROM. Nevertheless, this still does not match the natural torque curve of the muscle since the muscle is not equally strong in all parts of its ROM. Therefore, the muscle is really only stressed maximally at the weakest point of its ROM.

Cam varied resistance varies the torque throughout the ROM of the muscle and therefore strengthens the muscle at all parts of its ROM.

16. What is the overload principle?

To increase a muscle's performance, it must be taxed *beyond* its ordinary activities. This can be accomplished by manipulating frequency, intensity, duration, and mode of training.

17. Define $\dot{V}o_2$ and $\dot{V}o_2$ max?

The V in $\dot{V}o_2$ refers to the **rate**, and the O_2 refers to the **oxygen** being consumed. Put together, this is the **rate of oxygen consumption**. $\dot{V}o_2$max is the **maximum rate of oxygen consumption** and is a measure of the maximum intensity of exercise that can be sustained. $\dot{V}o_2$max is limited by the oxygen-carrying and utilization capacity of the body. Exceeding the $\dot{V}o_2$max for brief periods of time can be accomplished by reverting to glycolytic energy production; however, this creates a build-up of lactic acid and cannot be sustained.

18. Can a muscle's fiber type be changed by exercise?

Muscle fiber change is a controversial topic, and we may not have the definitive answers yet. However, Gollnick showed that the cross-sectional area of type I muscle fibers could be increased with aerobic training. The cross-sectional area of the type II fibers was not increased and so the relative proportion of type I and II was changed. Similarly, strength training results in hypertrophy of both type I and type II muscles; however, the type II fibers respond to a greater extent than the type I fibers, and so, again, this can cause a change in the cross-sectional proportions of the two muscle fiber types. There is felt to be minimal, if any, hyperplasia of either type I or type II fibers in human beings. Hyperplasia involves splitting fibers or growth of new muscle fibers. Rather than this occurring, what we see is an increase in the size of the existing fibers, not a growth of new fibers.

19. What are the "five P's" of exercise?

Kottke described "five P's" of exercise:

Perception (feedback)

Precision

Perpetual practice

Peak performance (do the activity as well as you can do it correctly),

Progression (break down the activity into subcomponents and later integrate them into a whole)

Practice doesn't make perfect. Perfect practice makes perfect.

20. What is the importance of warming up the muscles?

Warming up is generally accepted as a valid procedure prior to vigorous exercise. It is felt that the performer is better prepared both physiologically and psychologically for an activity and that the warm-up may reduce the chance of injury. Animal studies have shown that greater forces and increases in muscle length were required to injure a "warm" muscle than a "cold" muscle. It is suggested that warming up stretches the muscle tendon unit and allows for greater length and less tension at any given load on the unit.

Warm-up is classified two different ways:

- **General warm-up**—includes calisthenics, stretching, and general body movements usually unrelated to the specific neuromuscular action of the anticipated performance.
- **Specific warm-up**—specific rehearsal for the activity (i.e., swinging a golf club, throwing a baseball).

Specific ways in which warm-up may enhance performance include (a) increased speed of contraction and relaxation of muscles; (b) greater movement secondary to decreased viscous resistance within the muscles; (c) increased oxygen utilization because hemoglobin releases oxygen more readily at high temperatures; (d) may facilitate motor unit recruitment of motor units required for all-out effort; and (e) increased blood flow and temperature. There is no definitive evidence that warm-up actually improves performance. The possible physiological and strong psychological benefits are recommended until warm-up is proven to be harmful or not useful.

21. How do open and closed kinetic chain exercises differ?

This is best described in an example. Extending the leg with a free weight attached to the ankle is **open kinetic chain exercise**. The foot is not fixed. Squatting when the feet are anchored is a **closed kinetic chain exercise**. In general, it is felt that closed kinetic chain exercise causes less shear stress, especially on the knee.

22. What is the difference between upper-extremity and lower-extremity exercise?

Blood pressure (both systolic and diastolic) is considerably higher for a given level of upper-body exercise versus lower-body exercise. This is most likely due to the smaller muscle mass and vasculature of the upper extremities, which offers greater resistance to blood flow than the larger muscle mass and vasculature of the lower body/legs.

The highest oxygen uptake achieved by both men and women during arm exercise is generally about 70–80% of the Vo_2max during leg exercise. Maximum values for heart rate and pulmonary ventilation are lower with arm exercise. This inability to achieve similar maximum values when comparing upper- versus lower-body exercise is due to the smaller muscle mass of the arms as compared to the legs. The reverse pattern is seen during submaximal exercise. For a given level of exercise, the oxygen uptake is higher when exercising the arms as compared to the legs. This is an important distinction to be made in the context of exercise development and implementation.

23. What is Wolfe's law?

Wolfe's law is a statement that bone responds to exercise by increasing in mass (it also resorbs with a lack of exercise). It is generally felt that weight-bearing exercise is the most important exercise to maintain bone mass, although other effects of stress on bone have also been shown. For instance, tennis players have an increase in bone mass in the arm. In general, swimming is not considered to be particularly beneficial in maintaining bone mass.

24. How does aging affect muscle strength?

The effect of age on muscle strength is well documented: strength declines with age. This understanding is well supported but not clearly understood. Contributing factors can be the aging process, nutritional inadequacies, effects of disease, and a sedentary lifestyle. If strength decline is primarily due to the disuse of the muscles, then strength training would seem reasonable.

Fiatarone et al. conducted a study with ten subjects, average age 90.2 years, who participated in an 8-week resistance-training program. Both concentric and eccentric motions were used to train hamstring and quadricep muscles. Training was conducted 3 days a week and consisted of three sets of eight repetitions with 1–2-minute rest intervals. During the first week, the resistance equaled 50% of 1 RM; by the second week, the load was increased to 80% 1 RM. Strength gains were significant, averaging 174%. Strength increases were consistent throughout the 8 weeks and did not level off as training progressed.

Another finding of the study demonstrated that functional mobility, including walking speed and the ability to arise from a chair, also improved: two subjects stopped using a cane to walk. Following this resistance-training program, the subjects returned to their sedentary lifestyle. After only 4 weeks of the "detraining," a 32% loss of strength was noted. The study suggests that conventional resistance training is possible for older adults and could reverse the effects of aging on muscular strength.

25. How does sex affect muscle strength and the response to exercise? Ah, I mean gender.

Because they have lower levels of testosterone, women experience less hypertrophy of the muscles and have less of an increase in Vo_2max with exercise. In addition, since women on average have a greater amount of body fat (and therefore less lean muscle mass as a percentage of total body mass), they are less efficient in endurance exercise.

26. How does the cardiovascular system adapt to aerobic endurance-type exercise?

1. A decrease in resting heart rate, but no change in the maximum heart rate.
2. An increase in Vo_2 max and a decrease in Vo_2 for a given submaximal workload.
3. Increase in cardiac output and stroke volume and a decrease in heart rate response to submaximal exercise.

4. Decrease in systolic and diastolic blood pressure by 6 to 10 mmHg. In general, it is felt that isometric-like exercise (heavy weightl ifting) is contraindicated in hypertensive patients, as such exercise will elevate blood pressure. Moderate weight lifting exercise is felt to be safe.

5. Anginal threshold is unchanged, but there is less myocardial stress for a given workload, which can help to keep the subject working below the anginal threshold.

27. How does regular aerobic exercise affect diabetes?

For **non-insulin-dependent** diabetics, there is an increase in end-organ cell receptor sensitivity to insulin. Exercise will also decrease obesity, which will help in blood sugar control. Be careful to watch for the Somoygi effect when exercising, especially if exercise is performed late during the day. In addition, medication doses may need to be adjusted. Since diabetics may have silent cardiac ischemia, they should be monitored for this.

In **insulin-dependent** diabetics, exercise doesn't change the nature of their disease, but certainly will change their insulin requirements.

BIBLIOGRAPHY

1. Abernethy PJ, Jurimae J, Logan PA, et al: Acute and chronic response of skeletal muscle to resistance training. Sports Med 17:22–38, 1994.
2. Allerheiligen WB: Speed development and plyometric training. In Baechle TRM (ed): Essentials of Strength Training and Conditioning. Champaign, IL, Human Kinetics, 1994.
3. Alter MJ: Science of Stretching. Champaign, IL, Human Kinetics, 1988.
4. Anderson R, Anderson J: Stretching: 20th Anniversary. Shelter Publications, 2000.
5. Astrand PO, Rodahl K: Textbook of Work Physiology. New York, McGraw Hill, 1986.
6. Bacou F, Rouanet P, Barjot CP, et al: Expression of myosin isoforms in denervated, cross-reinnervated and electrically stimulated rabbit muscles. Eur J Biochem 236:539–547, 1996.
7. Crossman ERFW: A theory of the acquisition of speed-skill. Ergonomics 2:153–166, 1959.
8. deLateur BJ, Lehmann JF, Fordyce WE: A test of the DeLorme axiom. Arch Phys Med Rehabil 49: 245–248, 1968.
9. deLateur BJ, Lehmann JF: Therapeutic exercise to develop strength and endurance. In Kottke FJ, Lehmann JF (eds): Krusen's Handbook of Physical Medicine and Rehabilitation, 4th ed. Philadelphia, WB Saunders, 1990, p 512.
10. Dolkas CP, Rodnick KJ, Mondon CE: Effect of body weight gain on insulin sensitivity after retirement from exercise training. J Appl Physiol 68:520–526, 1990.
11. Edstrom L, Grimby L: Effect of exercise on the motor unit. Muscle Nerve 9:104–126, 1986.
12. Esselman PC, deLateur BJ, Alquist AD, et al: Torque development in isokinetic training. Arch Phys Med Rehabil 72:723–728, 1991 [erratum, p 970].
13. Fiatarone MA, Marks EC, Ryan ND, et al: High-intensity strength training in nonagenerians. Effects of skeletal muscle. JAMA 263:3029–3034, 1990.
14. Frontera WR, Hugh VA, Fielding RA, et al: Aging of skeletal muscle: 12 year longitudinal study. J Appl Physiol 88:1321–1326, 2000.
15. Frontera WR, Meredith CN, O'Reilly KP, et al: Strength conditioning in older men: Skeletal muscle hypertrophy and improved function. J Appl Physiol 64:1038–1044, 1988.
16. Galbo H: Hormonal and Metabolic Adaptation to Exercise. New York, G.T. Verlag, 1983.
17. Gollnick PD, Armstrong RB, Saltin B, et al: Effect of training on enzyme activity and fiber composition of human skeletal muscle. J Appl Physiol 34:107–111, 1973.
18. Kriska AM, Blair SN, Pereira MA: The potential role of physical activity in the prevention of non-insulin-dependent diabetes mellitus: the epidemiological evidence. Exerc Sport Sci Rev 22:121–143, 1994.
19. McArdle W, Katch F, Katch V: Essentials of Exercise Physiology. Baltimore, Williams & Willkins, 1994.
20. Moritani T, deVries HA: Neural factors versus hypertrophy in the time course of muscle strength gain. Am J Phys Med 58:115–130, 1979.
21. Moritani T, deVries HA: Potential for gross muscle hypertrophy in older men. J Gerontol 35:672–682, 1980.
22. Safran MR, Garrett WE Jr, Seaber AV, et al: The role of warm-up muscular injury prevention. Am J Sports Med 16:123–129, 1988.
23. Tesch PA: Skeletal muscle and adaptation consequent to long term heavy resistance exercise. Med Sci Sports Exerc 20 (5 Suppl):S132–S134, 1988.
24. Zinovieff AN: Heavy resistance exercises: The "Oxford" technique. Br J Phys Med 14: 129–132, 1957.

80. NUTRITION AND DIETARY ISSUES IN REHABILITATION

Marlene M. Young, B.A., Eli D. Ehrenpreis, M.D., and Mark A. Young, M.D.

1. Do rehabilitation patients really suffer from malnutrition?

Yes. Despite the ominous connotation, "malnourishment" can occur in otherwise healthy, unsuspecting patients. The incidence of malnutrition in hospitalized medical patients in the U.S. is between 30% and 50%. Dietary and nutritional deficiencies frequently occur in very subtle and insidious ways. Since rehabilitation patients often have chronic long-standing illnesses that require prolonged hospitalizations, malnutrition is often an inevitable consequence.

2. What is meant by the term *malnutrition*?

Malnutrition occurs when there is an imbalance between bodily intake and nutrient intake. Poor or inadequate nutrition occurs for a number of basic reasons, including malassimilation, insufficient food intake, and dietary indiscretion.

3. Name some common risk factors for malnutrition in older adults.

Sudden weight gain or weight loss, inadequate diet, underlying disease, multiple medications, economic hardship, oral pain, or tooth loss.

4. How can the physiatrist perform a simple bedside nutritional assessment?

1. **Review the medical record.**
   - Previous history of dietary or nutritional deficiency or systemic diseases (intestinal disease)
   - Documented weights from previous clinical visits
2. **Get a thorough nutritional history.**
   - Note changes in body weight, food diaries, GI symptoms, ability to obtain food, general mental status, and swallowing ability.
3. **Perform a focused clinical evaluation**.
   - Anthropometric measurements—i.e., height and weight
   - Physical examination—muscle strength, skin evaluation, neurologic exam

5. Name nine common serum markers that are diminished in malnourished patients.

1. Total protein	4. Cholesterol	7. Blood urea nitrogen
2. Albumin	5. Triglycerides	8. Total lymphocyte count
3. Pre-albumin	6. Creatinine	9. Beta-carotene

6. Name two common methods of assessing energy requirements of a rehabilitatiom patient by determining the basal metabolic rate (BMR).

1. **Harris-Benedict equation**
   Male kcal: $66 + (13.7 \times \text{weight in kg}) + (5 \times \text{height in cm}) - (6.8 \times \text{age})$
   Female kcal: $655 + (9.6 \times \text{weight in kg}) + (1.8 \times \text{height in cm}) - (4.7 \times \text{age})$
2. **Simple estimation**
   30 kcal/kg – 25%

7. What is ideal body weight (IBW) and how is it calculated?

The weight that is considered "normal" for a particular age, sex, and body frame is IBW. It is estimated from comparison tables, the most common of these being the Metropolitan Life Insurance Tables.

8. How does weight loss affect prognosis in malnourished patients?

Weight loss of > 20% is associated with significant deficits in organ function, resulting in increased morbidity and mortality. Weight of < 48% of IBW is considered to be incompatible with survival. This information is based on data from concentration camps in World War II and political prisoners voluntarily fasting in Northern Ireland.

9. How does distribution of body fat differ between men and women? What clinical implication does this have for drug bioavailability?

Distribution of excess body fat is generally higher in men (abdominal) than women (thighs and buttocks)—the old adage for this is apples (men) and pears (women). The percentage of fat in the body is greater in women than men in all age groups. This differing percentage of body fat has significant implications for drug metabolism and bioavailability and may explain why men and women show different responses to certain medication (e.g., analgesics and other pain medications).

10. What should rehabilitation professionals know about nutritional support?

Administered in two primary ways, enteral and parenteral, nutritional support is the provision of necessary nutrients (calories, protein, water, vitamins, and minerals) to patients who are unable to take in these nutrients on their own by eating.

11. What are the most frequent indications for total parenteral nutrition (TPN) in hospitalized patients unable to achieve adequate nutrition?

• Protracted nutrient losses with severe malnutrition
• Pre- and postsurgery with expected prolonged course prior to return to normal bowel function
• Preop patients who are malnourished
• Adjunctive therapy in patients with inflammatory bowel disease
• Inability to eat
• Nonfunctioning or poorly functioning GI tract
• Hypermetabolic conditions with decreased ability to take in nutrients

12. How is enteral nutrition support administered?

Oral intake of liquid supplements
Nasogastric feeding tubes
Gastrostomy or jejunostomy tubes (endoscopically or surgically placed)

13. What is the difference between a PEG and a PEJ?

The introduction of techniques for endoscopic placement of percutaneous feeding tubes has allowed administration of nutrients to a large number of patients who cannot eat but are poor surgical candidates. **Percutaneous endoscopic gastrostomy** (PEG) tubes are placed directly from the exterior of the abdominal wall into the stomach. **Percutaneous endoscopic jejunostomy** (PEJ) tubes, which may reduce the risk of aspiration, require a mature PEG tract. A thin tube is placed into a preexisting PEG. The tip of this tube is then dragged with an endoscope and deposited in the distal duodenum or proximal jejunum.

14. How does one choose the appropriate form of enteral nutritional support?

Initially, the length of time enteral support will be required is determined. Short-term nasogastric feedings or long-term PEG or PEJ feedings may be needed. Second, a formula based on the patient's capacity to absorb and digest nutrients is selected. A number of formulas are available that are specifically tailored to clinical conditions (e.g., malabsorption, diabetes, renal and hepatic diseases).

BIBLIOGRAPHY

1. Bendich A: Vitamin Intake and Health: A Scientific Review. New York, Marcel Dekker, 1999.
2. Heymsfield SB: Enteral solutions: Is there a solution? Nutr Clin Pract 10:4–7, 1995.
3. Whitney EN, Cataldo CB, Rolfes SR: Understanding Normal and Clinical Nutrition. Belmont, CA, Wadsworth Publishers, 1998.

81. PHARMACOLOGIC AGENTS IN REHABILITATION MEDICINE

Jennifer J. James, M.D., Steven A. Stiens, M.D., M.S., Karen Lew, PharmD, Stephen P. Burns, M.D., and Mark A. Young, M.D.

1. Why is a chapter on medications important to me as a physiatrist?

A wide variety of medications from different classes are used by the practicing physiatrist to enhance the rehabilitation process by decreasing impairment and improving function. Patients often present for rehab with a long list of medications, called **polypharmacy**. It is an essential component of rehabilitation for the physician to be knowledgeable about common physiatric applications, basic pharmacokinetics, side effects, drug interactions, and the mechanism of action of medications.

2. What is the "paper bag test"?

The clinician asks the patient to place all of his or her prescribed and over-the-counter medications in a paper bag and bring it to the clinic visit. Each bottle should be reviewed with the patient. The patient should be asked why he takes the particular medication, when it was last filled, and how many tablets and refills are left. The physiatrist will encounter many patients with multiple diagnoses and symptoms who receive treatment from a variety of clinicians and consultants. As a result, many prescribed medications can potentially interact and thus confound efforts to achieve therapeutic goals. Actual knowledge of which medications the patient takes, or does not take, is essential for safe and successful treatment.

3. Many medications have anticholinergic side effects. Name some of these effects.

Remember the phrase learned in medical school: "mad as a hatter, red as a beet, dry as a bone, blind as a bat"? Anticholinergic effects include altered mental status, sedation, confusion, memory impairment, fever, tachycardia, blurred vision, dry mouth, constipation, and urinary retention.

4. Can herbal "natural" supplements play a role in physiatric practice? Can these "natural" supplements do any harm to my patient?

Herbal preparations, minerals, vitamins, botanical phytomedicines, and nutraceuticals (supplements advertised as natural, derived from plants instead of chemicals) are increasing in popularity. Many of our pharmaceutical agents have herbal origins. Herbal supplements, however, are not regulated by the Food and Drug Administration (FDA). Examples include St. John's wort, gingko, ginseng, echinacea, glucosamine, and zinc. The potency and consistency of ingredients in these supplements is not known. Although there are a few scientific studies indicating possible efficacy, the clinician should inform their patient about many potential adverse side effects as well as drug-herb interactions.

5. List five mechanisms of potential drug interactions.

1. Increased or decreased renal excretion
2. Potentiation or inhibition of metabolic enzymes
3. Plasma protein binding affecting bioavailability
4. Gastrointestinal absorption and/or excretion effects
5. Pharmacodynamics

6. What are the major classes of antidepressants? What are their positive and negative side effect profiles?

Tricyclic antidepressants (TCAs) have anticholinergic, antihistaminic, and α-adrenergic effects. These include the anticholinergic side effects described above, plus orthostatic hypotension, weight gain, hyponatremia, and delayed ventricular conduction. TCAs are often used successfully in attenuating neurogenic pain but may have many drug interactions. Amitriptyline is still the second leading cause of death by overdose in the U.S. TCAs should never be used in bipolar depression and used with caution in populations with neurogenic bowel and bladder, orthostasis, polypharmacy, and the elderly. The tertiary amines (amitriptyline, imipramine) are associated with more side effects than the secondary amines (nortriptyline, desipramine).

Bupropion (Wellbutrin) is a weak inhibitor of serotonin, norepinephrine, and dopamine reuptake. It is also approved for use in smoking cessation. It appears to have no sedating effects and is not associated with weight changes or sexual dysfunction. At higher doses, it may lower the seizure threshold.

Selective serotonin reuptake inhibitors (SSRIs) may be associated with anxiety or agitation during treatment initiation and initially may have side effects of headache, nausea, and tremor. Persistent side effects of sexual dysfunction (e.g., erectile dysfunction, loss of libido) as well as insomnia and fatigue should be considered. There are some reports of SSRIs, as a class, increasing spasticity. Citalopram and sertraline have negligible drug interactions.

Serotonin/norepinephrine reuptake inhibitors (SNRIs), such as venlafaxine (Effexor), have no effect on norepinephrine reuptake at low doses and are essentially SSRIs. At higher doses, however, they have dual action as a SNRI. **Venlafaxine** is indicated for depression with or without comorbid anxiety disorder. At doses above 300 mg/day, it can cause supine hypertension. It does not have significant drug interactions. **Mirtazapine** (Remeron) is a dual action SNRI at all levels of dosing. It also possesses additional antihistaminergic effects from 5-HT$_2$ antagonism. It can be sedating.

7. What are the advantages and disadvantages of soporific agents (sleepers) prescribed by physicians?

Diphenhydramine (Benadryl) is frequently prescribed, but it has significant anticholinergic side effects. Due to its antihistaminergic mechanism, it also can cause sedation and confusion as well as gains in adipose tissue. Benadryl can also cause agitation in patients with brain injury. Because of the above side-effect profile, it is not the best agent of choice for a sleeper medication.

Antidepressants can be given for the side effect of sedation (see above selections).

Benzodiazepines, including temazepam (Restoril) and alprazolam (Xanax), can be used for management of insomnia and for their anxiolytic effect, but can alter normal EEG and sleep patterns. Prescribers must remember to warn patients that consumption of alcohol will potentiate "benzos" and chronic use may induce psychological dependence.

Hypnotics, such as chloral hydrate, are effective for some patients but can cause confusion, dizziness, and physical dependence.

Trazodone is a triazolopyridine, *not* a TCA, and therefore has much fewer side effects than the TCA class. It has a positive effect on sleep architecture but may cause vivid dreams and enhance appetite.

Zolpidem (Ambien) is a short-acting, nonbenzodiazepine hypnotic agent, acting through a variety of GABA receptors, and is less disruptive of normal sleep architecture (stage 3 and 4 "restorative" sleep) than benzos. It therefore produces a quality and pattern of sleep very similar to that of normal physiologic sleep.

Zalepon (Sonata) is a short-acting, nonbenzodiazepine agent similar to Ambien but with a better side-effect profile.

8. Explain some of the guidelines for anticoagulation in physiatry practice.

Aspirin inhibits aggregation by irreversible binding to the platelet for its 7–10-day lifetime and thus should be discontinued 10 days prior to any scheduled surgeries. Aspirin is an effective treatment for preventing thromboembolism in patients with stroke or atherosclerotic cardiovascular diseases, but is not effective in preventing deep venous thromboses (DVT).

Heparin works by inactivating coagulation factors and is dosed according to amount and route of administration depending on indication. It is the anticoagulant of choice when rapid intravenous anticoagulation is required, such as in acute myocardial infarction, stroke, pulmonary embolism, or DVT. Dosage is monitored by activated partial thromboplastin time (aPTT). Prevention of DVT usually requires 5000 units subcutaneously twice a day. Efficacy may be increased by titrating the aPTT ratio up to 1.2 after hip surgery and up to 1.5 after spinal cord injury. Heparin-induced thrombocytopenia is a well-known complication with significant sequellae.

Warfarin (Coumadin) interferes with vitamin K-dependent coagulation factors and is used in chronic treatment of many disorders. Dosage is monitored by the prothrombin (PT) test and international standardized ratio (INR). The American College of Chest Physicians recommends an INR of 2.0–3.0 for all indications except mechanical heart valves and acute myocardial infarction, for which an INR of 2.5–3.5 is recommended. Antiphospholipid antibody syndrome, an autoimmune coagulopathy, requires the highest INR of 3.0–4.0. The major risk of bleeding is increased when the patient is over 65 years of age, has history of stroke or GI bleed, has atrial fibrillation, renal insufficiency, or anemia, or is concurrently taking aspirin. Many medications interact with warfarin.

Low-molecular-weight-heparins (LMWHs) are derived from the depolymerization of heparin and thus have less risk of HIT or bleeding. LMWHs (e.g., Lovenox) are more effective in preventing DVT than subcutaneous or adjusted-dose heparin or warfarin in hip and knee surgery. LMWHs are also effective in preventing DVTs in stroke or spinal cord injury, as well as for treatment of DVTs.

9. Treatment of high blood pressure with medications clearly reduces the risk of cardiovascular morbidity and mortality, but which are considered as initial and supplemental agents?

Initial: diuretics, beta-blockers, ACE inhibitors, the dihydropyridine class of calcium channel blockers.

Supplemental: centrally acting α_2-agonists, peripheral-acting adrenergic antagonists.

10. What are the indications and precautions for diuretics?

Diuretics can be divided into three groups:

1. **Loop diuretics**, such as furosemide (Lasix), are more effective for patients with congestive heart failure and have been shown to decrease left ventricular hypertrophy without impairment of LV function. These agents can cause electrolyte disorders (hypokalemia, hyponatremia, hyperuricemia, hypercalcemia, hypomagnesemia) and should be used cautiously in patients with elevated creatinine.

2. **Potassium-sparing diuretics** are used to prevent hypokalemia and its resultant cardiac problems and decreased insulin release. If combined with ACE inhibitors or potassium supplements, the risk of hyperkalemia is increased.

3. **Thiazide diuretics** are considered first-line agents, but have possible side effects of hypokalemia, hyperuricemia, and hyperglycemia. Thiazides are not effective when creatinine clearance is < 30 mL/min.

11. What are the indications and precautions for other classes of antihypertensives?

1. **ACE inhibitors**, such as captopril, are associated with dry cough, angioedema, and hyperkalemia (if concomitant routine therapy with potassium or potassium-sparing diuretics). Their use should be avoided in patients who are volume-depleted (volume contraction) or have renal artery stenosis (exacerbate renal dysfunction). In the black patient, these are more effective if combined with a low-dose diuretic.

2. **Angiotensin receptor blockers**, such as candesartan, are less likely to cause cough and angioedema. They should be used with caution in volume-depletion and renal artery stenosis.

3. **Beta-blockers**, such as atenolol or metoprolol, are associated with decreased mortality following myocardial infarction. Side effects may include decreased heart rate, bronchospasm, and fatigue.

4. **Calcium channel blockers**, including the dihydropyridines such as amlodipine or felodipine, may be preferred because of their lack of negative inotropic effects. The other agents, such as diltiazem or verapamil, do have negative inotropic effects. All agents may cause headache and peripheral edema and should be used with caution in combination with a beta-blocker due to additive bradycardia.

5. **Peripheral α_1 antagonists**, such as prazosin or terazosin, are associated with first-dose syncope; therefore the first dose should be given at bedtime. These agents may improve male micturition due to binding to receptors in the prostatic urethra.

6. **Central α_2 antagonists**, such as clonidine, may cause rebound hypertensive crisis if stopped abruptly.

12. Are there any special considerations for using antihypertensives in the spinal cord injured (SCI) population?

Yes. Hypertension is prevalent in the SCI population. The incidence is related both to increasing age as well as lesion level. The lower the lesion, the more likely the need for antihypertensive agents. Although the optimal antihypertensive agent for the SCI population is unclear, there are certain considerations. Some **diuretics** (see above), nitrates, and clonidine may increase orthostatic hypotension, and all diuretics can cause various electrolyte abnormalities. **Beta-blockers** may decrease HDL, increase bronchospasm, and exacerbate insulin resistance. **ACE inhibitors** can lead to profound hypotension due to the dependence (tetraplegic > high paraplegic) on the renin-angiotensin system to maintain blood pressure. Although ACE inhibitors are also indicated as renal protective agents in diabetic SCI patients (a population much more prone to develop type II diabetes), the newer **angiotensin receptor blockers** may be preferable due to lesser effects on potassium. The dihydropyridine class of **calcium channel blockers** are a good choice because of the absence of negative inotropic effects.

13. Which medications can be used to attenuate orthostatic hypotension in the SCI population?

Ephedrine is a sympathomimetic with α and β properties, and may be given approximately ½ hour prior to arising from supine positioning.

Midodrine is also a sympathomimetic, but with predominant α receptor binding, and is preferred to ephedrine if patients have any concurrent cardiac problems.

Fludrocortisone is a very mild steroid and will cause fluid retention.

Salt tablets will also cause fluid retention but are not very palatable.

14. Name some medications that have potential deleterious implications for rehab patients.

Amiodarone has a high iodine content, and so patients must be monitored for development of hypothyroidism. It can cause pulmonary fibrosis, hepatotoxicity, peripheral neuropathy, and decreased vision (from corneal deposits) and has many drug interactions, most notably with digoxin and warfarin.

Meperidine (Demerol) produces a toxic active metabolite, normeperidine, that has a very long half-life and can accumulate with prolonged use (especially with compromised renal function). Normeperidine can provoke seizures, anxiety, tremors and myoclonus.

Cisapride (Propulsid) has been shown to produce fatal arrythmias from prolongation of the cardiac QT interval on ECG, and it has essentially been taken off the market.

Short-acting **nifedipine** may be detrimental in the setting of coronary heart disease because of rapid hypotension and reflex tachycardia, with a "coronary steal" phenomenon. Although the case reports were in non-SCI patients, it is a concern to use this medication for autonomic dysreflexia. In addition, the SCI population has a greater risk for atherosclerotic coronary disease.

15. Can any agent be administered to safely attenuate the diarrhea associated with pseudomembranous colitis?

Either **colestipol** or **cholestyramine** can bind *Clostridium difficile* toxin and be safely prescribed while awaiting the results of the stool sample, as well as during antibiotic therapy if the sample is positively confirmed for *Clostridium*. It is important to remember to discontinue the colestipol or cholestyramine once the diarrhea has resolved.

16. What are some important considerations for the physiatrist regarding management of the diabetic rehabilitation patient?

Certain characteristics of disabling etiologies may predispose to the development of increased endogenous insulin resistance of (already diagnosed) type II diabetes mellitus. This may be because of chronic corticosteroid use (as in rheumatoid arthritis), inactivity due to the disabling process, high prevalence of diabetes in amputees, and the development of syndrome X in the SCI population (triad of diabetes, hypertension, coronary artery disease).

17. Explain advantages and disadvantages of the drugs used to achieve glucose control in the diabetic rehab population.

1. **Oral sulfonylureas** increase endogenous pancreatic β-islet cell insulin secretion and may be used in synergistic combination with biguanides. This class has a higher incidence of hypoglycemia.

2. **Biguanides.** Metformin has three mechanisms of action: decreased hepatic glucose production, decreased intestinal glucose absorption, and increased insulin sensitivity by improving peripheral glucose uptake and utilization. It does not increase insulin secretion and is not associated with hypoglycemia at therapeutic doses except in special situations (inadequate caloric intake, strenuous exercise, and concurrent therapy with other hypoglycemics). Metformin does not cause weight gain. It is contraindicated in patients with renal dysfunction (serum creatinine > 1.5 in males and 1.4 in females) and should be avoided in liver disease. Metformin should be stopped prior to any radiologic studies using contrast media and may be restarted after 48 hrs or after renal function is in normal range.

3. **Thiazolidinediones**, such as pioglitazone and rosiglitazone, lower blood glucose by improving target cell response to insulin without increasing pancreatic insulin secretion. Absolute contraindications are liver impairment, hypersensitivity, and alcoholism. They are as effective as sulfonylureas as monotherapy and as effective as insulin in patients who have failed sulfonylureas. Caution is encouraged to temporarily discontinue this drug during episodes of systemic infection as well as significant hypoxia, as there is a possibility of developing lactic acidosis.

4. **Alpha-glucosidase inhibitors**, such as acarbose, decrease rate of absorption of carbohydrates and may create significant hepatic compromise (liver function tests should be monitored carefully). It is more widely used in Europe than in the U.S.

5. **Insulin** is not a benign intervention! It can perpetuate hyperinsulinemia and insulin resistance, accelerate atherosclerosis, increase plasma fibrinogen levels (thrombogenic), and lead to further adipose gain. It is also difficult to administer injections when patients are lacking in hand coordination or intrinsic innervation, compliance with blood sugar monitoring, or consistent attendants.

18. NSAIDs continue to be the most widely used drugs in musculoskeletal medicine. What are some of the newer agents?

COX II inhibitors. Preferential blocking of the second pathway of the cyclo-oxygenase enzyme provides more selective action against inflammatory prostaglandins, with less interference with the prostaglandins that protect the stomach. This results in greater potency and less toxicity, with studies demonstrating less ulceration. Patients with a sulfa allergy should use rofecoxib instead of celecoxib.

Tramadol (Ultram) bridges the gap between the opioid class and NSAIDs. Tramadol has a low affinity for the *mu* opioid receptor but is far less potent than narcotics. Analgesia can be attributed primarily to the active metabolite. It can be habit-forming and have adverse CNS and GI side-effects.

Ketoralac (Toradol) is used primarily as a postoperative analgesic in lieu of narcotics in patients sensitive to morphine and its derivatives.

19. Which agents can be used for effective topical analgesia?

1. **Capsaicin** is the most pungent ingredient of the red pepper, and its use for pain and pruritus has over a hundred years of historical documentation. Recent scientific evidence shows that, after the first application, it suppresses the release of neurotransmitters substance P and NMDA, which incite type C unmyelinated neurons. It must be applied at least two to three times a day to be effective.

2. **EMLA cream** (eutectic mixture of lidocaine analogs) is used frequently for localized topical analgesia prior to a procedure. It must be applied topically to the area, then covered with an occlusive hydrocolloid dressing, about 1 hour prior to the procedure.

3. **Topical lidocaine** can be very effective but must be applied several times a day.

4. **Jointritis**, a "natural" product, is a relatively new topical counterirritant ointment containing menthol, eucalyptus, copaiba extract, glucosamine, and chondroitin. It may be used to decrease pain in arthritic joints as well as in other benign musculoskeletal pain syndromes.

20. What should I tell my patient about the interaction of Viagra with medications containing nitrates?

Many forms of medications contain nitrates, including patches, pastes, sublinguals, and oral forms with varying half-lives. All nitrates dilate smooth muscle vasculature by increasing cGMP synthesis. Viagra (sildenafil) preferentially inhibits the enzyme that degrades cGMP within the vasculature of the penis, but it may have some systemic effects. Since Viagra and all nitrates essentially dilate blood vessels by the same mechanism (increasing cGMP levels), using both can have an additive effect. Patients could develop severe hypotension that progresses to cardiac or cerebral ischemia. There should be a 24-hour time span between the use of Viagra and any nitrate agent. Viagra should be relatively contraindicated in any SCI patient who has chronic hypotension or any chance of developing autonomic dysreflexia treated with nitropaste.

21. What are some important metabolic considerations in patients prone to repetitive or poorly healing pressure ulcers?

Nutrition. Adequate protein intake is imperative for the high-density collagen matrix protein synthesis required for wound healing. Because the very presence of an open wound causes a catabolic state, most sources recommend 1.5–2 mg/kg/day of protein.

Appetite. Although megestrol acetate (Megace) is FDA-approved for appetite stimulation, it is a progesterone and glucocorticoid analog and can therefore cause lean tissue catabolism, hyperglycemia, and adipose weight gain. It can also deplete testosterone levels, thus resulting in decreased endogenous anabolic stimulus for protein synthesis, poor skin turgor, and further risk of skin breakdown, osteoporosis, muscle wasting, and depression.

Anabolic hormone analog agent. Oxandrolone is the only FDA-approved medication for weight loss from a variety of etiologies and has been shown to increase lean body mass from enhancing protein synthesis. It also stimulates fibroblasts to produce the collagen that heals wounds. Low albumin is a marker for malnutrition, and low levels correlate with the presence, severity, and lack of healing of pressure ulcers. Oxandrolone is a testosterone analog (really has no steroid properties) with a higher anabolic profile and extremely low negative androgenic profile, but it should not be given with an elevated prostate-specific antigen (PSA). It also will potentiate coumadin and sulfonylureas.

Testosterone. Low levels can result from a multitude of etiologies such as SCI, advanced age, malnutrition, or catabolic stress from pressure ulcers or multitrauma. Supplements are now available as an injection, dermal patch, or topical cream. PSA must be checked prior to the decision to prescribe physiologic replacement.

22. Is there a difference between oral antispasmodics and antispasticity drugs? What are the best choices for my patient?

Medications such as Flexeril, Soma, or Robaxin are spasmolytic agents intended for transient muscle relaxation. These agents are not intended for centrally mediated, velocity-dependent spasticity. Antispasticity choices include the following:

1. **Tizanidine** is an α_2-agonist similar to clonidine, but it is formulated to produce negligible effects on lowering blood pressure. It has a short half-life and therefore should be dosed four times a day. Side effects may include sedation and headache.

2. **Gabapentin**, a GABA analog, is FDA-approved as an adjunct for partial seizures, but it is also used for neuropathic pain. It should be considered when a patient has neuropathic pain as well as spasticity. Because it is excreted unchanged in the urine, the side-effect profile is minimal and it has no known drug interactions.

3. **Baclofen** is also a GABA analog, dosed four times a day, and is usually the first choice for both spinal and centrally mediated spasticity. Although many clinicians prescribe more than the 80-mg/day recommended maximum, this is not without precautions. Higher doses may actually cause receptor up-regulation, creating the need for more baclofen to achieve the same effect. Recent literature also suggests that higher doses may exacerbate sleep apnea and respiratory depression. Baclofen side effects also include fatigue and clouded mental status. If the patient requires > 80 mg/day, consideration should be made to add another agent or to evaluate criteria for intrathecal baclofen delivery via a surgically implanted pump system.

4. **Valium** is a benzodiazepine effective for attenuating spasticity.

5. **Dantrolene** is the only peripherally acting antispasticity medication, which works by inhibiting calcium uptake at the sarcoplasmic reticulum. Liver function tests should be monitored regularly.

23. Name some classes of medications that can impair cognition.

Anticholinergic agents	Central-acting antihypertensive agents
Anticonvulsants	Gastric motility agents (e.g., metaclopramide)
Antiemetics	Cardiac glycosides
Antipsychotics	H_2 blockers
Beta-blockers	Hypnotics
Benzodiazepines	Opiates
Barbiturates	Xanthine derivatives (e.g., theophylline)

24. Which medications can be used to reverse respiratory pathophysiology in tetraplegics and higher level paraplegics?

Weakness of inspiratory and expiratory muscles is a primary reason that pneumonia and respiratory failure are common in acute SCI. Additionally, alterations of autonomic nervous system activity may contribute to respiratory dysfunction. With injuries rostral to the mid-thoracic level, sympathetic input to the bronchioles is interrupted, leading to unopposed parasympathetic activity with bronchoconstriction and increased production of pulmonary secretions.

Patients with acute tetraplegia frequently show airway hyperresponsiveness to methacholine during pulmonary function testing, even with no prior history of reactive airway disease. Inhaled β_2 **agonists**, such as albuterol, prevent bronchoconstriction.

Expiratory dysfunction diminishes the effectiveness of coughing in clearing pulmonary secretions. This problem is generally exacerbated if secretions are made more tenacious by anticholinergic agents. **Mucolytic agents** can facilitate secretion clearance when combined with appropriate assisted cough techniques, such as quad coughing or mechanical in-exsufflation. An example of an oral agent is guaifenesin. *N*-Acetylcysteine can be administered either orally or via inhalation but should be coupled with albuterol to reduce risk of bronchospasm. Purulent secretions may respond to inhaled recombinant human **DNase**, which breaks down DNA released by lysed neutrophils.

25. Explain the risks and benefits of neuroleptics for "chemical restraint" in an agitated patient recovering from TBI.

If behavioral or environmental management is not effective, the recommended first-line pharmacologic treatment for agitation and delirium in a TBI patient is the **short-acting benzodiazepine** class with no active metabolite (such as lorazepam). The use of **neuroleptics**, such as haldol, is considered second-line therapy, and minimal dosage is best. This class is postulated to disrupt neural recovery, cause extrapyramidal movement disorders, lower the seizure threshold, and place the patient at risk for neuroleptic malignant syndrome.

26. What are current recommendations for seizure prophylaxis after TBI?

Anticonvulsant prophylaxis is usually recommended only for the first week postinjury in those injuries without penetration or skull fracture. Long-term use of phenytoin has been shown to deter neural recovery, and therefore some authors suggest the alternative use of carbamazepine or valproic acid instead, due to fewer cognitive side effects.

27. What is the importance of medical informatics?

In our constantly evolving, high technology world, access to the computer network provides multiple resources via worldwide websites. Although these websites are a great resource, some do not have the peer-reviewed scrutiny and editing that is required of "hard copy" published journals and textbooks. Physicians should check pharmaceutical information obtained from websites with other references prior to prescribing any medications.

Computerized patient record systems have many advantages, including complete lists of the patient's medications for all practitioners to view. Pharmacy programs can provide "alerts" that appear on the screen to warn physicians about drug interactions as they attempt to prescribe a medication, or about laboratory results that need to be checked before medication renewals.

28. Why is it important to treat B_{12} deficiencies?

B_{12} deficiencies are much more prevalent that previously thought, especially in the SCI population and the elderly (up to 14.5%). Deficiencies can result in peripheral neuropathy, decreased memory and cognitive skills, poor wound healing (it is a protein synthesis cofactor), and pernicious anemia and may be associated with high homocysteine levels. Monthly intramuscular injections are known to be effective, however oral replacement therapy can be used in lieu of injections, with effective dosing of 1000 μg/day.

29. How can I regulate bowel function with medications?

Stool consistency modulation is first achieved with a bowel program that emphasizes exercise, fluid intake, and diet modifications. Agents to soften the stool for effective propulsion and elimination include docusate sodium, milk of magnesia, and sorbitol. For soft or liquid stools, bulking agents such as psyllium or colestipol (in chronic or extreme cases) are useful. Ideally, bowel care should be initiated with voluntary external anal sphincter relaxation or digital stimulation. If needed, pharmacologic agents can be used to trigger defecation.

The following agents are listed in the order of least to most potent: glycerine suppository, vegetable oil-based bisacodyl suppository, CeoTwo suppository, saline bisacodyl enemas, Therevac brand mini-enema, and the Magic Bullet (polyethylene glycol-based bisacodyl suppository).

BIBLIOGRAPHY

1. Jellin JM, et al: Pharmacist's Letter/Prescriber's Letter Natural Medicines Comprehensive Database, 3rd ed. Stockton, CA, Therapeutic Research Faculty Publishers, 2000.
2. Leipzig RM: Prescribing: Keys to maximizing benefit while avoiding adverse drug effects. Geriatrics 56:30–34, 2001.
3. Nance PW (ed): Rehabilitation Pharmacotherapy. Physical Medicine and Rehabilitation Clinics of North America. Philadelphia, W.B. Saunders, 1999.
4. Stitik T, Kleca R, Zafonte RO, Klein DS: Pharmacotherapy of disability. In DeLisa JA, Gans BM (eds): Rehabilitation Medicine: Principles and Practice, 3rd ed. Philadelphia, Lippincott-Raven, 1998.
5. Zorowitz RD, Robinson KM: Drugs used in rehabilitation. In Grabois M, et al (eds): Physical Medicine and Rehabilitation: The Complete Approach. Malden, MA, Blackwell Science Publishers, 2000.

82. ASSISTIVE TECHNOLOGY

Mark A. Young, M.D., Howard Choi, M.D., and Mary Macy, M.D.

1. What is the definition of assistive technology (AT)?

AT is defined in **Public Law 100-407** (the Technology-Related Assistance for Indivduals with Disabilities Act, 1988) as "any item, piece of equipment or product system whether commercially off the shelf, modified, or customized that is used to increase or improve functional capabilities of individuals with disabilities." This definition encompasses the simplest of items, such as a built-up fork or a single-point cane, to the most high-tech powered wheelchair, rigged with blink operated controls, laser-guided collision sensors, and a robot arm for taking out the trash. Whether low-tech or high, AT devices can help people overcome major barriers to participate fully in work, recreation, and family life.

2. Are employers required to provide AT in the workplace?

Employers with 15 or more employees are required by the **Americans with Disabilities Act** to make **reasonable accommodations** for persons with disabilities as long as the expense or maintenance of those accommodations do not put the entire existence of the business in jeopardy. Some examples of AT in the workplace might include extended levers for faucets, one-handed typewriters, or a power-assisted door.

3. What is a switch?

A switch is an object that can be triggered to operate a device. Any person capable of performing an isolated volitional muscle movement in a targeted way can trigger a switch. For some, it may mean pressing a button; for others it may mean blinking an eye. Switches can be adapted to all forms of body movement including foot, head, or tongue movement, sipping and puffing, voice control, EMG signals, or breath switches. There are even switches that respond to eye gaze, facial expression, or proximity of an extremity (without touch).

Modern switches have revolutionized the quality of life for many people with disabilities. For example, the simple, popular touch-activated switch (e.g., for lamps) has eased the daily routines of many arthritis sufferers. Using a sophisticated system of sip-and-puff commands, a ventilator-dependent complete tetraplegic can operate an adapted sailboat *solo* (with a motorized chase boat trailing close by for safety), something not even imaginable a few decades ago.

4. When is a sip-and-puff switch system indicated?

Sip and puff is generally indicated for persons with unreliable head movements and profound loss of motor control of the body. It may also be indicated if repetitive head movements are uncomfortable or cause overuse syndromes. Persons with C1 and C2 spinal cord injuries typically use sip and puff, while C3 and C4 spinal cord-injured persons may opt to use chin controls or mouthsticks.

5. How good are voice control (voice recognition) switches?

At present, voice control still requires a fair bit of user training. Reliability decreases considerably with fluctuations in voice quality. Also, a misinterpreted voice command or an extraneous environmental noise could potentially cause an inadvertent and possibly dangerous command to be executed. The demands of commercial industry and perpetual improvements in microprocessor technology, however, will ensure that voice recognition technology will continue to improve in the future.

6. What is an ECU?

An ECU, or **environmental control unit**, is a switch-operated device that controls an object or objects in a disabled person's environment. Commonly used ECUs include controls for doors, house lights, televisions, home appliances, and hospital-type beds, among others. (Always remember that AT and ECUs refer to the disabled population only. The same types of devices employed by a nondisabled person are not referred to by these terms.)

ECUs are comprised of five elements: the switch device, control device, connection, target device(s), and feedback device. The control device detects a signal from the switch, then transforms the signal and sends it through a connection to a target device to perform a function. The user is then alerted that the function has successfully been engaged or completed through a feedback, such as a light blinking on the control device. Note that infrared connections require a direct line of sight to the target device or a relay box, while standard copper wire, radiowave, and ultrasonic connections do not.

7. How have ECUs helped the disabled?

ECUs have improved the potential for independent living since the earliest units were devised in England in the 1960s for tetraplegics and disabled polio survivors. With the assistance of ECUs, many persons with severe mobility limitations and other disabilities have had the option to avoid institutionalization and live safely and comfortably in their own homes.

Outcome studies to document cost savings using ECUs, however, are for the most part nonexistent. Funding from medical insurance or public programs may be difficult to obtain, and support often comes from community groups, such as religious organizations or private foundations.

8. Will robots solve all of humanity's problems?

Perhaps eventually, but not necessarily in our lifetimes. There is certainly no lack of effort to make robotics work for the disabled. One ongoing project is the development of a robot arm for pick-and-place tasks. This arm has been applied to ADL workstations, wheelchairs, and mobile robots. Currently, the arms and terminal devices are still fairly crude, although more lightweight and dexterous models are under development.

The **HelpMate** mobile cart robot has been autonomously carrying lab supplies, medical records, and late patient meals in numerous hospitals throughout the U.S. for several years now. It is guided by radio transmitters planted in the hospital which help the robot triangulate its position with uncanny accuracy. It is also equipped with a speech synthesizer to warn people to get out of its way and a radio transmitter to call for elevators. With further improvements it is not far-fetched to imagine conceptually similar models adapted for home use in disabled populations.

Despite their technological glamour and mystique, however, robots have not lived up to expectations for people with physical impairments to date. Past and present generation robots do not seem to do well outside of very controlled environments and fail at some of the most basic of tasks. Some will recall the experiments a few years ago where the most sophisticated research robots were pitted against 2-year-old toddlers. The robots had great difficulty at tasks such as picking up a red ball out of a group of other objects, while the feisty little tykes accomplished the tasks with ease. In these days of cost cutting in medicine, cost-benefit analyses will have to demonstrate that routine use of advanced technologies such as robots is warranted. An alternative to consider for some limited tasks might be animal-assisted therapy.

9. What role does artificial intelligence (AI) play in AT?

Simple phrases that humans instinctively understand such as "*near* the edge of the table" or "pick up the glass *gently*" are difficult for digital systems to interpret. **Fuzzy logic** is an example of one AI system that handles the ambiguity and imprecision of human language in a quantitative way. Such systems must continue to improve in order for the interaction between humans and digital systems to become more seamless and practical. At the forefront of AI computing are systems like **genetic algorithms**. Genetic algorithms take random solutions generated by a computer and put them through a "fitness evaluation." Elements from the most successful or "fit" solutions are continuously bred, while unsuccessful solutions become extinct in Darwinian fashion. Eventually, an acceptable solution is reached. The algorithms are fast and efficient and can be used to determine an optimal pathway when a robot or other device is faced with a series of tasks.

10. Give some examples of AT devices for persons with special sensory impairments (e.g., hearing and/or visually impaired).

Amplification devices have been the mainstay for people who are hard of hearing. A relatively recent improvement is the directional microphone for selective listening in environments such as shopping malls or sporting events, where distortion due to ambient noise may render a traditional hearing aid useless. The deaf have long benefited from AT solutions such as vibrating or blinking light alerts to inform them of ringing phones, alarm clocks, crying babies, nearby sirens while driving an automobile, and other critical sounds in the environment.

TDD, or Telephone Devices for the Deaf, uses QWERTY keyboards outfitted with text displays for incoming messages which connect to standard phone lines. Two TDD users can communicate with each other independently. A deaf user wishing to "speak" with any non-TTD user can do so using a "Voice Carry Over Relay Service," which voices outgoing messages while textually displaying incoming messages.

Synthetic speech software aids blind people by reading text aloud. A variety of "speaking" devices exist, including watches, microwave ovens, glucometers, insulin dose readers, and money identifiers, just to name just a few. There are machines and computers that combine speech synthesis with **optical character recognition** (OCR) so that the blind can have access to all sorts of printed material. Computers can also be adapted with refreshable pin-screens for braille output or tactile displays that can chart graphs or pictures. Talking signs and ATMs are available, although they are not yet in wide usage. For those with low vision, **closed circuit television** (CCTV) can magnify text placed in view of a camcorder for display on a screen at home or even onto a virtual reality-style helmet.

11. What is augmentative and alternative communication (AAC)? Who uses it?

AAC is communication that involves something other than a person's own body. This includes everything from a pencil to the latest speech synthesizer. The most common congenital problems requiring AAC are cerebral palsy, mental retardation, autism, developmental verbal apraxia and developmental language disorders. Common acquired problems include brain injury, stroke, amyotrophic lateral sclerosis, tetraplegia, multiple sclerosis, and ventilator dependence.

12. Name some low- and high-tech examples of AAC.

A widely used low tech example is the basic **communication board**, which is an array of objects, letters, pictures, or symbols that can be selected by pointing, eye gaze, or other techniques. Advantages of this device include simplicity, low expense, portability, and negligible mechanical failure rate. They offer less independence, however, because they require more skill on the part of the communication partner and can be very slow. Often, for the sake of speed or due to impatience, the partner will dominate the conversation and reduce the participation of the person using the communication board.

More sophisticated devices, including those that use microprocessor technologies, have been developed over the last few decades. Vocabulary and the rate of output are expedited using symbol systems or word-prediction software, while gender and age-matched synthetic voices produce clear, efficient output. One example of a highly successful symbol-based device is the Liberator, which uses the **Minspeak** system. Many persons have developed superb fluency using these sorts of devices.

Incorporation of **orthographic symbols** (abstract symbols that can be combined to form infinite numbers of words or concepts—e.g., the alphabet, braille, morse code) is a important component in an AAC device for literate individuals. Systems that only allow for the most basic levels of output may lead to user frustration and AT intervention failure.

13. Why do AT devices sometimes fail or their users abandon them?

A patient's motivation and potential for use of an assistive device are often underestimated or overestimated by the caregiver(s) or rehab team. Often, a potential user will have very unrealistic expectations about a device, and these should be explored before committing to the device. If possible, equipment trials with adequate provisions for training are helpful. Specialized centers will often have sample devices that are adjustable for individual trials. They are also likely to have therapists or technicians familiar with the products who can train and comprehensively evaluate the device with the patient before a final commitment.

At all times, patient preference and self-image should be considered high priorities. Quite frequently, a device's aesthetic appearance may be the sole reason it is not used. Items that draw a lot of adverse attention, such as loud alarms used as reminders for pressure relief, rapidly fall into disuse. Whenever possible, encouragement for use of the device should be provided. Reassessments should be made at appropriate intervals. It is also important not to provide too many items at once.

It should not be forgotten that many devices simply do not accomplish their intended goals due to faulty design. Other devices are unreliable or prone to mechanical breakdown. A rule of thumb is that the more complicated a gizmo is, the more likely it will break down... and the more it will cost to fix it. Some devices can cause fatigue or overuse injury, even with optimal usage techniques.

14. What is an adverse technology reaction (ATR)?

You may be thinking of that churning feeling you had in your stomach the last time your computer crashed and ate up a precious document. According to the AMA, ATRs can be fitment problems, hygiene or safety issues related to the device, pain or excessive fatigue due to the device, or improper usage of the device by the user or caregiver.

15. What's in store for the future in AT?

As Yogi Berra once said, "Prediction is very hard, especially when it's about the future." Nobody knows what technological marvels will be introduced in 5 years or even tomorow. Miniaturized talking robots may be running around performing everyone's ADLs and jobs, while we all lie on the beach drinking MaiTais. Or the world may work much like it does today, with PM&R docs working hard (OK, *relatively* hard) to help our patients achieve functional independence and make sensible choices about their AT devices.

BIBLIOGRAPHY

1. American Medical Association: Candidates for the Use of Assistive Technology: Evaluation, Referral, Prescription. Chicago, AMA, 1994.
2. American Medical Association: Guidelines for the Use of Assistive Technology: Evaluation, Referral, Prescription. Chicago, AMA, 1994.
3. Garber S, et al: Adaptive systems: Adaptive seating and assistive technology. In Grabois M (ed): Physical Medicine & Rehabilitation: The Complete Approach. Malden, MA, Blackwell Science, 2000.
4. Monga T, Zimmerman K (eds): Advances in Rehabilitation Technology. Phys Med Rehabil State Art Rev 11(1):1, 1997.
5. Stiens SA: Personhood, disablement, and mobility technology: Personal control of development. In Gry DB, Quatrano LA, Lieberman M (eds): Designing and Using Assistive Technology: The Human Perspective. Towson, MD, Paul Brookes, 1998, pp 29–49.
6. Swenson J, et al: Assistive technology for rehabilitation and reduction of disability. In DeLisa J (ed): Rehabilitation Medicine: Principles and Practice, 3rd ed. Philadelphia, Lippincott-Raven, 1998.
7. Young M, et al: Independence for people with disabilities: A physician's primer on assistive technology. Maryl Med, Summer 2000.

83. COMMUNITY REINTEGRATION

*David Tostenrude, M.P.A., CTRS, Carrie Booker, CTRS,
and Steven A. Stiens, M.D., M.S.*

1. What is recreation therapy (RT)?

Therapeutic recreation is defined by the National Therapeutic Recreation Society as services "to facilitate leisure, recreation, and play for persons with physical, mental, emotional, or social limitations in order to promote their health and well-being." RT is further defined by the American Therapeutic Recreation Association as "treatment services which restore, remediate, or rehabilitate in order to improve functioning and independence."

RT was incorporated into the medical model in the veterans and military hospitals during World War II. Sports and recreation programs were included in the rehabilitation process to address the needs of the "whole"person. Since then, RT has developed national professional organizations and therapists have been incorporated in many other settings.

2. Define leisure.

Leisure is defined differently by each of us. No matter how active or inactive an individual is, leisure has a part in that person's life. **Leisure** is activity, apart from the obligations of work, family, and society, to which the individual turns at will for either relaxation, diversion, broadening his or her knowledge, or spontaneous social participation. Some people spend time outdoors hiking, boating, or mountain climbing, while others prefer working in the garden. In rehabilitation, it is critical to assess "what" leisure is to a person in order to identify the needs of the individual.

3. What is a recreation therapist?

A **Certified Therapeutic Recreation Specialist** (CTRS) is an individual who has fulfilled certification requirements through the National Council for Therapeutic Recreation Certification. To be awarded the CTRS certificate, an individual must meet eligibility requirements that include a professional internship and then pass the national exam. An RT is a skilled professional, with a baccalaureate, masters, or doctorate degree in Therapeutic Recreation or in Recreation, with a specialization in Therapeutic Recreation from an accredited college or university.

4. How does the recreation therapist interact with the interdisciplinary rehabilitation team?

The RT assesses the impact of the injury, disease, or disability on the patient's leisure lifestyle. The RT presents his or her assessment to the team, which then becomes part of the overall interdisciplinary plan. In addition, the role of the RT is to develop an individualized RT program that reflects not only the expressed needs of the patient but the treatment philosophy and the immediate goals of the other disciplines. The RT communicates with the other team members through documentation and charting, involvement in weekly team meetings, and coordination of interdisciplinary goals and interventions.

5. Is it just fun for the patients?

RT programs are fun. Additionally, they are designed to reflect not only the outcomes targeted for the patients but also the interests of the patients. If you are working with an individual who used to paint for self-expression and relaxation, then an effective approach may be to get them involved in painting during rehabilitation. This work could reflect then the state of coping and self-concept, as well as relationships to society.

Individuals demonstrate natural behaviors and skills when they are acting without prompting. A key aspect of RT is the ability to involve patients in situations in which they look past the long- or short-range goals associated with the activity, and thus the individual learns more and demonstrates the actual obtainment of a skill. An example is wheelchair mobility. The clinic provides an environment full of cues, scrutiny, and modification for accessibility. However, put that patient outdoors and they suddenly have to contend with natural distractions, traffic, other people, weather, and terrain. This unique equation forces problem-solving from the patient and draws on their creativity, judgment, and skill. During this experience, the RT will see whether a patient has learned the skill adequately or needs further attention.

6. What programs does a recreation therapist involve the patient in?

RTs design leisure activities to obtain functional outcomes. Patients are involved in activities depending on the benefits associated with the specific activity, level of supervision targeted by the team or goals, and assessed capabilities of the patient.

1. **Treatment services**—The provision of prescribed leisure activities that directly promote functional improvement of skills and independence.

2. **Leisure education**—Programs designed for the acquisition and enhancement of diverse leisure-related knowledge, skills, and attitudes.

3. **Recreation participation**—Activities allow for self-motivated leisure activities that provide the opportunity for leisure skill development, self-expression, creativity, and enjoyment.

In all of these programs, the social environment, supervision, and locus of control are dependent on the RT's assessment of the patient needs and the nature of the activity. The RT must be flexible and attentive to the needs of the patient population, while having competency at evaluating leisure activities for their participation requirements and potential benefits.

For example, **aquatic therapy** is a popular modality for treatment to address spasticity, tone reduction, endurance, and cardiovascular fitness. Additional benefits include relaxation, swimming stroke development, improved self-image, and socialization. The RT assists the patient in locating community resources at home to continue after discharge. Aquatics may be part of the initial therapy program, but as the patient progresses, swimming may become an optional activity. In this aspect of the program, goals for aquatics then become self-directed rather than rehab-discipline-supported.

7. What outcomes does a recreation therapist attempt to achieve?

The outcomes targeted by the RT are a reflection of those specific needs of the individual. RT outcomes reflect improved adjustment to disability/illness, successful independence in the community, increased awareness of community resources, or the obtainment of leisure skills. Outcomes are measured through demonstration of knowledge or skill, reports of satisfaction, or behavioral observation. The RT is challenged to develop behavioral outcomes that identify the abstract nature of competence, independence, self-determination, and quality of life.

8. What is community and why address it?

Community is the environment where the individual freely chooses to live, work, and play. The term *community* reflects the associations in our lives, including families, friends, and resources. Together, all of these internal and external factors constitute the individual's "community."

For a person to realize a meaningful life, regardless of disability, the following skills are necessary: negotiating community barriers (architectural and interpersonal), diverse recreation interests, financial planning, social skills training, managing an attendant, creative problem-solving, accessible community resources, assertiveness, vocational planning, sexual expression, and use of community transportation. For an individual who is confronted with a life-changing illness or disability, these specific needs in the community must be assessed and addressed to support the best outcomes for a patient.

9. How does community reintegration work?

Community reintegration is the ultimate goal of rehabilitation. The aim is that every person participating in rehab becomes happily situated, productively occupied, and effectively supported in their community. The RT, who assists the patients in the transition from the hospital to the community, facilitates community reintegration.

As part of this program, natural supports and native guides are identified and included in the training. **Natural supports** are family members, neighbors, coworkers, and friends who are already in the community where the patient would like to be. **Native guides** are people with disabilities who are successfully living in the community. They provide essential peer support for the patient and guidance through the environment which is "new territory" for those with new disabilities. Together, they provide necessary assistance to the patient to enable independent living and the fullest participation in community.

Community outings allow the patient to practice and reinforce critical skills in the "real" world. These are invaluable, essential experiences that convince the patient and others that they can satisfy their physical, social, emotional, and cognitive needs in the real world. Community reintegration tests and validates the interdisciplinary process as it specifically supports the individual's uniqueness.

10. How is community reintegration a part of the rehabilitation process?

The processes of rehabilitation should emphasize support of all activities that contribute to a sense of usefulness and life satisfaction, including a person's participation in community services, educational programs, gainful employment, and active leisure. The "whole" person perspective, or holistic approach, proposes that when a situation affects an individual, all of the aspects of that person's life be affected. Disability is emphasized when the needs of the "whole" person are not clearly addressed. The interdisciplinary team focuses on functional skills that contribute to minimizing disability. However, independence and mastery remain hypotheses until patients demonstrate skills in real world situations. Each community outing is an experiment that tests the level of preparedness of the patient for independent return to a community of choice.

11. How does the RT advocate the community reintegration needs of the individual into the treatment plan?

The RT assesses interests and history of the person, as well as the impact that the injury or illness has on the individual's life. First, this establishes a baseline of function by which progress can be measured. Second, this assessment identifies an appropriate direction in which to serve the individual. The treatment team then shares their discipline specific perspectives that establish an overall plan. This information is then assimilated into a community reintegration program that is reflective of the team's comprehensive, person-centered plan of care. The RT implements the community reintegration program while measuring the progress and needs of the individual in relation to the overall plan. Modifications are made to opportunities that continue to challenge and educate the person, their family, and caregivers. At discharge, the rehabilitation objectives are demonstrated as the individual returns home and relies on the skills that have been the focus throughout the process and necessary for a healthy and independent life.

12. What is play therapy?

In addition to the many goals addressed in leisure, an important aspect of "play" is **coping**. Play is effective therapy because patients perceive involvement as nonthreatening. They do not have to make decisions during the activity that may affect their lives or address possible dependency or disability. The requirement is that they focus on the activity, and the result is skill acquisition, enjoyment, social stimulation, and stress reduction.

13. What are these community reintegration outings?

Outings are opportunities designed for the patients to participate in leisure activities away from the facility. The program is developed in several parts:

1. First is the **planning phase**. The participant, or group, chooses an activity that is reflective of their interests. Education is focused towards the skills necessary to carry over the event at home. The patient must learn to communicate with other staff, family, or caregivers to line up equipment or care they need to go away from the facility. This includes management of needs that may arise, such as bowel or bladder issues.

2. Once away from the facility, the **outing** is executed. The person must demonstrate skills such as community mobility and negotiating architectural barriers, interacting with public, problem-solving, and directing care as needed.

3. On return to the facility, a comprehensive review of the experience is shared with the patients. This evaluation process includes assessment of transition skills and future programs as appropriate.

14. As a community outing, what value is there in going to the movies?

Movies allow for social participation, relaxation, and enjoyment. They allow the person to travel to distant places or take part in outrageous adventures. We dream and live vicariously through the arts. Simply going to a movie requires many tasks. First, in the planning stage, coordination and problem-solving regarding the scheduling of the movie time, location, transportation, and coordinating with family or friends are challenging. An individual must also prepare themselves to go. This includes self-care, medical management, and emergency preparedness. Secondly, the execution requires mobility challenges, community interaction with theatre employees, negotiating public restrooms, moving through dark theaters, managing money, and even advocating needs. Thirdly, during the comprehensive review, the individual acknowledges growth at many levels. There are both functional and emotional advantages of going to a movie. Finally, it is an important opportunity for the patient to get out and have fun and relax. This stress relief can help the patient overcome feelings of worthlessness and despair by showing them that they still have some control over their lives and that life after injury can be meaningful and rewarding.

15. Describe some examples of community reintegration outcomes.

RTs reinforce goals established by interdisciplinary team members by designing programs for use in the field. Short-term goals used in a community reintegration program help patients to establish spontaneous adaptive behaviors that effectively meet their needs in the communities of their choice.

PROBLEM	DIAGNOSIS	LONG-TERM GOAL	SHORT-TERM GOAL
Safety	TBI, with short-term attention deficits	Effective environmental scanning ability	Will idenytify 5 hazards while successfully avoiding during outing.
Fatigue	Multiple sclerosis	Management of endurance through strategic planning of schedule	Will describe duration and conditions ideal to meet a leisure interest with consideration of their physical capacity.
Expressive aphasia	Stroke	Communication of needs while in the community	Will successfully use communication board while purchasing 2 items at the grocery store.
Anger management related to adjustment issues	Bilateral below-knee amputation	Self-initiation of anger management techniques	Will initiate time-out in community as necessary
Mobility	SCI, tetraplegia	Management of access barriers through effective problem-solving	Will increase awareness of accommodation by identifying 4 architectural modifications.

16. Can you get the same results in the clinic?

No. The community offers an opportunity and element of risk that the clinic cannot. The clinic hosts a setting that is consistent and full of reinforcement and cues that the patient can become dependent on, but which limit independent behavior. Skills must be transferred to the community in order to observe true behaviors and for the patient to build self-reliance and experience the relevance of the skills they are learning. It is also essential for people to venture out-side the shelter of the clinic to an unpredictable environment, similar to what they will be faced with every day after discharge. This is the same interaction through life that we experience. This is how we grow, establish connections, and become self-actualized.

17. What risks are the patients exposed to and how are they managed?

"Do no harm" is a commitment that any community reintegration program must support. The first step of risk management is to assess the individual's emotional and physical readiness to leave the facility. The physician's responsibility is to authorize the individual readiness to partic-ipate in community outings. The primary guidelines are that the patient is able to tolerate sitting and endurance for a 3–4-hour activity, be medically stable, and orthopedically able to tolerate the movement associated with transportation. In the case of a cognitively impaired patient, he or she must also be able to follow simple commands to ensure safety during the outing. Readiness for involvement requires input and coordination from all disciplines.

Second, the outing must be reviewed. Obvious and unforeseen hazards must be anticipated and an action plan developed. For example, for an individual who has had a stroke with left ne-glect, the community reintegration plan is to address driving a scooter in the community safely. This person presents a hazard to him or herself and others due to the neglect. The action plan may involve increased supervision of the person, which may have implications on the staffing ratio.

Third, the patient needs to be informed and accept the risk. This heightened awareness in-creases responsibility, accountability, and personal growth.

18. How can patient outcomes in community reintegration be assessed? Can they be quan-tified?

The networking and exchange each patient has are unique and relate directly to who they are and what they hoped to do before and after the events that may have changed their function. The primary clinical outcome is the guided self-assessment by the patient of the community integration before disability and thereafter. Community integration must be understood in terms in consumer expectations and the quality of life perceived in integration. There are a variety of assessment in-struments: **Community Integration Questionnaire** (CIQ), **Reintegration to Normal Living Index** (RNLI), and the **Craig Handicapped Assessment and Reporting Tool** (CHART). The CHART estimates the person's ability to perform six community roles: orientation, physical inde-pendence, mobility, occupation, social integration, and economic self-sufficiency.

There are a variety of ways of subdividing the interaction that the person has with commu-nity, although none is particularly good for all populations. The World Health Organization de-scribes nine dimensions for **participation**: personal maintenance, mobility, exchange of information, social relationships, home-life, assistance to others, education and work, economic life, and community and civic life. Community integration has been organized into a theoretical model by McColl et al. that includes four categories: assimilation (acceptance), support (relation-ships), occupation (productivity and leisure), and independent living.

BIBLIOGRAPHY

1. Armstrong M, Lauzen S: Community Reintegration Program, 2nd ed. Ravensdale, WA, Idyll Arbor, 1994, p 5.
2. Craig A, Hancock K, Dickson H: Improving the long-term adjustment of spinal cord injured persons. Spinal Cord 37:345–350, 1999.
3. Kreuter M, Sullivan M, Dahllof AF, Siosteen A: Partner relationships, functioning, mood and global qual-ity of life in persons with spinal cord and traumatic brain injury. Spinal Cord 36:252–262, 1998.
4. McColl MA, Davies D, Carlson P, et al: The community integration measure: Development and prelimi-nary validation. Arch Phys Med Rehabil 82:429–434, 2001.
5. Sander AM, Fuchs KL, High WM Jr, et al: The community integration questionnaire revisited: An assess-ment of factor structure validity. Arch Phys Med Rehabil 80:1303–1308, 1999.
6. Stiens S, Biener Bergman S, Formal C: Spinal cord injury rehabilitation: Individual experience, personal adaptation, and social perspective. Arch Phys Med Rehabil 78(suppl):S65–S71, 1997.
7. Wood-Dauphinee S, Opzoomer A, Williams JI, et al: Assessment of global function: The reintegration to normal living index. Arch Phys Med Rehabil 69:583–590, 1988.

XIV. Physical Modalities

84. THE PHYSICAL AGENTS

Jeffrey R. Basford, M.D., Ph.D., and Veronika Fialka-Moser, M.D.

1. What is a physical agent?

A physical agent uses physical forces to speed healing and lessen pain. In theory, any physical phenomenon (e.g., pressure, heat, cold, electricity, sound, or light) may be utilized. In practice, only **heat, cold, water, ultrasound, shortwaves,** and **electricity** are widely used. Although these agents can seem esoteric, they are in essence quite simple and, for the most part, produce only a limited number of effects: heating, cooling, analgesia, muscle movement, and tissue healing. Although use of newer agents, such as ultrasound, shortwaves, and electrical stimulation, has increased, heat and cold remain the basis of most treatments.

2. Are the physical agents effective when used alone?

Physical agents are seldom used in isolation and are almost always used as adjuncts to a therapy program. As such, they supplement, but do not replace, exercise, stretching, massage, education, and medical or surgical interventions.

3. What are the limitations of the physical agents?

Although each agent has unique characteristics, many ultimately rely on heat or cold to gain their effects. As a result, they share common restrictions on their use based on the amount of energy that can be added to (heating) or taken away from (cooling) tissue. In particular, temperatures $\geq 45–50°C$ ($100–120°F$) or $< 0°C$ ($32°F$) can easily injure tissue. In practice, treatments involving these temperatures may be used for restricted portions of the body, but broader areas are treated less intensely.

HEAT AND COLD

4. How do physical agents heat or cool tissue?

There are only three ways that tissue temperature can be altered:

1. **Conduction** is defined as the transfer of heat between two bodies in contact at different temperatures. Examples include hot packs and paraffin baths.

2. **Convection** also involves contact between two objects at different temperatures but also requires that one flow past the other. This flow maximizes the temperature gradient between the objects (e.g., a whirlpool bath), so more intense heating and cooling are possible than by conduction alone.

3. **Conversive heating** utilizes the conversion of another form of energy to heat. Heat lamps and ultrasound diathermy, for example, rely on the conversion of infrared light and sound to heat.

5. What forms of heat therapy are available?

Superficial and deep. Superficial agents heat the skin and subcutaneous tissues. Deep heating agents, also known as **diathermies,** heat more deeply and can raise temperatures to therapeutic levels at depths of 3.5–7 cm. Hot packs and heat lamps characterize the superficial agents, whereas ultrasound and shortwave typify the diathermies.

6. What forms of cold therapy (cryotherapy) are available?

Cold is produced by the relative absence of thermal energy. Because a lack of energy cannot be projected, only superficial agents can be used. Conversive cooling is therefore not possible, and cooling therapies must rely on conduction and convection with agents such as ice packs and chilled whirlpools.

7. List five general goals of heat and cryotherapy.

Heat therapy	Cryotherapy
1. Analgesia	1. Analgesia
2. Muscle "spasm" relaxation	2. Muscle "spasm" relaxation
3. Hyperemia	3. Inflammation
4. Increased collagen extensibility	4. Spasticity
5. Acceleration of metabolic processes	5. Slowing of metabolic activity

8. Name the major contraindications to therapeutic heat.

Acute hemorrhage, inflammation, or trauma   Inability to respond to pain
Ischemia   Atrophic or scarred skin
Insensitivity   Bleeding dyscrasias
Malignancy

9. List four common superficial heating agents.

Hot packs, heat lamps, hot-water soaks/whirlpools, and paraffin baths.

10. Describe the use of hot packs.

Hot packs (such as Hydrocollator packs) consist of canvas bags filled with a silicon dioxide sand that can absorb many times its weight in water. The packs are hung on racks in water baths maintained at 70–80°C (168–175°F). During use, the packs are taken from the baths, excess water is drained off, and then the packs are wrapped in toweling or placed in an insulated cover. *Packs must be laid on, not under, the body* (see figure). Packs can maintain therapeutically useful temperatures for 20–30 minutes. Alternative forms of hot packs (e.g., mud packs) are used in a similar manner but contain materials that may have slightly different thermodynamic properties (or purported medicinal benefits) that result from the nature of the filling material itself. These packs are in relatively wide use in Europe but are uncommon in the U.S.

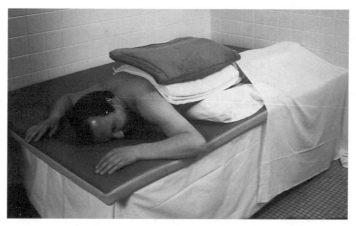

Hot pack treatment of the lower back. The pack is wrapped in an insulating cover and placed on, not under, the patient. (From Basford JR: Physical agents. In DeLisa JA, Gans BM (eds): Rehabilitation Medicine: Principles and Practice, 2nd ed. Philadelphia, J.B. Lippincott, 1993, pp 404–424, with permission.)

11. **What should I know about heat lamps?**
    - Although some heat lamps use special infrared (IR) heating elements, there is *no proof* that they are significantly more effective than other lamps that use regular incandescent bulbs.
    - Most lamps act as "point sources," and their heating effectiveness decreases with the square of their distance from the body (the $1/r^2$ law).
    - The patient should be warned that heat can produce reddish or brownish skin mottling (erythema ab igne), which may advance to permanent skin mottling with chronic use.
    - In practice, most heat lamps in the home and clinic use 100–150-W incandescent light bulbs and are placed 50–75 cm from the body.

12. **How are paraffin baths used?**
    Paraffin baths consist of 1:7 mixtures of mineral oil and paraffin maintained at about 52∞C. Paraffin treatments commonly take one of three forms. **Dipping** is the most common and involves placing the part to be treated (e.g., the hand) in the bath, removing it, pausing briefly to let the wax harden, and then repeating the cycle 10 times. The treated area is then covered with a plastic sheet and an insulating mitt for about 20 minutes. **Immersion** provides more vigorous heating than dipping and entails dipping the area into paraffin several times and then keeping it immersed for about 20 minutes. The third method uses a **brush** to paint paraffin onto portions of the body that cannot be easily placed in a bath.

    Paraffin baths are widely used to treat patients with rheumatoid arthritis of the hands who find simpler treatments, such as hot soaks or contrast baths, ineffective. These baths also are used to treat contractures, particularly in the hands and in those with scleroderma. Since paraffin baths are essentially filled with molten wax; bath temperatures must be monitored carefully to avoid burns.

13. **What are contrast baths and how are they used?**
    Contrast baths consist of two reservoirs filled with water, one warm (43°C) and one cool (16°C). Treatment typically begins with a 10-minute soak in the warm bath and then cycles between the warm and cool baths. Soaking durations vary but are often about 4 minutes in the warm bath and 1–2 minutes in the cool bath.

14. **Why are contrast baths used?**
    Contrast baths are used primarily for their purported desensitization and vasogenic reflex effects. In practice, the hands and feet are the most common sites of treatment, usually in patients with rheumatoid arthritis and neuropathic or sympathetically mediated pain (e.g., complex reginal pain syndrome [CRPS] type 1, reflex sympathetic dystrophy). Bath temperatures may be adjusted to the patient. In particular, the feet may be quite sensitive, and patients with sympathetically mediated pain may require less extreme initial temperatures.

15. **Which superficial heating agent is the most beneficial?**
    No agent is clearly the most beneficial. In specific situations, there may be reasons to choose one over another, but the choice ultimately depends on patient and therapist preference.

16. **When is cryotherapy appropriate? How is it performed?**
    Ice packs are probably the most common form of cryotherapy. Ice massage is frequently used for more intense treatment of localized areas of musculoskeletal pain, such as attachment syndromes (e.g., lateral epicondylitis). Ice slushes and whirlpools tend to be used mostly for motivated athletes who are willing to tolerate discomfort in the hope of a more rapid recovery. Chemical ice packs and vapocoolant sprays have varying levels of use, the former for acute injuries and the latter in the "spray and stretch" treatment of trigger points. Ice use is enshrined in the RICE (rest, ice, compression, elevation) approach to the treatment of acute musculoskeletal injury, spasms, and chronic musculoskeletal pain.

17. What are some of the physiologic effects of cryotherapy?

Analgesia, vasoconstriction, and control of the swelling associated with acute injury are the most obvious. However, spasticity can be reduced (if cooling is prolonged enough to reach the level of the muscle spindles), nerve conduction delayed, and metabolism slowed by cooling. Cryotherapy reduces blood flow in the area of treatment through its vasoconstrictive effects and may produce longer-lasting effects than heat.

18. Name the contraindications of cryotherapy.

Many of the contraindications for ice, like all physical agents, are relative. Thus, ice massage of a diabetic with neuropathy and atherosclerotic disease might be appropriate for trochanteric bursitis but not for a foot condition. The most common contraindications for ice include ischemia, Raynaud's syndrome, insensitivity, inability to respond to pain, cryoglobulinemia, cold allergy, and cold-induced pressor responses.

HYDROTHERAPY

19. What do I need to know about whirlpools?

Whirlpools use agitated water to produce convective heating or cooling, massage, and gentle debridement. Unit size, water temperature, agitation intensity, and solvent properties may all be adjusted to meet treatment goals. Water temperature is determined by the amount of the body submerged, the patient's health, and goals of treatment. A hand or limited portion of a limb with intact sensation may tolerate temperatures up to 45°C, but as more of the body is submerged, temperature should decrease—commonly to 40–41°C for immersion to the waist and 38–39°C if most of the body is submerged. The condition of the patient is important; an elderly diabetic patient would be treated more cautiously than a young athlete.

20. How are wounds treated with hydrotherapy?

Wounds treated with hydrotherapy typically have open areas with necrotic debris, adherent dressings, or contaminated or irregular surfaces. Wound sizes can range from small hand cuts and abrasions to large, secondarily infected, healing abdominal wounds. Dehiscence is not a contraindication, and, for example, exposed omentum or intestinal tissues do not prevent treatment if bath temperature, osmolality, and agitation parameters are chosen carefully. Agitation is adjusted to match patient preferences and treatment goals. Patients with large wounds may be fearful that treatment will be painful, but surprisingly, correctly adjusted baths are extraordinarily comfortable. Alternative hydrotherapy treatments are possible. When forceful debridement of large wounds is necessary, hand-held showerheads and sprays may be used. Small wounds may be treated with commercial footbaths or hand-held water jets, such as a WaterPik.

21. How can hydrotherapy solvent properties be manipulated? Why?

Warmed tap water (which is itself amazingly sterile) is usually used alone for hydrotherapy and debridement. Gentle detergents and antiseptic solutions may be added in the hopes of improving debridement and wound cleansing. Salt can be dissolved in a bath to produce a normal saline (0.9% NaCl) solution to improve comfort and reduce concerns about hemolysis and water intoxication in patients with large wounds.

22. List five common indications for hydrotherapy.
1. Open, contaminated wounds
2. Contractures
3. Muscle spasm
4. Burns
5. Morbidly obese, immobilized patients who cannot be cleansed in another manner

ULTRASOUND DIATHERMY

23. What is diathermy and what are the diathermy agents?

Diathermy means "heating through" (*thermy*, "heat"; *dia-*, "through"). Three diathermies have been used in the clinic: ultrasound, radio wave (shortwave and decimeter wave, in Europe), and microwave. All heat tissue conversively, sound being the energy source in the first case and electromagnetic energy in the latter. Microwave diathermy is still used in restrictive areas of medicine (e.g., some forms of prostate surgery and chemotherapy) but is now rarely used in therapy.

24. What are the important characteristics of ultrasound?

Ultrasound has all the characteristics of audible sound but is limited to frequencies above the nominal 20,000-Hz limit of human hearing. As such, ultrasound requires a medium for transmission and can be focused, reflected, or refracted (bent). Although a wide range of frequencies between 0.3 and 3 MHz are used, many feel that the best trade-off between focusing properties and tissue penetration occurs in the 0.8–1.0-MHz frequency range.

25. What effects does ultrasound have on the body?

Heating is the most important and best understood effect. **Nonthermal effects,** such as cavitation, media motion, and standing waves, also exist, but their therapeutic benefits are not understood as well. Cavitation, for example, produces bubbles, which, by their forced oscillation and bursting, are capable of disrupting tissue. Small-scale media motion may occur from ultrasound exposure. Standing-wave patterns in a stationary ultrasound field produce fixed areas of elevated pressure and rarefaction that have been found to have physiologic effects in the laboratory.

26. How deeply does ultrasound penetrate into tissue?

The depth of clinically beneficial heating depends on the power applied, nature of the tissue, direction of the beam, and frequency of the beam. For example, 50% of an ultrasound beam will penetrate 7–8 cm of fat but < 1 mm of bone. Direction is important in anisotropic tissue: a therapeutic ultrasound beam may penetrate 7 cm when travelling parallel to the fibers of a muscle, but only 2 cm when travelling perpendicularly. Frequency also has striking effects. Beam penetration in tissue may fall by about 85% as its frequency increases from 0.3 to 3.3 MHz. In practice, therapeutic ultrasound sources with frequencies of 0.8–1.0 MHz can produce 4–5°C temperature elevations at depths of 8 cm.

27. Where does the most intense heating take place during ultrasound treatment?

Ultrasound interacts with skin, fat, muscle, and bone during treatment. Heating occurs in all of these tissues due to beam attenuation but is most pronounced at tissue interfaces, where sound transmission discontinuities occur. **Bone–soft tissue interfaces** are where the most heating takes place. This tendency for bone–soft tissue heating provides added support for the practice of avoiding ultrasound treatment in the vicinity of laminectomy sites.

28. How is ultrasound applied?

The skin is usually coated with an acoustic gel or mineral oil to provide optimal acoustic coupling. Ultrasound is then applied by stroking the applicator (sound head) in a circular motion. Irregular body surfaces are sometimes submerged in degassed water, and the slightly separated applicator is moved over the surface. Ultrasound provides intense heating and requires the constant attention of the therapist. Treatments are relatively brief with durations of 7–10 minutes.

29. What is phonophoresis?

In phonophoresis, medication is mixed with the acoustic coupling medium in the expectation that the ultrasound beam will "drive" the pharmacologically active substance into the tissue. Penetration depths depend on the particular substance involved, and significant amounts of drug are picked up by the subcutaneous circulation. Claims of penetration to depths of several centimeters have been made. Clinical studies with topical anesthetics, corticosteroids, phenylbu-tazone, and chymotrypsin have suggested benefits, but more work is needed to establish the advantage of phonophoresis over injection or ultrasound alone.

30. What are some indications for therapeutic ultrasound?

Common	Less Established
Contractures	Wound healing
Tendinitis	Herpes zoster
Musculoskeletal pain	Plantar warts
Degenerative arthritis	
Carpal tunnel syndrome	
Subacute trauma	

SHORTWAVE AND MICROWAVE

31. What is shortwave diathermy?

Shortwave diathermy (SWD) conversively heats tissue by exposing it to radio waves produced by a machine that is essentially a shortwave radio. Although three frequencies—40.68, 27.12, and 13.56 MHz—have been allocated by the FCC for medical use in the United States, 27.12 MHz is the most commonly used frequency in both Europe and the U.S. Typical treatments involve output powers of several hundred watts.

32. How is shortwave diathermy administered?

Energy is delivered to the body by either capacitive or inductive electrodes. **Capacitive coupling** involves placing the portion of the body to be treated between two plates to which the shortwave output is applied (see figure). The body thus acts as a dielectric (insulator) in a series circuit. Heating is most marked in high-impedance, water-poor tissues such as fat. **Inductive coupling**, on the other hand, uses the body as a receiver and induces eddy currents in the tissues in its field. The highest currents, and therefore the most intense heating, occur in low-impedance, water-rich tissues, such as muscle. In practice, temperature elevations of 4–6°C can occur at depths of 4–5 cm in muscles.

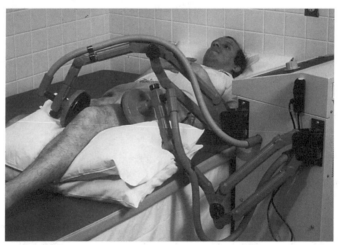

Capacitively coupled shortwave diathermy of the knee. The patient lies on an electrically nonconductive table. (From Bosford FR: Physical agents. In DeLisa JA, Gans BM (eds): Rehabilitation Medicine: Principles and Practice, 2nd ed. Philadelphia, J.B. Lippincott, 1993, pp 404–424, with permission.)

33. Discuss the limitations and contraindications of shortwave diathermy.

Water and metal are excellent electrical conductors and potentially can cause burns if present in SWD fields. Therefore, patients must remove jewelry, and perspiration should be absorbed by toweling or pads. In theory, metal implants and sutures might produce "hot spots," so most people avoid SWD when these are present. General precautions, with varying degrees of theoretical or established concern, include the avoidance of treating pregnant women, the menstruating uterus, or patients with implanted metal devices, pacemakers, defibrillators, pumps, or contact lenses.

34. What is microwave diathermy?

Microwave diathermy (MWD) is similar to shortwave diathermy in that electromagnetic waves are used to heat tissue. However, the FCC-approved frequencies for MWD are 915 and 2456 MHz, 30–100 times higher than those for SWD. MWD was once relatively common in the U.S. but is now rarely used as a therapeutic agent, having been supplanted by ultrasound and SWD. In Europe, 2450-MHz MWD is approved for treatment and is used to provide heating for superficial musculoskeletal pain. In both regions, however, MWD continues to have some medical use for localized hyperthermia in specific surgical and oncologic applications.

35. What are the characteristics of microwave diathermy?

Microwave beams, because of their higher frequencies (short wavelengths), are much more directable than SWD fields. Because tissue penetration decreases as frequency increases, MWD tends to heat more superficially than SWD and often delivers a large proportion of its energy to subcutaneous tissue.

36. What are the contraindications to microwave diathermy?

The contraindications of heat and SWD apply. In addition, microwaves produce cataracts and selectively heat fluid-filled cavities. There are also some concerns about its effect on growing bones.

ELECTRICAL STIMULATION

37. What is TENS?

Transcutaneous electrical nerve stimulation (TENS) is a form of analgesia that applies small electrical signals to the body with superficial skin electrodes. Electrodes may be placed over peripheral nerves, nerve roots, and acupuncture points, as well as proximal to, distal to, over, and (more controversially) contralateral to the areas of pain.

38. How does TENS produce analgesia?

A uniform mechanism is not well established. The "gate theory of pain," in which stimulation of large myelinated afferent fibers blocks the transmission of pain by small unmyelinated fibers at the level of the spinal cord, is often mentioned. Although it seems plausible in many ways, this theory does not explain all aspects of TENS analgesia (e.g., prolonged pain relief following use). Alteration of cerebrospinal endorphin concentrations is also reported following treatment (particularly for high-intensity TENS) but is difficult to correlate with therapeutic response.

39. Describe the characteristics of a TENS unit.

TENS units are usually programmable and small enough to fit in a pocket. Typically, they consist of a battery, one or more signal-generators, and two pairs of electrodes. Although clear benefits of one waveform over another are difficult to establish, a wide variety of continuous and modulated (e.g., pulsed, burst, ramped) signals are available. In practice, signal amplitudes are usually < 100 mA, pulse rates < 200 Hz, and pulse widths < 300 μsec. Biphasic and asymmetric waveforms are usually chosen, because they seem to be the most comfortable and should limit the tendency for a single polarity to produce electrolysis and skin irritation.

40. How many distinct TENS settings are possible?

In theory, an infinite number, but in practice, two. **High** (or conventional) TENS uses barely perceptible signal intensities with frequencies typically of 60–80 Hz. **Low** TENS uses larger-amplitude, low-frequency signals (< 4–8 Hz) that may be uncomfortable.

41. When is TENS therapy prescribed?

TENS is not a curative modality and should be used only in the absence of more effective alternatives. In addition, this is not an inexpensive treatment. In the U.S., a unit may cost $100 a month to rent and as much as $1000 to purchase. The cost in Europe is also significant (150–450 euros to purchase). As a result, the decision to prescribe a device requires careful assessment. Frequently, several therapy sessions are needed to establish electrode placement, stimulator settings, and benefits. Ideally, the unit can be used at home for a day or so before a final judgment is made. If the condition being treated has been refractory to other treatment, and TENS's benefits significant, rental is reasonable. Purchase is not considered until several months of stable, consistent use, and benefits have been documented.

42. Is TENS effective?

Systematic assessment of TENS's effectiveness is difficult because of the subjective nature of pain, varying study designs, diverse parameter choices (e.g., stimulation frequency, waveform), and the differing conditions evaluated. Studies in postsurgical, obstetric, and general musculoskeletal settings find benefits ranging from placebo levels to 95%. Other studies have reported elevated cutaneous perfusion and temperature in patients with neuropathy, accelerated wound healing, and elevated pain thresholds following treatment. In the end, success is sporadic and seems to depend on the individual patient.

43. List seven common uses for TENS.
1. Musculoskeletal pain
2. Post-traumatic pain
3. Postsurgical pain
4. Peripheral nerve injury
5. Peripheral neuropathy
6. Phantom limb pain
7. Sympathetically mediated pain (reflex sympathetic dystrophy, causalgia)

44. List six contraindications for TENS use.
1. Stimulation over the carotid sinuses
2. Cardiac pacemakers or implanted cardiac defibrillators
3. Pregnancy (although the risk from distal treatment seems small)
4. Inability to report effects or discomfort
5. Atrophic skin
6. Allergies to the electrodes or gels

45. What is iontophoresis?

Electric fields can accelerate the movement of charged atoms or molecules (ions) through the skin. Iontophoresis, operating on this principle, uses charged electrodes (positive or negative) to drive medically active, charged (polar) substances into the skin. Any charged or polar substance can theoretically be iontophoresed, and medications have included lidocaine, iodine, salicylate, gentamicin, cefoxitin, and silver.

46. What is iontophoresis used for?

Iontophoresis with tap water (referred to as *galvanization* in Europe) is an effective treatment of hyperhidrosis of the hands, feet, and axilla. It has also been used to deliver antibiotics to poorly vascularized tissue, such as cartilage, to produce local anesthesia, to speed wound healing, and to treat musculoskeletal pain. Although there is evidence that treatment can be effective, many feel that an injection can provide higher concentrations of an active medication with more speed and less difficulty.

47. What is low-intensity electrical stimulation?

TENS is one form of low-intensity electrical stimulation. In addition, a variety of milliampere- and even microampere-current generators have been studied for > 30 years. Although benefits are well established in the treatment of nonhealing fractures, their use for other indications (such as wound healing) remains mostly investigational.

48. Can electrical stimulation increase muscle strength?

Electrical stimulation can be used to maintain muscle bulk and strength, but there is little evidence that it can strengthen healthy active muscle more effectively than exercise alone. Applications of this technique are relatively limited to maintaining strength in immobilized limbs and training of paretic muscles following stroke or peripheral nerve or spinal injury.

49. What is functional neuromuscular stimulation?

Functional neuromuscular stimulation (FNS), also known as functional electrical stimulation (FES), utilizes electrical stimulation to provide functional movement of paretic muscles. Stimulation may be done in conjunction with orthoses and may involve the complex programming and coordinated stimulation of many muscles. In theory, FNS might benefit anyone with a neuromuscular impairment, but in practice, limitations imposed by its complexity, cost, reliability, electrode positioning, donning, and safety have restricted its use. Foot-drop orthoses and exercise and ambulation devices for spinal cord injury are the best-known applications of this approach. With time, FNS may supply simple and unobtrusive help for people with stroke and other neurologic deficits.

50. What is interferential current?

Electrical waves that differ slightly in frequency but are otherwise identical can interact with each other and produce **product waveforms** with frequencies equal to the sum or differences of the original waves. Interferential current machines take advantage of this phenomena and generate waves at different frequencies—e.g., 2000 and 2040 Hz—which can penetrate tissue without discomfort. Pairs of electrodes associated with each wave are placed so that the waves cross at the area to be treated. The waves *interfere* at this crossing point and produce a "difference" wave (here, 40 Hz—in the clinical situation, only the low-frequency "difference" waves are important) that can be used to produce TENS effects or stimulate muscle contraction. It turns out that modulated high-frequency carrier waves alone may be able to provide many of these benefits without the need for the interaction of two beams.

PRESSURE

51. How are pneumatic pumps used?

Numerous pneumatic devices are available with varying cycling modes (e.g., fixed or associated with heart beat) and construction (e.g., single or multicompartment). These pumps are often effective in controlling edema but should be used only if elevation and compressive wraps alone are ineffective. Pressure settings depend on the device but are often set between the venous and arterial pressures. Treatment durations are prolonged, sometimes involving hours per day. Between treatments, the limb is kept elevated and wrapped in compressive dressings. There are also many reports that pneumatic pumping can improve arterial perfusion in the distal extremities, but their value and usage are still under investigation.

52. What do I need to know about using compressive garments?

Compressive garments are measured and applied once limb edema has been minimized. Pressures are maximal at the wrist or ankle and lessen proximally in a graduated manner.

Garments are specified by their maximal pressures (e.g., 20, 30, 40, and at times, 50 mmHg). Stocking pressures and style (e.g., calf-high, thigh-high, leotard) are dictated by edema severity and the patient's ability to doff and don the garment. Most lower-extremity stockings are in the 30–40-mmHg range, with allowances made for sensation, perfusion, and patient compliance. In most cases, off-the-shelf garments are suitable, although custom-measured garments are often necessary for people who are obese, difficult to fit, or need compression for less common applications such as post-burn treatment..

53. List six common indications for compression garments.
1. Treated deep venous thrombosis
2. Venous incompetence
3. Postmastectomy edema
4. Edema due to congestive heart failure
5. Lymphedema
6. Orthostatic blood pressure resistant to medical treatment (garments must be thigh-length or a leotard to be effective)

54. List four contraindications to pneumatic pumping.
Active deep venous thrombosis, cellulitis, compromised perfusion, or severely impaired sensation.

55. What are some simple rules of thumb about compressive garments?
• Use the shortest garment possible.
• Thigh-length garments slide down the leg without the use of straps or adhesive.
• Men tend to resist leotards.
• Garments are more effective with slender people.
• Obese people tolerate garments poorly.
• Most patients can be fitted with off-the-shelf garments.

ALTERNATIVE AND NEW PHYSICAL AGENTS

56. How is laser therapy used in physical medicine?
Low-intensity laser irradiation has been used for > 30 years to promote wound healing and to lessen pain and speed recovery from musculoskeletal injury. Many devices have been used, but most have powers < 100 mW and utilize red (0.6 μm) or infrared (0.82–1.06 μm) wavelengths. Irradiation produces striking effects on cellular processes, immune function, and collagen formation in the laboratory. Unfortunately, translation of these findings into the clinic has been difficult. Despite widespread use in Europe and Asia, laser therapy has not yet gained FDA approval for clinical use in the U.S.

57. Are there other new physical agents or new applications of older agents?
Yes, laser therapy and shock wave therapy perhaps have had the most attention, but other agents, and old agents with new uses, exist. For example, ultrasound and low-intensity electromagnetic fields accelerate fracture healing. In addition, there are a number of newer agents with, thus far, limited proof of effectiveness. Among these is the use of dynamic magnetic field stimulation to treat painful musculoskeletal conditions and stress incontinence and the use of "micro"-electromagnetic and static magnetic fields are felt by some to have beneficial effects.

BIBLIOGRAPHY

1. Balmaseda MT, Fatehi MT, Koozekanani SH, Lee AL: Ultrasound therapy: A comparative study of different coupling media. Arch Phys Med Rehabil 67:149–152, 1986.
2. Banga AK, Bose S, Ghosh TK: Iontophoresis and electroporation: Comparisons and contrasts. Int J Pharm 179:1–19, 1999.

3. Basford JR: Low intensity laser therapy: still not an established clinical tool. Lasers Surg Med 16:31–42, 1995.
4. Basford JR: Physical agents. In DeLisa JA, Gans BM (eds): Rehabilitation Medicine: Principles and Practice, 3rd ed. Philadelphia, Lippincott Williams & Wilkins, 1998, pp 483–504.
5. Chantraine A, Ludy JP, Berger D: Is cortisone iontophoresis possible? Arch Phys Med Rehabil 67:38–40, 1986.
6. Downing DS, Weinstein A: Ultrasound therapy of subcranial bursitis: A double-blind trial. Phys Ther 66:194–199, 1986.
7. Ebenbichler GR, Erdogmus CB, Resch KL, et al: Ultrasound therapy for calcific tendinitis of the shoulder. N Engl J Med 340:1533-1538, 1999.
8. Ebenbichler G, Resch KL, Nicolakis P, et al: Ultrasound therapy is effective in treating carpal tunnel syndrome: Results of a randomised "sham"-controlled trial. BMJ 316:731–735, 1998.
9. Franchimont P, Juchmes I, Lecomite J: Hydrotherapy: Mechanisms and indications. Pharmacol Ther 20:79–93, 1983.
10. Hammer DS, Rupp ST, Ensslin ST, et al: Extracorporal shock wave therapy in patients with tennis elbow and painful heel. Arch Orthop Trauma Surg 120:304–307, 2000.
11. Hunt JW: Applications of microwave, ultrasound, and radiofrequency heating. Natl Cancer Inst Monogr 61:447–456, 1982.
12. Knight KL: Cryotherapy: Theory, Technique and Physiology. Chattanooga, TN, Chattanooga Corp., 1985.
13. Lake DA: Neuromuscular electrical stimulation: An overview and its application in the treatment of sports injuries. Sports Med 13:320–336, 1992.
14. Lehman JF, de Lateur BJ: Diathermy and superficial heat, laser and cold therapy. In Krusen's Handbook of Physical Medicine and Rehabilitation, 4th ed. Philadelphia, W.B. Saunders, 1990, pp 283–367.
15. Melzack R, Jeans ME, Stratford JG, Monks RC: Ice massage and transcutaneous electrical stimulation: Comparison of treatment for low back pain. Pain 9:209–217, 1980.
16. Quittan M, Sochor A, Wiesinger GF, et al: Strength improvement of knee extensor muscles in patients with chronic heart failure by neuromuscular electrical stimulation. Artif Org 23:432–435, 1999.

85. ELECTROTHERAPY

Peter H. Gorman, M.D., M.S., Norman Shealy, M.D., Ph.D., Saul Liss, Ph.D., Stanley H. Kornhauser, Ph.D., and Charles Cannizzaro, M.D., P.T.

1. What is functional electrical stimulation (FES)?

FES is the technique of applying safe levels of electric current to activate the damaged or disabled nervous system. FES is sometimes referred to as **functional neuromuscular stimulation** or **neuromuscular electrical stimulation**. Depending on one's perspective, neuromuscular electrical stimulation may be considered a more general or more specific term, because it includes both therapeutic and functional purposes but excludes use in sensory systems, such as cochlear prostheses.

2. Do FES systems for muscle activation stimulate nerve or muscle?

Motor units are activated electrically by depolarization of motor axons or their terminal nerve branches at the neuromuscular junction. A muscle can be directly depolarized by electrical current, but the amount of current necessary for this to occur is considerably greater than that for the nerve. Therefore, for practical purposes, FES systems stimulate nerves, not muscles.

3. What happens to FES-stimulated muscles over time?

Just like muscles undergoing voluntary exercise, FES-stimulated muscles will change morphologically and physiologically. Type II glycolytic fibers will convert to type I oxidative fibers over weeks to months, depending on the intensity and frequency of stimulation. This phenomenon is associated with changes in vascular supply and increases the fatigue resistance of the muscle.

4. What are the clinical applications of FES in rehabilitation?
1. Muscle strengthening
2. Improvement in range of motion (ROM)
3. Facilitation and re-education of voluntary motor function
4. Orthotic training, restoration of functional movement or activity
5. Inhibition of spasticity or muscle spasm

5. What are the contraindications to FES?
Although there are **no absolute contraindications** for use of FES, patients with a cardiac demand pacemaker should be approached with extreme caution. Electrical stimulation applied anywhere on the body has the potential to interfere with the sensing portion of the demand pacemaker. **Relative contraindications** include patients with cardiac arrhythmias, congestive heart failure, pregnancy, electrode sensitivity, or healing wounds (muscle stimulation may adversely move healing tissues). For the most part, implantable FES devices are MRI compatible, but each device must be assessed individually before imaging is performed.

6. What conditions may benefit from FES technology?
• Paralysis, spasticity, and cardiovascular deconditioning
• Neurogenic bowel, bladder, and sexual dysfunction resulting from spinal cord injury (SCI), stroke, multiple sclerosis, or closed head injury
• Epilepsy, scoliosis, tremor, restoration of hearing, and restoration of vision
• Pain control (TENS), iontophoresis, and wound healing

7. List the uses of FES in spinal cord injury.
Therapeutic uses. Muscle strengthening and cardiac conditioning. Possible other benefits include improvement in venous return from the legs, reduction of osteoporosis, improvement in bowel function, and psychological benefits.
Functional uses. Standing, walking, hand grasp (and release), bladder, bowel and sexual function, respiratory assist, and electroejaculation for fertility.

8. Explain the rationale behind use of FES-induced exercise in patients with spinal cord injury.
Persons with SCI are generally forced to become more sedentary. Paralysis is compounded by impaired autonomic nervous system function, which limits the cardiovascular response to exercise, especially in individuals with lesions at or above T5. Muscle bulk, strength, and endurance all decrease after SCI, and muscle fibers convert primarily to anaerobic metabolism after injury. Paralysis of intracostal musculature reduces vital capacity. In addition, there is reduced peripheral circulation, lean body mass, and bone density and an altered endocrine response.

9. What systems are available for therapeutic electrical stimulation in persons with SCI?
The most common system for lower-extremity FES exercise is the **bicycle ergometer**. The most common commercially available ergometer in use is the ERGYS Clinical Rehabilitation System made by Therapeutic Technologies, Inc. (Tampa, FL). This computer-controlled FES exercise ergometer uses six channels and surface electrodes to sequentially stimulate quadriceps, hamstring, and glutei bilaterally. Some systems also include the capacity for simultaneous voluntary arm-crank exercise by paraplegics, permitting hybrid exercise.

10. What benefits can be anticipated in subjects involved in FES bicycle ergometry?
Cardiac capacity and muscle oxidative capacity both improve with FES ergometry. Some patients can train with FES ergometry up to a similar aerobic metabolic rate (measured by peak VO_2) as is achieved in the able-bodied population. Electrical exercise also increases peripheral venous return and fibrinolysis, and in one study, FES in conjunction with heparin therapy was more effective in preventing deep venous thrombosis than heparin alone. There are limits to the

cardiovascular benefits of FES ergometry, however, especially in those with lesions at or above T5. In those patients, there is loss of supraspinal sympathetic control, which in turn limits the body's ability to increase heart rate, stroke volume, and cardiac output.

11. What about FES for standing and walking in paraplegia?

At least 17 laboratories worldwide have or are investigating the use of FES for lower-extremity standing and walking in paraplegia. Several different approaches are being researched. Hybrid approaches, such as the **reciprocating gait orthosis** (RGO), use both mechanical bracing and surface FES. Specifically, FES hip extension on one side provides contralateral leg swing through the RGO mechanism. Quadriceps stimulation then provides knee lock.

Only one surface FES walking system is FDA-approved for use in the U.S. The **Parastep System** (Sigmetics, Inc.) uses the triple flexion response elicited by peroneal nerve stimulation as well as knee and hip extensor surface stimulation to construct the gait cycle. The patient controls the gait with switches integrated into a rolling walker (which is also needed for stability and safety).

Implantable lower-extremity FES has also been developed to aid in activating deep musculature. Both percutaneous electrodes and implantable stimulator-receivers with epimysial or intramuscular electrodes have been tested, although neither is currently available commercially. A multicenter trial of implantable FES standing systems is currently underway.

12. What about FES for restoration of hand grasp in tetraplegia?

Tetraplegic hand grasp systems have focused on the C5- and C6-level SCI populations. Patients with C4-level injury (i.e., those without biceps or deltoid strength) have participated in limited laboratory investigations of FES systems. Patients injured at the C7 and lower levels have multiple voluntary active forearm muscles (e.g., brachioradialis, extensor carpi radialis longus and brevis, pronator teres), which can be used to motor new functions without sacrificing current function through techniques of tendon transfer surgery Physiologically, patients considered for implantable hand grasp systems need to have adequate motor innervation of forearm and hand muscles to allow for FES grasp synthesis. Best results occur with motivated people who have good social support systems to reinforce use.

13. What are the components of the implantable FES hand grasp system? How does it work?

The Neuroprosthetic Hand Grasp System, commercially known as the Freehand System, initially developed at Case Western Reserve University, consists of (1) an external joint position transducer/controller, (2) a rechargeable programmable external control unit (ECU), and (3) an implantable eight-channel stimulator/receiver attached via flexible wires to epimysial disc electrodes. The user controls the system through small movements of either the shoulder or wrist. The joint position transducer, which operates somewhat like a computer joystick, typically is mounted on the skin from sternum to contralateral shoulder or across the ipsilateral wrist, and senses these movements. The ECU uses this signal to proportionally control hand grasp and release. Communication between the ECU and the implantable stimulator, which is located in a surgical pocket created in the upper chest, occurs through radio frequency coupling. The system can be programmed through a personal computer interface by a trained therapist to individualize the grasps as well as the shoulder control for each patient.

Future improvements in tetraplegic hand grasp systems likely will include implantable controllers, greater number of stimulation channels, closed-loop feedback, proximal muscle control (i.e., triceps or biceps) in C4 and C5 patients, and bilateral implementation of grasp in C6-level tetraplegic individuals.

14. How do bladder stimulation systems work in spinal cord injury?

Electrical stimulation to control bladder function after suprasacral SCI is now commercially available both in the U.S. and Europe. The most experience and success has occurred with a device termed the Vocare System (in the U.S.), which provides S2 through S4 anterior sacral nerve root stimulation. This system is surgically implanted through lumbar laminectomy, employs either epidural or intradural electrodes, and usually is done in conjunction with a dorsal rhizotomy. The electrodes are connected via cable to an implanted radio receiver, which couples to an external stimulator/transmitter. Pulsed stimulation is used to take advantage of the differences between activation of the slow-response smooth musculature of the detrusor and activation of the fast-twitch striated sphincter musculature. This produces short spurts of urination but can result in nearly complete bladder emptying. The sacral anterior root stimulators have also been shown to improve bowel care (i.e., increased defecation, reduced constipation) in those patients using them. Approximately 60% of men can also produce penile erection with the device.

15. What is the role of FES in respiratory assistance?

In a high-level tetraplegic individual injured at C1 or C2, the use of the phrenic pacemaker has become a standard part of the clinical armamentarium and an alternative to chronic ventilator dependence. Those with lower level injuries (i.e., C3 and C4) who do not have adequate voluntary respiration may have phrenic nerve denervation precluding the use of phrenic pacing techniques. Therefore, phrenic nerve conduction studies must be performed before considering this type of FES device.

16. What is TENS?

TENS is a form of electrical analgesia whose mechanism of action is based partially on the **gate theory of pain** popularized by Melzack and Wall in 1965. That theory explains TENS analgesia as resulting from a blocking mechanism via non-nociceptive receptors carrying the TENS signal on faster-conducting, myelinated fibers, inhibiting the nociceptive stimuli caused by smaller, myelinated, slower A-delta and small, unmyelinated C-fibers in subthalamic nuclei. It is also postulated that TENS effects are partially secondary to release of endogenous opiates (neuropeptides), possibly endorphins in higher CNS centers and enkephalins in the dorsal horns of the spinal cord.

TENS is a single therapeutic modality and is best utilized as part of a comprehensive individualized rehab program.

17. Is there an optimal waveform employed in the use of TENS for pain management?

Some studies claim that there is a stronger endorphin release at low-frequency (< 10 Hz), high-amplitude stimulation than with higher-frequency (60–100 Hz), lower-intensity stimulation ("conventional" TENS); however, experimental findings are mixed.

18. What other effects besides analgesia have been noted with the use of TENS?

Although these effects are controversial, and results remain poorly confirmed, some authors report TENS affecting vasodilatation in subjects with chronic skin ulcers, diabetic neuropathy, and Raynaud's phenomena. Low-frequency TENS has been reported to raise pain thresholds, but pain thresholds are not altered or increased according to other authors. The relative effects of low- and high-frequency TENS are not well understood and may be related to the intensity of the stimulation.

19. What applications are commonly used for TENS in pain management?

TENS is appropriate in the treatment of both acute and chronic pain. Success rates vary, from placebo rates to approximately 30–95%. The reasons for the difference in outcomes probably result from differences in stimulating parameters, electrode placement, type and duration of pain, concurrent medication, previous treatment, choice of controls, length of follow-up, and patient expectations.

20. Is there an optimal placement of TENS electrodes on the skin?

Determination of stimulation parameters and patterns of electrode placement remains more an art than a science. Generally, a painful area is sandwiched between a pair or pairs of electrodes. (Most TENS units have dual-channel capability with independent stimulation para-meter settings for each pair of electrodes.) However, electrodes can be placed paravertebrally or proximal and distal to a nerve feeding a site of pain. Some applications are placed over acupuncture sites on the body or auricular points via small clip electrodes as a form of elec-troacupuncture.

21. Does one know immediately whether a TENS placement provides adequate analgesia?

A single session usually will not indicate the success or failure of a TENS application. The patient usually requires at least an overnight trial or even several days to establish efficacy. A rea-sonable period of evaluation (1 week) also allows elimination of placebo effect as well as opti-mization of stimulation parameters, such as pulse width, duration, and intensity. Too often, TENS may be considered a failure, not for lack of physiologic effect, but for lack of adequate patient in-struction, less-than-optimal electrode placement montage or stimulation parameter setting, or failure of the clinician to get a detailed description from the patient on what effect was derived, and the patient's opinion as to the success of the trial.

22. Is TENS used continuously for pain management when it has been determined to be beneficial in a subject?

No optimal utilization time of TENS has been determined. Usage is individualized and usu-ally is determined with an adequate trial-and-error period.

High-frequency TENS ("conventional" TENS, 60–100 Hz) is applied at barely perceptible levels to two to three times the sensory threshold and can usually be tolerated for many hours daily. Low-frequency TENS (~0.5–10 Hz) usually involves stronger intensities at three to five times the sensory threshold and is comfortably tolerated for 20–30-minute periods for several short sessions daily. An often-used approach is to initiate TENS therapy at high-frequency levels and then switch to low-frequency only if the higher frequency is not effective. Most patients find the low-frequency uncomfortable at the higher intensity and additionally complain of the annoy-ing perception of "beating."

23. What is the key to successful use of TENS?

If TENS is to be successful, it directly reflects the patience, time, and anatomic knowledge of the therapist. TENS should never be employed solely in the treatment of low back pain. The Quebec Task Force concluded that decreased pain relief has been demonstrated, but the sole use of TENS has not been shown to accelerate return to work or to a usual level of function. TENS contributes most effectively to a carefully developed comprehensive rehab program with close physiatric monitoring.

24. What are the contraindications for TENS use?

TENS should best be viewed as an ancillary device utilized for the symptomatic control of pain to facilitate exercise training and functional restoration.
• Avoid TENS in the presence of a pacemaker, particularly a demand one.
• Placement over the carotid sinus may produce a vasovagal response.
• Safety in pregnancy has not been established.
• Skin sensitivity to the electrode or tape may occur but is sometimes avoidable with skin barrier preparation.

25. What are the precautions for TENS?

1. TENS should be used with caution for undiagnosed pain syndromes in which the etiology has not been established.
2. TENS is less effective for pain of central origin than pain of peripheral origin.
3. TENS devices should be used only under the supervision of a physician.
4. TENS devices should be kept out of reach of children.

BIBLIOGRAPHY

1. Baker LL, McNeal DR, Benton LA, et al: Neuromuscular Electrical Stimulation: A Practical Guide, 3rd ed. Downey, CA, Rancho Los Amigos Medical Center, 1993.
2. Creasey GH: Restoration of bladder, bowel and sexual function. Top Spinal Cord Inj Rehabil 5:21–32, 1999.
3. Faghri PD, Rodgers MM, Glaser RM, et al: The effects of functional electrical stimulation on shoulder subluxation, arm function recovery, and shoulder pain in hemiplegic stroke patients. Arch Phys Med Rehabil 75:73–79, 1994.
4. Glaser RM: Physiology of functional electrical stimulation-induced exercise: Basic science perspective. J Neurol Rehabil 5:49–61, 1991.
5. Glenn WWL, Brouillette RT, Dentz B, et al: Fundamental considerations in pacing of the diaphragm for chronic ventilatory insufficiency: A multi-center study. Pacing Clin Electrophysiol 11:2121–2127, 1988.
6. Gorman PH: An update on functional electrical stimulation after spinal cord injury. J Neurorehabil Neural Repair 14:251–263, 2000.
7. Keith MW, Lacey SH: Surgical rehabilitation of the tetraplegic upper extremity. J Neurol Rehabil 5:75–87, 1991.
8. Mannheimer J, Lampe G: Pain and TENS management. In Mannheimer J, Lampe G (eds): Clinical Transcutaenous Electrical Nerve Stimulation. Philadelphia, F.A. Davis, 1985, pp 7–27.
9. Peckham PH, Creasey GH: Neural prostheses: Clinical applications of functional electrical stimulation in spinal cord injury. Paraplegia 30:96–101, 1992.
10. Ragnarsson KT, Pollack SF, Twist D: Lower limb endurance exercise after spinal cord injury: Implications for health and functional ambulation. J Neurol Rehabil 5:37–48, 1991.
11. Spitzer W, et al: Scientific approach to the assessment and management of activity-related spinal disorders: A monograph for clinicians. Report of the Quebec Task Force on Spinal Disorders. Spine 12(suppl):S1–S57, 1987.
12. Yarkony GM, et al: Neuromuscular stimulation in spinal cord injury: I. Restoration of functional movement of the extremities. Arch Phys Med Rehabil 73:78–86, 1992.

ADDITIONAL RESOURCE

Additional information about many of the emerging technologies within the FES field can be obtained from FES Information Center, 11000 Cedar Avenue, Cleveland, Ohio 44106-3052. Telephone: (800) 666-2352 or (216) 231-3257. Web site: http://feswww.fes.cwru.edu

86. TRACTION, MANIPULATION, AND MASSAGE

Steven R. Hinderer, M.D., M.S., P.T., and Peter E. Biglin, D.O.

1. What physiologic effect(s) does traction have?

Most studies have concluded that elongation of the cervical spine, of 2–20 mm, can be achieved with 25 lbs or more of tractive force. Ten pounds is needed to counterbalance the weight of the head (less in some persons, more in others). It is proposed that prolonged pull on the cervical spine with adequate force leads to fatigue of cervical paraspinal muscles, which is potentially of therapeutic value when muscle spasm is present.

It has been less consistently demonstrated that traction on the lumbar spine also causes elongation when the effects of friction are overcome by adequate pull or a split table. Retraction of herniated disc material is another potential effect of lumbar traction.

2. What techniques are available for applying traction?

1. **Manual**—cervical traction performed by the physician or therapist, usually to gauge the effectiveness of mechanical or motorized methods of application
2. **Mechanical**—administered using a pulley and free weight system

3. **Motorized**—mechanical traction applied by a motorized system, administered in continuous or intermittent periods

4. **Gravity**—hanging upside down

5. **Autotraction**—uses a specially designed device that self-administers lumbar traction by pulling with the arms

3. Describe the advantages of mechanical traction administered at home versus in the clinic.

Mechanical traction can be administered at home using a pulley and free weight system. **Home cervical traction** units typically consist of a bag filled with 20 lbs or more of water or sand and a pulley system mounted on top of a door. Improper head or neck position, along with inadequate weight (< 20 lbs) are the most common reasons home cervical traction fails. Initial instruction and weekly follow-up by the therapist or physician greatly improve the chances for success.

Administration of continuous or intermittent (timed on-and-off periods) mechanical traction applied with a motorized device is commonly limited to physical therapy clinics due to the need for close monitoring of position and its effect on symptoms. Most patients tolerate greater forces of pull with intermittent administration. It is common to prescribe mechanical traction initially in the treatment course and, if benefit ensues, to continue treatment with a home unit.

4. For which patients is gravity traction recommended?

Gravity (inversion) traction was marketed extensively a few years ago. Its theoretical basis is that body weight, when inverted (by hanging upside down), will distract the lumbar spine. Numerous side effects have been reported, including persistent headaches, blurred vision, petechiae, and numerous musculoskeletal complaints. Along with the potential implications of contraindications associated with these symptoms, one should probably reserve this method for use only with nonhuman primates having back pain.

5. What parameters need to be specified in a prescription of traction?

Positioning

Intermittent or continuous administration

Amount of pull

Duration

Other modalities to be used concurrent to traction also should be specified and may include methods to facilitate muscle relaxation, which is essential to maximize the therapeutic effects from traction. Hotpacks are most commonly prescribed.

6. Discuss positioning.

Positioning is a key element of a traction prescription. For **cervical traction**, specification of sitting or supine should be based on patient comfort in different positions. If cervical traction is being administered to relieve symptoms of nerve root compression, 20–30° of flexion will optimally open the intervertebral foramina. Less flexion is required for treatment of muscle spasm in the absence of radicular symptoms.

The supine position with 90° of hip and knee flexion is the most common position for **lumbar traction**. In this position, the lumbar lordosis is maximally reduced with the low back well supported on the traction table and the spine in a relatively flexed position to facilitate optimal vertebral separation.

7. When is intermittent traction prescribed? When continuous?

It is thought that a greater force of pull can be tolerated with intermittent as opposed to continuous administration. Selection is based on the desired therapeutic effect. If distraction of the spine is desired to open neural foramina or retract herniated disc material, then the greater forces of pull that can be tolerated by intermittent application are more desirable. If the goal is muscle relaxation, then it may be more beneficial to provide the prolonged stretch of continuous traction.

8. How much pull is usually used and for how long?

The amount of pull should be specified in the traction prescription. For cervical spine distraction, forces > 25 lbs need to be achieved, but forces > 50 lbs probably do not provide any additional advantage. Forces above 50 lbs are required with lumbar traction to achieve posterior vertebral separation, and forces > 100 lbs are required for anterior separation. The countertraction on the chest and shoulders to provide tractive forces over 100 lbs is often poorly tolerated by patients.

The duration of treatment sessions is usually specified as 20 minutes. Studies seem to support that therapeutic effects are achieved over this time period.

9. What are the contraindications to prescribing or administering traction?

The potential for cervical ligamentous instability, as might occur with rheumatoid arthritis, Down's syndrome, achondroplastic dwarfism, Marfan syndrome, or previous trauma, are absolute contraindications. Cervical extension during traction should be avoided, especially in the presence of vertebrobasilar insufficiency. Documented or suspected tumor in the region of the spine, osteopenia, infectious process of the spine or surrounding soft tissue, and pregnancy are absolute contraindications. Old age is a relative contraindication due to degenerative spine changes.

10. What is manipulation?

The definition of manipulation is the use of hands in the patient management process using instructions and maneuvers to maintain maximal, painless movement of the musculoskeletal system in postural balance.

11. What are the goals of manipulation?

The primary goal is to optimize physical function in areas such as gait, ADLs, and transfers by maintaining body symmetry, improving motion in restricted areas, and enhancing pain-free motion.

12. When do you use manipulation?

Manipulation is used in the presence of a **somatic dysfunction**, which is defined as impaired or altered function of related components of the somatic system, including skeletal, ligamentous, myofacial, related vascular, neural, and lymphatic elements. Somatic dysfunction can be detected on physical exam as **t**enderness, **a**symmetric structure, **r**ange of motion abnormalities, and **t**issue texture changes (TART). Manipulation can be helpful, when appropriate, in the following conditions:

Acute or chronic back and neck pain	Piriformis syndrome
Rib pain	Sciatica
Bulging intervertebral discs	Headaches
Facet syndrome	Sacroiliac syndrome

13. What are some of the most common types of manipulation used by practitioners?

The differences in the following techniques are defined by the following parameters: thrusting versus nonthrusting force, intrinsic versus extrinsic forces, passive versus active motion, indirect versus direct engagement of the restrictive barrier.

- **Thrusting**

    High-velocity, low-amplitude mobilization—the classic "crack" type (audible or palpable crack not manditory for success)

- **Nonthrusting**

Articulatory	Myofacial release
Muscle energy	Soft tissue
Counterstrain	Craniosacral

14. Is manipulation dangerous, and what are the absolute and relative contraindications?

There are very few risks with the application of spinal manipulation. No complications have been reported in the literature with the nonthrusting techniques. The most severe complications following manipulation were associated with cervical thrust techniques, in which the neck was extended during the procedure resulting in vascular compromise of the vertebrobasilar system or the spinal cord. These complcations are rare, given the frequency with which these procedures are performed.

Contraindications to Manipulation When Using Thrust Technique

ABSOLUTE CONTRAINDICATIONS	RELATIVE CONTRAINDICATIONS
Vertebral malignancy	Spinal deformity or anomalies
Infection of inflammation	Systemic anticoagulation (disease-related or pharmacologic)
Cauda equina syndrome	Severe diabetes
Myelopathy or spondylosis	Atherosclerosis
Multiple adjacent radiculopathies	Severe degenerative joint disease
Vertebral bone diseases	Vertigo or symptoms of vertebrobasilar disease
Vertebral bony joint instability	Inactive rheumatoid disease
(fractures, dislocations)	Ligamentous joint instability
Rheumatoid disease in the cervical	Congenital laxity syndromes (Marfan's or Ehlers-Danlos)
region	Aseptic necrosis
	Local aneurysm
	Osteomalacia
	Osteoporosis

15. Who does manipulation?

Licensed osteopathic physicians, chiropractors, physical therapists (with special training), and medical doctors with additional training (CME course).

16. What are some of the current theories behind the mechanisms of manipulation?

- Restoration of joint, disc, or facet symmetry
- Restoration of muscular and myofacial range of motion
- Manipulation-induced reduction of afferent pain signals
- Manipulation-induced endorphin release
- Placebo effect

17. When is a massage medium required?

A massage medium is used to reduce friction over the skin. Examples include mineral oil, glycerin, coconut oil, cocoa butter, Nivea cream, and baby powder. Such media are used when the massage is intended for edema reduction, relaxation/sedation, or relief of muscle spasm/tightness. When the massage is used to loosen or stretch scar tissue, fascia, or subcutaneous tissue, no medium is used, allowing the therapist to gain purchase on and move appropriate tissue structures.

18. What are commonly used techniques of therapeutic massage?

Classical massage involves stroking and gliding movements (**effleurage**), kneading (**petrissage**), and percussion (**tapotement**). Stroking, gliding, and friction movements are helpful for locating areas of muscle spasm or focal pain. Stroking can help produce muscle relaxation in locations where spasm exists. Kneading techniques are performed on muscle and subcutaneous tissue for the purposes of muscle relaxation, improving circulation, and reducing edema. Percussion is primarily used for chest therapy in conjunction with postural drainage.

19. What physical parameters of massage can be altered depending on the desired therapeutic effect?

Deep friction massage is used to prevent adhesions in acute muscle injuries and to break up adhesions in subacute and chronic injuries. Deep friction is applied transverse across the muscle fiber, tendon, or ligament.

Soft-tissue mobilization is a forceful massage of the muscle-fascial system element and differs from most massage in that it is done with fascia and muscle in a stretched position rather than relaxed or shortened. It is particularly effective as an adjunct to passive stretching for reduction of contractures.

Myofascial release has been defined as "a hands-on technique that applies prolonged light pressure in specific directions into the fascia system." It is applied in conjunction with passive ROM with the purpose of stretching focal areas of muscle or fascial tightness.

Accupressure is the application of sustained deep pressure over trigger points, as defined by Travell. Accupressure is often done in conjunction with application of other therapeutic modalities to the trigger points (e.g., ice, ultrasound, electrical stimulation).

20. Are there any contraindications to massage?

Yes, there can be potential harm from massage. It is contraindicated over malignancies, open wounds, thrombophlebitis, and infected tissues. Peripheral nerve compression from hematoma formation has been reported when accupressure was applied too vigorously.

BIBLIOGRAPHY

1. Atchinson JW, Stoll ST, Cotter AC: Traction, manipulation, and massage. In Braddom RL (ed): Physical Medicine and Rehabilitation, 2nd ed. Philadelphia, W.B. Saunders, 2000, pp 413–439.
2. Bourdillon JF: Spinal Manipulation, 3rd ed. New York, Appleton-Century-Crofts, 1983.
3. Bridger RS, Ossey S, Gourie G: Effect of lumbar traction on stature. Spine 14:82–90, 1989.
4. Cyriax JH: Textbook of Orthopaedic Medicine: Treatment by Manipulation, Massage and Injection, 10th ed. London, Bailliere-Tindall, 1982.
5. Gianakopoulos G, Waylonis GW, Grant PA, et al: Inversion devices: Their role in producing lumbar distraction. Arch Phys Med Rehabil 66:100–102, 1985.
6. Greenman PE: Principles of Manual Medicine. Baltimore, Williams &Wilkins, 1989.
7. Onel D, Tukzlaci M, Sari H, Demir K: Computed tomographic investigation of the effect of traction on lumbar disc herniations. Spine 14:82–90, 1989.
8. Rechtien JJ, Andary M, Holmes TG, Wieting JM: Manipulation, massage, and traction. In DeLisa JA, Gans BM (eds): Rehabilitation Medicine: Principles and Practice, 3rd ed. Philadelphia, Lippincott-Raven, 1998, pp 521–552.
9. Sherman DG, Hart RG, Easton JD: Abrupt change in head position and cerebral infarction. Stroke 12:2–6, 1981.
10. Travell J: Myofascial Pain and Dysfunction. Baltimore, Williams & Wilkins, 1983.
11. Twomey LT: Sustained lumbar traction: An experimental study of long spine segments. Spine 10:146–149, 1985.

XV. *Interventional Physiatry*

87. EPIDURAL BLOCKS, FACET INJECTIONS, AND SPINAL THERAPEUTICS

Frank J. E. Falco, M.D., Charles M. Narrow, M.D., John R. Carbon, D.O., M.S., Gabriel Martinez, M.D., and Michael E. Frey, M.D.

1. What is interventional physiatry?

Interventional physiatry takes place primarily as a curative phase of medicine; focusing on diagnosis and treatment regarding the spine. This may involve procedures such as nerve blocks, interarticular injections, epidural injections, intradiscal electrothermal annuloplasty, sacroiliac joint injections, nerve ablations, lumbar discography, and sympathetic blocks.

2. Describe the innervation of the lumbar intervertebral disc.

The sinuvertebral nerve, gray rami communicans, and ventral rami innervate the lumbar intervertebral discs. The gray ramus communicans from the sympathetic trunks supplies the ipsilateral anterior, lateral, and posterolateral annulus. The ventral ramus directly branches as it exits the intervertebral foramen to supply the ipsilateral outer third to half of the lateral annulus. The sinuvertebral nerve, formed by the gray ramus communicans and a branch from the segmental ventral ramus, innervates the posterior annular fibers of the segmental and cephalad intervertebral discs.

3. Are lumbar and cervical facet joints true joints?

Spinal facet joints, zygapophyseal joints, are true diarthrodial synovial joints with a joint space, hyaline cartilage, synovial membrane, and fibrous capsule. These joints possess nociceptive fibers and therefore can be pain generators. Each facet joint receives innervation from two different medial branch nerves, one to the superior and the other to the inferior aspect of the joint. Facet joint arthropathy or hypertrophy may result in central or lateral canal stenosis, which can eventually cause radicular pain.

4. What are the clinical indications for lumbar or cervical epidural steroid injections in the treatment of low back pain?

Epidural steroid injections are used for the treatment of **radicular pain**, not axial or referred limb pain. Constant radicular pain is typically achy and affects the proximal portion of the limb with distal numbness or paresthesias. Intermittent radicular pain is described as shooting or lancinating pain that travels down the affected limb in a specific nerve root distribution. Spinal epidurals are efficacious in treating cervical, thoracic, or lumbar radiculopathy.

5. Which injection techniques are utilized in performing lumbar epidurals?

The **caudal, translaminar** (also known as interlaminar), and **transforaminal** are the different injection routes for lumbar epidurals. These injections are ideally performed under fluoroscopic visualization, which allows precise needle placement. Injection of radiopaque contrast confirms needle position and ensures that the tip has not entered a vascular structure or the thecal sac prior to injecting medication.

The **caudal** approach is accomplished by passing a spinal needle through the sacral cornu and sacrococcygeal ligament into the sacral hiatus. Caution is taken not to advance the spinal needle above the S2 level and risk intrathecal puncture. Caudal epidurals are helpful in treating lower lumbar and sacral lumbar radiculopathies, as well as patients with a radiculopathy who have had previous lower lumbar surgery in whom there is epidural scarring or obliteration of the epidural space at the surgical site.

Translaminar injections are performed by passing an epidural needle between the lamina using either a median (between the spinous processes) or paramedian (oblique to the spinous processes) approach. The needle is advanced through the ligamentum flavum into the posterior epidural space using a "loss of resistance" technique. This method allows the injectionist to place the medication at the site of pathology.

The **transforaminal** epidural injection is achieved by placing a spinal needle into the antero-lateral portion of the lumbar foramen. Care is taken not to advance the needle tip too far medially and risk puncturing the dural sleeve, which can lead to an inadvertent intrathecal injection. This epidural injection technique is useful for patients with previous lumbar spine surgery and can provide diagnostic information when evaluating for the presence of a radiculopathy by only blocking a specific nerve root.

6. What is the most common potential complication associated with a translaminar epidural injection? What are other complications?

The most common complication is **thecal sac puncture**, occurring in 5% of lumbar epidurals. The most notable side effect is a **spinal headache**, with a prevalence of 0.4% according to the obstetric population. Infection, direct trauma to the spinal cord, and epidural hematomas (extremely rare) may occur. Severe cases of epidural hematomas present with profound weakness and usually occur in the immediate postsurgical procedure. These complications may result in devastating sequelae in the cervical or thoracic spine.

7. What is the prevalence of lumbar facet pain in the patient with chronic low back pain?

In the past, lumbar facet syndrome has typically been characterized as axial back pain only made worse by lumbar spine extension. Lumbar facet dysfunction accounts for 15% of chronic low back pain and can actually cause referred lower extremity symptoms as well as axial pain.

8. Which medial branch nerves are blocked in order to anesthetize the L4/5 facet joint?

The L4–5 facet joint is anesthetized by blocking the **medial branch nerve** at the facet joint and the L3 and L4 medial branch nerves. The adjacent medial branch nerve travels proximally over the L5 transverse process to join the intermediate and lateral branch nerves, forming the dorsal ramus of the L4 segmental nerve. Therefore, the medial branch nerve blocked at the L5 transverse process level is actually by nomenclature the L4 medial branch nerve. Therefore, the L4–5 facet joint is anesthetized by blocking the L3 and L4 medial branch nerves.

9. When would you consider medial branch nerve blocks versus intra-articular facet injections to treat lumbar or cervical facet syndrome?

Medial branch nerve blocks are performed to locate the source of low back or neck pain or determine candidates for denervation by radiofrequency, cryoanalgesia, or alcohol injections. Medial branch nerve blocks carry a 30% false-positive rate, which must be considered before proceeding with a denervation procedure.

10. What relationship, if any, exists between the SI joint and leg pain?

Prior to the description of the herniated disc and sciatica in 1934 by Mixter and Barr, SI joint dysfunction was considered as the primary cause of lower extremity pain. Today, lower extremity symptoms in the presence of SI joint dyfunction are felt to be secondary to capsular irritation. Recently, it has been suggested that there may actually be a relationship between the SI joint and radicular leg pain. In some individuals with "leaky" SI joint capsules, contrast extravasation has been documented to flow between the SI joint and one of three different nearby neural structures. Contrast extravasation has been observed to flow to specific neural structures according to the location of capsular disruption. These three pathways have been described to involve the dorsal sacral foramina from the posterior capsule, the fifth lumbar nerve root from the capsular superior recess, and the lumbosacral plexus from the ventral capsule.

11. What is the prevalence of discogenic low back pain? What are its symptoms?

Internal disc disruption was first used by H.V. Crock to describe the internal pathologic changes of intervertebral disc structure. Annular fiber deterioration can lead to radial fissuring, which can extend into the outer innervated disc margin resulting in low back pain. The prevalence of discogenic pain is approximately **40%** in chronic low back pain sufferers.

Pain is typically described as centralized, nonradicular pain produced during certain activities. Patients can also have diffuse, nondermatomal lower limb pain associated with low back pain, but not typically in isolation. Symptoms are increased with axial-loading activities such as sitting, lifting, and standing. Physical examination findings are usually unremarkable except for restricted ROM, pain with flexion or extension, and pain with mobilization at discogenic segments.

12. When is provocative lumbar discography used?

Lumbar discography was first introduced to aid in the diagnosis of disc pathology, particularly disc prolapse, prior to the advent of sophisticated imaging techniques such as MRI and CT. Provocative discography became of interest when injection of contrast into ruptured discs exacerbated low back symptoms in certain individuals. Over time, lumbar discography became the standard (although with continued controversy) for identifying discogenic low back pain from internal disc disruption as seen, for example, with radial annular tears. The indications for provocative lumbar discography have been refined to surgical planning for a lumbar fusion; evaluating structural integrity of a disc adjacent to a fusion or spine abnormality, such as spondylolisthesis, as part of percutaneous disc procedures; and in identifying symptomatic internal disc disruption.

13. What complications are associated with lumbar discography?

Risk of complications from lumbar discography is low. Potential risks include discitis, subarachnoid puncture, nerve root injury, meningitis, bleeding, and allergic reaction. Risks can be minimized by excluding individuals with contrast dye allergies, using nonionic contrast, and employing sterile technique.

14. What is discitis?

Discitis is the most feared complication of lumbar discography, with a reported incidence of 0.05–4% for each evaluated disc level. The most common pathogen is *Staphylococcus epidermidis*. Prophylactic and intradiscal antibiotics may decrease risks.

Individuals who develop discitis typically present with severe back pain and spasms 2–4 weeks after the procedure. Back pain is increased by any activity and relieved by rest. Patients may report fever and chills, but documented temperature elevations or elevated white blood cell counts are unusual. Bone scan, sedimentation rate, and MRI are often normal within the first 3 weeks. MRI is considered the best means for early detection.

15. Define intradiscal electrothermal (IDET) annuloplasty. How does it work?

IDET is a percutaneous procedure designed to treat symptomatic lumbar internal disc disruption, as determined by provocative lumbar discography. The procedure employs a navigable catheter inserted into the disc via a large-bore needle. The distal portion of the catheter incorporates an active electrothermal tip placed within the posterior annulus. The thermal resistive coil generates heat that is directly transferred to the annular tissues from the active tip to modify collagen fibers and coagulate nociceptors.

16. What are the indications for lumbar facet joint radiofrequency neurotomy in the treatment of chronic pain?

Patients selected for lumbar facet joint radiofrequency neurotomy should have failed conservative care, been given a reasonable period of recovery time, and have an accurate diagnosis of facet joint syndrome. The only method of making this diagnosis and minimizing the large percentage of placebo responders (approx. 30% false-positive rate) is to use diagnostic injections with a double-block paradigm. A comparative blockade of the medial branch nerve using two different anesthetics significantly reduces the chance of a false-positive response. Patients are considered for radiofrequency neurotomy of the medial branch nerves when there is a significant degree of pain relief from the diagnostic injections.

17. Which patients can benefit from spinal endoscopy?

Spinal endoscopy is commonly used in the treatment of chronic radiculopathy and, in particular, the postoperative spine patient who has developed perineural epidural fibrosis. The endoscope is used in the same way as catheters are used for neurolysis of adhesions. The distinct advantage of using the spinal endoscope is the direct optical visualization and the maneuverability of the scope. It is a minimally invasive means of treating chronic radiculopathy from postsurgical scarring.

The fiberoptic endoscope is placed into the epidural space via the caudal canal and advanced cephalad under fluoroscopic control to the site of pathology. Adhesions are then treated under direct optical visualization with a combination of mechanical blunt and pressurized saline debridement. Success probably depends on early intervention before the scar tissue has hardened.

18. What is vertebroplasty and who does it benefit?

Osteoporosis is inevitable in the elderly. When the vertebral bodies weaken and fracture, it can cause significant pain. Metastatic disease also causes compression fractures due to the osteolytic nature of the tumor. Vertebroplasty is a percutaneous injection of polymethylmethacrylate into the vertebral body.

19. How does the role an interventional physiatrist differ from that of an anesthesiologist?

The physiatrist focuses on function and is usually engaged in preprocedure evaluation. This includes history and physical examination, but PT, OT, imaging, and functional capacity evaluations are often used as well. Postinjection procedure therapeutics such as exercise prescription, manipulation, and traction are often used to increase function, not to just treat pain.

BIBLIOGRAPHY

1. Bedder MD: Spinal cord stimulation and intractable pain: Patient selection. In Waldman SD, Winnie AP (eds): Interventional Pain Management. Philadelphia, W.B. Saunders, 1996, pp 412–418.
2. Bogduk N, Brazenor G, Christophidis N, et al: Epidural Use of Steroids in the Management of Back Pain. Canberra, Australia, National Health and Medical Research Council, 1994.
3. Brown FW: Management of diskogenic pain using epidural and intrathecal steroids. Clin Orthop 129:72–78, 1977.
4. Derby R, Eek B, Chen Y, et al: Intradiscal electrothermal annuloplasty (IDET): A novel approach for treating chronic discogenic back pain. Neuromodulation 3:82–88, 2000.
5. Fortin JD, Washington WJ, Falco FJE: Three pathways between the sacroiliac joint and neural structures. Am J Neuroradiol 20:1429–1434, 1999.
6. Fraser RD, Osti OL, Vernon-Roberts B: Discitis after discography. J Bone Joint Surg 69B:26–35, 1987.
7. Kirkaldy-Willis WH, Burton CV (eds): Managing Low Back Pain, 3rd ed. New York, Churchill Livingstone, 1992.
8. Schwarzer AC, Aprill CN, Derby R, et al: Clinical features of patients with pain stemming from the zygapophysial joints: Is the lumbar facet syndrome a clinical entity? Spine 19:1132–1137, 1994.
9. Schwarzer AC, Aprill CN, Derby R, et al: The false-positive rate of single lumbar zygapophysial joint blocks. Pain 58:195–200, 1994.
10. Schwarzer AC, Aprill CN, Derby R, et al: The relative contributions of the disc and zygapophyseal joint in chronic low back pain. Spine 19:801–806, 1994.
11. Schwarzer AC, Aprill CN, Derby R, et al: The sacroiliac joint in chronic low back pain. Spine 20:31–37, 1995.
12. Young M, Lavin R (eds): Spinal Rehabilitation. Physical Medicine and Rehabilitation; State of the Art Reviews, vol. 9, no. 3. Philadelphia, Hanley & Belfus, 1995.

88. LOCAL INJECTIONS FOR MUSCLE SPASTICITY (NERVE BLOCKS)

Thomas J. Cava, M.D., and Christopher O'Brien, M.D.

1. What are the clinical indications for local injection techniques to reduce spasticity?

Localized muscle spasticity that is poorly responsive to systemic medications and physical therapy treatment, and that causes pain or interferes with mobility, sleep, or activities of daily living (ADLs). Specific examples include limb spasticity resulting in joint contracture and adversely affecting body positioning or orthosis fit to improve hygiene of the palm or perineum.

2. What are the most common diagnoses of patients treated with local injections for spasticity?

Upper motor neuron lesions, which include stroke, head injury, multiple sclerosis, spinal cord injury, and cerebral palsy.

3. Which drugs are locally injected to treat patients with spasticity?

Phenol (carbolic acid) is commonly prepared in a 5–6% aqueous solution for adults and 3–5% for children. It has been injected adjacent to peripheral nerves and as intramuscular nerve blocks since the 1960s.

Ethyl alcohol is prepared in concentrations of 35–100%. Although it has been injected to treat spasticity since the 1950s, recent literature regarding its use in spasticity is limited.

Botulinum toxin. Botulinum toxin is one of the most potent biologic toxins known to man—6 million times more toxic than snake venom! There are seven distinct neurotoxins produced by the anaerobic bacteria *Clostridium botulinum*, labeled A through G. The only commercially available serotypes are types A and B. There are two type A preparations described in the world literature; Botox (Allergan) is the only one available in the U.S. Botulinum toxin type B (Myobloc, Elan Pharm.) was approved by the FDA in 2000 for the treatment of cervical dystonia. It should be noted that the dose of neurotoxin used is not comparable among the various preparations. Additionally, use of type A or B for spasticity is currently considered by the FDA to be "off-label."

Botulinum toxin has been used in the past decade with dramatic results when injected intramuscularly to treat strabismus, blepharospasm, and cervical dystonia (spasmodic torticollis). In the past several years, its effectiveness in the treatment of limb muscle spasticity has become established largely through investigator-driven clinical trials.

4. How do these agents work to reduce spasticity?

Each has a different specific mechanism of action, but their final effect is chemodenervation, or the chemical disconnection of a nerve from the muscle that it innervates. This results in a localized, focal muscle relaxation. **Phenol** and **alcohol** are neurolytic agents, that cause immediate axonal protein denaturation. **Botulinum toxin** is a potent neurotoxin that inhibits the release of acetylcholine at the neuromuscular junction via a complex mechanism of action.

5. What is so complex about the action of botulinum toxin?

Plenty. There are three steps involved in botulinum toxin-mediated muscle paralysis:
(1) **binding** to the cholinergic, presynaptic nerve terminal;
(2) **internalization** into the acetylcholine vesicle; and
(3) **inhibition** of neurotransmitter release into the synapse.

The neurotoxin cleaves one of the synaptic fusion proteins, thereby preventing the "chemical handshake" that occurs when the acetylcholine vesicle docks and fuses to the presynaptic membrane. Without acetylcholine, the propagation of the action potential is terminated, resulting in a partial muscle paralysis. The seven botulinum neurotoxins cleave different intracellular targets. The type A neurotoxin cleaves SNAP-25 and type B cleaves synaptobrevin.

6. With such complex pharmacology among the antispasmodics, accurate treatment dose must be important, right?

The treatment dose varies with each agent and is dependent on the type of block, size of muscle or nerve injected, degree of spasticity reduction desired, and toxicity profile of the drug chosen. For **phenol nerve block** (phenol neurolysis), a dose of 0.5 to 2 mL of 5% aqueous solution is typically injected adjacent to a single motor nerve. For **phenol motor point block** (phenol intramuscular neurolysis), a total dose of 1–15 mL is commonly given in multiple 0.2–0.5-mL injections into the belly of the target muscle. The recommended maximum total dose per treatment sessions is 1 gm, which is equivalent to 20 mL of 5% solution. Phenol has systemic toxicity at doses > 8.5 gm, which can result in tremors, seizures, CNS depression, and cardiac failure.

Alcohol nerve blocks and **motor point blocks** (intramuscular alcohol wash) are performed less commonly than those with phenol and botulinum toxin, and typical doses injected range from 1 to 30 mL of a 45–100% solution of ethanol. **Botulinum toxin** dosing is altogether different than dosing with the other agents, and the different serotypes require different doses.

7. How is the dosage of botulinum toxin determined?

Botulinum toxin dosage is measured in units of **biologic activity** instead of quantity. The amount of botulinum toxin required to kill 50% of a colony of female, Swiss-Webster mice is referred to as the **LD_{50}** in mice and is equal to **1 mouse unit**. While no PM&R residents have yet volunteered for the human LD_{50} study, the extrapolated lethal dose in humans is 3000 units of Botox and 150,000 units of Myobloc!

For the **type A preparation** (Botox), typical **adult treatment** doses are 30–40 units/muscle for small, distal limb muscles and 100–300 units/muscle for large proximal muscles. General recommendations set a total maximum body dosage of 400–600 unit/visit, which is an order of magnitude below the estimated LD_{50} in humans. The **pediatric dosage** guideline for total maximum body dose per visit is the lesser of 12 units/kg or 400 units.

For the **type B preparation** (Myobloc), dosage guidelines are emerging but appear to be in the 5000–15,000-unit range for adults with limb spasticity.

8. How is botulinum toxin supplied?

In the U.S., botulinum toxin is available as two different serotypes, A or B. The A serotype is available as Botox in 100-unit vials of lyophilized toxin, which must be reconstituted with sterile, preservative-free, 0.9% NaCl solution. Botox is an FDA-approved drug for treatment of strabismus, blepharospasm, and cervical dystonia.

The type B toxin is available as Myobloc, which is a liquid solution available in three vial sizes at a standard concentration of 5000 units/mL.

9. Describe the technique for phenol motor point block.

Skin surface stimulation is used to identify sites that produce low threshold muscle twitches. These motor points are marked and prepared with betadine or alcohol for sterile injection. A 27-gauge Teflon-coated cathode simulator needle is attached by flexible tubing to a 3- to 5-mL syringe containing 5% aqueous phenol. The cathode is attached to a stimulator with the following settings: a square wave pulse duration of 0.1 ms, a pulse rate of 1 Hz, and a stimulus intensity of 0.2–30 mA. The motor nerve is located with needle advancement and maximization of muscle twitch response. Stimulus intensity is then reduced and needle placement refined to produce the largest twitch with the lowest amperage (0.5–1 mA). The syringe should be aspirated to avoid intravascular injection, and phenol is injected, 0.1–0.5 mL at a time. The needle is advanced or the position adjusted to redirect the dose if the muscle twitch does not disappear. The process is repeated at multiple motor points until the desired clinical effect is achieved. The procedure for alcohol is similar to phenol injection.

10. How does the technique for botulinum toxin injection differ from phenol injection?

Botulinum toxin type A must be reconstituted with preservative-free normal saline; botulinum toxin type B is available as a ready to use solution. Because minute quantities are injected, a tuberculin syringe is needed for measurement. A needle stimulation technique may be used to identify and confirm the designated muscle belly; however, precise motor point identification by reduction of stimulus intensity is not necessary. Suggested needle size is 25 to 27 gauge, with a needle length of 37–75 mm. The onset of action of botulinum toxin is not immediate and typically occurs in 12–72 hours, with a peak effect occurring in 2–4 weeks. Reinjection may be safely performed when spasticity returns. It is suggested to wait at least 3 months between injections to reduce the risk of antibody formation.

11. How do you choose which muscle(s) to inject?

Carefully. Clinical and functional examination is indispensable, and gait lab analysis is at times advantageous for lower-extremity spasticity patients. Careful attention to the balance of forces about the involved joint is critical. Attention should be directed to distinguishing primary versus compensatory muscle overactivity. Hypertonic muscles should be chosen if spasticity limits function. Potential benefits may include spasm and pain relief, prevention of joint contracture, improved gait, improved seating position, improved perineal hygiene, potential for greater voluntary antagonist muscle activity, and improved ADLs. Clinical success can be quantified with the Modified Ashworth Scale, hand-held myometry, goniometry, function measures, and gait analysis.

12. What are the advantages of botulinum toxin injection in the treatment of spasticity?
- Botulinum toxin is locally applied.
- Effect can be titrated with stepwise, incremental dosing after appropriate interdose intervals (typically 3–4 months).
- Botulinum toxin affects only motor function and acts selectively on the peripheral cholinergic nerve endings.
- There is no risk of sensory dysesthesias.
- Effect is sustained but clinically reversible.
- Procedure is relatively quick to perform.
- Patient tolerance is excellent.

13. How long does the effect of the injections last?

The duration of action varies with the agent injected, dosage, anatomic localization, and severity of spasticity. Phenol blocks typically last from 3–6 months, although longer periods have been reported in unblinded studies. Alcohol blocks have been reported to last for 1–36 months, but clinical consensus is that alcohol generally has a shorter duration of action than phenol. The duration of action of botulinum toxin is 2–6 months. Comprehensive physical and occupational therapy programs after the blocks may optimize functional outcome.

14. Can spasticity return after the block?

Yes. Indirect evidence suggests that reinnvervation of the muscle occurs initially by temporary axon terminal sprouting. This sprouting begins in a few days, and eventually the microterminals retract. The original terminal reactivates as the sprouts regress, re-establishing endplate function and reversing the denervation over subsequent months. The effect typically allows greater movement, permitting better success with stretching and new functional routines. If new capabilities are regularly exercised, spasticity may have less severe effects despite reinnervation.

15. What are the side effects of injections for spasticity?

A potential side effect of all spasticity injections is **loss of motor function**, which is dependent on the affected muscle spasticity. Each agent has its own adverse effect profile. **Phenol** may cause sensory dysesthesias when injected into mixed sensory-motor nerves, but this is rarely reported in its use in motor point blocks. It may also cause transient muscle swelling, induration, and tenderness. **Alcohol** may cause hyperemia and a transient burning sensation. The most common side effects of **botulinum toxin** are transient injection site discomfort, mild denervation in adjacent nontarget muscles, or excessive weakness of target muscles.

An infrequent result of therapy with botulinum toxin injection is the formation of **antibodies** that block neurotoxin binding to nerve acceptor sites. While this presents no dangerous clinical effects, it may render a patient unresponsive to future treatment. To date, cervical dystonia patients with secondary nonresponsiveness to type A botulinum toxin have responded to treatment with type B toxin. Cases of antibody development have primarily been reported in studies of patients with dystonia and not spasticity. The exact clinical significance of abnormal serologic tests remains to be determined.

16. What are some common spasticity patterns that may benefit from local therapeutic injection?

UPPER EXTREMITIES	LOWER EXTREMITIES
Clenched fist	Equinovarus foot
Flexed wrist	Flexed knee
Flexed elbow	Hyperextended hallux
Thumb in palm	Adducted hip
Adducted arm	

17. List some typical injections with phenol, alcohol, and botulinum toxin.
Phenol
   Obturator, musculocutaneous, sciatic, thoracodorsal, and tibial nerve blocks
   Gastrocnemius, posterior tibialis, biceps and triceps motor point blocks
Alcohol
   Tibial nerve block
   Gastrocnemius, soleus, and biceps motor point blocks
Botulinum toxin
   Biceps, wrist flexor, finger flexor, and thenar muscle injections (upper extremities)
   Adductor, quadriceps, gastrocnemius, soleus, tibialis posterior, toe flexor, and toe extensor injections (lower extremities)

18. Can botulinum toxin injection be used simultaneously with phenol blocks to treat spasticity?
   Yes, botulinum toxin and phenol blocks can be used at the same treatment session, in an attempt to overcome the dose limits of each respective agent and to achieve an additive benefit in the comprehensive management of severe spasticity.

19. What are the contraindications to local injections for spasticity?
   Absolute contraindications
      • Allergy to the proposed agent
      • Infection or inflammation at the planned injection site
      • Pregnancy
   Relative contraindications
      • Coagulopathy
   Specific precautions for botulinum toxin injection
      • Preexisting disorders of the neuromuscular junction
      • Concurrent use of aminoglycosides or other drugs that may potentiate neuromuscular blockade

BIBLIOGRAPHY

1. American Academy of Neurology, Therapeutics and Technology Assessment Subcommittee: The clinical usefulness of botulinum toxin-A in treating neurologic disorders. Neurology 40:1332–1336, 1990.
2. Brashear A, Lew MF, Dykstra DD, et al: Safety and efficacy of NeuroBloc (botulinum toxin type B) in type A responsive cervical dystonia. Neurology 53:1430–1446, 1999.
3. Brin MF, Lew MF, Adler CH, et al: Safety and efficacy of NeuroBloc (botulinum toxin type B) in type A resistant cervical dystonia. Neurology 53:1431–1438, 1999.
4. Brin MF: Interventional neurology: Treatment of neurological conditions with local injections of botulinum toxin. Arch Neurol 54(suppl):1–23, 1991.
5. Cava TJ: Botulinum toxin management of spasticity in upper motor neuron lesions. Eur J Neurol 2(suppl 3):57–60, 1995.
6. Cosgrove AP, Graham HK: Botulinum toxin-A in the management of children with cerebral palsy. J Bone Joint Surg 74B:135–136, 1992.
7. Glenn MB: Nerve blocks. In Whyte J (ed): The Practical Management of Spasticity in Children and Adults. Philadelphia, Lea & Febiger, 1990, pp 227–259.
8. Halpern DM, Meelhysen FE: Phenol motor point block in the management of muscular hypertonia. Arch Phys Med Rehabil 47:659–664, 1966.
9. Koman LA, Mooney JF 3d, Smith BP, et al: Management of spasticity in cerebral palsy with botulinum-A toxin: Repeat of preliminary randomized, double-blind trial. J Pediatr Orthop 14:299–303, 1994.
10. NIH Consensus Development Statement: Clinical use of botulinum toxin. Arch Neurol 48:1294–1298, 1991.
11. Simpson DM, Alexander DN, O'Brien CF, et al: Botulinum type A in the treatment of upper extremity spasticity: A randomized, double-blind placebo-controlled trial. Neurology 46:1306–1310, 1996.
12. Snow BJ, et al: Treatment of spasticity with botulinum toxin: A double-blind study. Ann Neurol 28:512–515, 1990.
13. Yablon SA, Agana BT, Ivanhoe CB, Boake C: Botulinum toxin in severe upper extremity spasticity among patients with traumatic brain injury: An open-labeled trial. Neurology 47:939–944, 1996.

89. ACUPUNCTURE

John Giusto, M.D., and Joseph M. Helms, M.D.

1. What is acupuncture?

Acupuncture is the use of fine needles inserted through the skin at various points on the body to treat illnesses of all kinds. The basic idea is that the stimulation provided by the needles assists the body's mechanisms of physiologic regulation and repair.

2. When and where did acupuncture begin? How long has it been used in western medicine?

Acupuncture is a traditional treatment that dates back over 2000 years in China. As a tradition, it has spread to other cultures, being adapted to local needs and customs. As a medical art, it has evolved with the passage of time. Acupuncture has been used for 1500 years in Japan and 200 years in Europe, but it has only been used to any significant extent in the U.S. for 30 years. Comparatively recent developments include the use of electrical stimulation and treatments solely based on neuroanatomic principles. **Medical acupuncture** is a hybrid approach that "respects our contemporary understanding of neuromuscular anatomy and pain physiology while embracing the classical Chinese perception of a subtle circulation network of a vivifying force called *qi*."

3. Explain the classical Chinese conception of acupuncture.

"Acupuncture is one discipline extracted from a complex heritage of Chinese medicine—a tradition that also includes massage and manipulation, stretching and breathing exercises, and herbal formulae, as well as exorcism of demons and magical correspondences. … The language in classical Chinese medicine texts reflects nature and agrarian village metaphors and describes a philosophy of man functioning harmoniously within an orderly universe. The models of health, disease, and treatment are presented in terms of patients' harmony or disharmony within this larger order, and involve their responses to external extremes of wind, heat, damp, dryness, and cold, as well as to internal extremes of anger, excitement, worry, sadness, and fear. Illnesses likewise are described and defined poetically, by divisions of the yin and yang polar opposites (interior or exterior, cold or hot, deficient or excessive), by descriptors attached to elemental qualities (wood, fire, earth, metal, and water), and by the functional influences traditionally associated with each of the internal organs. The classical anatomy of acupuncture consists of energy channels traversing the body. The principle energy pathways are named for the organs whose realms of influence are expanded from their conventional biomedical physiology to include functional, energetic, and metaphorical qualities (e.g., kidney supervises bones, marrow, joints, hearing, head hair, will, and motivation …)." [J.M. Helms, 1995]

4. What disorders can acupuncture treat?

The clinical literature of **controlled trials** includes treatment of low back pain, headaches, arthritic pain, extremity pain, postoperative pain, respiratory problems, urologic problems, and substance abuse. **Uncontrolled reports** include claims of effective application in almost every discipline of medicine. The World Health Organization maintains a list of conditions recommended for treatment by acupuncture and, in 1997, the National Institutes of Health issued a consensus statement dealing with the rational basis for acupuncture treatment. Both reports are available over the internet.

5. How big are the needles, and how deep do they go?

Acupuncture needles are much thinner than needles to draw blood or give injections. They are available in sizes from 30–36 gauge. The needles are usually 1–1.5 inches long but range from 0.5–5 inches for special applications. The depth of insertion depends on the type of treatment and location of the point as well as the size of the patient. Most points on the extremities are needled to a depth of 0.25–0.5 inch, while points on the low back are routinely needled 1–1.5 inches. Points on the buttocks may require insertion of 3 inches or more.

6. How many needles are used in a treatment?

The usual range is 10–20 needles in any given treatment. Often fewer needles (5–10) are used in the initial treatment of someone who has not had acupuncture before. Many needles (25–40) may be used when superficial (< ⅛ inch) needling techniques are employed to treat large areas of chronic myofascial pain.

7. Does it hurt?

There may be a pinching sensation when the needle first breaks the skin. This sensation is minimized through the use of proper insertion techniques or guide tubes. Most patients report a mild but deep ache lasting for several seconds when the acupuncture needle reaches the depth of the point. Occasionally, fleeting, sharp, or electric sensations occur when a sensory nerve is stimulated. These are not dangerous and do not last.

8. How many treatments are needed, and how often are they given?

A typical course of treatments will number 6–12 sessions, with the first 2–4 treatments done twice weekly, the next 4 to 6 done weekly, and the remainder at 2–4-week intervals. While some recent problems (< 3 months' duration) can be resolved in as few as 3 visits, most long-standing conditions (> 1 year's duration) need a full course of 10–12 sessions. A reasonable clinical trial would be 6 treatments; it is unlikely that significant results will be obtained if a response has not occurred in this period.

9. What effects can one expect after receiving acupuncture?

The most common effect after the first few treatments is a global feeling of **euphoria** and mild disorientation that can last several hours. It is more pronounced after the use of electrical stimulation and is attributed to endorphin release. At times, patients experience intermittent residual **achiness** at the points that were needled. This achiness rarely lasts > 12 hours and can be relieved with nonprescription analgesics.

With respect to the underlying condition, there are three possible **treatment outcomes**—no response, improvement, or worsening. The last response, treatment aggravation, is not necessarily a bad sign. Often, it is simply the result of too vigorous or too extensive an input. It should not last > 3 days and may be addressed with anti-inflammatory or analgesic medications, including prescription-strength drugs.

10. Have studies been done to show the analgesic effects of acupuncture?

Acupuncture for purposes of analgesia is one of the most thoroughly researched areas in medicine. Animal and human experiments started in China in the 1960s and since have been pursued in Europe and the U.S.

Two types of analgesia have been identified. One is **endorphin-dependent** and is induced by manual twirling of the needle or electrical stimulation that is of low frequency (2–4 Hz) and high intensity (> 10 mA). Characteristics of this response include slow onset with peak response at 30 minutes; long duration with effects usually lasting many hours; potentiation, with a second treatment in a few hours having a greater effect than the first one; cumulative effects after several treatments; and systemic reactions.

The other type of acupuncture analgesia is **monoamine-dependent** and is induced by electrical stimulation that is of high frequency (> 70 Hz) and relatively low intensity (< 10 mA). Its characteristics include rapid onset and local/segmental effects only.

11. How is the brain stimulated by acupuncture?

"Acupuncture actuates nerve fibers (type II and type III) in the muscle which send impulses to the spinal cord and activate three centers (spinal cord, midbrain, and hypothalamus-pituitary) to cause analgesia. The **spinal** site uses enkephalin and dynorphin to block incoming messages with stimulation at low frequency, and other transmitters (perhaps GABA) with high-frequency stimulation. The **midbrain** uses enkephalin to activate the raphe descending system, which inhibits spinal cord pain transmission by a synergistic effect of the monoamines, serotonin, and norepinephrine. The midbrain also has a circuit which bypasses the endorphinergic links at high-frequency stimulation. Finally, at the third center, the **hypothalamus-pituitary**, the pituitary releases beta-endorphin into the blood and CSF to cause analgesia at a distance (e.g., the midbrain). Also, the hypothalamus sends long axons to the midbrain and via beta-endorphin activates the descending analgesia system. This third center is not activated at high frequency, only a low-frequency stimulation." [B. Pomeranz, 1987]

12. Has research shown any other effects?

Research has investigated the **circulatory** and **autonomic** influences of acupuncture. Inserting a needle into a muscle in spasm dilates the blood vessels in that muscle via a reflex action involving sympathetic nerve fibers. Needles inserted into paravertebral muscles result in dilatation of blood vessels in peripheral spastic ischemic muscles at the same segmental level through a somato-autonomic reflex whose center is located in the contralateral anterior hypothalamus. Both the local and segmental needling result in decreased muscle spasm in the symptomatic area. A generalized decrease in peripheral sympathetic tone also has been noted after acupuncture. The above findings may help explain thermographic studies that show a normalizing increase in the temperature of chronic pain areas from acupuncture treatments given local or distant to the painful site.

Also of note are studies on **tissue healing** that have found a measurable current of injury emanating from acupuncture points after needling. This current has been shown to modulate neurohormonal activity and activate tissue-repair mechanisms. An area of intense speculation is whether acupuncture has its main effect on an electromagnetic bioinformational system in the body.

13. How effective is acupuncture?

Effectiveness of Analgesia for Chronic Pain

Placebo	30–35%
Sham acupunture (needles inserted in wrong location)	33–50%
True acupuncture	55–85%
Morphine	70%

14. Explain the physiology of acupuncture's effectiveness in myofascial pain.

Myofascial pain syndromes of neuropathic origin seem to be uniquely qualified for acupuncture therapy. C. Chan Gunn has introduced a physiologic theory of these syndromes and developed a specialized form of intramuscular needle stimulation to treat them.

Neuropathic pain is distinguished by either chronic dysesthetic or deep aching pain in the absence of ongoing injury or inflammation. This pain is typically accompanied by sensorimotor and autonomic manifestations, such as disuse supersensitivity (hyperexcitability, increased susceptibility, and super-reactivity), vasomotor changes (decreased temperature), sudomotor changes (increased sweating), pilomotor changes (goosebumps), and trophedema (local subcutaneous edema caused by increased tone in lymphatic vessel smooth muscle and increased blood vessel permeability).

Gunn considers the most common cause of neuropathic pain in any location to be **spondylosis** of all gradations. This phenomenon increases with age because of an accumulation of minor and sometimes major injuries to a segment. If neuropathy arises from pressure on a nerve root, the stage is set for a vicious cycle: neuropathy (radiculopathy) leads to pain and spasm in segmentally innervated muscles, including paraspinal muscles, both directly and indirectly from supersensitivity to minor trauma. The spasm in the paraspinal muscles compresses the intervertebral disc and narrows the intervertebral foramina, which further compresses the nerve root and worsens the neuropathy. Increased pressure on facet joints can also cause arthralgia (i.e., **facet syndrome**). Even in solitary peripheral lesions, there often is asymptomatic segmental paraspinal muscle spasm precipitating or aggravating the symptomatic peripheral neuromuscular dysfunction.

The key to treating neuropathic dysfunction is to release the muscle spasm, especially in the deep paraspinal muscles, and desensitize the involved nerves by reflex-stimulation. Acupuncture seems to be uniquely qualified for safely accessing the anatomic locations involved in myofascial pain of neuropathic origin while addressing the causative physiologic mechanisms. It should be noted that if fibrotic changes have replaced most striated muscle tissue so that spasm can no longer be considered a major component of the pain syndrome, acupuncture is unlikely to be of benefit. Extreme fibrosis would be evidenced by a lack of "needle grasp."

15. Is acupuncture safe? What about risks of infection, pneumothorax, and other complications?

Infection is an uncommon consequence of acupuncture treatment, though bacterial skin abscesses and ear chondritis can occur. Hepatitis B transmission is extremely rare and the only reported incidences in the U.S. literature involve non-physicians re-using unsterilized needles. There have been no responsible reports of HIV transmission. **Pneumothorax** is an infrequent complication. Deep needling of the thoracic cage and hilar areas is discouraged. The small size of the acupuncture needles makes a significant pneumothorax unlikely in any case. While **ecchymoses** are occasionally seen, significant **hematomata** are not. This is probably because of the torpedo shape of an acupuncture needle, as opposed to the beveled cutting edge of a hypodermic needle. The needle shape is also probably responsible for the lack of enduring damage to nerves or other tissues and structures. One phenomenon to be aware of is "**needle shock**." It is a vasovagal response to needling that may occur in initial treatments. It responds readily to standard maneuvers.

16. Are there any contraindications to acupuncture?

Contraindications are similar but less restrictive than those for injection techniques: overlying cellulitis, severe coagulopathy, and uncontrolled anticoagulation. Therapeutic anticoagulation does not in general present any difficulties, although ecchymoses are more common. Vigorous or deep needling and repetitive needle-pecking techniques should be avoided. Pregnancy is not a contraindication to acupuncture. Certain points, however, are avoided on practical or theoretical grounds, such as points overlying the pregnant uterus and those stimulating the lumbosacral nerve plexes.

Contraindications to **electrical stimulation** of acupuncture needles are the same as those for electrical stimulation in general: stimulation of the thorax in patients with pacemakers, pregnancy (safety not established), and carcinoma (unknown effects).

17. Is there any standardized training in acupuncture?

There are not yet nationally recognized standards for physician training in acupuncture. Each state establishes its own requirements for licensure, and those requirements vary widely. The most comprehensive training available for physicians is given through the Office of Continuing Medical Education at the UCLA School of Medicine. It is a 300-hour CME I program entitled "Medical Acupuncture for Physicians." Shorter courses are offered at other teaching centers. It should be noted that licensed nonphysician acupuncturists are not generally familiar with the principles and techniques of medical acupuncture.

18. Where does one get more information and find a qualified practitioner?

The most important resource for general information and referrals to qualified practitioners is:
American Academy of Medical Acupuncture (AAMA)
4929 Wilshire Boulevard
Los Angeles, CA 90010
Tel: 323-937-5514 (general information) or 800-521-5016 (referrals)
Fax: 323-937-0959
Internet @ www.medicalacupuncture.org

19. How many acupuncture points are there? Where are they located?

There are 361 classically described channel points and almost as many nonchannel points. General anatomic characteristics of acupuncture points include:
- Proximity to the neurovascular hilus of the muscle, probably equivalent to motor or trigger points
- Passage of peripheral nerves through bone foramina
- Penetration of deep fascia by peripheral nerves
- Bifurcation points of peripheral nerves
- Nerve plexes
- Sagittal plane where superficial nerves from both sides of the body meet
- Areas of dense fibrous connective tissue that are richly innervated
- Suture lines of the skull

As all of the above points generally show a decrease in electrical resistance when compared to the surrounding tissue, especially when they are tender to palpation, any point of lowered electrical resistance can be considered a potential acupuncture point.

20. What are the most common problems treated by acupuncture in outpatient pain management?

The most common problem is pain of >3 months' duration that has not responded to pharmacologic, surgical, or traditional physical therapies. By location, low back and neck/shoulder pain are the most common, followed by appendicular joint pains and headaches. By physiologic pathology, myofascial mechanisms are the most common, followed by neurologic, degenerative, and inflammatory processes.

21. Are there specialized needle techniques used with musculoskeletal problems?

Apart from the use of electrical stimulation and obtaining needle grasp in the classical acupuncture points, there are three major techniques for musculoskeletal problems. They are distinguished by the location and depth of needle insertion:

1. In the **surface technique**, many needles are employed and a repetitive pecking motion is utilized to free up palpable restrictions in the superficial fascia of entire zones of the body.

2 **Intramuscular needling** is used for treating trigger points anywhere in the body and generally makes use of a four quadrant fanning technique.

3. **Deep needling** of fascia or even periosteum is used when these tissues or adjacent neurovascular structures are implicated in the pain syndrome, e.g., by tenderness to palpation or analysis of pain distribution patterns.

One highly effective method for treating recalcitrant chronic pain combines elements from all three techniques for its local treatment. In its purest form, these local (symptomatic) points are accompanied by paravertebral points to address the spinal segments responsible for dermatomal (skin), myotomal (muscle), sclerotomal (bone), and even sympathetic nervous system pain-referral zones.

22. How is electrical stimulation used?

Electrical stimulation can be used with intramuscular or deep needling techniques. For most chronic pain problems, treatment is begun at low frequencies (2–4 Hz) at an intensity that is strong enough to be felt but is not uncomfortable. If there is no satisfactory response after two to three treatments, intermediate (10–30 Hz) and then high (75–200 Hz) frequencies may be tried. Some stimulation devices allow for an alternation of stimulation frequencies at intervals of a few seconds, presumably to prevent accommodation and tolerance. Usually alternating 2 Hz and 15 Hz can help if low-frequency treatment alone has not been successful. More acute problems or flare-ups of chronic conditions may be treated solely with high-frequency stimulation, a combination of low- followed by high-frequency stimulation, or alternating low- and high-frequency stimulation.

23. What is the role of ear acupuncture?

In acupuncture, the ear is considered a microsystem, or somatotopic system, an area of the body that registers and can be used to treat pathology occurring anywhere in the body. The other popular microsystem approaches are Korean hand acupuncture and scalp acupuncture. (For justification of the somatoptopic claim for the ear, see Helms and Oleson in the bibliography.) Clinically, the ear can be needled as an entire treatment in itself, especially in needle-sensitive patients, or used to reinforce the body acupuncture treatment. Points on the ear generally are located with the aid of a point-locating device that detects areas of decreased resistance (increased conductivity) with respect to the surrounding skin. Ear points commonly are used in treatment protocols for substance abuse management.

24. How can acupuncture be integrated into the therapeutic armamentarium of the physiatrist?

Acupuncture can be seen as lying on a continuum of available treatment options. In terms of increasing invasiveness, we might consider the following order: conventional physical therapy modalities, acupuncture, therapeutic injections, and then surgery. For electrical stimulation procedures, the following breakdown may be useful: transcutaneous electrical nerve stimulation (TENS), interferential current, neuromuscular stimulation (NMS), and then electro-acupuncture.

One method of integration is simply to proceed across the spectrum, increasing the invasiveness if the starting treatment regimen is not successful. Another method is to follow the continuum in the opposite direction as part of an effort at progressive rehabilitation and decreased reliance on invasive procedures. Perhaps the best method is to gain experience with acupuncture and apply it where it seems most indicated and effective in your hands, e.g., myofascial pain of neuropathic origin.

BIBLIOGRAPHY

1. Greenman PE: Principles of Manual Medicine. Baltimore, Williams & Wilkins, 1989.
2. Gunn CC: Treating Myofascial Pain: Intramuscular Stimulation (IMS) for Myofascial Pain Syndromes of Neuropathic Origin. Seattle, University of Washington, 1989.
3. Helms JM: Acupuncture Energetics: A Clinical Approach for Physicians. Berkeley, Medical Acupuncture Publishers, 1995.
4. Helms JM: An overview of medical acupuncture. In Jonas WB, Levin JS (eds): Essentials of Complimentary and Alternative Medicine. Baltimore, Williams & Wilkins, in press.
5. Lee MHM, Liao SJ: Acupuncture in physiatry. In Kottke FJ, Lehmann JF (eds): Krusen's Handbook of Physical Medicine and Rehabilitation. Philadelphia, W.B. Saunders, 1990.
6. Ng LKY, Katims JJ, Lee MHM: Acupuncture: A neuromodulation technique for pain control. In Aronoff GM (ed): Evaluation and Treatment of Chronic Pain, 2nd ed. Baltimore, Williams & Wilkins, 1992, pp 291–298.
7. Oleson TD, Kroening RJ, Bresler DE: An experimental evaluation of auricular diagnosis: The somatotopic mapping of musculoskeletal pain at ear acupuncture points. Pain 8:217–229, 1980.
8. Pomeranz B: Scientific basis of acupuncture. In Stux G, Pomeranz B: Acupuncture: Textbook and Atlas. Heidelberg, Springer-Verlag, 1987, pp 1–34.
9. Rotchford JK: Overview: Adverse events of acupuncture. Medical Acupuncture 11(2) fall 1999/winter 2000.
10. Seem M: The New American Acupuncture: Acupuncture Osteopathy: The Myofascial Release of the Bodymind's Holding Patterns. Boulder, CO, Blue Poppy Press, 1993.
11. Travell JG, Simons DG: Myofascial Pain and Dysfunction: The Trigger Point Manual. Baltimore, Williams & Wilkins, 1983.
12. Travell JG, Simons DG: Myofascial Pain and Dysfunction: The Trigger Point Manual: Vol 2. The Lower Extremities. Baltimore, Williams & Wilkins, 1992.
13. Walsh NE, Dumitru D, et al: Treatment of the patient with chronic pain. In DeLisa J (ed): Rehabilitation Medicine: Principles and Practice. Philadelphia, J.B. Lippincott, 1988, pp 708–864.

90. INJECTIONS OF PERIPHERAL JOINTS, BURSAE, AND TENDON SHEATHS

Mark G. Greenbaum, M.D., and Stuart A. Rubin, M.D.

1. What conditions can be treated with corticosteriod injections?

Intra-articular corticosteroid injection is a widely accepted adjunctive therapy in patients with rheumatoid arthritis, osteoarthritis, traumatic synovitis, crystalline arthrosis, and seronegative spondyloarthropathies. Nonarticular disorders, such as entrapment neuropathies, periarthritis, bursitis, and tendinitis, are also commonly treated with corticosteroid injections.

2. How do local (intra-articular) corticosteroid injections achieve their effects?

The proposed mechanism of actions for these injections includes:

Decreased synovial fluid complement

Decreased neutrophil number

Decreased synovial membrane/vascular permeability

Decreased synovial fluid acid hydrolases

Stimulation of synovial lining cell lysosomes

Decreased synovial cell mast cell numbers

The injections decrease pain and swelling and increase function. In rheumatoid arthritis, injection of intermediate or long-acting glucocorticoids aids in suppression of rheumatoid synovitis. Intra-articular corticosteroids are useful in treating acute exacerbations of osteoarthritis associated with significant effusions.

3. List the absolute and relative contraindications for intra-articular and nonarticular corticosteroid injections.

ABSOLUTE CONTRAINDICATIONS	RELATIVE CONTRAINDICATIONS
Infectious arthritis	Juxta-articular osteopenia
Bacteremia	Anticoagulant therapy
Peri-articular cellulitis	Joint instability
Acute injury	Poorly controlled diabetes mellitus
Osteochondral fracture	Hemarthrosis
Adjacent osteomyelitis	Joint prosthesis
Uncontrolled bleeding or clotting disorder	Questionable therapeutic benefit from prior injections

4. What are the possible adverse effects of corticosteroid injections?

1. **Systemic absorption**—significant with repeated injections.
   Suppression of the hypothalamic-pituitary-adrenal axis.
   Iatrogenic Cushing's syndrome
   Occasional transient, but dramatic, increase in blood sugar level and glucosuria in diabetic patients
   Glucocorticoid-induced osteoporosis.

2. **Local effect on articular cartilage**—steroid arthropathy.
   Many animal studies, chiefly on rabbits, showing cartilage injury from intra-articular glucocorticoids.
   Destructive arthropathy may be from post-injection pain relief and overuse of a damaged joint, rather than direct steroid cartilage toxicity. Therefore, the joint or non-articular structures injected should not be put under undue stress for 1 week after injection.

3. **Other rare local effects**
   Iatrogenic joint inflammation—extremely rare if injection site is prepared with alcohol solution and disposable instruments are used.
   Tendon and ligament rupture—usually occur with systemic steroid use, frequent injections of weight-bearing joint or peri-articular soft tissue, injection directly into tendon or ligament, or injection of inappropriately high dose of corticosteroid.
   Postinjection flare—a true crystal-induced arthritis. Steroid crystals precipitate in the presence of certain paraben preservatives used in local anesthetic preparations. The acute synovitis is self-limited and responds well to ice, rest, and NSAIDs. It can be avoided by using single-dose vials of lidocaine or by using longer-acting bupivacaine that do not contain the paraben preservative. It is more common after use of microcrystalline steroid preparation, such as triamcinolone hexacetonide.
   Skin hypopigmentation and subcutaneous atrophy and degeneration—unusual if needle depth before injection is > 5 mm and if steroid is not tracked to the skin on needle withdrawal.

5. How should injections be integrated into treatment of patients?

Conservative, nonprocedural treatments should be done initially if symptoms are not disabling. This includes correction of underlying biomechanical disorders, activity modification in the workplace and at home, and technique changes in athletics. When deciding to proceed with therapeutic injection, it should be performed within the context of a well-designed, comprehensive rehabilitation program, including physical therapy for mobilization, stretching and strengthening, and a home exercise program.

6. How many bursae are there in the body? What is bursitis?

Bursae are closed filled sacs lined by synovial cells which facilitate motion of tendons, muscles and skin over bones. There are more than 80 bursae on each side of the body. Inflammation of the bursal wall (bursitis) may be caused by excessive friction or trauma, as well as septic, metabolic, hematologic, and inflammatory connective tissue diseases.

7. Which bursa is located at the "foot of the goose"?

The **pes anserinus**—the conjoined tendon of the semitendinosus, sartorius, and gracilis (pneumonic: STSG, as in "split-thickness skin graft")—lies above the anserine bursa. The bursa lies above the medial collateral ligament of the tibia. Pes anserine bursitis is very common, especially in women with heavy thighs and osteoarthritis of the knees. Often, there is pain on stair climbing. Corticosteroid injection is easy and quite effective in this superficial bursa.

8. Which is the most common bursitis of the shoulder?

Subacromial or subdeltoid bursae are the most commonly affected bursae of the shoulder. These rest on the supraspinatus tendon and are covered by the acromion, coracoacromial ligament, and deltoid muscle. They are often associated with rotator cuff tendinitis or tear or with shoulder impingement syndrome. The subacromial bursa is the one that facilitates passage of the rotator cuff under the subacromial arch. Corticosteroid injections into the bursa, as well as injection into the biceps tendon sheath for bicipital tendinitis and into the glenohumeral joint for adhesive capsulitis, are frequently used for shoulder problems.

9. Name a common cause of hip pain.

Trochanteric bursitis is a common cause of hip pain. The bursa of the greater trochanter lies beneath the tendon of the gluteus maximus and posterolateral to the greater trochanter. It is common in the elderly and in patients with a pelvic obliquity (leg-length discrepancy, scoliosis). Because of its deep location, superficial modalities such as hot packs and ultrasound usually do not suffice, and corticosteroid injection (using a long needle) is useful.

10. Which bursitis can present as "pump bumps"?

Subcutaneous or **Achilles' bursitis** lies subcutaneous to the posterior surface of the Achilles' tendon. It can present as "pump bumps," caused by closely contoured heel counters. Neither the deep bursa nor the Achilles' tendon sheath should be routinely injected because of the possibility of rupture of this heavily stressed tendon.

11. What is weavers' bottom bursitis?

A tailor's or weaver's bottom bursitis is an **ischial bursitis**. The ischial bursa lies between the ischial tuberosity and the gluteus maximus. Not a very common bursitis, it usually occurs due to prolonged sitting on a hard surface. It may occur in adolescent runners, often in conjunction with ischial apoplysitis.

12. What is tendinitis and what causes it?

Tendinitis is an inflammation of tendon, tendon sheath, or its attachment to bone. It is usually caused by excessive repetitive trauma and/or muscular or systemic disorders. Nodular hypertrophy of the tendon (as in trigger-fingers) and stenosis of its sheath (as in stenosing tenosynovitis of deQuervain's disease) can result. Simultaneous deposition of calcium, usually at the shoulder and occasionally at the wrist and ankle, can result in calcific tendinitis.

13. Do you have to play tennis to have tennis elbow?

Tennis elbow is **lateral epicondylitis**. It is an inflammation of the tendinous origin of the wrist and finger extensors at the lateral epicondyle. There is pain on resisted wrist extension and supination. It can be common in tennis players (usually from a faulty backhand), but it can also occur in anyone with repetitive overuse of the involved tendon. If refractory to modalities, splinting (tennis elbow strap), and anti-inflammatory drugs, a local corticosteroid injection is usually curative.

14. What is golfer's elbow? Do you have to be a golfer to have it?

Golfer's elbow is **medial epicondylitis**. It is inflammation of the tendinous origin of the wrist and finger flexors at the medial epicondyle. There is pain on resisted wrist flexion and pronation. It can be common in golfers but can also occur in anyone with repetitive overuse of the involved tendon. If refractory to modalities and anti-inflammatory drugs, local corticosteroid injection is usually curative.

Wearing a golfing glove can help cushion the impact when the club head hits the golf ball and thereby diminish referred tension to the medial epicondyle region. An overtight grip can also cause undue tension in this region. Improving in golfing mechanics and skills can help decrease a medial epicondylitis.

15. Why is cubital tunnel syndrome often seen with golfer's elbow?

Medial epicondylitis can often present with cubital tunnel syndrome of the ulnar nerve. The cubital tunnel is formed by the aponeurosis connecting the two heads of the flexor carpi ulnaris. It arises from the medial epicondyle of the humerus and attaches to the medial border of the olecranon and forms the gateway through which the ulnar nerve travels distally. This area, also known as the "**funny bone**," can be confused with golfer's elbow. In the latter, however, there are usually no ulnar-related symptoms into the forearm or hand. Care must be given not to inject into the cubital tunnel so as not to affect the ulnar nerve.

16. What is the Finkelstein's sign? In what type of tendinitis is it found?

Finkelstein's sign is elicited by placing the thumb in the palm and grasping it with the fingers. Ulnar deviation of the wrist causes sharp pain at the radial aspect of the wrist. This sign is pathognomonic for **deQuervain's disease**—a stenosing tenosynovitis of the abductor pollicis longus and extensor pollicis brevis at the radial styloid. It is common with repetitive grasping movements of the hand in an ulnar direction. Avoiding the provoking activity and splinting with a thumb-Spica splint is sometimes curative. Local corticosteroid injection into the tendon sheath at the anatomic snuffbox often results in improvement. Observation of filling of the tendon sheath confirms adequate placement. Due to the close relationship of the superficial radial nerve to the first dorsal compartment, any symptoms of paresthesias in the thumb while placing the needle indicate a need for needle repositioning.

17. Are injections useful for sacroiliac (SI) joint dysfunction?

The SI joint may be a primary source of back pain, and it may also be a secondary site of pain when dysfunction occurs anywhere along its kinetic chain. Anesthetic and steroid injection into the posterior ligamentous (extracapsular) structure of the SI joint done "blindly" (without fluoroscopic guidance) can be very effective, especially when combined with manipulation. These injections are thought to provide an anti-inflammatory effect and blockade of the posterior primary rami (likely L5–S3). If this injection is not helpful, then fluoroscopically guided, contrast-enhanced intra-articular injection of the SI joint should be considered.

18. What relatively new intra-articular injection technique is useful for osteoarthritis of the knee?

The hyaluronidase polymers sodium hyaluronate (Hyalgan) and hyaline G-F 20 (Synvisc) are composed of various fractions of hyaluronate and are approved by the FDA for the treatment of pain associated with osteoarthritis of the knee in patients who fail to respond adequately to conservative, nonpharmacologic therapy and simple analgesics. Under sterile technique, the synovial fluid in the knee joint is aspirated and the hyaluronate derivative is injected. A series of three weekly injections for hyaline G-F 20 and five weekly injections for sodium hyaluronate are required.

Clinical studies have demonstrated that injection of these agents into the joint space of osteoarthritic knees is followed by significant reduction of pain and improvement in function capacity in a majority of patients. The beneficial results may persist for 6–12 months. A repeat series may be done if the original series achieved a significant improvement in pain and functional capacity or a significant reduction in the dose of NSAIDs taken, and at least 6 months has elapsed since the prior series of injections.

19. Is corticosteroid injection useful in the management of carpal tunnel syndrome (CTS)?

First, a trial of noninvasive treatment should be attempted in the treatment of carpal tunnel syndrome. Splinting (including daytime wear), ergonomic modifications, physical therapy (including wrist traction), vitamin B_6, and NSAIDs are sometimes curative. If symptoms persist, corticosteroid injection may be useful and may help avoid surgical intervention. Injection should be at the wrist flexion crease, slightly ulnar to the palmaris longus tendon to avoid needling the median nerve itself. The needle should be directed at a 30° angle, beneath the transverse carpal ligament and oriented radially, until the carpal tunnel is entered. If the patient feels paresthesias, the needle should be withdrawn and repositioned.

20. What is prolotherapy and how does it work?

Prolotherapy is the injection of a solution for the purpose of tightening and strengthening loose or weak tendons, ligaments, or joint capsules. A proliferant (usually 15% dextrose solution) is injected and causes multiplication and activation of fibroblasts, which synthesize precursors to mature collagen, resulting in thicker, stronger, and tighter connective tissue. It has been used successfully to treat degenerative tendinosis and ligamentosis in chronic sprain/strain and overload injury, as well as joint laxity and instability. It is also useful in myofascial pain and fibromyalgia.

BIBLIOGRAPHY

1. Dreyfuss P, Cole AJ, Pauza K: Sacroiliac joint injection techniques. Phys Med Rehabil Clin North Am 6:785–813, 1995.
2. Greenbaum MG, Rubin SA: Non-articular and myofascial pain syndromes. In Lefkowitz M, Lebovits AH (eds): A Practical Approach to Pain Management, Boston. Little, Brown, 1996.
3. Lennard TA (ed): Pain Procedures in Clinical Practice, 2nd ed. Philadelphia. Hanley & Belfus, 2000.
4. Mazanee DJ: Pharmacology of corticosteroids in synoval joints. Phys Med Rehabil Clin North Am 6:815–831, 1995.
5. Micheo WF, Rodriques RA, Amy E: Joint and soft-tissue injections of the upper extremity. Phys Med Rehabil Clin North Am 6:823–840, 1995.
6. Milard RS, Dillingham MF: Peripheral joint injections: Lower extremity. Phys Med Rehabil Clin North Am 6:841–849, 1995.
7. Reeves KD: Prolotherapy: Present and future applications in soft-tissue pain and disability. Phys Med Rehabil Clin North Am 6:917–926, 1995.
8. Sheon RP, Moskowitz RW, Goldberg VM: Soft Tissue Rheumatic Pain: Recognition, Management, Prevention, 3rd ed. Philadelphia, Lea & Febiger, 1996.

XVI. Orthotics, Prosthetics, and Wheelchairs

91. AMPUTATION REHABILITATION

Nasser Eftekhari, M.D.

1. How common is limb loss in the U.S.?

The incidence of major amputations is estimated to be at least 70,000 new cases annually. Prevalence is estimated to be over 500,000 cases for major amputation and nearly 2 million for finger and toe amputations. The majority of new amputations involve the lower extremity related to diabetes, with an average cost of $40,000 each!

2. What are the major reasons for amputation in the United States?

The greatest cause of limb loss is **peripheral vascular disease** (65%), often associated with diabetes. These patients are generally in the 60–75-year age group, with mean age of 62. Nearly half of diabetic lower-extremity amputees will lose the other leg within 5 years.

Trauma accounts for 25% of all amputations and occurs most commonly in the 17–55-year age group, with most cases involving the lower extremity. **Malignancy** accounts for 5% of all amputations and is frequently seen among 10–20-year-olds. Approximately 5% of amputations are due to **congenital limb deficiency**, which accounts for 60% of all amputations in children.

3. Which limb is amputated more often, the upper or lower?

Lower-extremity amputations (excluding digits) account for 80–85% of major limb amputations. More than two-thirds of cases are caused by vascular and infectious complications, with or without diabetes. Right and left occurrence is about equal.

4. What special concerns are faced in the elderly patient undergoing an amputation?

Geriatric amputation deserves special attention due to their higher incidence of diabetes and peripheral vascular diseases. Elderly patients also are more likely to require higher levels of amputation. About 80% of all amputations performed at age 80 or later are above the knee. Long-term survival for elderly amputees has been increasing in the past few decades, but elderly amputees continue to remain at considerable risk. In most major series, the 2-year survival rate after bilateral amputation is < 50% and decreases steadily with age at the time of amputation. As expected, the common causes of death are coronary, stroke, and malignancy. The more proximal the amputation, the higher the mortality rate.

5. How common are amputations due to peripheral vascular disease among patients with diabetes mellitus?

Many of the estimated 14 million persons in the U.S. with diagnosed or undiagnosed diabetes will experience pathologic changes in their lower extremities, which when combined with minor trauma or infection may lead to serious foot problems. The most commonly described diabetic foot conditions include neuropathy, structural deformities, calluses, skin and nail changes, foot ulcers, infection, and vascular disease (See figure, question 6).

An estimated 20% of diabetic patients will develop an ulcer on the feet or ankles at some time during the disease course. At least 50% of diabetic patients with peripheral vascular disease in the U.S. population eventually undergo nontraumatic lower-limb amputation. With the increasing incidence of diabetes, it is estimated that the total number of patients could exceed 20 million by the year 2000.

6. Is there a link between glycemic control and amputation risk in diabetics?

Many investigations have postulated that the presence of chronic hyperglycemia accelerates development of chronic complications of diabetes. The relationship between glycemic control and amputation was addressed by West, who found among patients with diabetes and higher blood glucose levels, a twofold increased risk for leg lesions, including gangrene, than in those with lower blood glucose concentrations. In the population-based Rochester study, amputation risk was higher for non-insulin-dependent diabetics than for insulin-dependent diabetics (35.6 vs. 28.3 per 10,000 patients).

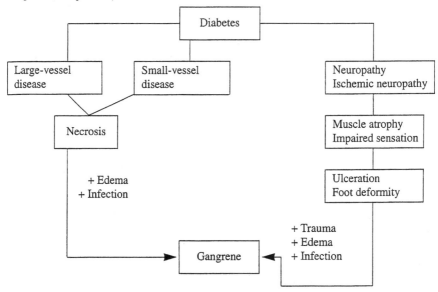

7. Name the most significant signs and symptoms of acute arterial occlusion in diabetic patients.

In the diabetic patient, most ischemic changes occur slowly, although sudden occlusion from emboli or acute complete thrombosis can occur with atherosclerosis as the underlying cause. More than 70% of the emboli originate in the heart (underlying conditions such as atrial fibrillation or myocardial infarction with mural thrombi usually exist). The signs and symptoms of acute arterial occlusion are commonly referred to as the **five Ps**:

1. **Pain** (sudden onset)
2. **Pallor** (waxy)
3. **Paresthesia** (numbness)
4. **Pulselessness** (no pulse below the block)
5. **Paresis** (sudden weakness)

8. What are the levels of amputation for the lower extremities?

In 1974, the Task Force on Standardization of Prosthetic-Orthotic Terminology developed an international classification system to define amputation level. The major terms in common use today are as follows:

Levels of Amputation

Partal toe—Excision of any part of one or more toes	Short below-knee (transtibial)—< 20% of femoral length
Toe disarticulation—Disarticulation at the MTP joint	Knee disarticulation—Amputation through the knee joint, femur intact
Partial foot/ray resection—Resection of the 3rd, 4th, 5th, metarsals, and digits	Long above-knee (transfemoral)—> 60% of femoral length

Table continued on following page

Levels of Amputation (Continued)

Transmetatarsal—Amputation through the midsection of all metarsals	Above-knee (transfemoral)—35–60% of femoral length
Syme's—Ankle disarticulation with attachment of heel pad to distal end of tibia; may include removal of all maleoli and distal tibial/fibular flares	Short above-knee (transfemoral)—< 35% of femoral length
	Hip disarticulation—Amputation through hip joint, pelvis intact
Long below-knee (transtibial)—> 50% of tibial length	Hemipelvectomy—Resection of lower half of the pelvis
Below-knee (transtibial)—20–50% of tibial length	Hemicorpectomy—Amputation of both lower limbs and pelvis below L4,5 level

9. How many types of transtibial below-knee amputations are performed?

1. **Closed amputation**
   - Long posterior flap (Burgess technique)
   - Equal anterior and posterior flaps (fishmouth)
   - Equal medial and lateral (sagittal) flaps
   - Skew flaps

2. **End-weight-bearing amputations** (osteomyoplasty, Ertl procedure)

3. **Open amputations**
   - Guillotine
   - Open circumferential
   - Open flap(s)

10. Describe the major criteria in determining amputation level in the dysvascular limb.

Patients about to undergo an amputation are informed that the amputation will be performed at the lowest possible level, but the exact level will have to be determined in the operating room. Clinical features that have bearing on the selection of the amputation level include:

1. Palpable pulses at the next more-proximal joint have clinical significance only when present, and their presence is a very positive indication of the likelihood of healing at any given level.

2. Skin temperature is a representative measure of collateral circulation. Skin temperature should always be compared to the opposite limb and evaluated throughout the diseased limb.

3. Dependent rubor indicates marginal viability of the skin. Incision through ruborous tissue may not heal, and dependent rubor should be considered an absolute contraindication to amputation at that level.

4. Degree of sensory loss is of significance in the diabetic patient whose ischemic process is frequently accompanied by peripheral neuropathy. The etiology of the diabetic ulcer or infection frequently involves neuropathic as well as ischemic factors.

5. Bleeding of the skin edges at the time of surgical incision is probably the best clinical sign available to predict healing at the intended level.

11. What are the limb-salvage decision-making variables?

Certain criteria can predict amputation of the limb in patients with severe skeletal or soft tissue injuries of the lower extremities with vascular compromise. These data might discriminate the salvageable from the unsalvageable limb.

Patient variables
  Age (usually unfavorable result after age 50)
  Occupational considerations
  Patient and family desires
  Underlying chronic disease (e.g., diabetes)

Extremity variables
  Mechanism of injury (soft tissue injury kinetics; massive crush or high-energy soft tissue injuries have poor prognosis)
  Arterial/venous injury location (e.g., poor prognosis with infrapopliteal arterial injury)
  Neurologic (anatomic) status
  Injury status of ipsilateral limb
  Intercalary ischemic zone after revascularization

Associated variables
Magnitude of associated injury
Severity and duration of shock (poor prognosis with prolonged severe hypovolemic shock)
Warm ischemia time (unfavorable prognosis if warm ischemia time is > 6 hrs)

12. How does etiology differ between wet and dry gangrene of the foot?
The most common cause for foot amputation is infection (**wet gangrene**) in patients with diabetes mellitus. The initiating cause is often a normal bony prominence combined with sensory neuropathy and inappropriate shoewear producing penetrating ulcerations.

Dry gangrene, in contrast, is frequently seen as a result of dysvascularity with or without diabetes mellitus and attendant sensory neuropathy. Smoking is often an aggravating factor. Dry gangrene of the forefoot may also develop in collagen diseases such as lupus erythematosus or from showers of microemboli settling in the end arteries of the toes following cardiac surgery.

13. What is myoplasty?
In **myoplasty**, opposing muscle groups are simply joined to each other by sutures through myofascia and investing fascia over the end of the bone. In a severely dysvascular residual limb with marginal muscle viability, myoplasty is probably the preferable method, but it should be done with little closure tension. Tapering of the muscle mass avoids excessive distal bulk.

14. What is myodesis?
The most structurally stable residual limbs are achieved with **myodesis**, in which the surrounding muscles and their fasciae are sutured directly to the bone through drill holes. In the case of transfemoral amputation, the additional advantages of myodesis are stabilization of the femur in adduction by the adductor magnus, enhanced hip flexion by the rectus femoris, and enhanced hip extension by the biceps femoris, all three being muscles that cross the hip joint. In this method, tapering of the muscle mass prevents excessive distal bulk. Myodesis is contraindicated in cases of severe dysvascularity in which the blood supply to the muscle appears compromised. In patients with normal blood supply to the stump, myodesis may be combined with myoplasty.

15. What are the options in postoperative dressing in lower-extremity amputation?
Immediate postoperative fitting prosthesis (IPOP) or **rigid dressing** using elastic plaster bandage with minimal tension starting on the distal lateral aspect of the residual limb. In below-knee amputation, IPOP is done easier than at the above-knee level, since the use of rigid spica, particularly in elderly people, causes physical difficulties and hygienic problems.

Semirigid postoperative dressing. A variety of semirigid dressings have been used to provide wound support and pressure. The **Unna paste dressing**, a compound of zinc oxide, gelatin, glycerin, and calamine, may be used as a wrapping over conventional soft dressings. It allows limited joint movement.

Controlled environment and air bags. The equipment for controlled environment treatment is designed to provide a controlled wound-healing environment. Pressure, humidity, temperature, gas, sterility, visualizations of the wound, and some degree of immobilizing are obtained with a flow-through air bag attached to a portable mechanical console unit. There will be no dressing directly over the wound or operative site, which can be inspected until the bag is removed (usually 10–14 days postoperatively).

Soft dressing is the oldest method of postoperative residual limb management and includes two forms: elastic shrinker and elastic bandages. Soft dressings are inexpensive and lightweight, and they can be reapplied several times daily. Their disadvantages include poor control of edema; they require a skilled individual to wrap the residual limb properly.

16. List the benefits of IPOP.
1. Rapid wound healing by controlling postoperative edema without restricting circulation
2. Earlier ambulation and shorter hospital stay
3. Minimizing inflammatory reaction
4. Reducing phantom pain
5. Psychological benefit

17. What are the major factors in prognosis of a dysvascular limb?

SYMPTOMS	BETTER PROGNOSIS	POOR PROGNOSIS
Pain	Slow onset	Rapid onset
Vibratory sensation	Present	Absent
Deep tendon reflexes	Present	Absent
Gangrene	Slow onset	Rapid onset
Infection	Absent	Present and spreading
Edema	Absent	Present
Diabetes	Absent or well-controlled	Present
Smoking	Nonsmoker	Smoker

18. Name the major vascular complications of smoking.
Acceleration of atherosclerosis
Increased blood viscosity and clotting factors
Inhibition of prostacyclin production
Increased VLDL and decreased HDL cholesterol
Increased platelet aggregation, fibrinogen, and von Willebrand factor
Decreased plasminogen
Increased carboxyhemoglobin and carbon monoxide

19. What is the ischemic index?
The pulse signal can indicate the degree of collateral circulation by pulsatility. An **ischemic index** is calculated for each level by dividing the **systolic pressure** measured in the limb by the **brachial artery pressure**. For example, the systolic pressure may be 120 mmHg at the arm and thigh, 90 mmHg at the calf, 60 mmHg at the ankle, and 20 mmHg at midfoot. The ischemic index would be 1 at the arm and thigh, 0.75 at the calf, 0.50 at the ankle, and 0.17 at the midfoot. The lowest level of healing is at 0.45 in the diabetic and at 0.35 in nondiabetics.

20. Define phantom limb pain.
Phantom pain can be defined as pain referred to a surgically removed limb or portion of the limb. **Stump pain** is a different entity and should be distinguished from phantom pain.
The three most commonly described painful sensations include postural type of cramping or squeezing sensation; burning pain; and sharp, shooting pain. Many patients may complain of a mixed type of pain, but often the major sensation falls into one of the above three categories. Other unpleasant sensory occurrences, such as paresthesia, hypothesia, and dysesthesia, should be excluded from the definition (they may coexist with phantom pain).

21. What is phantom sensation?
This term is usually reserved for individuals who have an awareness of the missing portion of their limb in which the only subjective sensation is **mild tingling**. It is rarely unpleasant or painful. The incidence of phantom sensation is 80–100% in amputees immediately after amputation. Only 10% develop it after 1 month. Phantom sensation may appear in children with congenitally missing limbs and those who had amputations in early childhood.
Most of the available data indicate that nonpainful phantom sensation seems to be the normal experience of the body, encoded (neurosignature) over a precise brain region (neuromatrix) from birth. Phantom sensation experience is produced by networks in the brain that are normally triggered by the continuous incoming modulated flow from the periphery. As soon as this flow ceases, nonpainful phantom sensation replaces the lost organ. To most patients, the limb feels perfectly normal or somewhat shortened. Patients can "move" this phantom limb normally into various positions. Sometimes, the phantom limb stays in a single position, the position of the limb at the time of the accident and before the amputation (e.g., in the case of prior peroneal palsy the patient may experience phantom dropfoot!).

22. How common is phantom pain?

Recent studies show rates of at least 50%. Older studies show a lower incidence (0.5–10%), but they seem to be flawed by sampling bias and by difficulties in clinical differentiation between phantom and stump pain.

Interestingly, in a surveyed population of 2700 veterans, 69% were told by their physicians that the pain was just "in their heads," and only 20% were offered any treatment for their pain. However, in a survey of 5000 veteran amputees, phantom pain prevented 18% from working and interfered with the work of 33.5% who were employed; 36% found it hard to concentrate due to pain, 82% had sleep disturbances, and 45% could not carry out social activity. All this implies that the true reported incidence could be higher than 50% (maybe up to 85%). Many patients are afraid to tell their physician about the phantom pain for fear that physician will think them "insane."

23. Is phantom pain more common with war injuries?

The incidence of phantom pain is the same in civilian and war-related amputations. Pain may occur immediately after the amputations, and 50–75% of patients have pain within 1 week post-operatively. Pain may be delayed weeks, months, or years after the amputation.

24. Is there any treatment for phantom pain?

Therapeutic regimens have had < 30% long-term efficacy. Although at least 68 methods of treatment have been identified, most report varying success. Treatment methods include TENS, tricyclic antidepressants, anticonvulsants, beta-blockers, chlorpromazine, chemical sympathectomy, neurosurgical procedures, analgesics, anesthetic procedures, and sedative/hypnotic medications. Usually, treatments reducing stump problems (neuroma, infection, etc.) also decrease phantom pain.

Treatment measures that create increased peripheral control input may provide at least temporary relief of the phantom pain. One of the more effective adjuncts is extensive use of the prosthesis. Other treatments include gentle manipulation of the stump by massage or a vibrator, stump wrapping, baths, ultrasound, and application of hot packs if sensation is intact. No single drug has been proved effective in long-term control of phantom pain (narcotics should be avoided). Trigger point injection on or near the stump may be useful (aqueous steroid and local anesthetic agents).

25. What are the common skin problems of amputees?

Amputation at any level is accompanied by distinct problems of functional loss, prosthetic fitting and alignment problems, and medical conditions such as skin disorders. Skin lesions, however minute they may appear, are nevertheless of great importance since they can be the beginning of an extensive skin disorder that may be physically, mentally, socially, and economically disastrous.

Skin Problems in Amputee Stumps and their Treatment

PROBLEM	CAUSE	TREATMENT
Poor hygiene	Bacterial and fungal infections, dermatitis, odor	Wash stump and socket, and wash stump socks, with sudsing detergent or soap containing bacteriostatic agent, at night.
Contact dermatitis and edema	Proximal choking of stump by socket, sensitivity to stump socks, plastic resins	Patch test, modification of prosthesis. Cool compress, topical topical steroid and antipruritic creams.
Maceration	Moist skin	Cornstarch in socket and on stump. Absorbent stump socks, more frequent change of socks
Friction and skin stretch	Secondary to socket design	Elasto-Gel. Thin nylon stump sock.

Table continued on following page

Skin Problems in Amputee Stumps and their Treatment (Continued)

PROBLEM	CAUSE	TREATMENT
Excessive sweating	Lack of evaporation	Antiperspirants
Nonspecific eczema	Associated with chronic edema and congestion of distal part of stump, characterized by weeping and itching	Modification of prosthesis, topical steroids
Fungal infection	Secondary to increased moisture	Fungistatic creams
Skin adherence	Constant rubbing of scar tissue on on prosthesis, may cause skin breakdown and ulceration	Massage to soften scar tissue, modification of prosthetic socket
Folliculitis, cysts, furuncles	Hair follicle and sweat gland occlusion with staphyloccal infection	Discontinue wearing prosthesis, eliminate high pressure points in socket, wearing nylon sheath between skin and stump sock. Furuncles often require incision, drainage and systemic antibiotics
Open ulcer	Multiple causes: e.g., high pressure area, excessive socket pressure, or motion of limb in socket	Discontinue wearing prosthesis until ulcer is healed, modification of socket, wound care
Epidermoid cysts	Follicular keratin plugs, very sensitve (usually found along upper margins of prosthesis, common in transfemoral amputees)	Surgical incision and drainage, systematic antibiotics, discontinue wearing prosthesis until stump is healed.
Painful neuromas and hypersensitivity	A natural repair phenomenon that occurs in any transection of a peripheral nerve	Desensitize by tapping, local injection, surgical excision
Choked stump syndrome, painful verrucous hyperplasia with cracking and weeping of stump	Insecure suspension and lack of total contact distally stretching the skin over the end of the bone with each step. Underlying vascular disorder usually present.	Refitting with new total contact socket usually solves the problem and skin gradually changes to normal. Proximal pressure must be avoided.

26. Does energy expenditure differ between dysvascular and traumatic amputees during ambulation?

Older dysvascular amputees use more energy during walking than their younger, usually traumatic counterparts. A comparison of the two etiologies of amputation at the below-knee (BK) and above-knee (AK) levels reveals that comfortable walking speed is slower and the O_2 consumption higher for the dysvascular BK amputee than for the traumatic BK amputee (45 m/min and 0.20 mL/kg/m vs. 71 m/min and 0.16 mL/kg/m, respectively).

The same differences were observed at the AK level between dysvascular and traumatic amputees (36 m/min and 0.28 mL/kg/m vs. 52 m/min and 0.20 mL/kg/m). Most older patients who have AK or higher amputations for vascular disease are not successful prosthetic ambulators. Very few are able to walk with a prosthesis without crutch assistance. If able to walk, they have a very slow walking speed and an elevated heart rate if crutch assistance is required.

27. How does energy expenditure differ between crutch and prosthetic ambulation?

Direct comparison of walking in unilateral traumatic and dysvascular amputees at the Syme's, BK, and AK levels using a prosthesis or a swing-through crutch-assisted gait without a prosthesis reveals that almost all amputees have a lower rate of energy expenditure, heart rate, and O_2 cost when using a prosthesis. This difference is insignificant in dysvascular AK patients and is related to the fact that even with a prosthesis, most of these patients require crutches for some support, thereby increasing the O_2 rate and heart rate. It can be concluded that a well-fitted prosthesis that results in a satisfactory gait not requiring crutches significantly reduces the physiologic energy demand. Since crutch-walking requires more exertion than walking with a prosthesis, crutch-walking without a prosthesis should not be considered an absolute requirement for prosthetic prescription and training.

28. What is the goal in rehabilitation of the geriatric bilateral amputee?
The great majority of bilateral lower-limb amputees today are elderly who lose their limbs secondary to diabetes and peripheral vascular disease. In general, dismissing these patients as poor prosthetic candidates is a grave mistake, and it compromises their rehabilitation potential when immediate postsurgical treatment is delayed. Lack of exercise and mobility will encourage joint contractures, weaken the patient, cause loss of independence, bring on depression, and maybe even become life-threatening. Unfortunately, the challenge of rehabilitating these patients is frequently complicated by the presence of other illnesses, such as diabetes, chronic infection, kidney disease, cardiovascular disease, respiratory disease, arthritis, impaired vision, delayed wound healing, and neuropathy. These coexisting diseases warrant additional consideration and precautions, but chronologic age *alone* should not determine whether an amputee is a prosthetic candidate.

29. What is the segmental weight of the limbs and its percentage of total body weight?
In a typical rehab setting, knowing the approximate segmental weight of each limb at different levels can be helpful in managing various clinical situations, including nutritional assessment of an amputee. Following are segmental weights of the limbs and percentage of the total body weight for a 150-lb man:

Lower limb (entire length)	23.4 lb	15.6%	Upper limb (entire length)	7.3 lb	4.9%
Thigh	14.5 lb	9.7%	Arm	4.0 lb	2.7%
Leg	6.8 lb	4.5%	Forearm	2.4 lb	1.6%
Foot	2.1 lb	1.4%	Hand	0.9 lb	0.6%

30. To what degree does malnutrition affect the healing of lower-extremity amputations?
The significant incidence of malnutrition in hospitalized patients has been well documented. Patients undergoing lower-limb amputations are frequently elderly and debilitated. Diabetics with dysvascular limbs often have open wounds and systemic sepsis, causing increased metabolic demands and an increased energy requirement 30–55% above basal values. Protein malnutrition, in general, has an adverse effect on mortality in hospital patients.

Dickhaut demonstrated that in Syme's amputations, even subclinical malnutrition makes wound healing almost impossible. Despite the technical expertise that yielded an 86% success rate in his nourished patients, Dickhaut had an 85% failure rate in malnourished amputees (Syme's).

Serum albumin levels and total lymphocyte counts are excellent ways to gauge the nutritional status of the patient. They are easy to obtain and have great predictive value for complications in the hospitalized patient. Serum albumin of < 3.4 g/dL and total lymphocyte counts < 1,500 cells/mm³ are considered abnormal. Surgical procedures on these patients should be delayed until their nutritional status is improved.

31. Why is preoperative amputee assessment an important part of the rehab program?
Amputees at various levels have distinctive problems of anatomic and functional loss, fitting and alignment of the prosthesis, gait abnormalities, and medical issues that require continued care for the remainder of their lives. A neglected part of total patient management is the pre-amputation stage. When amputation is anticipated or planned, rehabilitation clinicians have the opportunity to help prepare the patient physically and psychologically.

Questions can be answered and instructions given to alleviate anxieties of the unknown. Patients want to know what a prosthesis looks like, what it is made of, and how much it costs. The patient should be shown what type of exercise program is expected and how ambulation is performed with crutches or a walker on flat surfaces and stairs. Addressing these issues *before amputation* not only shortens the recovery time but also gives the patient a psychologic edge.

32. What is the risk categorization for injury prevention of insensate foot?

Risk and Management Categories

RISK	MANAGEMENT
Category 0	
Protective sensation present	Foot clinic once/year
No history of plantar ulcer	Patient education to include proper shoe style
May have foot deformity	selection
Has a disease the could lead to insensitivity	
Category 1	
Protective sensation absent	Foot clinic every 6 months
No history of plantar ulceration	Review all footwear the patient wears
No foot deformity	Add soft insoles
	Also consider leprosy
Category 2	
Protection sensation absent	Foot clinic every 3–4 months
No history of planter ulcer	Custom-molded orthotic devices are usually
Foot deformity present	necessary
	Prescription footwear often required
Category 3	
Protective sensation absent	Foot clinic every 1–2 months
There is a history of foot ulceration and/or	Custom orthotic devices are necessary
vascular laboratory findings indicate	Prescription shoes are often required
significant vascular disease	

BIBLIOGRAPHY

1. Bowker J: Atlas of Limb Prosthetics. St. Louis, Mosby, 1993.
2. Kostnik J: Amputation Surgery and Rehabilitation. New York, Churchill Livingstone, 1981.
3. Lange R: Limb reconstruction versus amputation: Decision making in massive lower-extremity trauma. Clin Orthop 96:1–243, 1989.
4. Levin M, O'Neal L, Bowker J (eds): The Diabetic Foot. St. Louis, Mosby, 1993.
5. O'Sullivan S, Schmitz T: Physical Rehabilitation: Assessment and Treatment. Philadelphia, F.A. Davis, 1994.
6. Sherman R, Arena J: Phantom limb pain. Crit Rev Phys Med Rehabil 4:1–26, 1992.
7. Varda G, Friedmann L: Postamputation phantoms. Phys Med Rehabil Clin North Am 1:334, 1991.
8. Waters R: Energy expenditure. In Perry J (ed): Gait Analysis: Normal and Pathological Function. Thorofare, NJ, Slack, 1992, p 477.

92. UPPER-LIMB ORTHOSES

John B. Redford, M.D., Abna A. Ogle, M.D., and Richard C. Robinson, M.D.

A complex system that works is invariably found to have evolved from a simple system that works.
                                                                    —John Gaule

1. What is an orthosis?

An orthosis is an external apparatus worn to restrict or assist movement. An orthosis can be used to transfer load from one area to another. The terms **brace** and **splint** are used interchangeably with orthosis.

2. State three general reasons why orthotics are prescribed.

The mnemonic **SAP** highlights the three broad cardinal indications for the orthotic prescription:
S—Support
A—Alignment
P—Protection
By supporting, aligning, and protecting body parts, orthotics can enhance the function of movable body regions and prevent or correct deformities. Orthotics can be used to enhance functionality.

3. State four functions of upper limb movement that must be considered in the orthotic prescription.

1. **Reach:** Primarily accomplished by shoulder and elbow positioning and function. Severe loss of shoulder function is devastating to reach, yet hard to treat with orthoses.
2. **Carry:** The action of transporting a load. Orthotic substitutions are of little consequence.
3. **Prehension pattern:** All the functional aspects of holding objects in the hand. This aspect is very important in orthotic prescription and follow-up.
4. **Release:** Active digital extension accompanied by relaxation of digital flexors. This is an essential reverse action in all prehensile function, and it may need special orthotic attention.

4. They say that monkeys cannot use their hands like humans. What does that mean?

Hook prehension (such as carrying a suitcase) or **cylindrical grasp** (such as grabbing a rail) are tasks monkeys can do as easily as humans. However, only humans have an **opposable thumb**, and so monkeys cannot compare with humans for fine motions such as **fingertip pinch**, **lateral pinch** (holding a key), and **palmar prehension** (three jaw-chuck prehension or opposition between the thumb and second and third digits). Monkeys cannot be baseball pitchers; they cannot hold balls well because they lack **spherical grasp**. These observations imply that for any hand orthosis to work—in conjunction with hand therapy—it must restore these unique human functions as closely to normal as possible.

5. Why are upper limb splints used?

1. **To rest the body part** so that the patient does not hurt inflamed joints or further injure muscles, ligaments, or fractured bones.
2. **To prevent contractures**—i.e., to prevent patients from losing adjoining joint motion as the result of untreated burns, injury to nerves, or spasticity.
3. **To correct deformity**, in conjunction with surgery and occupational or physical therapy—a splint will be formed to keep the treated parts on a stretch.
4. **To promote exercise** for recovery of weak muscles or to correct muscle imbalances—splints are worn to strengthen certain key muscles.
5. **To substitute for lost function**—if the patient has lost a certain muscle action, it may be partly restored or retrained with an orthosis.

6. How do static and dynamic orthoses differ?

Static orthoses keep underlying segments from moving. They are often used to rest body parts during healing, to reduce tone in spastic muscles, or to decrease or prevent deformity. In some cases, they can substitute for lost joint function (e.g., an orthotic thumb post makes the thumb rigid to oppose the fingers).

Dynamic orthoses move. They have external or internal power sources and encourage restoration and control of joint movements. External power means providing motion primarily by elastics, springs, or, rarely, pneumatic or electrical systems; internal power means providing motion through action of another body part, such as using wrist extension or a shoulder motion via harness and cable to operate finger grasp and release. The prescription should always indicate which motion a dynamic orthosis is to assist: for example, the phrase *finger flexion assist* would be part of the prescription for an orthosis to restore prehension.

7. How long should patients expect to wear an orthosis?

Generally no more than a month or two. Most upper limb orthoses are to be worn only during postoperative recovery or until the useful effects of medication, physical modality, or exercise to improve mobility and strength evidently have overcome the acute problem. At first, orthoses are applied 2–3 hours once or twice a day. Gradually, patients wear them longer, depending on the condition. Some are worn mainly at night.

8. When are upper limb orthoses most likely to be used?

Indications include:
* Trauma and surgery
  Tendon repair
  Postreconstructive surgery (Dupuytren's contracture release)
  Joint injuries
* Nerve injuries
* Painful disorders (rheumatoid arthritis, carpal tunnel syndrome)
* Improve function after disease (poststroke, neuromuscular disease, peripheral nerve disorders)

9. What are static shoulder orthoses?

We rely so much on free unrestricted motion for shoulder function that static orthoses to immobilize fractures of the upper arm can only be used for short periods. Effective immobilization is hard to achieve unless the orthosis applies most of the force through the longitudinal axis of the upper arm and combines this with a force in the frontal plane to hold the humerus into the glenoid cavity.

Most varieties of static or partly dynamic shoulder slings do not really perform well biomechanically. Many orthoses tried for the subluxed paralyzed shoulder, a frequent sequela of stroke, do help to relieve pain but do little to promote function. An **airplane splint** holds the arm out like a wing (see figure on following page). It is designed to promote healing of fractures or immobilizing the shoulder in abduction after reconstructive surgery or injury. However, it is an example of a good mechanical or orthotic idea, but a bad human interactive idea, because patients tolerate them so poorly. Nevertheless, an airplane splint may be the only useful device to prevent an axillary burn from causing a contracture or to ensure healing of a shoulder fusion.

10. Is a ballbearing feeder used to feed patients ball bearings?

No! A ballbearing feeder is an old name for the dynamic shoulder orthosis called a **balanced forearm orthosis** (BFO). This device attaches to the upright of a wheelchair and supports the forearm with a freely moving rod located beneath the forearm trough. The BFO works to modify the effects of gravity so that persons confined to a wheelchair and with slight use of the shoulder or elbow (grade 2 at least in area muscles) may be more functional in a wheelchair. A BFO is not useful unless some hand function remains and the patient really wants to feed himself or do other activities requiring reach. An occupational therapist must make the necessary adjustments before conducting training. The patient should have a trial of a dynamic overhead sling suspension orthosis before applying the BFO because the sling is much easier to set up and use for evaluation.

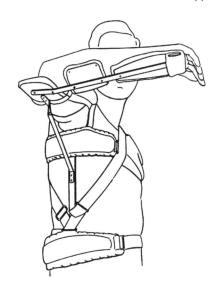

Airplane splint. A static shoulder orthosis. (From Long C, Shutt AH: Upper limb orthotics. In Redford JB (ed): Orthotics Etcetera, 3rd ed. Baltimore, Williams & Wilkins, 1986, pp 198–277, with permission.)

11. What are some purposes for elbow orthoses?

Elbow orthoses are used most commonly to **reduce flexion contractures**, employing a static type with hinged bars attached by Velcro to the upper arm and forearm cuffs. Single-axis elbow joints can be sequentially adjusted to extend the elbow further. A tension spring to extend the elbow joint dynamically, or a turnbuckle applied between the upper arm and the lower forearm cuffs, can provide steady stretch to reduce the contracture. Less commonly, a static or dynamic orthosis is used to **reduce an extension contracture**. Dynamic elbow orthoses are rarely used to substitute for muscle loss, such as lost elbow flexion, because they lack cosmetic appeal and are just not very effective.

12. What special problems must be considered when splinting the wrist or hand?

1. After any surgery or injury to the hand, it will swell. Unless this **edema** is properly approached, joints may become stiff as a result of the subsequent overactivity of fibroblasts. It has been said, "Hand therapy is behavior modification of fibroblasts during the healing response." As part of this hand therapy, you do not want hand splints applied incorrectly during recovery. Orthoses may aggravate edema. Their use must be carefully monitored, especially in patients with limited cognition or inappropriate emotional reactions to using splints.

2. The hand has great **sensibility**, and any sensory loss results in significant effects on function. Unfortunately, sensory loss is very common. Its extent must be mapped carefully and orthotic pressure over insensate areas kept to a minimum. Because the hand is the organ of touch, the orthosis must be designed to avoid blocking sensation to critical areas, such as the fingertips. The hand is so sensitive that fitting must be exact; any discomfort will result in rejection of the orthosis.

3. There is a multiplicity of joints in the hand. It may be necessary to make an orthosis that immobilizes one or more joints to allow movement in others. Deciding how to do this requires good judgment and wide experience with the various materials needed for fabrication. A good example is the MCP block orthosis: The MCP joints are held in flexion to block the action of the long finger extensors and allow the PIP and DIP joints to extend.

13. What is a SEWHO?

Upper limb orthoses are all named for the parts that they incorporate, and these are then usually abbreviated. Some examples are:

Shoulder-elbow-wrist-hand orthosis—SEWHO   Hand orthosis—HO
Wrist-hand orthosis—WHO   Finger orthosis—FO

14. Hand therapists, like all specialists, have their own language. Define some of the more common terms.

Assist: Any dynamic component designed to provide a certain motion.

Block or stop: Any part of an orthosis designed to block a given motion as in the MCP block orthosis. The block is sometimes in the form of a lock (e.g., an elbow lock).

C-bar: A C-shaped strip of plastic or metal applied in the thumb/index finger webspace to prevent thumb adduction against the palm.

Dorsal wrist/hand orthosis *(WHO)*: An orthosis applied to the superior surface of the hand and wrist; it contrasts with the more common palmar or volar WHO.

Finger deviation splint: A hand orthosis with components to prevent abduction or adduction of the fingers, as incorporated in splints for the rheumatoid arthritic hand to prevent ulnar drift. Whether they really help prevent drift is controversial.

Opponens bar: A component for positioning the thumb, such as a bar outside the thumb to prevent it from extending.

Opponens splint: An orthosis that holds the thumb in opposition to the fingers; sometimes described as "short" (below the wrist) or "long" (incorporating the wrist and hand).

Outrigger: A component applied above or below an orthosis to provide a platform from which various dynamic components can pull against the digits with elastics and cuffs or springs.

15. How should you order and classify orthoses for the wrist and hand?

The easiest way to describe a hand orthosis is to state whether it is static or dynamic and the main area it encompasses or immobilizes. In any orthosis, the prescriber should also say if it is to mobilize, assist, or apply traction to a certain joint or movement. The authors of the American Society of Hand Therapists Splint/Orthotic Classification System recommend further distinction between static and dynamic orthoses by clarifying the purpose of an orthosis as immobilizing, mobilizing, restricting, or a combination of several of these terms.

Common Kinds of Hand Orthoses

TYPE	DESCRIPTION
Wrist orthosis	Ends in the palm
Wrist-hand orthosis	Ends over digits
Wrist-thumb orthosis	Extends into webspace of thumb
Wrist-MCP orthosis	Extends just distal to PIP crease
Forearm-wrist-finger orthosis	Many variations, but must end on fingers
Hand orthosis	Starts below the wrist
Thumb orthosis	Incorporates the thumb in some way
Finger orthosis	One finger only
Tenodesis orthosis	A special class of orthosis prescribed mainly in tetraplegic patients, employing the natural tendency of the fingers to close when the wrist is extended and open when it is flexed

16. What are some design categories of upper limb splints?

Nonarticular—provides support for a body part without crossing any joints (e.g., the humeral fracture splint with circumferential support to the upper arm).

Static motor blocking—permits motion in one direction by blocking motion in another (e.g., a swan neck finger orthosis that allows flexion in a PIP joint but blocks hyperextension of that same joint).

Serial static—splint that is periodically changed to alter joint angle and generally used to regain motion.

Static progressive—splinting to regain motion using a static line of pull that is tightened periodically to regain tissue length. One such splint (available commercially) has a MERiT component that resembles a tuning screw on a guitar; tension increases on the static line length as the MERiT is turned, thus increasing the motion into flexion of a digit.

Dynamic traction—offers traction to joints while allowing controlled motion (e.g., using longitudinal traction across an intra-articular fracture while gently flexing and extending the joint).

Tenodesis—improves function in a hand that has lost motion from injury to the nervous system (e.g., the RIC tenodesis splint, in which active extension of the wrist produces, through tenodesis action of the finger flexors, a controlled passive flexion of the fingers against a static thumb post in a patient with C6 tetraplegia).

Continuous passive motion orthosis—an electrically powered device that by moving joints mechanically through a wanted ROM over a set time keeps joints supple and mobile in the hand during healing after injury or surgery.

17. Making splints is expensive. Why not just buy off-the-shelf orthoses?

Many static splints and a few dynamic ones can be prefabricated and kept in stock. A common WHO, for example, is the Futuro line of products. However, like army clothing designed to fit everyone but really fitting no one, prefabricated orthoses may produce unexpected problems if poorly fitted. Custom-made orthoses used to be more expensive when they were made from metal or polyester resins. Almost all now are made from low-temperature thermoplastic and take much less time to make than the older ones. Hands differ so much in size, shape, and even innervation that only custom-made orthoses can be used in many situations.

18. What are the main considerations in prescribing upper limb orthoses?

- **Patient cooperation.** The patient must understand the purpose of the splint, and the therapist must judge the likelihood of patient use.
- **Comfort and cosmesis.** The splint must be comfortable to the wearer and as light as possible. In addition, the patient should be able to choose the color and suggest cosmetic considerations to satisfy concerns about appearance.
- **Wearing schedule.** This requires discussion of the times to be worn to meet the goals of the patient and therapist. Most splints are used only temporarily and are only part of any treatment plan.
- **Design.** The splint must be biomechanically suited to reach optimum goals, and prescriber follow-up is needed to make design alterations as condition improves or changes.

BIBLIOGRAPHY

1. Baily JM, Cannon NM, Casanova J, et al: Splint Classification System. Chicago, American Society of Hand Therapists, 1992.
2. Carcis D, Lamb J, Johnson: Upper limb orthoses. In Bowker P, Condie DN, Bader DL, Pratt DJ (eds): Biomechanical Basis of Orthotics Management. Oxford, Butterworth-Heineman, 1993, pp 191–218.
3. Irani KD: Wrist and hand orthoses. Phys Med Rehabil State Art Rev 1:137–160, 1987.
4. Hunter JM, Mackin EJ, Callahan AD: Rehabilitation of the Hand: Surgery and Therapy, 4th ed. St. Louis, Mosby, 1995.
5. Long C, Schutt AH: Upper limb orthotics. In Redford JB (ed): Orthotics Etcetera, 3rd ed. Baltimore, Williams & Wilkins, 1986, pp 198–277.
6. Malick MH: Manual on Dynamic Hand Splinting with Thermoplastic Materials, 3rd ed. Pittsburgh, American Rehabilitation Education Network, 1982.
7. McKee P, Morgan L: Orthotics in Rehabilitation: Splinting the Hand and Body. Philadelphia, F.A. Davis, 1998.
8. Miner LJ, Nelson VS: Upper limb orthoses. In Redford JB, Basmajian JV, Trautman P (eds): Orthotics: Clinical Practice and Rehabilitation Technology. New York, Churchill Livingstone, 1995, pp 103–132.
9. Schutt AH: Upper extremity and hand orthotics. Phys Med Rehabil Clin North Am 3:223–241, 1992.
10. Shurr DG, Cook TM: Upper-extremity orthotics. In Shurr DG, Cook TM (eds): Prosthetics and Orthotics. East Norwalk, CT, Appleton & Lange, 1990, pp 173–181.

93. UPPER-LIMB PROSTHESES

Atul T. Patel, M.D., Anthony S. Salzano, M.D.,
and Subhadra Lakshmi Nori, M.D.

> *When you do the common things in life in an uncommon way, you will command the attention of the world.* —George Washington Carver (1864–1943)

1. What is the most common congenital upper-extremity limb deficiency?

A unilateral, short, below-elbow deficiency, with absence of the forearm, wrist, and hand (terminal tranverse radial limb deficiency).

2. What is the prevalence of upper-limb amputations among all amputees in the U.S.?

Approximately 10% of all amputations involve the upper limb, most frequently below the elbow. The ratio of lower- to upper-extremity amputations is approximately 5:1.

3. Describe the most common upper-extremity prosthetic patient.

A male, 20–50 years old, who has suffered a traumatic injury to his right arm. The dominant upper limb is often injured in operating heavy machinery. The second most common cause of an upper-limb amputation is cancer.

4. How are congenital upper limb deficiencies classified?

The International Terminology for the Classification of Congenital Limb Deficiencies defines limb deficiencies as either terminal or intercalary. **Terminal** is used to define a deficiency in which a limb has developed normally to a certain level, beyond which no further skeletal elements exist (e.g., terminal transverse radial limb deficiency). **Intercalary** is used to define deficiencies in the long axis where normal skeletal elements may be present distal to the affected segment (e.g., partial reduction of the ulna with normal radius and hand elements).

5. At what age should an infant with a congenital limb deficiency be fitted with an upper-extremity prosthesis?

From 3–6 months of age, when the child begins to sit and needs the arms for prop support. At first, a passive-type prosthesis is provided; active components are added as motor landmarks are reached.

6. How are upper-extremity amputations classified?

For **below-elbow amputations**, the length of the stump remaining below the elbow is measured from the medial epicondyle of the humerus to the end of the longer residual bone (the radius or ulna). For **above-elbow amputations**, the length of the stump remaining above the elbow is measured from the tip of the acromion to the end of the residual humerus. This length is expressed as a percentage of the distance from the acromion to the lateral humeral epicondyle of the sound limb. (See figure on following page.)

7. Why is it so important to preserve as much of the limb as possible during surgical amputation?

A longer residual limb provides more stump to prosthesis contact, more proprioceptive sensation, and a longer lever arm to power the prosthesis.

8. In child amputees, the disarticulation level of amputation is preferred. Why?

The goal is the preservation of the epiphyses to allow maximum limb growth and to avoid bony overgrowth that can occur in amputations performed through the shaft of a long bone.

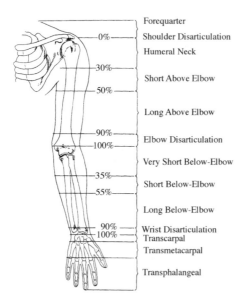

Forequarter

Shoulder Disarticulation

Humeral Neck

—0%—

—30%—

Short Above Elbow

—50%—

Long Above Elbow

—90%—

Elbow Disarticulation

—100%—

Very Short Below-Elbow

—35%—

Short Below-Elbow

—55%—

Long Below-Elbow

90% —

Wrist Disarticulation

100% —

Transcarpal

Transmetacarpal

Transphalangeal

From Kottke FJ, Lehmann JF (eds): Krusen's Handbook of Physical Medicine and Rehabilitation, 4th ed. Philadelphia, W.B. Saunders, 1990; with permission.

9. What are the goals of upper-extremity stump care?

To control pain and swelling, maintain strength and range of motion (ROM), and promote wound healing and residual limb maturation.

10. What is the foremost goal of the pre-prosthetic training period?

To help the patient achieve functional independence in ADL skills using the remaining normal arm. This promotes self-esteem and encourages the patient to realize that he or she can accomplish more than was thought possible prior to training.

11. What are the essential goals of prosthetic training?

During early prosthetic training, the patient wears the prosthesis for short periods of time, usually not longer than 15 minutes. Skin integrity is carefully monitored. The amputee progresses from learning to put on (don) and take off (doff) the prosthesis, to executing and controlling ROM of the prosthetic joints, to developing basic essential prehension movements. The final step is learning terminal-device dexterity in various elbow and shoulder positions. Bilateral amputees must have one functional prosthesis as soon as possible; ideally, this should be provided to the dominant limb.

12. What requirements must an amputee meet before he or she can be fitted with a permanent upper-extremity prosthesis?

1. The stump must be free of edema and skin breakdown for comfortable fitting.

2. The patient must have adequate active ROM and motor strength to operate the prosthetic control system.

3. The patient must demonstrate adequate cognitive ability to participate successfully in prosthetic training.

13. Name the most important things to keep in mind when developing the prescription for an upper-extremity prosthesis.

Function and comfort, rather than cosmesis. The patient's vocational and avocational habits must be evaluated to determine the combination of components that will best meet his or her needs—e.g., the requirements of a farmer who operates heavy equipment will differ substantially from those of a secretary.

14. How soon should a person with an upper limb amputation be fitted with a prosthesis?

There is a 3–6 month window of opportunity to fit an amputee with a prosthesis to significantly increase the likelihood of long-term prosthetic use. It is thought that once a person achieves independence in performing activities of daily living (ADLs) with the preserved upper limb, then the chance of fully incorporating the prosthesis in routine activities is reduced.

15. After successful fitting of the definitive prosthesis, is further medical follow-up needed?

Yes. Usually within 4–6 weeks. But this depends on several factors, including how well the patient functions at home and whether medical problems develop, such as phantom limb pain, neuroma, diminished joint mobility, bony overgrowth, and—the most common problem—skin complications such as blisters, ulcers, infections, or stasis eczema.

16. What are the essential components of every prescription for a functional upper-limb prosthesis?

Suspension system (cuffs and harness), socket, control system (cables for a body-powered prosthesis, batteries for an externally powered prosthesis), elbow hinge, wrist component, and terminal device (hook or hand). A nonfunctional or cosmetic prosthesis is usually indicated when the patient is unable to operate a functional prosthesis for his or her level of amputation.

17. A 30-year-old right-hand-dominant man has a right below-elbow amputation secondary to a farm accident. His forearm stump is about 50% in length, and his wounds are well healed with sensation loss limited to the scar. Name the most commonly prescribed components of a below-elbow prosthesis for this type of patient.

Figure-eight harness with a triceps pad/cuff; plastic laminate double-walled socket; Bowden single control cable system; flexible elbow hinges; friction wrist unit; and voluntary opening (VO) split hook.

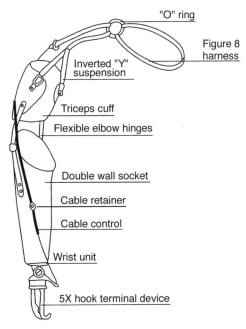

A body-powered transradial prosthesis with components identified. (From Esquenazi A: Upper limb amputee rehabilitation and prosthetic restoration. In Braddom RL (ed): Physical Medicine and Rehabilitation, 2nd ed. Philadelphia, W.B. Saunders, 2000, p 270, with permission.)

18. A 60-year-old left-hand-dominant man has an above-elbow amputation secondary to burns. The wounds over the entire distal stump are healed with a significant amount of

**scarring and decreased sensation. The stump is about 50% in length. Name the most
commonly prescribed components of an above-elbow prosthesis for this type of patient.**

Figure-eight harness; double-walled plastic laminant socket; internal locking elbow; dual-
control cable system; friction wrist unit; and VO split hook.

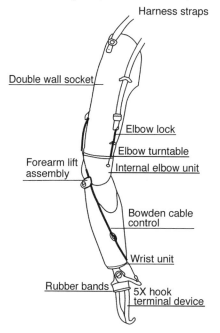

Harness straps

Double wall socket

Elbow lock

Elbow turntable

Forearm lift
assembly

Internal elbow unit

Bowden cable
control

Wrist unit

Rubber bands

5X hook
terminal device

A body-powered transhumeral prosthesis with components identified. (From Esquenazi A: Upper limb
amputee rehabilitation and prosthetic restoration. In
Braddom RL (ed): Physical Medicine and Rehabilitation, 2nd ed. Philadelphia, W.B. Saunders, 2000, p
269, with permission.)

19. What is the purpose of the terminal device?

To provide prehension (the ability to grasp objects). The human hand is capable of six types
of prehension: lateral, palmar, tip, cylindrical grasp, spherical grasp, and hook or snap. The terminal device replaces the types of prehension that allow the amputee to perform ADL skills
either with one device or, at most, two.

20. What are the advantages of a hook terminal device compared to a prosthetic hand?

Normal lateral prehension or pinch is grasping an object between the pad of the thumb and
the lateral surface of the index finger. The **hook** provides this function and is better suited for
tasks requiring manual dexterity than a prosthetic hand. It is lighter in weight and easier to maintain, and its simple design allows for maximal visualizaton of objects manipulated to compensate
for touch sensation loss.

Normal palmar prehension, or three-jaw chuck pinch, is grasping an object between the pad of
the thumb and the pads of the index and middle fingers. The **prosthetic hand** provides this function
and can be used to grasp larger objects and rounded ones. It also provides better cosmesis. The selection of a hook or a prosthetic hand is determined by the needs and preferences of the amputee.

21. What is the most commonly used terminal device?

The Dorrance VO split hook. This device was patented in 1912 by D.W. Dorrance, who was
a bilateral upper-extremity amputee. Prior to this "split" hook, terminal devices were actually
hooks and provided no prehension at all.

22. What functions do wrist units provide?

Both the friction and locking types of wrist units serve as the attachment point for the terminal device, and thus, they do not function as true wrist joints. They provide passive pronation and
supination which the patient controls by using the normal hand to rotate the wrist.

23. Explain the advantages of the epicondyle suspension prosthesis (Muenster-type below-elbow prosthesis).

Used with very short below-elbow amputations, the socket of this prosthesis is set at 30° of elbow flexion. Since this shortens the lever arm during flexion movements, it requires much less effort to operate. Because the socket is securely fitted above the humeral epicondyles, a high degree of retention is attained without the use of suspension devices, such as elbow hinges, cuffs, or pads.

24. What suction type of suspension system can be used in upper-limb prostheses?

Silicon suction suspension. This type of system has been found to be useful in patients with delicate or sensitive skin—e.g., burn patients or those with degloving-type injuries. It has also worked well in patients who play sports and are very active.

25. Name the three basic types of below-elbow hinges. What are their indications?

Flexible, rigid, and step-up hinge. The selection of the type of hinge depends on the level of amputation and on the functional status of the residual limb. A long below-elbow amputee will use the **flexible hinge**; the short below-elbow amputee requires more stability and needs the **rigid hinge**. When the below-elbow stump is very short and flexion is severely limited, the gear arrangement of the **step-up hinge** permits the socket to flex through a greater range than the residual elbow joint would otherwise allow. Keep in mind that with short below-elbow stumps, the supracondylar suspension prosthesis is often a good alternative to hinges.

26. How does the amputee operate the body-powered upper-extremity prosthesis?

An amputee is trained to perform coordinated body movements that transmit tension along a cable system that slides inside one or more flexible housings. The stainless-steel cable is attached proximally to the harness and distally to the terminal device. With an above-elbow prosthesis, the cable is also attached to the elbow unit.

An amputee with a below-elbow prosthesis uses a single-control system (**Bowden control system**) to operate the terminal device through coordinated arm flexion and shoulder abduction.

An amputee with an above-elbow or very short below-elbow prosthesis needs a dual-control system (**fair-lead system**) in which arm flexion operates the terminal device and controls forearm flexion, and arm extension operates the elbow lock. When the elbow is locked between 90–135°, the terminal device is operated by biscapular abduction (shoulder shrug).

27. Why is the figure-eight harness the most commonly used? What are some other types?

It provides the widest range of everyday activities with the least restrictions of the body. Other harness types meet more specific requirements of an amputee. The **figure-nine harness**, for example, affords more freedom of movement of the prosthetic limb and is used in the supracondylar prosthesis. The **triple-control system harness**, which separates terminal-device operation from forearm flexion and replaces the dual-control system, is useful for people with above-elbow amputations. The **modified shoulder saddle harness** provides a larger weight-bearing area and permits the amputee to lift heavy objects without transmitting excessive pressure to the sound axilla.

28. How much weight can be typically lifted with the upper limb fitted with a prosthesis?

A person with a transradial amputation can typically lift about 20–30 lbs, while a person with a transhumeral amputation can be expected to lift 10–15 lbs.

29. How does the myoelectric-type prosthesis work?

When this type of prosthesis is worn by a patient with an upper-extremity amputation, surface electrodes housed in the socket are brought into contact with muscles that have been trained to contract and to generate a minimum signal of 10 µV. This voltage, which is amplified 20,000–40,000 times, activates a rechargeable nickel-cadmium battery that then operates the small reversible electric motors in the terminal device and prosthetic joints.

30. What is the value of the myometric evaluation?

This evaluation uses a myotester to measure the action potentials of the amputee's stump muscles and to determine whether the muscles are capable of activating the surface electrodes of the prosthesis that operate the terminal device.

31. Which type of prosthesis requires more time for training—externally powered or body-powered?

Generally the control training for an externally powered prosthesis is more complex and requires more time to learn the appropriate muscle motions and contractions needed to operate the device precisely.

32. What particular difficulties does a patient with a shoulder disarticulation or forequarter amputation face?

These patients have no residual stumps and therefore cannot easily mobilize their shoulder girdle strength to operate the control systems. In the forequarter amputation (interthoracoscapular amputation), the problem is even more difficult, since there is no residual shoulder girdle. Thus, an amputee must expend great effort and be highly motivated to operate a body-powered shoulder disarticulation prosthesis.

33. What are the essential components of the body-powered shoulder disarticulation prosthesis?

This appliance, also called the active prehensile arm, consists of the shoulder component, arm section, elbow unit, forearm section, wrist unit, and terminal device. All these are operated by shoulder girdle movements.

BIBLIOGRAPHY

1. Atkins DJ, Meier RH 3d: Comprehensive Management of the Upper-Limb Amputee. New York, Springer-Verlag, 1989.
2. Esquenazi A: Upper limb amputee rehabilitation and prosthetic restoration. In Braddom RL (ed): Physical Medicine and Rehabilitation, 2nd ed. Philadelphia, W. B. Saunders, 2000, pp 263–278.
3. Nader EHM (ed): Otto Bock Prosthetic Compendium—Upper-Extremity Prostheses. Berlin, Schliele & Schon GmbH, 1990.
4. New York University Post-Graduate Medical School: Upper-Limb Prosthetics. New York, NYU, 1986.
5. Schmidl H: Protesi per arto superiore. Riv Chir Mano 20(1):53–58, 1983.

94. LOWER-LIMB ORTHOSES

Kristjan T. Ragnarsson, M.D., Jay Schechtman, M.D., and Richard A. Frieden, M.D.

1. What are the indications for use of an ankle-foot orthosis (AFO) to improve a patient's gait?

1. Mediolateral instability at the ankle
2. "Foot-drop," passive plantar flexion in swing phase
3. "Foot-drop" at heel strike due to weak ankle dorsiflexors
4. Weak push-off at late stance phase

2. What requirement must the patient meet in order to use an AFO effectively?

1. Knee extension strength > 3/5
2. Stable limb size without fluctuating edema for use of a plastic AFO
3. Skin pressure tolerance and patient compliance with skin checks

3. What are posterior and anterior stops on an AFO?

Anterior and posterior stops are used to control ankle dorsiflexion and plantar flexion on a jointed AFO. A posterior stop limits plantar flexion in swing phase; an anterior stop limits dorsiflexion following midstance. Limiting dorsiflexion at the ankle allows less knee flexion moment during stance and stabilizes it. Limitation in dorsiflexion at late stance replaces push off and passively raises the center of gravity. This improves the energy efficiency of gait. A posterior stop is also helpful when moderate spasticity is present to control plantar flexion spasms and to prevent equinus deformity from developing.

4. How do AFO stops differ from AFO assists?

An anterior stop limits dorsiflexion. An anterior assist (spring) aids in plantar flexion, substituting for a weak gastrocsoleus muscle. A posterior stop limits plantar flexion. A posterior assist (spring) aids in dorsiflexion, substituting for a weak tibialis anterior muscle.

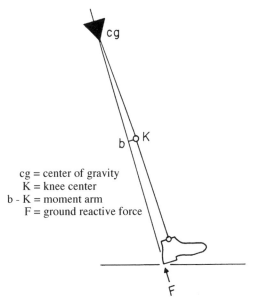

Knee bending moment at heel strike. (From Lehmann JF: The biomechanics of ankle foot orthoses: Prescription and design. Arch Phys Med Rehabil 60:200–207, 1979; with permission.)

cg = center of gravity
K = knee center
b - K = moment arm
F = ground reactive force

5. How is the AFO altered to stabilize the knee?

An AFO can be adjusted to alter the forces that are transmitted from ground reaction through the closed kinetic chain of the limb to the knee. When the AFO is set into plantar flexion, the knee is provided with a stabilizing extension moment during stance in foot-flat and push-off. The opposite result can occur if the AFO is set in dorsiflexion, causing a destabilizing knee flexion moment at heel strike.

6. Which type of AFO is used when clonus is present at the ankle?

When a patient has severe clonus at the ankle, the foot should usually be locked in a **solid AFO**. In a patient with significant spasticity, an AFO with any form of spring action may permit movement to trigger and perpetuate clonus.

7. What is a spiral brace? How does it work?

A **spiral brace** is a thermoplastic AFO that is made in a spiral design to control both dorsiflexion and plantar flexion. The spiral winds around the patient's calf from the medial footplate in a full spiral to the anterior tibial area at the level of the tibial condyles. The spiral unwinds with weight-bearing to allow plantar flexion. When the body weight is removed, the spiral rewinds and provides a dorsiflexion assist.

A **hemi-spiral brace**, in contrast, has only a half-spiral winding up the leg from the lateral footplate and provides a better control of equinus and varus forces at the ankle; i.e., it limits inversion and plantar flexion.

The spiral brace uses the **three-point pressure system** common to all orthotics to provide eversion and inversion control at the ankle. Spiral braces are most useful in patients with flaccid weakness of all the ankle muscles (i.e., both dorsiflexors or plantarflexors), but these orthoses are contraindicated in the presence of significant spasticity.

8. What is a floor-reaction orthosis?

The biomechanics of the floor-reaction orthosis are based on the same principles that were discussed regarding AFOs and knee stability (see question 4), because in essence the floor reaction orthosis is an AFO with the footplate set in slight plantar flexion. The extension moment created by plantar-flexing the orthosis is transferred to the patellar tendon by a band of material on the top of the orthosis. The extension moment helps to stabilize the knee. Floor reaction orthoses are prescribed to help with knee extension in patients who have at least fair (3/5) quadriceps motor strength.

9. What is a Klenzack joint?

Klenzack ankle joints are (or were) used in a jointed metal AFO. The joint has a spring assist for ankle dorsiflexion. This brace should generally not be used in the presence of significant spasticity, as the spring may amplify clonus.

10. Explain the considerations necessary when ordering an AFO.

A patient who has weakness of the ankle dorsiflexors without spasticity or mediolateral instability can be prescribed a plastic AFO. A posterior-leaf-spring AFO, however, provides limited mediolateral stability and does not compensate for weak plantar flexors. If the patient has both weak dorsiflexors and plantar flexors with no or very little spasticity, the most appropriate orthoses would be a custom-molded plastic AFO with an anterior trimline cut just anterior to the malleoli. To provide maximal mediolateral stability, toe pick-up and push-off require the use of a solid ankle double-upright AFO with a T-strap medially for eversion control and laterally for inversion control. For a person with mild spasticity and a tendency for equinus, a hemi-spiral AFO or a plastic AFO with a posterior trimline could suffice.

11. Does prophylactic knee bracing prevent knee injuries in football?

There is some controversy on this issue. A study of college football players at West Point found a statistically significant decline in medial collateral injuries in defensive players who used prophylactic knee braces. A larger study on NCAA collegiate football players actually showed more knee injuries in those using prophylactic knee orthoses. Currently, it appears that there is no compelling evidence to recommend prophylactic knee bracing to football players.

12. What should be checked when a patient receives a new AFO?

If the orthosis is jointed, the anatomical ankle joint which runs through the malleoli should be in the same axis as the orthotic joint. In stance, the knee should be fully extended and the sole of the shoe should be flat on the floor. In swing, there should be adequate toe clearance. The knee should flex slightly immediately following heel strike. There should be a 1- or 2-inch clearance from the upper brim of the orthosis to the fibular head in order to prevent pressure on the peroneal nerve.

13. Which type of orthosis is used in Legg-Calvé-Perthes disease?

Legg-Calvé-Perthes disease is a childhood disorder with avascular necrosis of the capital femoral epiphysis. The goal of bracing in this disorder is to maintain the femoral head completely within the acetabulum in order to maintain its sphericity. Both plaster casts and orthoses of different designs, such as the Toronto, Newington, and Atlanta Scottish Rite orthoses, have been used to place the **hip in hyperabduction and external rotation**. It is not necessary to remember the names of all the different designs of such orthoses, as long as the hyperabduction concept is understood.

14. What type of orthosis is used for persons with spina bifida who are community ambulators?

Persons with spina bifida who can ambulate successfully in the community generally must be intact, to at least the L3 neurologic level, and have fair (3/5) quadriceps strength. The child should be braced in bilateral solid AFO. It is unwise to extend the orthoses to the knee, as the child may not be able to advance the limb with the knee locked in extension. An assistive device for balance is often needed.

15. Should you prescribe knee-ankle-foot orthoses (KAFOs) for a patient with thoracic paraplegia?

Clinical experience has shown that few persons with thoracic paraplegia use KAFOs (long-leg braces) for functional ambulation. This has been attributed to the high energy expenditure and the slow speed of such gait. A study of persons with high thoracic paraplegia using Scott-Craig KAFOs to ambulate has shown that energy expenditure was similar regardless of the exact neurologic level. These individuals were found to decrease their energy expenditure by decreasing ambulation speed in order to reach a comfortable power output level.

There are, however, significant psychologic and functional benefits for persons who achieve the ability to be able to stand erect and perform some ADLs upright. There may also be considerable physiologic benefits from regularly assuming the standing position and performing the physical exercise associated with KAFOs (swing-to or swing-through) ambulation. Therefore, KAFOs should not be denied to a person based only on the SCI level and the poor prospects for functional ambulation. However, the person with paraplegia must be advised that KAFOs are only an adjunct to, and not a replacement for, the wheelchair as primary means of locomotion.

16. Why is ambulation with bilateral KAFOs and crutches so much more energy-consuming than wheelchair propulsion?

Ambulation requires moving the center of gravity up and down as well as side to side, and along with it the whole weight of the body. Bilateral KAFO ambulation requires lifting the limbs with shoulder depressors and swinging them forward while on crutches. This tripod or swing-through gait is energy-consuming. A wheelchair translates the center of gravity horizontally and in a straight line without the energy cost associated with moving the center of gravity vertically or laterally.

17. What is the difference between the reciprocating gait orthosis (RGO) and other types of hip-knee-ankle-foot orthoses (HKAFO)?

The **RGO** is designed to include a custom-molded pelvic girdle with a thoracic extension (as required by the patient for balance) which is attached with ballbearing hip joints to bilateral KAFO components. The unique characteristic mechanism consists of two cables with conduits that translate hip extension movement on one side into hip flexion on the other. The RGO is usually used with a walker and infrequently crutches. The unloaded limb is thereby advanced forward with forces transmitted from the loaded side, thus providing a "reciprocating" gait. Experimental work continues to focus on enhancement of ambulation efficiency, i.e., reduction of both energy expenditure over distance and energy cost over time, by using the RGO in combination with functional electrical stimulation (see Chapter 85).

18. Can orthotics correct in-toeing in children?

In-toeing in children may be caused by metatarsus adductus, internal tibial torsion, or femoral anteversion. In-toeing due to any of these causes generally improves or resolves as the child grows older and rarely causes long-term impairment or disability. Orthoses, such as Dennis-Browne splints, are no longer recommended for this condition.

19. How are shoes modified to correct leg-length discrepancy?

Minor leg-length discrepancies of up to $\frac{1}{2}$ inch may be left uncompensated or are corrected by placing $\frac{1}{4}$-inch heel pads inside the heel only of the shoe. Any lift > $\frac{1}{2}$ inch should be added externally to both the heel and sole of the shoe. The outer sole elevation should be approximately half of the heel elevation and taper forward from the ball of the shoe to the toe.

20. How can shoes be modified to control knee, foot, and ankle motions?

Shaving the heel of a shoe can bring the ground reaction force closer to the axis of knee rotation, thus stabilizing the joint. A cushioned heel can reduce the flexion moment at the knee by permitting faster ankle plantar flexion. A medial wedge can limit pronation caused by a weak tibialis posterior muscle. A lateral wedge can limit supination caused by a weak peroneus longus muscle. A rigid sole and a rocker bar can take pressure off the metatarsal heads and reduce hyperextension of the metatarsophalangeal joints.

21. What is the impact of footwear on orthotics?

In order for an orthosis to transmit and modify applied forces in the desired manner, the footplate of the orthosis must maintain proper contact with the foot. The shoe must hold the footplate in the correct position. If the upper (of the shoe) is too soft or the counter is too flexible, the patient will ride over or roll over the shoe during the stance phase of gait. This may decrease the efficacy of the AFO, especially to control medio-lateral stability. A shock absorbing material built into the soles of the shoes may reduce the forces imparted to the legs during ambulation with KAFOs.

BIBLIOGRAPHY

1. Biering-Sorensen F, Ryde H, Bojscn-Moller F, Lyquist E: Shock absorbing material on the shoes of long leg braces for paraplegic walking. Prosthet Orthot Int 14:27–32, 1990.
2. Dietz FR: Intoeing—fact, fiction and opinion. Am Fam Physician 5:1249–1259, 1994.
3. Douglas R, Larson PF, D'Ambrosia R, McCall RE: The LSU reciprocating gait orthosis. Orthopaedics 6:834–839, 1983.
4. Hirokawa S, Grimm M, Le T, et al: Energy consumption in paraplegic ambulation using the reciprocating gait orthosis and electric stimulation of thigh muscles. Arch Phys Med Rehabil 71:687–694, 1990.
5. Lehneis HR: Plastic spiral ankle-foot orthoses. Orthot Prosthet 28:3–13, 1974.
6. Lehmann JF: Biomechanics of ankle-foot orthosis: Prescription and design. Arch Phys Med Rehabil 60:200–207, 1979.
7. Loke M: New concepts in lower limb orthotics. Phys Med Rehabil Clin North Am 11:477–496, 2000.
8. Merkel KD: Energy expenditure in patients with low, mid, or high thoracic paraplegia using Scott-Craig knee-ankle-foot orthoses. Mayo Clin Proc 60:165–168, 1985.
9. Ragnarsson KT: Lower extremity orthotics, shoes, and gait aids. In DeLisa JA, Gans BM (eds): Rehabilitation Medicine: Principles and Practice, 3rd ed. Philadelphia, J.B. Lippincott, 1998, pp 651–667.
10. Sitler M, Ryan J, Hopkinson W, et al: The efficacy of a prophylactic knee brace to reduce knee injuries in football: A prospective, randomized study at West Point. Am J Sports Med 18:310–315, 1990.
11. Stauffer ES, Hussey RW: Spinal cord injury: Requirements for ambulation. Arch Phys Med Rehabil 54:544–547, 1973.
12. Tan JC: Practical Manual of Physical Medicine and Rehabilitation: Diagnostics, Therapeutics and Basic Problems. St. Louis, Mosby, 1998, pp 178–228.
13. Teitz CC, Hermanson BK, Kronmal RA, Diehr PH: Evaluation of the use of braces to prevent injury to the knee in collegiate football players. J Bone Joint Surg 69A:2, 1987.

95. LOWER-LIMB PROSTHETICS AND GAIT DEVIATIONS

Joan E. Edelstein, M.A., P.T., FISPO, and Norman Berger, M.S.

1. What is the most common prosthesis for a patient with transtibial (below-knee) amputation?

A prosthesis with a SACH foot-ankle assembly, endoskeletal shank with foam cover, plastic total contact socket with polyethylene foam liner, and cuff suspension suits most patients who have transtibial amputation. The socket is sometimes called **patellar-tendon bearing**; in fact, all portions of the amputation limb support weight, although a major site of loading is the patellar ligament (i.e., the connective tissue between the patella and the tibial tubercle). The foam liner accommodates changes in limb volume and distributes forces through the gait cycle. The endoskeletal shank can be adjusted to length and alignment; the cover contributes to the look and feel of the prosthesis. The cuff is readily adjustable. The **SACH** (**s**olid **a**nkle **c**ushion **h**eel) foot absorbs energy at heel strike and has a rigid keel that supports the body during the stance phase.

2. When should the transtibial prosthetic prescription differ from the basic prescription?

The individual who can be expected to walk rapidly and engage in vigorous sports will benefit from an energy-storing foot, such as the Flex-Foot, Seattle foot, or Springlite foot. Someone who will engage in very heavy labor may need an exoskeletal shank; this shank is less expensive and more durable than the endoskeletal one. If the amputation limb volume has stabilized, the prosthesis need not have a foam liner. Alternative liners are available, including those made with silicone or oil-filled chambers to distribute pressure hydraulically. Cuff suspension may not be adequate for the person with a very short amputation limb; supracondylar suprapatellar suspension is more suitable. Supracondylar suspension eliminates the need to buckle a strap and thus is more streamlined, particularly when the wearer sits. Corset suspension should be reserved for the patient who has knee instability.

3. What is the most usual prosthesis for a patient with transfemoral (above-knee) amputation?

Most patients benefit from a prosthesis which has a SACH foot-ankle assembly, endoskeletal shank, single axis knee unit with constant sliding friction and an extension aid, plastic total contact socket, and partial suction suspension with Silesian bandage as auxiliary suspension. The endoskeletal shank is appreciably lighter than the exoskeletal one for transfemoral prostheses. Socket contour may be **quadrilateral** (high anterior and lateral walls, relatively narrow anteroposteriorly) or **ischial containment** (high posterior and medial walls, relatively narrow mediolaterally).

4. When should the transfemoral prosthetic prescription differ from the basic prescription?

Patients who are expected to ambulate at a variety of speeds are good candidates for fluid friction in the knee joint, either pneumatic or hydraulic. Those with poor coordination require a knee unit that has a friction weight-bearing brake or a manual lock. The individual with stable limb volume can manage with total suction suspension, eliminating the Silesian bandage. A pelvic band provides maximum hip stabilization.

5. How do energy-storing feet work? What effect do they have on gait?

Energy-storing feet, such as Springlite, Flex-Foot, Carbon-Copy, or Seattle Foot, have a flexible keel made of carbon fiber or nylon. The **keel** is the longitudinal structural support of the foot. Depending on the particular design, during early, mid, or late stance on the prosthesis, the load applied by the patient bends the keel, thereby storing energy. During late stance, the keel recoils, producing a ground reaction force from below and behind, propelling the patient up and forward. Prosthetic foot action imitates the propulsive force normally provided by gastrocnemius-soleus contraction. Anecdotal evidence favors energy-storing feet, with patients liking the springy action. If, however, the patient is too feeble to apply substantial force to the foot, the energy-storing effect will be minimal.

6. What factors influence the patient's energy consumption during walking?

Residual limb length and etiology of the amputation are the principal factors. Individuals with transtibial amputations consume less energy per distance walked than those with trans-femoral amputation. Those with longer residual limbs are more energy-efficient. Systemic disease that affects cardiovascular, pulmonary, nervous, or muscle function obviously impacts on the safety, quality, and efficiency of gait.

7. What patients are not candidates for a prosthesis?

Individuals with moderate or severe cognitive impairment and those with exercise-limiting cardiopulmonary disease do not benefit from prosthetic rehabilitation. Severe arthritis, obesity, and neurologic disease do not specifically contraindicate prosthetic fitting, but patients can be expected to experience considerable difficulty ambulating with a prosthesis. Specific patient-centered functional goals need to be considered in each patient. Some patients may benefit from a prosthesis for transfers, standing, short-distance ambulation, or enhanced appearance when sitting in a wheelchair.

8. What anatomic factors interfere with the gait of patients with amputation?

Hip and knee contractures compromise prosthetic stability, even when the prosthesis is aligned to compensate for the joint deformity. A short residual limb limits surface for prosthetic contact and presents a sort of lever arm for transmission of force.

9. How do you evaluate the gait of a patient with amputation?

Select an unobstructed walkway at least 4 meters (12 ft) long. Ask the patient to walk at a comfortable pace (80 m/min) along the walkway. Stand behind the patient to observe the width of the walking base and movements in the frontal and transverse planes. Stand on the side of the prosthesis to observe sagittal movements. From each observation position, systematically note the action of the foot, knee, hip, and trunk in comparison with joint action in gait of people without amputation and full limb function. Observation focuses on the knee for individuals wearing transtibial prostheses, while those wearing transfemoral prostheses may have difficulty in the lower-limb or trunk.

Other means of assessing gait clinically include recording step length, cadence (steps per minute), and walking velocity.

10. When watching the knee joint from the side, what specifically should be looked for?

When a nonamputee walks at a comfortable speed (approx. 80 m/min), the knee flexes about 15° between heel strike and foot-flat. At the slower comfortable walking speed of the unilateral transtibial amputee, the knee flexes only about 10° following heel strike. The observer must note whether the knee flexion on the amputated side is significantly more or significantly less than the expected 10°.

11. Excessive knee flexion in early stance is termed "buckling." What might cause this excessive knee flexion?

Heel cushion or bumper too hard or too stiff: Normally, as a result of ankle plantarflexion and knee flexion, the ball of the foot descends to the floor very quickly after heel strike. However, if plantarflexion is restricted by too hard a prosthetic heel, the knee will flex excessively (> 10°) after heel strike to allow the forefoot to reach the floor rapidly and ungracefully. Also, an overly hard or stiff heel will not absorb the impact force as the prosthetic heel strikes the floor. Absorption must then be accomplished by rapid and excessive flexion of the knee.

Foot in dorsiflexion: If the foot is attached to the shank in an excessive dorsiflexed position, the ball of the foot is so far from the floor at heel strike that it cannot descend to foot-flat without excessive knee flexion.

Socket too far forward over the foot: The force transmitted through the socket (Force A in figure) and the reaction force from the floor (Force B) constitute a force couple that tends to rotate the prosthesis in the clockwise direction around the heel as a fulcrum. Clearly, the farther forward of the heel the socket force occurs, the greater will be the moment causing the clockwise rotation. This rotation will be seen by the observer as an abrupt and excessive flexion of the knee immediately after heel strike. Also, the quadriceps, which is eccentrically contracted at this time to prevent knee buckling, will contract much more forcefully to resist the increased flexion moment. Fatigue and overloading may result. Also, it is important to remember that as the quadriceps contracts to control the flexing knee, compression and shear between the socket and residual limb increase dramatically, particularly at the anterior-distal tibia. (No wonder that this area is a common site of discomfort and complaint.)

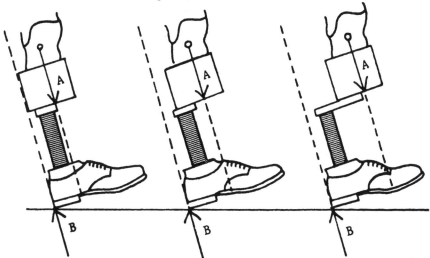

Knee flexion contracture, uncompensated: If the tibial remnant is flexed on the femur because of tight hamstrings, the socket of an uncompensated prosthesis will be considerably forward of the foot. An increased knee flexion moment, excessive knee flexion, and increased anterior-distal tibial pressure will all be present. If the residual limb is short and the contracture is not large, the prosthetist can move the foot forward underneath the socket. The shorter the residual limb, the greater the degree of contracture that can be accommodated by this compensating realignment.

12. What happens to gait during late-stance phase?

At heel-off, the body's center of gravity passes over the metatarsophalangeal (MTP) joints, and the knee, which had been extending, begins to flex. If the weight of the body were to pass over the MTP joints too soon (e.g., if the foot were very short), the resulting early loss of anterior support would allow the knee to flex prematurely, and the body would drop fairly abruptly until arrested by heel strike on the other side. Note that the last three causes discussed in question 11 each have the effect of moving the weight forward with respect to the foot. Thus, the distance that the weight must travel forward before anterior support is lost is minimized, and premature knee flexion ("**drop off**") will likely be seen in the latter part of stance phase.

13. If there is too little or no knee flexion, what might cause this deviation?

Heel cushion or bumper too soft or too flexible: The soft heel absorbs so much of the floor reaction force that little remains to cause knee flexion.

Prosthetic foot in excessive plantarflexion: The foot reaches the floor too quickly after heel-strike, with no need for knee flexion to contribute to the process.

Socket too far posterior over foot: The clockwise rotation of the prosthesis (flexion moment) produced by the force couple is reduced as the socket force moves closer to the floor reaction. In fact, if the force transmitted through the socket is coincident with the floor reaction force, there would be no flexion moment at all.

Quadriceps weakness: Supporting body weight over a flexed knee is possible only if the quadriceps is sufficiently powerful to prevent the knee from buckling. The individual with weak knee extensors avoids the danger of collapse by walking over a fully extended knee, with the gluteus maximus largely responsible for maintaining knee extension against the knee flexion moment normally present at heel-strike.

Anterior-distal tibial discomfort: Increased pressure between the anterodistal tibia and the socket stems primarily from the activity of the quadriceps controlling the rate and extent of knee flexion after heel-strike. To alleviate any resulting discomfort, the amputee may develop a habit of holding the knee in full extension. Thus, the gait may be the same as the weak quadriceps pattern, even though examination reveals normal strength. Differentiation between these two causes requires muscle testing, residuum and socket inspection for evidence of high-pressure injury, and careful questioning of the patient.

14. What is "climbing the hill"?

A patient with transtibial amputation may complain of "**climbing the hill**" during late stance if the prosthesis is excessively stable. Such factors as a foot that is malaligned too far anteriorly or is plantarflexed, a socket that is set too far posteriorly or is insufficiently flexed, or a suspension cuff or thigh corset attached too far anteriorly contribute to this effect. Quadriceps weakness may be compensated by keeping the knee extended; this maneuver may produce or aggravate pain at the anterodistal aspect of the amputation limb. Hyperactive quadriceps, such as occurs in extensor synergy following stroke, also produces the sensation of climbing the hill.

15. What is "lateral thrust"?

Midstance on the prosthesis is the period of single support on the prosthesis. Because the prosthetic socket surrounds soft tissue, some shifting or thrusting of the proximal portion of the socket relative to the amputation limb is apt to occur. The transtibial prosthesis is aligned to maximize load on pressure-tolerant tissue, namely the proximomedial aspect over the pes anserinus, and to minimize pressure on the proximolateral aspect over the fibular head and peroneal nerve. A properly aligned prosthesis thrusts laterally at midstance. Excessive lateral thrust, usually produced by aligning the prosthetic foot too far medial to produce a walking base < 10 cm (4 in) between the heel centers, is undesirable because high pressure is felt at the distolateral portions of the amputation limb at the distal end of the fibula as well as proximomedially.

16. When observing the transtibial amputee from the rear to see frontal-plane knee motion, what specifically should you see?

Excessive lateral thrust—i.e., a fairly sudden lateral motion of the socket that occurs at about midstance. This lateral thrust results from an alignment in which the supporting foot on the floor is medial to the force line extending through the weight-bearing socket. The foot is "**in-set.**" The resulting force couple tends to rotate the prosthesis laterally, so that the medial socket brim presses against the residuum (increases pressure), and the lateral socket brim moves away from the residuum (decreases pressure).

Considering that the medial side of the residuum is quite tolerant of pressure (medial tibial flare) and that the lateral side is quite sensitive to pressure (fibular head), this would seem to be an excellent arrangement. And it is! The foot should be slightly medial to the socket. But if the foot is excessively "in-set," an excessive lateral thrust results. The observer will see this lateral motion, the amputee may complain of discomfort on the medioproximal aspect, and skin and lateral collateral knee ligaments may be irritated.

17. Describe the gait of the transfemoral (above-knee) amputee.

As compared to the transtibial amputee, the transfemoral amputee walks more slowly, expends more energy, is more likely to use a cane or other supports, and exhibits more deviation from a normal pattern. These are among the consequences of loss of the anatomic knee.

To be more specific, the loss of the quadriceps necessitates a fully extended or stable prosthetic knee throughout stance phase to avoid the danger of buckling under weight-bearing. Maintaining full extension requires strength of the gluteus maximus, prosthetic alignment that brings the force line anterior to the knee very early in stance enhancing stability, a relatively soft prosthetic heel to absorb heel-strike impact and limit the knee flexion moment, and in some cases, special knee unit designs that inhibit or prevent flexion.

During swing phase, the quadriceps normally functions to limit knee flexion immediately after toe-off, while the hamstrings act to decelerate the foot prior to heel-strike. In the absence of these muscular controls, both the speed and direction of the swinging shank are difficult for the amputee to regulate.

18. What are the more common deviations seen when observing the transfemoral amputee from the rear?

Lateral trunk bend   Circumduction
Abducted gait (wide walking base)   Whips, medial or lateral

19. Describe the mechanics and causes of lateral trunk bend.

As soon as the sound limb lifts off the floor and begins its swing phase, the pelvis tends to drop or dip on the unsupported side. The hip abductors on the prosthetic, stance-phase side contract strongly to control the pelvic dip. In the absence of hip abductor control, the trunk must lean toward the prosthetic side to counteract the instability toward the swing-phase side (**Trendelenburg sign**). Among the conditions that interfere with pelvic control by the hip abductors and thus are causes of lateral trunk bend are:

a. Weak hip abductors
b. Hip abduction contracture or abducted socket. The effectiveness of the shortened hip abductors is considerably reduced.
c. Poor fit of lateral socket wall. When the gluteus medius contracts, it exerts force at both its origin and its insertion, i.e., on the pelvis and femur. For it to stabilize the pelvis, the femur must be prevented from moving. This is the primary function of the lateral socket wall, which must fit snugly to prevent femoral abduction.
d. Lateral-distal femoral discomfort. If femoral abduction against the lateral wall results in discomfort, the amputee may adopt a lateral trunk bend to reduce pressure.
e. Lack of distal stabilization of the femur.

20. What causes abducted gait (wide walking base)?

In this deviation, the walking base is > 10 cm between heel centers. The prosthetic foot is held away from the midline throughout the gait cycle and is associated with lateral trunk bending and wide-based gait. The major causes include:

1. Perineal discomfort. When the amputee experiences pain in the crotch area, the prosthesis is abducted to move the medial socket brim away from the sensitive spot.

2. Prosthesis problems. It is difficult for an excessively long prosthesis to clear the floor during swing phase and to be placed directly under the hip during stance phase. Both problems are solved by holding the prosthesis out to the side.

3. Abduction contracture, uncompensated. Other problems include poor socket fit, locked knee, too low a medial socket wall.

4. Short amputation limb
5. Hip arthritis
6. Hip dislocation
7. Inguinal hernia

A cane, preferably held in the contralateral hand, minimizes lateral bending and may enable the patient to walk with a more narrow base.

21. What causes the knee on a transfemoral prosthesis to swing through an excessively large range?

Swing-phase biomechanics depend on the wearer's walking speed and the adjustment of the knee unit. At a given walking speed, the patient will exhibit high heel rise (excessively acute knee flexion) during early swing phase if the friction mechanism, the extension aid, or both components are relatively loose. During late-swing phase, a loose friction mechanism or a tight extension aid will cause terminal impact. Some patients like the sound at impact because it indicates that the knee is extended and will be stable during early stance phase. A person who walks rapidly while wearing a prosthesis that has a sliding friction knee unit will experience high heel rise and terminal impact. A fluid controlled knee unit adjusts automatically to changes in walking speed, thus minimizing high heel rise and terminal impact.

22. How does circumduction manifest?

This swing-phase deviation is characterized by a laterally curved line of progression—i.e., the prosthesis is swung out to the side but brought back to the midline for the next heel strike. Amputees who are fearful of stubbing the toe adopt this maneuver to ensure that the prosthetic foot clears the floor. Because prosthetists rarely fabricate a prosthesis of excessive length, it becomes necessary to examine the patient for conditions that create a "functionally long" prosthesis:
  a. Foot in plantarflexion: toe tends to scuff floor.
  b. Socket too small: residuum cannot enter fully.
  c. Inadequate suspension: socket slips down during swing.
  d. Insufficient or no knee flexion during swing because the knee unit includes a manual lock, excessive friction, or too tight an extension aid.
  e. Amputee is reluctant to flex the knee during swing because of poor balance or fear.

23. What are whips? Why do they occur?

A whip is a sudden, abrupt rotation of the prosthesis that occurs at the end of stance phase, as the knee is flexed to begin swing. If the prosthetic heel is seen to move medially, a **medial whip** is noted, while lateral rotation of the heel denotes a **lateral whip**.

Mechanically, flexion and extension of the prosthetic knee (i.e., motion of the shank and foot) can take place only in a plane perpendicular to the knee axis. Thus, for the shank to swing along a sagittal line, the knee axis must be perpendicular to that line. If the knee axis were externally or internally rotated, the shank could only swing diagonally. Keeping this in mind, major causes of whips are:
  a. **Improper alignment of the knee axis:** An externally rotated axis produces a medial whip, because at initial flexion of the knee, the prosthesis rotates to a position perpendicular to the axis. Similarly, an internally rotated axis produces a lateral whip.
  b. **Flabby, weak musculature that rotates freely around the femur.** The prosthesis rotates with this underlying soft tissue unless a suspension component, such as a Silesian bandage, is used to control rotation.

24. Which deviations in the gait of the transfemoral amputee are best observed from the side?

Short step on sound side
Uneven heel rise
Terminal impact

25. What is vaulting? What are its causes, and who is most apt to vault?

Vaulting refers to exaggerated plantarflexion on the contralateral intact leg during swing phase of the prosthesis. Vaulting increases the distance between the prosthetic foot and the floor, thus reducing the likelihood of tripping on the prosthesis. Because this deviation is arduous, it is primarily seen in children and young adults. Older adults who formed the habit years earlier may persistently vault.

26. What causes a short step on the sound side?

a. **Hip flexion contracture:** In order for the sound limb to take a normal length step, the prosthetic side must assume a hyperextended position. When a hip flexion contracture on the amputated side prevents this, the sound side step-length must decrease.

b. **Insufficient socket flexion:** In the presence of any restriction of hip extension range, the socket should be aligned in compensatory flexion so that the prosthesis may still reach a position of hyperextension though the femur cannot. Whether this can be accomplished depends on the degree of extension limitation and the length of the residuum. The shorter the residual limb, the more compensatory socket flexion can be introduced.

c. **Pain, insecurity, fear:** Discomfort from an ill-fitting socket or fear of balancing on an in-sensate, jointed stilt will cause the amputee to spend as little time as possible in pros-thetic-stance phase. Body weight is shifted quickly back to the sound side, which has taken a rapid, short step so as to be prepared to accept the weight.

27. Describe the mechanics of uneven heel rise.

Normally, the quadriceps is responsible for limiting knee flexion in early swing. Without a quadriceps, the transfemoral amputee must depend on resistance to motion provided by the pros-thetic knee unit through friction mechanisms, pneumatic or hydraulic cylinders, or extension aids. If these produce too little resistance to motion, there will be excessive heel rise in early swing as the knee flexes too much. Conversely, if there is too much resistance to motion, there will be insufficient heel rise as the knee flexes too little.

28. How do you recognize terminal impact?

Toward the end of swing phase, the hamstrings are responsible for decelerating the rapidly moving shank—i.e., controlling the rate of knee extension. Without hamstrings, the transfemoral amputee must depend again on resistance to motion from the prosthetic knee unit. If there is too little resistance from the friction or cylinders, the forward inertia will swing the shank forward too quickly and produce a forceful impact into full extension—clunk!

A small amount of terminal impact is often considered useful and beneficial by the above-knee prosthesis wearer. The impact provides important feedback information, signaling that the knee is fully extended and that it is now safe to put the prosthesis on the floor and transfer body weight to it. This is a good example of the general proposition that gait deviations are seldom ac-cidents but habitual compromises that make the amputee reluctant to walk without them.

29. What effect does the shoe have on the gait of patients who wear prostheses?

The shoe is an integral part of the prosthesis. A loose shoe will slip from the prosthetic foot during late stance. A tight shoe will interfere with toe break action during late stance. A shoe with an excessively high heel will reduce knee stability, both in the anatomic knee of the person wear-ing a transtibial prosthesis and the knee unit in a transfemoral prosthesis. A shoe that has too low a heel or a heel that is excessively compressible will make the knee on the prosthetic side overly stable. A stiff boot restrains knee flexion during late stance.

BIBLIOGRAPHY

1. Berger N: Analysis of amputee gait. In Bowker JH, Michael JW (eds): Atlas of Limb Prosthetics, 2nd ed. St. Louis, Mosby, 1992, pp 371–379.
2. Chiu C-C, Chen C-E, Wang T-G, et al: Influencing factors and ambulation outcome in patients with dual disabilities of hemiplegia and amputation. Arch Phys Med Rehabil 81:14–17, 2000.
3. Edelstein JE: Prosthetic assessment and management. In O'Sullivan SB, Schmitz TJ. Physical Rehabilitation: Assessment and Treatment, 4th ed. Philadelphia, F.A. Davis, 2000.
4. Gauthier-Gagnon C, Grise M-C, Potvin D: Predisposing factors related to prosthetic use by people with a transtibial and transfemoral amputation. J Prosthet Orthot 10:99–109, 1998.
5. Gonzalez EG, Edelstein JE: Energy expenditure during ambulation. In Gonzalez EG, Myers SJ, Edelstein JE, et al (eds): Downey and Darling's Physiological Basis of Rehabilitation Medicine, 3rd ed. Woburn, MA, Butterworth Heinemann, 2000.

6. Huang ME, Levy CE, Webster JB: Acquired limb deficiencies: 3. Prosthetic components, prescriptions, and indications. Arch Phys Med Rehabil 82(Suppl 1):S17–S24, 2001.
7. Legro MW, Reiber G, del Aguila M, et al: Issues of importance reported by persons with lower limb amputations and prostheses. J Rehabil Res Dev 36:155–163, 1999.
8. Lehmann JF, Price R, Okumura R, et al: Mass and mass distribution of below-knee prostheses: Effects on gait efficiency and self-selected walking speed. Arch Phys Med Rehabil 79:162–168, 1998.
9. Levy CE, Bryant PR, Spires MC, Duffy DA: Acquired limb deficiencies: 4. Troubleshooting. Arch Phys Med Rehabil 82(Suppl 1):S25–S30, 2001.
10. Murray MP, Drought AB, Kory RC: Walking patterns of normal man. J Bone Joint Surg 46A:335, 1964.
11. Nissen SJ, Newman WP: Factors influencing reintegration to normal living after amputation. Arch Phys Med Rehabil 73:548–551, 1992.
12. Saunders JB, Inman VT, Eberhart HD: Major determinants in normal and pathological gait. J Bone Joint Surg 35A:543, 1953.
13. Snyder RD, Powers CM, Fontaine C, et al: The effects of five prosthetic feet on the gait and loading of the sound limb in dysvascular below knee amputees. J Rehabil Res Dev 32:309–315, 1995.

96. SPINAL ORTHOSES

John B. Redford, M.D., Abna A. Ogle, M.D., and Richard C. Robinson, M.D.

An undefined problem has an infinite number of solutions.—Robert A. Humphrey

1. What is a spinal orthosis?

The word *orthosis* derives from the Greek word meaning "making straight." Spinal orthoses or braces are appliances used in an attempt to correct and support the spine. Their use has been extensively documented in human history, predating Christ until the present day.

2. What does the functional unit consist of in the human spine?

Two vertebral bodies, their articulating joints, and an interposed fibroelastic disc. The human spine is an aggregate of superimposed segments, each segment being a self-contained functional unit, with the sum total of all the units forming the vertebral column.

3. List the three principal functions of the vertebral column.

1. Protect the spinal cord and its nerve roots
2. Absorb axial compressive forces
3. Provide a base for mobility of the human skeleton

4. What is the purpose of a spinal orthosis?

1. Prevention and correction of deformities
2. Reduction of axial loading
3. Stabilization of a vertebral segment
4. Relief of pain by limiting motion or weight-bearing
5. Improvement of spinal function
6. Provision of effects such as heat, massage, and kinesthetic feedback

5. How do spinal orthoses work?

Spinal orthoses, when applied to the body, exert forces on the spine. This is accomplished in one or more of the following ways:

1. **Three-point pressure system.** (see figure)
2. **Fluid compression.** When the brace encompasses the trunk, it forms a semirigid cylinder surrounding the vertebral column. This results in an increase in intra-abdominal pressure, which

measurably decreases intervertebral disc pressure and decreases shearing forces across the lowest functional units.

3. **Irritant.** The brace is constructed so that the wearer is forced into the desired posture to avoid discomfort (kinesthetic feedback).

4. **Skeletal fixation.** The scientific basis for orthotic use is well delineated in the correction of certain progressive spine deformities. However, as orthopedic surgery has advanced, the use of external corrective devices has declined. They are commonly used in nonsurgical musculoskeletal complaints, such as back or neck strains. It is in this arena that empirical evidence is incomplete. However, clinical experience and patient report provide justification for their continued use.

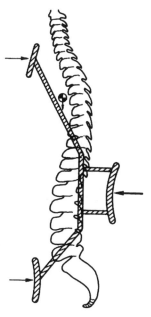

Three-point pressure system as applied in a hyperextension TLSO.

6. What are the potential complications of spinal orthoses?

- Loss of skin integrity due to compressive forces
- Weakening of axial muscles
- Soft-tissue contractures
- Increased movement at the ends of immobilized segments
- Physical and psychological dependence
- Osteopenia

7. There are so many different orthoses, how can I remember their names?

There is a bewildering variety of devices, several even sporting the name or hometown of the creator. To avoid confusion and aid in classification of braces, the American Academy of Orthopaedic Surgeons and the American Academy of Prosthetists and Orthotists together have devised a uniform naming system. *The orthosis is named for the segments of the body and/or spine that it covers.* Thus, a CO is a cervical orthosis covering only the neck. A CTO is a cervicothoracic orthosis encompassing the neck and thoracic spine.

Commonly Used Spinal Orthoses

Cervical orthosis	CO
Cervicothoracic orthosis	CTO
Cervicothoracolumbosacral orthosis	CTLSO
Thoracolumbosacral orthosis	TLSO
Lumbosacral orthosis	LSO
Sacroiliac orthosis	SIO

8. What are initial considerations in prescribing spinal orthoses?

- **Compliance.** The prescribing physician may have to judge the likelihood of the patient wearing an orthosis before the expense is incurred.
- **Purpose.** The ultimate goal of the orthosis should be described and understood by the patient.
- **Length of use.** With few exceptions, use of restrictive neck and back supports should be temporary and length of time for wear on both a daily and long-term basis should be proposed.
- **Alternative treatment.** Whenever feasible the aim should be to restore physiologic forces acting on the spine through correcting postural habits or voluntary muscular action, rather than relying upon a passive external orthotic device.

9. Describe the movement possible in the cervical spine.

The cervical segment is the most mobile portion of the spine. It is capable of movement in three planes: flexion and extension, lateral rotation, and side-bending. Most cervical rotation occurs between C1 and C2. The greatest amount of flexion and extension is between C5 and C6. Because of extensive innate mobility, the cervical spine is very difficult to immobilize or stabilize.

10. Your patient has an acute but uncomplicated cervical strain. What orthosis do you prescribe?

The **soft collar** is probably the most commonly used orthosis. It is made of a firm foam covered with cotton and fastened posteriorly with Velcro. It is usually prescribed for a **cervical muscle strain**. It provides little restriction of cervical movement (only reduction of flexion and extension by approximately one-fourth, and virtually no reduction of lateral bending or rotation) but allows soft tissues to rest, provides warmth to strained muscles, and reminds the patient to avoid extremes of neck movement.

11. When is a Philadelphia collar used?

This type of cervical orthosis provides more restriction to movement than does the soft collar, but less than a halo vest or custom-made plastic CTO. The Philadelphia collar is made of a foam reinforced by firm thermoplastic material. It has anterior and posterior portions that conform to the chin and occiput.

A Philadelphia collar is frequently prescribed after **cervical surgery** when very strict neck immobilization is not necessary. It may also be used in cases with **cervical ligament rupture** and in some relatively **stable cervical spine fractures**. It provides more limitation in flexion and extension and side-bending than a soft collar but does not significantly limit rotation. Patients frequently complain of feeling hot and sweaty under this collar, but it is generally well-tolerated.

The Philadeplphia collar is relatively ineffective in controlling rotation and lateral bending according to radiographic and goniometric studies. It shares this feature with other "off-the-shelf" COs, such as the Aspen, Stiff-neck, and Miami J.

12. What is a halo vest orthosis?

This CTO consists of two parts: The halo portion is a circular band of steel attached to the skull via metal screws. Adjustable rods connect the halo to a vest that encircles the trunk (see figure on following page). This device provides the most rigid fixation of the cervical spine and is the orthosis most widely used in **unstable cervical fractures**. Some intervertebral movement is still possible, however, as evidenced by the "snaking" phenomenon (slight movement between the individual cervical segments, which can be seen on plain films of the neck). This brace makes possible early mobilization and rehabilitation of the patient following spinal surgery, while maintaining a stable spine. The disadvantage of the halo vest orthosis is that it is subject to slipping and infection at the screw sites over the skull.

The thermoplastic Minerva body jacket with a halo portion secured by lateral extensions arising from the neck portion provides immobility equal to the metal halo. It is lighter, noninvasive and more comfortable than the metal halo and used much more in children.

13. When are thoracic orthoses used?

The thoracic spine is the most stable and least mobile portion of the spine. It owes its stability, at least in part, to the thoracic cage with its connecting ribs and sternum. Problems such as **compression fractures**, **fracture-dislocations**, and **scoliotic** or **kyphotic** deformities of the spine are the most common reasons for prescription of a **thoracolumbar sacral orthosis** (TLSO). It is important to know that to limit motion in one segment of the spine, the orthosis must extend proximally and distally to adjacent segments.

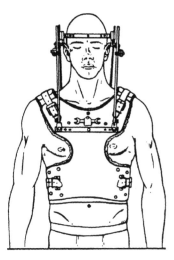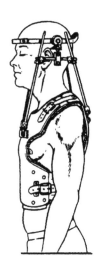

Halo vest orthosis, front and
side views.

14. What braces are used for thoracic deformities?

For low thoracic scoliosis, there appears to be a real and predictable effect from bracing. For mid and high thoracic scoliosis, the efficacy of corrective orthoses remains debatable. **Milwaukee bracing** (CTLSO) for progressive spinal curvature is a complex system of dynamic bracing advocated for many years to treat idiopathic scoliosis. The pressure and discomfort necessary for correcting posture are frequently so great as to diminish compliance in use of the brace. Brace wearers must be followed for years and checked every 3–4 months.

Idiopathic or paralytic scolioses are amenable to surgery if bracing proves ineffective. The **Taylor brace** is prescribed for counteracting kyphosis. It has high thoracic uprights and shoulder straps. These straps must be tightened (often to the discomfort of the patient) to provide adequate antideformity forces.

The **CASH** (cruciform anterior spinal hyperextension) orthosis is also used to decrease kyphosis. It has an anterior cross-bar with pads at the four ends of the cross. This orthosis adjusts posteriorly with straps held closed with Velcro. It is lightweight and easy to put on but may require frequent repositioning.

The **Jewett** (hyperextension TLSO) orthosis uses the three-point system to facilitate thoracic hyperextension. The two anterior pads are positioned over the sternum and pubic symphysis, while the third opposing posterior pad lies over the thoracolumbar junction. It does not limit spine rotation but is fairly comfortable to wear and more easily adjusted than the CASH orthosis.

If a TLSO for increased angle kyphosis is not well tolerated, a thoracic weighted kyphosis-orthosis as described by Sinaki for osteoporosis may be helpful.

15. How is a painful nondisplaced thoracic compression fracture treated?

There is clinical experience that orthoses can alleviate acute pain, but no scientific evidence exists of how this may occur. Short-term use of a brace is acceptable in the first 7–10 days following a fracture. The patient should also receive back protection and posture education, as well as trunk-strengthening exercises.

16. How are unstable thoracic fractures treated?

Surgical stabilization is usually indicated, but postoperative bracing may be recommended by the surgeon. The brace is usually a custom molded thermoplastic TLSO.

17. When are lumbosacral orthoses used?

They are frequently prescribed for **uncomplicated low back pain** but are primarily used for support and immobilization of the spine after **trauma** or **surgery**. Application of these orthoses for low back pain is controversial. Some clinicians cite the lack of consistent scientific evidence to support their use, especially in chronic low back pain. Others would agree with their limited use during high-impact activities, along with patient education and an exercise program.

18. There are so many LSOs on the market. How can I choose appropriately?

One way to keep straight the ever-increasing multitude of LSOs is to consider them in order from the least to the most immobilizing:

1. **Corsets** provide the least restriction in spinal movement. These can be made of canvas or elasticized material and can be reinforced with metal or plastic stays or even a thermomolded plastic pad. Corsets are more comfortable than rigid metal orthoses, such as the chair-back brace, and achieve lumbar support by increasing intra-abdominal pressure. They also provide some warmth to extensor muscles of the spine and can remind the wearer to avoid extremes of movement.

2. **Spinal braces,** reinforced with rigid metal bars and rigid plastic jackets, are more restrictive than corsets and vary in length: the greater the length, the more immobilizing the effect. An example is the short flexion jacket (Raney orthosis) that has been advocated by some for preventing extension in the lumbar spine; it is used in low back pain, particularly that caused by spondylolisthesis. This orthosis is made of thermomolded plastic anterior and posterior parts, fastened with Velcro. The anterior portion presses into the abdomen, causing increased intra-abdominal pressure. The forced flexion of the lumbar spine may also alleviate pressure in the posterior elements of the vertebral column.

3. **Lumbosacral spicas** provide the most effective way of immobilizing the lower lumbar spine. They are made of thermomolded plastic extending from 2 cm below the inferior angle of the scapulae to the sacrum. A unilateral side piece is extended distally, usually immobilizing the hip in 15–20° of flexion. Investigation of lumbosacral movements has demonstrated that the lower lumbar vertebrae are best immobilized when there is fixation of the pelvis (via the extended thigh piece). This orthosis is useful for postoperative immobilization and unstable lower spine fractures.

BIBLIOGRAPHY

1. Anderson CW, Redford JB: Orthotic treatment for injuries and diseases of the spinal column. Phys Med Rehabil State Art Rev 14:471–484, 2000.
2. Askins V, Eismont FJ: Efficacy of five cervical orthoses in restricting cervical motion. A comparison study. Spine 22:1193–1198, 1997.
3. Fisher SV: Spinal orthoses. In Kottke F, Lehmann J (eds): Krusen's Handbook of Physical Medicine and Rehabilitation, 4th ed. Philadelphia, W.B. Saunders, 1990, pp 593–601.
4. Fisher SV, Winter RB: Spinal orthoses in rehabilitation. In Braddom R (ed): Physical Medicine and Rehabilitation, 2nd ed. Philadelphia, W.B. Saunders, 2000, pp 353–369.
5. McLain RF, Karol L: Conservative treatment of the scoliotic and kyphotic patient. Arch Pediatr Adolesc Med 148:646–665, 1994.
6. Nachemson AL: Orthotic treatment for injuries and disease of the spinal column. Phys Med Rehabil State Art Rev 1:11–24, 1987.
7. Noonan KJ, Weinstein SL, et al: Use of the Milwaukee brace for progressive idiopathic scoliosis. J Bone Joint Surg 78A:557–567, 1996.
8. Plaisier B; Gabram SG, Schwartz RJ, Jacobs LM: Prospective evaluation of craniofacial pressure in four different cervical orthoses. J Trauma 37:714–720, 1994.
9. Sandler AJ, Dvorak J, et al: The effectiveness of variouis cervical orthoses: An in vivo comparison of the mechanical stability provided by several widely used models. Spine 21:1624–1629, 1996.
10. Sinaki M: Rehabilitation of osteoporatic fractures of the spine. Phys Med Rehabil State Art Rev 9:105–123, 1995.
11. Sypert GW: External spinal orthotics. Neurosurgery 20:642–649, 1987.

Resource
American Orthotic and Prosthetic Association www.oandp.org

97. MANUAL WHEELCHAIRS

R. Lee Kirby, M.D.

1. Discuss briefly the importance and prevalence of wheelchair use.

The wheelchair is arguably the most important therapeutic tool in rehabilitation, equivalent in importance to vaccination in preventive medicine or antibiotics in curative medicine. The wheelchair acts as an interface between the person and the environment, establishing mobility and enhancing independence in role performance in many life venues. In 1992, there were 1.4 million wheelchair users in the U.S., about 75% of whom were using manually propelled wheelchairs. This figure is expected to have increased to approx. 2.0 million by 2000. The prevalence is about fivefold greater among the elderly than for the general population.

2. How safe are wheelchairs?

The long-term use of wheelchairs can adversely affect the health of users due to chronic or repetitive stresses—for instance, affecting shoulders, peripheral nerves, and skin. In the U.S., there are about 50 wheelchair-related deaths per year and about 70,000 wheelchair-related injuries per year that are serious enough to require attention at an emergency department. The majority (approx. 75%) of these deaths and injuries are because the wheelchair users tip over and/or fall from their chairs.

3. Compare the ride of folding- and rigid-frame wheelchairs.

The flexibility of the folding frame leads to a more comfortable ride and makes it more likely that all four wheels will remain in contact with uneven terrain. Rigidity provides a responsive feel to wheelchair propulsion and turning because the applied forces are not damped by the chair flexing. A rigid frame also allows more precise wheel alignment.

4. Why is seat depth important?
- If the seat is too short, the thighs are not fully supported. The weight of the body must be distributed over the buttocks, raising pressure under bony prominences (ischia and sacrum).
- A seat that is too long can cause pressure sores in the popliteal space or may force the user to scoot forward into a slumped (lumbar-kyphotic) position and cause sacral shear and pressure.
- Ideal seating is achieved by specifying seat size, height, plane angle, and cushion surface.

5. How might you lower the seat height?
- Use drop hooks to lower a rigid seat surface below the level of the side rails.
- Select a higher axle position for the rear wheel.
- Use a rear wheel with a smaller diameter.

The latter two actions will tilt the seat backwards unless the casters are also modified.

6. What are the pros and cons to increasing the seat-plane angle?

Pros: The seat-plane angle (the angle of the seat plane relative to the horizontal, usually 1–4° higher in front) may be accentuated to reduce (1) spasticity, (2) the tendency for the user to slide forward on the seat, or (3) lumbar lordosis.

Cons: the accentuated angle makes transfers more difficult and puts more weight on the ischial tuberosities.

7. What are the considerations in choosing a wheelchair cushion?

1. Virtually all personal wheelchairs should be fitted with a removable cushion, for pressure distribution, shock absorption, and/or positioning.

2. Very flexible cushions should be supported fully by the seat surface (preferably rigid) so that they do not fold over the seat margins.

3. In choosing the cushion materials (e.g., foam, air, gel), their distribution, and the shape of the cushion, one needs to consider such issues as sensation, pressure distribution, presence of spasticity/flaccidity, and incontinence. For instance, a user with spasticity may benefit from an anterior wedge and a slight pommel between the thighs; a user with flaccidity, who rests with the knees apart, may benefit from more lateral support.

4. Decisions about the cushion should be made early, because the dimensions of the compressed cushion affect a number of wheelchair dimensions (e.g., backrest, armrest, seat height).

8. How high should the backrest be?
- The upper border of the backrest should be 1–2 inches lower than the scapulae for users who propel their own wheelchairs, to minimize irritation from rubbing during propulsion.
- Higher backrests (sometimes with an added headrest) provide more support and more area for pressure distribution for the user who does not propel the wheelchair independently or who uses a recliner.
- Backrests that do not extend above the lumbar region are increasingly common and are surprisingly well tolerated if the lumbosacral area is supported. Such low backrests have the advantage of permitting great freedom of upper body and trunk movement.

9. What should the backrest angle be?
The angle of the backrest is commonly tilted back about 8° from vertical (i.e., approx. 95° from the seat plane).

Users of lightweight wheelchairs may prefer to increase the seat-plane angle and reduce the backrest-to-seatplane angle. Such a snug fit (often called "squeeze") can assist the user in applying force to the wheels by preventing the trunk from being pushed backwards with each arm thrust.

For the user with weak trunk muscles, increasing the backrest-to-seatplane angle ("recline") can decrease the likelihood of falling forward onto the lap, obviating the need for a chest strap in some cases. Recline reduces the pressure on the ischial tuberosities in proportion to the extent of the recline. However, because the mechanical axis of a backrest with variable recline is usually below and behind the anatomical axis of the user's hip joint, there are shear forces produced due to the relative movement of the chair and user's backs.

10. What is "tilt" and why is it used?
Tilt is a change in the seat's position or attitude rather than a change in the posture (relative position of body parts). Tilt obviates the shear problem of recliners and is less likely to trigger spasms. It also reduces the pressure on the ischial tuberosities, in proportion to the extent of the tilt.

11. What are the pros and cons of desk-length armrests?
Short armrests (those without their forward one-third) allow a closer approach to a desk or table. However, they may not provide enough length to be useful for sit-to-stand transfers. This limitation can be circumvented if the armrests are reversible.

12. What is the principal advantage of a "wrap-around" armrest?
The rear attachment of the wrap-around armrest is behind the frame rather than beside it. This allows the rear wheels to be placed closer to the frame, narrowing the outside width of the wheelchair without narrowing the seat width.

13. What are the considerations in choosing the footrest height?
1. The lowest point on the footrests should be at least 2 inches above the floor to avoid being caught on obstacles and incline transitions.

2. If the footrests are too high, the thighs are lifted from the seat, increasing the pressure on the ischial tuberosities.

3. If the footrests are too low (or removed), the front edge of the seat will bear more weight than appropriate, with the potential for pressure ulceration under the distal thighs. Also, there will be less support for forward leans.

14. What should the knee-flexion angle be?

The usual "**hanger angle**" is 60–70° (0° being full knee extension). Elevating the footrests (extending the knees) reduces edema and knee-flexion contractures but decreases forward stability, both because the center of gravity is altered and because footrests serve as forward antitippers. This latter effect can lead to a violent yawing tip when only a single footrest is elevated. Also, there can be relative movement between the elevating footrest and the user if the axes of the mechanical and anatomical joints are not colinear. Some elevating footrests compensate to prevent for shear by either a gooseneck attachment (to raise the mechanical axis) or a telescoping mechanism that lengthens the footrest as it is elevated.

Some wheelchairs set the knees in flexion of > 90°. This has several benefits: closer access to objects, protection of the feet, ease of transport of the wheelchair, inhibition of spasticity, tighter turns due to the reduced overall length, better traction, and, by bringing the limb segments closer to the yaw axis, faster turns can be due to reduced moment of inertia (analogous to a spinning skater who speeds up when bringing the arms closer to the body). However, users with long legs may be difficult to accommodate; a small caster diameter and caster trail may be needed to avoid having the caster swivel into the footrests/heels when changing direction; and the footrests are less effective as forward antitip devices.

15. Describe the pros and cons of front-rigging "taper."

Pros: Some manufacturers provide models that are narrower in front, with a tapered (or wedge) configuration to permit tighter cornering and to hold the legs together.

Cons: Taper may aggravate hip deformities (e.g., chronic or recurrent dislocation of the hip), may produce pressure lesions on the lateral aspects of the lower legs, may interfere with side transfers if the legs are tightly jammed in place, and may interfere with floor-to-seat transfers if the pelvis is too wide for the user to sit on the footrests.

16. How does rear-axle position affect the wheelchair?

- Raising the axle lowers the seat height, tilts the wheelchair backwards, lowers rear stability, raises forward stability, and causes a cambered wheel to toe out.
- Moving the axle back raises rear stability, decreases the ease of doing wheelies, limits the ability of a wheelchair user or an attendant to lift the front wheels, reduces traction, lengthens the wheelbase, raises rolling resistance, and raises downhill-turning tendency.

17. How does grasping the rear wheels affect the likelihood and violence of a rear-tipping accident?

The static rear stability of a wheelchair with the wheel locks (or brakes) on (or equivalently grasped) is less stable than with the rear wheels free to roll, because the axis of rotation is at the wheel-ground interface in the former situation and at the level of the rear-wheel axle in the latter. Furthermore, once a wheelchair has tipped beyond the stability limits, the ensuing rear tip is slower and less violent if the wheels are grasped.

18. What is camber and how does it affect the wheelchair?

Camber, usually 3–9°, is present when the distance between the tops of the rear wheels is less than the distance at the bottoms. Camber provides a natural angle for the arms to address the wheels during propulsion, protects the user's hands from doorways or from other players in sports, reduces downhill-turning tendency on side slopes, increases the ease of turning, and increases lateral stability.

However, changing the camber induces many mechanical effects that may need to be compensated for, including lengthening of the wheelbase, tilting the wheelchair backwards, toe-out, and altering the caster-stem angle and the caster-trail distance. Camber causes more wear on wheel bearings, more rolling resistance, and creates a wider track (causing more difficulty in tight spaces), and a cambered wheel, even if perfectly aligned when all four wheels are on the ground, will toe out during a wheelie, in proportion to the wheelie angle. Unless compensations are made, camber increases forward and reduces rear stability as well, due to some of the above-noted effects that are coupled to camber angle.

19. What is "toeing error" and how can it be corrected?

The rear wheels are "**toed in**" when the fronts of the rear wheels are closer to each other than the backs; the opposite is "**toe out**." Symmetrical toeing error increases the rolling resistance, quite dramatically even for a malalignment of as little as 2°. Asymmetrical toeing can cause the wheelchair to persistently deviate to one side. If the wheelchair has an axle-adjustment plate, toeing error can be eliminated by adding washers under the front or back bolts. If the axle is housed in a tube of fixed alignment, the tube can be rotated.

20. What are caster "trail" and "flutter"?

Caster trail is the distance on the ground between two points: one obtained by dropping a vertical from the caster axle, the other by projecting the caster-swivel axis to the ground. The greater the trail, the greater the diameter that must be kept free (of the rear wheels, footrests, and heels) if the caster is to swivel freely.

Caster flutter (or shimmy) is the tendency for the casters to oscillate from side to side at a certain speed. This can be annoying, can increase rolling resistance, and can cause an unintentional change in direction. To decrease flutter at normal rolling speeds, one can reduce the size and weight of the caster, increase the caster trial, or increase the proportion of the weight on the casters.

21. Why should the caster stems be vertical?

If the caster stems (and therefore the axes around which the swivel occurs) are not vertical, the caster axle will be lower at one swivel extreme than the other. This may cause the wheelchair to "settle" after the wheelchair has come to a halt. When starting up, there may be some resistance to overcome to get the caster "uphill."

22. Why do many wheelchair users remove conventional rear anti-tip devices or adjust them into ineffective positions?

Most rear anti-tip devices have a limited range of adjustability and, when adjusted in a way that makes them effective in preventing full rear tips, they interfere with maneuverability (e.g., by "grounding out" during incline transitions, or by preventing the wheelchair from being tipped back sufficiently to get the casters up a curb).

23. Where should a wheelchair user carry a load to maximize or minimize the effect on stability?

To raise rear stability, the footrest position should be the first choice of location for an added load; to lower rear stability, use the high-rear position. To raise forward stability, use the low-rear position; to lower forward stability, use the footrest position. To minimize the effect that added loads have on stability, use the lap or low-anterior position (under the seat).

24. Aside from showing off, when is a "wheelie" useful?

A wheelie is when a manual wheelchair user lifts the front wheels from the ground by applying forward force to the handrims and then maintains balance on the rear wheels by forward and backward forces on the handrims. The wheelie position is useful for transiently reducing the loads on the ischial tuberosities, to decrease neck discomfort when talking to a standing person, for turning in tight spaces, and to negotiate obstacles such as rough or soft ground, inclines, and curbs.

25. How much input should the wheelchair user have in the prescription process?

Lots. The prescription process should fully involve the user (and, if appropriate, the family or other caregivers). For the first wheelchair, the limited experience of users will mean that they will need to rely heavily on the clinical team. However, as users develop more experience, they are able to participate more fully in the process.

26. What are the steps in the prescription process?

1. The clinical team assesses the user, particularly his or her impairments, diagnoses, prognosis, residual abilities, extent of social participation, goals of wheelchair use, financial resources, priorities (because tradeoffs will invariably be necessary), and the user's dimensions.

2. The clinical team and user develop a generic list of the ideal wheelchair and seating features for the user.

3. The ideal-feature list is then compared with what is available in the user's price range from a reputable manufacturer and for which prompt service will be available.

4. The user test-drives the chairs under consideration, preferably with a member of the clinical team present.

5. Once the appropriate wheelchair has been selected, the user is trained in its optimal use (including static, indoor and outdoor challenges, or simulations thereof) and the results of training are documented.

6. After the user has used the wheelchair for a few months (and periodically thereafter), the situation should be reviewed and adjustments made.

BIBLIOGRAPHY

1. Axelson P, Minkel J, Chesney D: A Guide to Wheelchair Selection: How to Use the ANSI/RESNA Wheelchair Standards to Buy a Wheelchair. Washington, DC, Paralyzed Veterans of America, 1994.
2. Bergen AF, Presperin J, Tallman T: Positioning for function: Wheelchairs and other assistive technologies. Valhalla, NY, Valhalla Rehabilitation Publications, Ltd, 1990.
3. Brubaker C: Ergonometric considerations: Choosing a wheelchair system. J Rehabil Res Dev Clin Suppl 2:37–48, 1990.
4. Cooper R: Wheelchair Selection and Configuration. New York, Demos Medical Publishing, Inc., 1998.
5. Denison I, Shaw J, Zuyderhoff R: Wheelchair Selection Manual: The Effect of Components on Manual Wheelchair Performance. Vancouver, BC, British Columbia Rehabilitation Society. [4255 Laurel St, Vancouver, BC V5Z 2G9]
6. Kirby RL: Principles of wheelchair design and prescription. In Lazar RB (ed): Principles of Neurologic Rehabilitation. New York, McGraw-Hill, 1997, pp 465–481.
7. Kirby RL: Wheelchair stability: Important, measurable and modifiable. Technol Disabil 5:75–80, 1996.
8. Wilson AB Jr: How to Select and Use Manual Wheelchairs. Topping VA, Rehabilitation Press, 1992.

EPILOGUE

Martin Grabois, M.D., and Thomas E. Strax, M.D.

When the editors asked us to write this epilogue for *Physical Medicine and Rehabilitation Secrets, 2nd Edition*, it gave us time not only to reflect on the past and present, but also to focus on the future. Both of us have been in the field since the early 1970s and have seen the field grow and mature from its official beginnings in 1948. We have known and been taught by the giants of our field, who have influenced us and the field as a whole.

THE PAST

The roots of physical medicine and rehabilitation (PM&R) can be traced back to ancient times when heat, water, and light were the modalities used to treat patients. Later, the advent of electric-powered modalities expanded the variety of physical interventions. Modern rehabilitation medicine is an outgrowth of World War I and, to a greater extent, World War II. In the 1940s, antibiotics and new surgical techniques were successfully used to treat the casualties of war, but these medical innovations alone did not adequately meet the needs of all disabled survivors. A group of physicians recognized and developed a special body of knowledge, along with certain procedural skills, that could benefit these patients, and the specialty of PM&R was established. The specialty of PM&R continues to help patients, adding years to life and life to years by improving quality of life.

The specialty of PM&R has not been always been readily accepted. An eclectic medical specialty that diagnoses and treats neurologic and muscle conditions and does rehabilitation as well is difficult to conceptualize. Furthermore, rehabilitation is a process in the medical continuum (prevention, acute care, rehabilitation) and is not particularly related to a system of the body or a period of human development (pediatrics, geriatrics). The emphasis on personal enablement and diminishing disablement transcends the medical model and can be perplexing. We physiatrists have had to overcome the prejudices of our colleagues, and occasionally it is still difficult to convince some medical colleagues of our value—that is until their family or friends are in need of our services.

Stillwell compared and contrasted PM&R with orthopedic surgery, which in its infancy was not well received or accepted as a subspecialty. It was only in and after World War I that orthopedic surgery became accepted, when orthopedic surgeons clearly demonstrated their superiority in the management of injuries of the bones and joints.

Arthur Sulzburger published a commentary on PM&R in the *New York Times* that read: "If there is any good about a war, it is taking the good things developed because of it and making them available to all people." Unfortunately, after most wars, the impetus for rehabilitation falls prey to lack of governmental support, and disabled veterans are provided with pensions and dependency rather than programs to achieve and maintain independence. Fortunately, in the United States after World War II, leaders such as Krusen and Rusk, along with the support of Bernard Baruch, would not let the concept of PM&R die. Later, the half a million active, intelligent, young individuals with disabilities from the Vietnam War benefited from the work of these PM&R pioneers.

THE FUTURE

There are two themes for the future that we would like to emphasize. The first theme is the importance physiatrists have always placed on **providing the highest quality of care for our patients**.

Embedded in that theme are the issues of medical ethics, research, patient education, and quality of life. Even in the current era of health care reform, we all know that patient care should remain our top priority. Eugene Moskowitz, in his 1975 presidential address, noted, "We must not dislocate the patient from the nucleus of the every-growing complex circle of care to the extent that he becomes a peripheral problem, with the medical superstructure and its affiliates occupying the center of the arena." To accomplish this goal, medical rehabilitation professionals have to work in partnership with one another and with consumer organizations. There is precedent for joining forces. When rehabilitation medicine organizations joined with the community of people with disabilities to support passage of the American with Disabilities Act (ADA), they were successful and enjoyed one of the their finest hours.

We all recognize as Cole did that patients are becoming increasingly active participants in their own health care. In this new era, consumers want physicians to make them well and keep them well, and they want employers and government to pay their expenses. On the other hand, providers want to exercise their skills while remaining free from external intrusions. Cole argued that by working *with* consumers we have a better chance of achieving both goals. He urged us never to forget that rehabilitation requires the patient to be an active participant of the health care team.

DeJong noted in 1993 that the use of special interest groups is among the more important and powerful ways by which individual and professional needs and desires are expressed in the political process. The relationship between medical rehabilitation professionals and consumers is interdependent. DeJong urged medical rehabilitation professionals to work toward a new compact and alliance with people with disabilities to forge a new sense of community. Medical rehabilitationists alone cannot break the political gridlock and policy stalemate in this country, but we can be leaders in this arena. We already have a value system and professional orientation in place that are perhaps more consumer friendly than that of most other medical disciplines.

The second theme is that we need to **reinvent ourselves and plan for the future**. Avner Griver, M.D., while a senior resident in PM&R at Baylor College of Medicine, in a Grand Rounds presentation entitled "Health Care in Transition," noted, "Every so often in the collective unconscious of our nation, a movement arises from reform. This movement is usually based on an idea that a crisis has developed that needs to be dealt with. Whether these crises are related to political opportunism, the mass media, or the awakening of a nation to truths never before discussed is the topic of another discussion. Nevertheless, in the last few years, this nation has begun to grapple with a health care crisis, which, whether real or perceived, is a fact of life."

During the last few years, we have witnessed a great deal of action in the area of health care reform. What began as a national initiative has become an initiative at the state and local levels. We are seeing changes in our communities in the way medical care is being provided and paid for. Managed care companies are looking principally at the bottom line, and with that view, it is often the patient who suffers through lack of adequate attention to his or her medical and rehabilitation needs. We believe that we can and must work with managed care organizations to improve the care their members receive in a cost-effective manner.

The fastest growing groups in our society are the elderly and people with disabilities. We must find a way to encourage and reward outcomes as the basis of medical reimbursement instead of cost-shifting as a method to reduce health care cost. Because we know that managed care is not going away for now, we must create new strategies to work with managed care companies to ensure the highest quality patient care that is cost-effective. This will mean collaborating with payors and educating patients about how to work within the managed care system to achieve the best outcomes possible. This is going to require changes in how we conduct business. It is going to mean that we spend more time explaining to payors the rationale behind our treatment recommendations. To compete better with managed care organizations, we need to provide cost-effective and competitive care, produce effective outcomes, consider vertical integration and becoming part of a health care network, provide consumer satisfaction, be available, and finally, become known as the place to go for treatment.

However, for the field and the physiatrist to prosper, it will take time and commitment. This is not the time to sit back and hope someone else will do it. Each of us should adopt the philosphy, ask not what the field has done for me but what I can do for the field and the patients I serve.

We have challenges before us that many of us never thought we would face. We believe that we must face these new realities and aggressively pursue strategies for change. Change is hard for both individuals and organizations. We become set in our ways of doing things, but if we are to prosper, we must embrace change and steer a course that will be beneficial to our patients and to our profession.

We hope we have given you the keys to open the door. Now you must open it and walk through to embrace the changes and opportunities available. We urge you to do it now.

INDEX

Page numbers in **boldface type** indicate complete chapters.

Abdomen, acute, in spinal cord injury patients, 209
Abdominal reflex, absence of, in cervical spinal cord
    lesion patients, 107
Abducens nerve
    diabetic palsy of, 161
    function of, 25
Abduction pillows, 286
Abscess, acupuncture-related, 544
Access Board, 85
Accessory nerve, function of, 26
Acetylcholine, 35, 156, 157
Acetylcholinesterase inhibitors, as Alzheimer's disease
    therapy, 228
Achilles tendon lengthening, 446
Acquired immunodeficiency syndrome (AIDS), 333,
    334
    dementia complex of, 335
    differentiated from human immunodeficiency virus
    (HIV) infection, 333
Acromioclavicular joint
    ligamentous support for, 47
    pain in, 261
Acromioplasty, rehabilitation after, 262
Actin, 37
Action potentials, 32, 33
Activities of daily living
    cancer-related impairments of, 325
    functional assessment of, 9–14
    self-care skills of, 10
Acupressure, 351, 532
Acupuncture, **541–547**
Addiction, in burn patients, 356
Adductor muscle sprains, in ballet dancers, 395
Adenosine triphosphate, role in muscle contraction, 37
ADFR (activation, depression, free, repetition)
    mnemonic, for coherence therapy, 454
Adiposis dolorosa (Dercum's disease), 291
Adson's test, 146
Advance care directives, for motor neuron disease
    patients, 219
Adverse technology reaction, 507
Ages and Stages Questionnaire, 417
Aggression
    sexual, 75
    by traumatic brain injury patients, 200
Aging. *See also* Elderly patients
    effect of exercise on, 441
    effect on muscle strength, 492
"Aging in place," 88
Agitated patients, chemical restraint of, 502–503
Agnosia, 481
Agrammatism, 481
Air bags
    as postoperative dressings, 556
    in vehicles, effect on traumatic brain injury risk, 194
Air conduction threshold testing, 70
Airway secretions, elimination of
    in chronic obstructive pulmonary disease patients,
    239
    in ventilatory impairment patients, 235

Alcohol abuse/use
    as avascular necrosis risk factor, 280, 288
    as stroke risk factor, 167
    as traumatic brain injury risk factor, 194
Alcohol injections, as spasticity treatment, in cerebral
    palsy patients, 421
Alendronate, as osteoporosis treatment, 452
Algometer, pressure, 370
Allis sign, 418
Allodynia, 373
Alpha$_2$ adrenergic agonists, as brain injury-related
    spasticity treatment, 198
Alpha$_2$ adrenergic antagonists, central and peripheral,
    499
Alpha-glucosidase inhibitors, 500
Alzheimer's disease, acetylcholinesterase inhibitor
    therapy for, 228
Amantadine, as Parkinson's disease treatment, 184
Ambulation, 10. *See also* Gait; Running; Walking
    community, muscle function required for, 208
    energy expenditure during, in amputees, 559–560
    by hip fracture patients, 287
    by meningomyelocele patients, 426
    by multiple sclerosis patients, 179–180
    by spinal cord injury patients, 230–231
Ambulation assistive devices
    for the elderly, 119
    for multiple sclerosis patients, 180
    for total hip arthroplasty patients, 286
    for total knee arthroplasty patients, 295
American Academy of Medical Acupuncture, 545
American Academy of Physical Medicine and
    Rehabilitation, 2, 13
American Association of Cardiovascular and
    Pulmonary Rehabilitation, 241
American Board of Medical Specialties, 3
American Board of Physical Medicine and
    Rehabilitation, 2
American College of Sports Medicine, 245
American Hospital Association, 3
American Medical Association, 3
American Medical Association Guides to the
    Evaluation of Permanent Impairment, 122
American Sign Language (ASL), 59
American Spinal Cord Injury Association, 203
Americans with Disabilities Act, 53, 54, 55, 56, 82,
    90–91, 92
    disability definition of, 90–91
    reasonable accommodation provision of, 91, 122, 504
Amiodarone, side effects of, 499
Amphetamines, 225–227
Amplification devices, for hearing-impaired persons,
    87, 506
Amputation, **553–561**
    atherosclerotic peripheral vascular disease-related, 247
    in burn patients, 356
    forequarter, 329, 572
    lower-extremity, 553–561
    levels of, 554–555
    postoperative dressings for, 556

Amputation (*cont.*)
upper-extremity, 553, 567–568
in children, 567
Amputees
ambulation-related energy expenditure by, 559–560
cancer patients as, 328
geriatric, 120–121, 553, 560
lower-extremity
gait of, 578, 580, 581, 582
prosthetics for, 577, 578
phantom limb pain in, 557–558
skin problems of, 558–559
upper-extremity, prostheses for, **567–572**
Amyotrophic lateral sclerosis, 212–213, 216
Amyotrophy
diabetic, 151–152
neuralgic, as brachial plexopathy cause, 154
Anabolic hormone analogs, as pressure ulcer
preventive, 501
Anabolic steroids, as osteoporosis treatment, 453
Analgesia
acupuncture-related, 543
topical, 501
transcutaneous electrical nerve stimulation-induced,
519, 526–527
Anal sphincter
examination of, 472
internal, 467
Analysis of covariance, 19
Analysis of variance (ANOVA), 19
Anastomosis, Martin-Gruber, 129–130, 141
Anatomic snuff box, 273
Anemia
iron-deficiency, 431
as pressure ulcer risk factor, 461
renal failure-related, 323
Angina, as dyspnea cause, 435
Anginal threshold, 243–244
Angiotensin-converting enzyme inhibitors, 498, 499
Angiotensin receptor blockers, 498, 499
Ankle, **300–305**
anatomy of, 297
clonus at, 107, 573
dorsiflexor muscles of, 51
equinus state and deformity of, 303
injuries to, 298
kinesiology of, 50–51
rheumatoid arthritis of, 297–298
sprains of, 298, 299, 300
lingering pain associated with, 304
vascular status of, 298
Ankle-brachial index, 298
Ankle-foot orthoses (AFOs), 113, 422–423, 572–573, 574
Ankle joint, secondary, 303
Ankle ligament complex, injury and instability
evaluation of, 299
Ankylosing spondylitis, 286, 346–347
Annuloplasty, intradiscal electrothermal, 535
Anomia, 103, 180
Anomic aphasia, 103
ANOVA (analysis of variance), 19
Anterior cord syndrome, 205–206
Anterior cruciate ligament
function of, 290
tears/injuries of, 289, 290, 291, 387
implication for sports participation, 388

Anterior interosseous syndrome, 144, 147
Anthraquinone derivatives, 469
Anticholinergic drugs, as Parkinson's disease treatment,
184
Anticholinergic effects, of drugs, 496
Anticoagulants, 497–498
Anticonvulsants
as neuropathic pain treatment, 153–154
as traumatic brain injury treatment, 198
Antidepressants. *See also* Tricyclic antidepressants
soporific effect of, 497
Antihypertensive agents, 498–499
Antiparkinson drugs, 183–184
side effects of, 184, 191
Antiplatelet agents, as stroke prophylaxis, 167
Antispasmodic drugs
local injections of, 537–541
oral, compared with antispasticity drugs, 501–502
Anulus fibrosus, 45
Apartments, accessibility of, 85–86
Apgar scores, 411
Aphasia, 28, 103–104, 481
classification of, 479
differentiated from dysarthria, 103
multiple sclerosis-related, 180
nonfluent, 479–480
differentiated from fluent, 479–480
gesture-facilitated speech in, 231
stroke-related, 168, 173–174
terminology associated with, 481
Apley's test, 290, 292
Apoptosis, brain injury-related, 195–196
Apraxia, 480–481
limb, 229–230
multiple sclerosis-related, 180
stroke-related, 174
types of, 174
Aquatic exercise/therapy, 509
by rheumatic disease patients, 342
Arachnoid membrane, 24
Arcuate premotor area, 43
Argyll-Robertson pupil, 26
Arm. *See also* Upper extremity
coordination testing of, 108
muscle weakness of, 106
segmental weight of, 560
Arnold-Chiari malformation, 425, 426
Arterial occlusion, diabetes-related, 554
Artery of Adamkiewicz, 205
Arthralgias, systemic lupus erythematosus-related, 350
Arthritis. *See also* Rheumatoid arthritis
degenerative, ultrasound therapy for, 518
HIV infection-related, 335
inflammatory, 338
differentiated from noninflammatory, 337–338
noninfectious, of the hip, 284
Reiter's syndrome-related, 346
of the shoulder, 262–263
Arthroplasty
of thumb carpometacarpal joint, 279
total elbow, 269–270
total hip, 120, 283–284, 285–286, 287, 289, 343
total knee, 119–120, 293–296
volar plate, 278
Artificial intelligence (AI), 505–506
ASIA Impairment Scale, of spinal cord injuries, 206

Aspiration
  excessive, 484
  in stroke patients, 170–171
Aspirin
  action mechanisms of, 338
  anticoagulant activity of, 497–498
  as cancer pain treatment, 327
  as stroke prophylaxis, 167
Assistive devices/technology, **504–507**
  for the elderly, 119
  effect on energy expenditure, 113
  failure of, 507
  federal government's promotion of, 95
  for the hearing-impaired, 68–69, 70, 71, 506
  use in vocational rehabilitation, 402
Association of American Medical Colleges, 3
Asymmetric tonic neck reflex, 417
Ataxia, 108, 168, 191
Athetosis, 191
Athletes. *See also* Sports participation
  spondylolysis and spondylolisthesis in, 409–410
Audiologists, 71
Audiology evaluation, 70
  of delayed language development, 416
Audiometry, brainstem evoked response, 73
Auditory system, 34
Auerbach's plexus, 466
Aural rehabilitation, 70, 72
Autonomic nervous system
  anatomy of, 20–21
  functions of, 34
Axillary nerve, injuries to, 21, 22
Axonal lesions, clinical features of, 129
Axonopathy, distal sensory and motor, 152
Axonotmesis, 130, 144
Axons, 31

Babinski sign, 107
Back pain. *See also* Low back pain
  bed rest (immobilization-related), 440
  ergonomic modifications for management of, 406
  vertebral compression fracture-related, 451, 452
Baclofen, as spasticity treatment, 444, 445, 502
  intrathecal administration of, 368, 422, 445, 502
Baker, William Morrant, 292
Balanced Budget Act of 1997, 92
Balanced forearm orthosis, 563
Ballismus, 191
Ball-valve effect, 430–431
Bankart repair, of shoulder instability, 263–264
Barthel Index, 13
Basal ganglia
  injuries to, 25
  role in voluntary movement control, 40, 41–42
Basal metabolic rate (BMR), 494
Bathroom
  accidents and falls in, 88
  environmental adaptations in, 86
Bayley Infant Neurodevelopment Screen, 417
Bed mobility, 10
Bed rest
  contraindication as low back pain treatment, 256
  detrimental effects of, 341
  prevention of, **438–442**
  by organ transplant recipients, 318
  recovery from, 440

Bed rest (*cont.*)
  as rheumatic disease treatment, 341
  short-term beneficial effects of, 439
  as vertebral compression fracture treatment, 452
Behavioral disorders, traumatic brain injury-related,
  199, 200
Bell's palsy, 27, 130, 151, 275
Bennett's fractures, 275
Benzodiazepines
  as "chemical restraint," 502
  as Gilles de la Tourette syndrome treatment, 188
  soporific effect of, 497
  effect on stroke recovery, 228
  as tardive dyskinesia treatment, 191
Benzotropine mesylate, interaction with acetylcholine,
  35
Beta$_2$-adrenergic agonists, as airway
  hyperresponsiveness treatment, 502
Beta-blockers, 498
  use by spinal cord injury patients, 499
"Between-subjects" research design, 16–17
Bicycle ergometry, functional electrical stimulation,
  524–525
Bier block, 382
Biguanides, 500
Biker's palsy, 389
Bi-level positive airway pressure (BiPAP),
  differentiated from continuous positive airway
  pressure (CPAP), 237
Biofeedback, as Gilles de la Tourette syndrome
  treatment, 188
Biomedical model, of illness, 6
Biopsychosocial model, of illness, 6
Bisphosphonates, as osteoporosis treatment, 452, 453
BITE mnemonic, for contracture formation, 439
Bladder, innervation of, 471, 472
Bladder dysfunction
  in multiple sclerosis patients, 179
  neurogenic bladder
    long-term drainage of, 475
    in meningomyelocele patients, 426
    in stroke patients, 171
    urinary tract complications of, 476
  pharmacologic management of, 476–477
  in spinal cord injury patients, 472, 474–475
Bladder neck, sympathetic innervation of, 472
Bladder stimulation systems, in spinal cord injury,
  525–526
Blepharospasm, 188, 189
Blindness, legal, 65
Blind patients. *See also* Visually impaired patients
  rehabilitation of, **65–68**
Blink response, 129
Blood circulation, cerebral, 28–29
Body fat, distribution of, gender differences in, 495
Body image, effect of disability or illness on, 75
Body jacket, as vertebral compression fracture
  treatment, 451
Body ventilators, 235
Body weight, ideal (IBW), 494
Bone, as metastases site, 306, 327, 329–330
Bone conduction threshold testing, 70
Bone disease
  metabolic, **447–456**
  renal, dialysis-related, 322

Bone formation, stimulation of, 453
Bone mass measurement, indications for, 449–450
Bone mineral density, effect of weightlessness on, 450
Bone scans, 307
    for complex regional pain syndrome evaluation, 381
    for heterotopic ossification diagnosis, 458
Botulinum toxin, action mechanism of, 537–538
Botulinum toxin injections
    as dystonia treatment, 190
    as spasticity treatment, 421, 446, 537–538, 539, 540
Botulism, 157
Boutonnière deformity, 275, 345
Bowel care, 467–469
    in lower motor neuron bowel, 468
    in upper motor neuron bowel, 467–468
Bowel dysfunction
    bowel incontinence
        in multiple sclerosis patients, 180
        in stroke patients, 171
    neurogenic bowel, **465–470**
        in meningomyelocele patients, 426
    in stroke patients, 171
Bowel function, pharmacologic regulation of, 503
Bowel programs, 467
Bowel resection, effect on patients' nutritional status, 325
Bowler's thumb, 276
Boxer's elbow, 268
Boxer's fractures, 275
Brachial artery pressure, 557
Brachial plexus
    anatomy of, 21
    injuries/lesions of, 154
        complete disruption, 260
        differentiated from radial nerve palsy, 148
        microsurgical reconstruction of, 410–411
Brachioradialis muscle, 266
Bracing
    as fracture treatment, 310
    prophylactic knee, in football players, 574
    in rheumatic disease, 343
    spinal, 588
    spiral, 573–574
    as thoracic deformity treatment, 587
    as vertebral compression fracture treatment, 451
Bragard's test, 290
Brain
    acupuncture-related stimulation of, 543
    blood supply of, 28–29
    cerebrospinal fluid flow in, 30
    descending tracts from, 38–39
"Brain death," 162
Brain injury
    adverse drug effects in, 434
    bladder dysfunction associated with, 475–476
    in children, outcome of, 413
    cognitive deficits associated with
        pharmacologic therapy for, 225–229
        stimulant therapy for, 225–227
    diaschisis associated with, 224–225
    mental status changes in, 434
    sepsis associated with, 430
    synapse unmasking after, 224
    traumatic, **194–202**
        vocational rehabilitation in, 401
Brain injury patients, compared with brain tumor
    patients, 331

Brainstem, anatomy of, 25, 26, 27
Brainstem auditory evoked potential/auditory brainstem
    response studies, 162–164
Brainstem auditory evoked response audiometry, 73
Brain tumor patients, compared with brain injury
    patients, 331
Brain tumors, 331–332
Breast cancer, 331, 332
Brisement, as "frozen" shoulder treatment, 263
Broca's aphasia, 103, 173
Bromocriptine, interaction with dopamine, 35
Bronchitis, differentiated from emphysema, 237–238
Brown-Séquard syndrome, 206
Bruininks-Oseretsky scale, 417
Bulbocavernous reflex, 472, 474
Bunion, 297, 347
Bunionette, 297
Bunnell-Littler test, 274
Bunnstrom treatment method, for hemiplegia, 171
Bupropion, 497
"Burners," 387
Burn rehabilitation, **352–361**
Burns
    classification of, 352
    as disfigurement cause, 357, 360
    to the hand, contracture prevention in, 278
Bursae, 548
Bursitis, 548–549
    prepatellar, 292
    subacromial, 549
    subcutaneous/Achilles', 549
    subdeltoid, 549
        differentiated from supraspinatus bursitis, 258
    trochanteric, 281–282, 549

Cadence, 111
Calcitonin, as osteoporosis treatment, 452, 453
Calcium, daily requirements for, 455
Calcium channel blockers, 188, 499
Calcium ions
    role in action potentials, 33
    role in muscle contraction, 37–38
Callus, plantar, differentiated from warts, 304
Camel's sign, 289
Cam varied resistance, during range-of-motion, 490
Cancer. *See also specific types of cancer*
    information sources about, 333
    as limb loss cause, 553
    metastatic, 306
    as motor neuron disease cause, 214
Cancer rehabilitation, **325–333**
Canes
    for multiple sclerosis patients, 180
    for visually impaired patients, 67
Capillary filling pressure, 441
Capsaicin, 501
Capsular shift, 263–264
Capsulorrhaphy, thermal, 263–264
Capute Scale, 417
Carbamazepine
    as cancer pain treatment, 327
    as traumatic brain injury treatment, 198
Carbidopa, as Parkinson's disease treatment, 183
Cardiac output, 243
Cardiac rehabilitation, **241–246**
    contraindications to, 243

Cardiac steal phenomenon, 244
Cardiac stress tests, 244
Cardiovascular system, effect of aerobic endurance-type exercise on, 492–493
Carotid artery, internal, first branch of, 29
Carpal bones, 272
  fractures and dislocations of, 48
Carpal compression test, 140
Carpal tunnel, anatomy of, 137, 138
Carpal tunnel syndrome, **137–143**, 144
  differentiated from cervical radiculopathy, 147
  differentiated from media neuropathy, 139
    false-positive results in, 140–141
  "flick sign" of, 138
  in musicians, 392
  resistant, 405
  treatment of, 142–143
    corticosteroid injections, 551
    open release *versus* endoscopic release, 279
    ultrasound therapy, 518
Cartilage transplantation, in the osteoarthritic knee, 293
Case, definition of, 4–5
Case managers, 398–399
CASH (cruciform anterior spinal hyperextension) orthosis, 587
Cast disease, 307
Casting
  serial, in burn patients, 359
  as spasticity treatment, 446
Cataracts, 65
CAT (Clinical Adaptive Test) scale, 417
Categorical measurement, 16
Catheterization, intermittent urinary, in multiple sclerosis patients, 179
Cauda equina, location of, 24
Caudal epidural injections, 533–534
Causalgia, 379
Cavus foot, 304, 426
Central cord syndrome, 206
Central fluid shift, 440
Central nervous system
  anatomy of, 20
  connection with brainstem, 26
  extrathalamic ascending neuromodulatory systems of, 34–35
  lesions of, differentiated from peripheral nervous system lesions, 21
  motivational subsystem of, 34
Central nervous system evoked potential studies, **160–165**
Central pattern generation, 230
Central slip extensor tendon injury, short arc motion protocol for, 277
Central somatosensory conduction time, 161
Cerebellar dysfunction, 108, 109, 191
Cerebellar testing, 108–109
Cerebellum
  blood supply of, 29
  injury to, 25
    as motor dysfunction cause, 41
    role in voluntary movement control, 40, 41
Cerebral arteries, 28–29
Cerebral cortex, role in planning and control of movement, 42, 43
Cerebral hemispheric injury, right, as communication deficits cause, 480

Cerebral palsy, 411–412, **418–424**
  dorsal rhizotomy treatment for, 421, 422, 446
  spinal curvature in, 410
Cerebrospinal fluid, 30
Cerebrum, functions and lesions of, 28
Certified Therapeutic Recreation Specialist (CTRS), 508
Cerumen, impacted, 73
Cervical spine
  functional anatomy of, 251
  ligamentous instability of, as contraindication to traction, 530
  movement of, 586
  pain in, **251–253**
Cervical thrust techniques, 531–532
Cervical traction, 529
Charcot, Jean M., 209
Charcot-Marie-Tooth disease, 214, 304
Charcot neuroarthropathy, 299
Charcot's spine, 209
Chemical burns, 352–353, 354
Child abuse, as fracture cause, 412–413
Child Development Inventory, 417
Children, **409–414**
  brainstem auditory evoked potential/auditory brainstem response studies in, 162
  as burn patients, 357
    return to school by, 361
  complex regional pain syndrome in, 381
  disabled, education of, 94–95
  Duchenne muscular dystrophy in, 409
  fractures in, 310
  hearing loss in, 73–74
  HIV infection in, 336
  motor neuron disease in, 213–214
  pain assessment of, 357
  painful hip in, 282
  pushed or pulled elbows in, 267
  spinal cord injury without radiologic abnormality (SCIWORA) in, 203, 412
Children's Orientation and Amnesia Test (COAT), 413
Chinese medicine, 541–542
Cholecystitis, in spinal cord injury patients, 432
Cholelithiasis, in spinal cord injury patients, 432
Cholestyramine, 431, 499–500
Chondromalacia patella, 289, 290
Chorea, 191
  Huntington's disease-related, 192
Chrondritis, acupuncture-related, 544
Chronic graft-versus-host disease, 319–320
Chronic obstructive pulmonary disease (COPD), 237–240
Chronic pain syndrome, 363–367
Cingulate cortex, anterior, 42, 43
Circle of Willis, 29
Circumduction, 582
Cisparide, side effects of, 499
Civil rights, of disabled persons, 90
Civil Rights Act of 1964, 90
CLAM (Clinical Linguistic Auditory Milestones) scale, 417
Claudication, intermittent, 247
Claw toe, 297
Clients
  definition of, 5
  patients as, 54

"Climbing the hill," 580
Clinical care map, 101
Clinical pathway, 101
Clonazepam
    as essential tremor treatment, 188
    as tardive dyskinesia treatment, 191
Clonidine, as spasticity treatment, 444, 445
Clonus, 106
    at ankle, 107, 573
Clostridium difficile infections, 431, 470, 499–500
Clozapine, as tardive dyskinesia-related psychosis
    treatment, 191
COAT (Children's Orientation and Amnesia Test), 413
Cocaine abuse, as stroke risk factor, 167
Cochlear implants, 70, 73
    as contraindication to magnetic resonance imaging, 59
Codeine, as cancer pain treatment, 327
"Codfish" vertebrae, 453
Codman's exercises, 259
Cognitive deficits
    brain injury-related, 199
        pharmacologic therapy for, 225–229
        stimulant therapy for, 225–227
    drug-induced, 502
    in the elderly, 118
    HIV infection-related, 335
    meningomyelocele-related, 426
    multiple sclerosis-related, 180
    stroke-related, 168
Cognitive remediation therapy, for traumatic brain
    injury patients, 200
Cognitive status testing, bedside, 102
Cogwheel sign, of rigidity, 105
Coherence therapy, 454
Cold allergy, as cryotherapy contraindication, 516
Cold-induced injuries, 354
Cold therapy. See Cryotherapy
Colestipol, 499–500
Colitis, 431
Collagen fibers, length of, 439
Collars
    Philadelphia, 586
    soft cervical, 312–313, 586
Colon, innervation of, 465–466
Colostomy, 469
Coma
    barbiturate, 162
    traumatic brain injury-related, 200–201
Coma/Near-Coma Scale, 197
Coma Recovery Scale, 197
Communication
    with aphasic patients, 104
    augmentative and alternative, 506
    with disabled people
        invalidating statements in, 62–63
        terminology for, 61–62
    disorders of, 478–483
    with the elderly, 119
    with sexual partner, 76
    strategies in, for rehabilitation professionals, 53–64
Communication board, 506
Community, definition of, 509
Community Integration Questionnaire (CIQ), 512
Community reintegration, 508–512
COMO ESTAS mnemonic, for mental status testing,
    102

Complex regional pain syndrome, 260, 314, 379–383
Complex repetitive discharges, 126
Compliance, by patients, 5
Compound motor action potentials
    in Bell's palsy, 130
    effect of temperature on, 128
Compression garments, 521–522
    for burn patients, 358
Compression stockings, 250
Computed tomography, quantitative, for osteoporosis
    diagnosis, 449
Computer use
    by cerebral palsy patients, 423
    as headache cause, 253
Conceptual apraxia, 229
Concrete Change, 87
Concurrent validity, of functional assessment scales, 11
Conduction, 513
Conduction aphasia, 103, 173
Conduction apraxia, 229
Confusion, Parkinson's disease therapy-related, 184
Congenital limb deficiency, as limb loss cause, 553
Congestive heart failure patients, cardiac rehabilitation
    of, 246
Conjunctivitis, 346
Constipation
    in bed-confined patients, 440
    as diarrhea cause, 430–431
    in multiple sclerosis patients, 180
    in stroke patients, 171
Constraint-induced movement therapy (CIMT),
    220–222
Constructional apraxia, 174
Construct validity, of functional assessment scales, 11
Consultations, physiatric, 97–102
Consumer, patients as, 54
Contextual factors, 5
Continuous passive motion machines, 294, 360
Continuous positive airway pressure (CPAP),
    differentiated from bi-level positive airway
    pressure (BiPAP), 237
Contractures
    burn-related, 278, 358–359
    cerebral palsy-related, 420
    definition of, 439
    of the elbow, 270, 564
    equinus, 299
    flexion, differentiated from extensor lag, 296
    of the hip, 280–281, 583
    in immobilized limbs, 438, 439
    knee flexion, 115, 579
    meningomyelocele-related, 426
    rheumatoid arthritis-related, 345
    treatment for, 218
    ultrasound therapy for, 518
    Volkmann's, 278
Contrast baths, 515
Convection, 513
Conversion heating, 513
Cool-down periods, in cardiac rehabilitation exercise
    programs, 245, 246
Cooling, of tissue, mechanisms of, 513
Coordination testing, 99
Coprolalia, 188
Coproraxia, 188
Coracoclavicular ligament, 47

Coronary artery disease
  incidence and significance of, 241–242
  modifiable risk factors for, 244, 245
  in spinal cord injury patients, 210
Correlational studies, 16
Corsets, 588
Corticospinal tract, 24, 38
  lesions of, 25
  role in muscle tone, 39
Corticosteroid injections, 547–551
Corticosteroids
  as cancer pain treatment, 327
  low-dose, as muscle atrophy cause, 338
  as osteoporosis cause, 450
  as radiculopathy treatment, 367
Costoclavicular syndrome, 147
Council on Medical Education, 3
Countertransference, in physician-patient relationship,
    54
Coxa saltans, 281
Craig Handicapped Assessment and Reporting Tool
    (CHART), 512
Cramps
  abdominal
    immobilization hypercalcemia-related, 209
    Parkinson's disease therapy-related, 184
  writer's, 188, 189
Cranial nerves. *See also specific cranial nerves*
  of autonomic nervous system, 20–21
  diabetes-related mononeuropathies of, 151
  evaluation of, 104–105
  functions of, 25–26
Creatinine clearance, 321
Credé, 473
Cremasteric reflex, absence of, in cervical spinal cord
    lesion patients, 107
Criterion validity, of functional assessment scales,
    11
Cruciform anterior spinal hyperextension (CASH)
    orthosis, 587
Crutch-assisted ambulation, energy expenditure during,
    559–560
Crying, pathologic, 218
Cryotherapy, 513, 514, 515–516, 340
Cubital tunnel syndrome, 268, 272, 392, 550
Cumulative trauma syndromes, in workers, 403–405
Cuneate tract, 204
Cunnilingus, 80
Customer, definition of, 5
Cyst
  Baker's (popliteal), 291, 292
  epidermoid, in amputees, 559
Cystometry, 473
Cystoscopic examination, 475

Dancers
  female athletic triad in, 394
  groin pain in, 394
  physical examination of, 392
  turnout in, 393–394, 395
Dance screening, 393
Dandy-Walker syndrome, 425
Dantrolene, as spasticity treatment, 198, 444, 445, 502
Deafness. *See also* Hearing-impaired patients; Hearing
    loss
  definition of, 68

Debridement
  arthroscopic, of the osteoarthritic knee, 293
  of pressure ulcers, 462–463
  with warmed tap water, 516
Deconditioning, as focal muscle weakness cause, 110
Deep brain stimulator, as Parkinson's disease treatment,
    184
Defecation
  in bed-confined patients, 440
  physiolgic sequence of, 466
  in upper motor neuron bowel, 467–468
Degenerative disc disease, of the neck, 253
Dejerine-Roussy syndrome, 173
Delorme technique and axiom, 490
Deltoid ligament, injuries to, 299
Deltoid muscle, 47–48
Dementia, 103
  HIV/AIDS-related, 335
  vascular, 118
Dementia patients, environmental adaptations for, 88
Demyelinating lesions, clinical features of, 129
Dendrites, 31
Denver Development Screening Test, 417
Depersonalization, hospitalization-related, 81
Deprenyl, as Parkinson's disease treatment, 184
Depression
  in cancer patiens, 325
  in multiple sclerosis patients, 180
  in Parkinson's disease patients, 185
  in stroke patients, 168, 171, 174
deQuervain's disease, 274, 550
Dercum's disease (adiposis dolorosa), 291
Dermatologic disorders, in amputees, 558–559
Dermatome-like sensory deficits, peripheral nerve
    lesion-related, 21
Dermatomes
  anatomic landmarks of, 108
  innervation of, 21
Desensitization, as reflex sympathetic dystrophy
    treatment, 382
Detrusor compliance, 473
Detrusor hyperreflexia, multiple sclerosis-related, 179
Detrusor-sphincter dyssnergia, 472, 473–474
Developmental milestones, **415–418**
  in cerebral palsy, 419
Dextroamphetamine, 225–226
Diabetes mellitus
  effect of aerobic exercise on, 493
  conditions associated with
    amyotrophy, 151–152
    foot biomechanical disorders, 304
    insulin resistance, 500
    limb loss, 553, 554
    neuropathy, 150–151
    peripheral vascular disease, 247, 553, 554
  glucose control in, 500
  in inpatient rehabilitation unit patients, 433
Diagnosis, components of, 5
Diagnosis-related group (DRG)-exempt status, of
    rehabilitation hospitals and rehabilitation units, 13
Diagnostic and Statistical Manual-IV, pain
    classification of, 364
Diagnostic tools, in physiatry, 3
Dialysis, 321–322, 323–324
Diaphragmatic breathing exercises, for Parkinson's
    disease patients, 187

Diarrhea
  in constipated patients, 430–431
  HIV infection-related, 334
  neurogenic bowel-related, 470
  Parkinson's disease therapy-related, 184
  pseudomembranous colitis-related, 499–500
Diaschisis, 195, 224–225
Diathermy, 513, 517–519
Diazepam, as spasticity treatment, 444–445
Diencephalic fits, 197
Diffuse idiopathic skeletal hyperostosis (DISH), 286
Digital rectal stimulation, 467
Diphenylhydramine, soporific effect of, 497
Diplegia, cerebral palsy-related, 419
Diplopia, 105
Disability
  definitions of, 6, 11, 90–91, 121–122
  determination of severity of, 399
  differentiated from impairment and handicap, 11, 121
  HIV infection-related, 334
  incidence and prevalence of, 90
  low back pain-related, 255–256, 257
  in organ transplant recipients, 320
  permanent, 122–123
Disability benefits, effect of return to work on, 400
Disability etiquette, 61
Disability rating, 121–124
  in traumatic brain injury, 197
Disability studies, 59–60
"Disability syndrome," 255–256
Disabled Manifesto (Woodward), 53
Disabled persons
  alternative employment for, 399
  communication with, 53–64
  as patients, 53–54
Disablement, 5
Disadvantage, definition of, 5
Discitis, 535
Discography, 368
  lumbar provocative, 535
Disc pain, 251
Disease
  classification of consequences of, 5
  definition of, 4
  functional presentation of, 118
Disease-modifying antirheumatic drugs, 338
Dislocation, differentiated from subluxation, 313
Disruptive behavior, of traumatic brain injury patients, 200
Dissociative apraxia, 229
Diuretics, 498, 499
Dobutamine HCl echocardiography, 244
Door openers, automatic, 86
Doors, accessibility of, 86
Doorways, for disabled persons, 86
L-Dopa
  interaction with dopamine, 35
  as Parkinson's disease treatment, 183, 184, 185
Dopamine, 35
  role in motor recovery, 226
Dopamine agonists, as traumatic brain injury treatment, 227–228
Dopamine antagonists, as Parkinson's disease treatment, 184
Dopamine-blocking medications, as parkinsonism cause, 183

Dopaminergic system, of basal ganglia, failure of, 42
Dorsal scapular nerve, 21
"Double-crush syndrome," 147
Draftsman's elbow, 266
Drawer sign
  anterior, 299
  posterior, 291
Dressing apraxia, 174
Dressings
  postoperative, for lower-extremity amputations, 556
  for pressure ulcers, 463–464
Driving skills, of Parkinson's disease patients, 187
Drooling
  cerebral palsy-related, 423
  Parkinson's disease-related, 185
"Drop arm test," 259
Drug abuse, as traumatic brain injury risk factor, 194
Drug bioavailability, effect of body fat distribution patterns on, 495
Drugs. See also specific drugs
  as cognitive impairment cause, 502
  interactions of, 496
  as mental status change cause, 434
  as parkinsonism cause, 183
  as peripheral neuropathy cause, 154–155
  pyogenic, 430
  use in rehabilitation medicine, 496–503
Dual energy x-ray absorptiometry, 449
Dual photon absorptiometry, 449
Duchenne muscular dystrophy, 409
Dura, 24
Dynamometers, hand-held, 110
Dysarthrias
  classification of, 481
  differentiated from aphasia, 103
  multiple sclerosis-related, 180
  stroke-related, 168
Dysautonomia, central, traumatic brain injury-related, 197
Dysdiadochokinesis, 41
Dyskinesia, Parkinson's disease-related, 185
Dysphagia, 105, 478
  cerebral palsy-related, 423
  compensations for, 484–485
  exercises for management of, 484–485
  motor neuron disease-related, 219
  multiple sclerosis-related, 180
  Parkinson's disease-related, 185
  stroke-related, 168, 170–171
Dyspnea, in inpatient rehabilitation unit patients, 434–436
Dysreflexia, autonomic, 208, 209, 469, 437, 475
Dysrhythmias, cardiac stress test evaluation of, 244
Dystonia, 188–190
  oromandibular, 188, 190
  psychogenic, 192, 193
Dystonia musculorum deformans, 189, 190
Dystrophin, 409

Ear, as acupuncture site, 544, 546
Ear, nose, throat (ENT) evaluations, referrals for, 72–73
Ecchymoses, acupuncture-related, 544
Echocardiography, dobutamine HCl, 244
Echolalia, 481
Ectopic membrane potential, 32
Eczema, in amputees, 559

Edema
    in amputees, 558
    central spinal cord, 206–207
Edinger-Westphal nucleus, 26
Education for All Handicapped Children Act,
    94
Effect size, 18
Effleurage, 531
Ejaculation, 77
Elastic binders, as vertebral compression fracture
    treatment, 451
Elbow
    anatomy of, 265–266
    articulations of, 265
    boxer's, 268
    carrying angle of, 265–266
    contractures of, 270, 564
    disarticulation of, 271
    dislocation of, 270–271
    draftsman's, 266
    fractures of, 270–271
    fusion of, 271
    golfer's (medial epicondylitis), 267, 550
    little leaguer's, 268, 389
    muscles of, 266
    osteochondritis dissecans of, 268–269
    pulled or pushed, in children, 267
    replacement prostheses for, 269
    stability of, 48
    tennis (lateral epicondylitis), 267, 269, 389,
        549
    total arthroplasty of, 269–270
Elderly patients
    amputations in, 120–121, 553, 560
    evaluation of, **116–121**
    falls by, 115, 119, 288, 305
    fractures in, 119, 307, 310
    hearing aid use in, 72
    lower-extremity joint parameters in, 115
    malnutrition in, 494
    neurologic changes in, 116–117
    pain management in, 121
    physical activity of, 441
    spinal cord injury without radiologic abnormality
        (SCIWORA) in, 203
    strokes in, 175–176
Elderly population, characteristics of, 116
Electrical injuries, 354
Electrical stimulation, 519–521
    of acupuncture needles, 542–543, 545, 546
    functional, 523–526
    low-intensity, 521
    neuromuscular, 523
    as pressure ulcer treatment, 464–465
Electric outlets, ground fault intercept, 86
Electrocardiogram (EKG) stress test, 244
Electrodiagnosis, **125–132**
    of carpal tunnel syndrome, 139, 140–142
    of fibromyalgia, 372–373
    of median neuropathy of the wrist, 140, 142
        false-positive results in, 140–141
    of myofascial pain syndrome, 372–373
    of spinal muscular atrophy, 409
Electrolyte disorders, in inpatient rehabilitation unit
    patients, 432–433
Electromagnetic fields, therapeutic use of, 522

Electromyography
    needle, 125–127
        for carpal tunnel syndrome evaluation, 141
        for median neuropathy evaluation, 141
        for radiculopathy evaluation, 135–136
        single-fiber, for neuromuscular transmission
            disorder evaluation, 157
        effect of temperature on, 128
Electromyography-triggered neuromuscular electrical
    stimulation, 222–223
Electrotherapy, **523–528**
Ely's test, 281
Embolism, pulmonary, 434
    deep vein thrombosis-related, 249
    stroke-related, 170
    as sudden unexpected death cause, 441
    total hip replacement-related, 283
Emergency, definition of, 429
Emission, 77
EMLA (eutectic mixture of lidocaine analogs) cream, 501
Emphysema, differentiated from bronchitis, 237–238
Employment, of disabled persons, 91, 92. *See also*
    Vocational rehabilitation
    individualized plans for, 94
Empowerment medicine, 63–64
En bloc upper humeral interscapulothoracic resection,
    329
Encephalopathy
    HIV infection-related, 335–336
    metabolic/toxic, 103
End-of-life care, for motor neuron disease patients, 219
Endorphins, acupuncture-induced release of, 542–543
Endoscopy, spinal, 536
Endotracheal intubation
    in respiratory distress distress, 236
    use in ventilatory failure rehabilitation, 237
Endplate spikes, 126
Enemas, 469, 503
Energy expenditure
    effect of assistive devices on, 113
    by rheumatic disease patients, 342–343
    during walking, 578
Energy requirements, of rehabilitation patients, 494
ENIGMA mnemonic, for sexual history-taking, 78
En pointe dance position, 394
Entacapone, as Parkinson's disease treatment, 184
Enteral support, 495
Enthesitis, 346
Entrance ways, accessibility of, 85
Environment, components of, 81–82
Environmental adaptations, 7, **81–89**
    for the elderly, 119
    for hearing-impaired persons, 87–88
    for Parkinson's disease patients, 186–187
    for visually-impaired persons, 87
Environmental barriers, assessment of, 82
Environmental control units (ECUs), 505
Ephedrine, 499
Epicondyle suspension prosthesis, 571
Epicondylitis
    lateral (tennis elbow), 267, 269, 389, 549
    medial (golfer's elbow), 267, 550
Epidural injections, 533–534
Epidural spinal cord compression, 330–331
Equal Employment Opportunities Commission
    (EEOC), 91

Equinovarus deformity, 298, 299, 419
Equinus, in swing, 114
Equinus deformity, 303
Equinus state, 303
Erectile dysfunction, neurologic injury-related, 77
Erections, 76–77
Erogenous zones, relocation of, following central
    nervous system injury, 80
Errors, type I and type II, 17–18
Erythropoietin, as anemia of renal failure treatment, 323
Eschar, 358
Estrogen replacement therapy, 454–455
Ethane hydroxydiphosphate, as heterotopic ossification
    treatment, 458
Ethyl alcohol injections, as spasticity treatment, 537,
    540
Etidronate, as osteoporosis treatment, 452
Etiquette, with disabled people, 61
Evaluation, of patients, 5, 7
Evoked potential studies, of central nervous system
    disorders, **160–165**
Executive attention network, 42
Exercise, therapeutic, 7, **487–493**
    aerobic
        cardiovascular effects of, 492–493
        by diabetic patients, 493
        as fibromyalgia treatment, 351
        by polymyositis patients, 348
        by spinal cord injury patients, 246
    effect on aging, 441
    aquatic, 509
        by rheumatic disease patients, 342
    as atherosclerotic peripheral vascular disease
        preventive, 248
    "five P's" of, 491
    flexibility, 489–490
    gender-related differences in response to, 492
    by inflammatory arthritis patiens, 341
    isokinetic, as joint inflammation cause, 342
    isometric
        as joint inflammation cause, 342
        by polymyositis patients, 348
        by rheumatic disease patients, 342
    isotonic
        as joint inflammation cause, 342
        by rheumatic disease patients, 342
    by multiple sclerosis patients, 178
    open and closed kinetic chain, 390, 491–492
    by osteoporosis patients, 450–451
    passive, by inflammatory arthritis patients, 341
    plyometric, 489
    range-of-motion, 110–111
    by renal failure patients, 323–324
    strengthening, for motor neuron disease patients, 219
    stretching, 489–490
        Achilles tendon, 300
        by polymyositis patients, 348
    upper-extremity, differentiated from lower-extremity,
        492
Exercise prescription, in cardiac rehabilitation, 245
Exercise testing, of pulmonary disease patients, 238
Exercise tolerance, in renal disease, 323
Expanded Disability Status Scale, 178
Experiments, design of, 16
Extensor digitorum muscle, isolation of, in extensor
    indicis testing, 49

Extensor indicis muscle, testing of, 49
"Extensor lag," 295, 296
Extensor lurch, 114
Extensor tendons, rheumatoid disease-related rupture
    of, 343

FABER test, 281
Face masks, for burn patients, 360
Facet blocks, for low back pain, 367
Facet joints, 251, 533
Facet joint syndrome, 534, 544
    pain management in, 367–368, 535–536
Face validity, of functional assessment scales,
    11
Facial nerve
    evaluation of, 105
    function of, 25, 27
    lesion of, as facial weakness cause, 27
Fair Housing Act of 1988, 85
Falls
    in bathrooms, 88, 286
    by elderly persons, 115, 119, 288, 305
    by hip surgery patients, 286
    prevention of, in the home, 451–452
Family scenario mapping, 84
Fasciculation, 33
    amyotrophic lateral sclerosis-related, 213
Fasciculation potentials, 126–127
Fatigue
    dialysis-related, 322, 324
    fibromyalgia-related, 350
    HIV infection-related, 334
    multiple sclerosis-related, 178–179
    neuromuscular disease-related, 106
    renal disease-related, 322, 324
    rheumatic disease-related, 342
    systemic lupus erythematosus-related,
        350
Fazio-Londe disease, 214
Fecal impaction
    in bed-confined patients, 440
    in stroke patients, 171
Federal Communications Commission, 92
Fellatio, 80
Female athletic triad, in dancers, 394
Femoral circumflex artery, 280
Femoral head, avascular necrosis of, 288
Femoral neck
    anatomy of, 50
    fractures of, 282–283, 284, 287, 305
Femoral nerve, 280
    injuries to, 24
    neuropathy of, differentiated from L3 radiculopathy,
        149
Femur, intertrochanteric line of, 49
Fertility, in spinal cord injury patients, 76, 77–78
Fetal nigral cell transplantation, as Parkinson's disease
    treatment, 184
Fever
    drug-induced, 430
    in inpatient rehabilitation unit patients, 429–430
Fiberoptic endoscopic evaluation of swallowing
    (FEES), 484
Fiber supplements, 469
Fibrillation, neuromuscular, 33
Fibrillation potentials, 126

Fibromyalgia, 350–351, 366, **369–378**
  differentiated from myofascial pain syndrome, 371–372
  post-traumatic, 314
Fibrosis, perineural epidural, 536
Fingers
  balance mechanisms of, 49
  flexion injuries of, 276–277
  little and index, numbness of, 146
  ulnar deviation of, 275
Finger-to-chin test, 108
Finkelstein's sign/test, 274, 550
Fire extinguishers, 87
Fistula, cerebrospinal fluid, traumatic brain injury-related, 199
Fitness, endurance, 489
Flaps, myocutaneous, for pressure ulcer closure, 461
Flexor digitorum profundus muscle
  in flexor digitorum superficialis testing, 48
  integrity testing of, 273
Flexor digitorum profundus tendon, lumbrical plus deformity of, 277
Flexor digitorum superficialis tendon
  integrity testing of, 273
  testing of, in isolation, 48
Flexor pollicis longus tendon, rheumatoid arthritis-related rupture of, 275
Flexor tendons, of the fingers, rehabilitation of, 276
Floor-reaction orthosis, 574
Fludrocortisone, 499
Fluoxetine, interaction with serotonin, 35
Folic acid deficiency, chemotherapy-related, 326
Folliculitis, in amputees, 559
Foot, **300–305**
  anatomy of, 297
  diabetes-related disorders of, 553
  energy-storing, 577–578
  fractures of, 298
  gangrene of, 556
  insensate, injury prevention for, 561
  kinesiology of, 51
  pronation and supination of, 51
  rheumatoid arthritis of, 297–298, 345
  segmental weight of, 560
  tendons of, 299
  ulcers of, 298
  vascular status of, 298
Football players, prophylactic knee bracing in, 574
Foot care, 248
"Foot of the goose," 549
Forced use. *See* Constraint-induced movement therapy (CIMT)
"Forced-use paradigm," of stroke treatment, 172
Forearm, pronation and supination axis of, 48
Forefoot, equinus deformity of, 303
Fractures, **305–311**
  avulsion-type, 298
  Bennett's, 275
  boxer's, 275
  cervical, unstable, 586
  child abuse-related, 412–413
  closed, 305
  complications of, 305, 307
  distal radius, 277, 278
  of the elbow, 270–271
  of femoral neck, 282–283, 284, 287, 305

Fractures (*cont.*)
  Galeazzi's, 268
  healing of, 305–306
  of the hip, 119, 282–283, 311, 455
  injury mechanisms of, 305
  intertrochanteric, 283, 287
  joint dislocations associated with, 311
  Jones, 298
  Maissoneuve, 300
  march, 311
  Monteggia's, 267
  open, 305
  pathologic, 306–307, 311, 329–330
  scaphoid, 48, 275–276, 307
  of the shoulder, 263–264
  stress, 311
  subtrochanteric, 287
  thoracic, 587
  traumatic brain injuries associated with, 194
  vertebral compression, 120, 305, 451–452
Frankel classification, of spinal cord injuries, 206
Free weights, 490
Friction massage, 531
Froment's sign, 274
Frontal cortex, 40
Frontal lobe
  function of, 28
  ventrolateral, 42
Functional assessment, **9–14**
  functional assessment scales for, 11–13
  multidimensional, 339–340
  of rheumatoid arthritis patients, 339–340
Functional Assessment Measure scores, in traumatic brain injury, 197
Functional capacity evaluations (FCEs), 406, of low back pain, 122
Functional electrical stimulation, 523–526
  contraindications to, 524
Functional home assessment, 84–85
Functional Independence Measure (FIM), 13, 120, 197
Functional motor testing, 99
Functional musculoskeletal rehabilitation, 389
Functional neuromuscular stimulation (FNS), 521
Fungal infections, in amputees, 559
"Funny bone," 550
Furuncles, in amputees, 559
Fuzzy logic, 505
F-wave, 135
  differentiated from H-reflex, 129

Gabapentin
  as cancer pain treatment, 327
  as neuropathic pain treatment, 153–154, 502
  as spasticity treatment, 445, 502
  as traumatic brain injury treatment, 198
Gadget tolerance, 98
Gag reflex, 483
Gait
  abducted, 581
  of amputees, 578
  antalgic, 113–114
  apraxia of, 174
  of cancer patients, 325
  of cerebellar dysfunction patients, 108
  of cerebral palsy patients, 419, 422
  determinants of, 112

Gait (*cont.*)
  effect of lower-limb prostheses on, **577–584**
  of multiple sclerosis patients, 179–180
  of Parkinson's disease patients, 183, 185, 186
  of rheumatoid arthritis patients, 346
  steppage, 114
  of toddler's, 114–115
  Trendelenburg, 114
Gait analysis, 108, **111–116**
  of cerebral palsy patients, 422
  in multiple sclerosis, 179–180
Gait cycle, 111
  gluteus maximus and iliopsoas muscles in, 50
Galeazzi's sign, 418
Gallstones, in spinal cord injury patients, 432
Gamekeeper's thumb, 276
Gangrene, 247, 554, 556
Gastrectomy, 325
Gastrocnemius muscle, position during standing, 50
Gastrocolic response, 468
Gastrointestinal disorders, in inpatient rehabilitation
    unit patients, 430–432
Gastrostomy, percutaneous endoscopic (PEG), 495
Gate control theory, of pain, 379, 519, 526
Gehrig, Lou, 212–213
Gender identity, 75
Gene therapy, 63
Genetic algorithms, 505–506
Genitofemoral nerve, 24
Genu recurvatum, 114, 290
Genu valgus, 289
Genu varum, 290
Gerstmann's syndrome, 174
Gilles de la Tourette syndrome, 188
Glasgow Outcome Scale scores, in traumatic brain
    injury, 197
Glatiramer acetate, as multiple sclerosis treatment, 181
Glenohumeral joint
  in abduction, 47–48
  active-passive motion initiation in, 259
  anatomy of, 259
  mobility and instability of, 47
  range of motion of, 110
Glenoid labral injury, 388–389
Glioma, 331
Global aphasia, 103, 173
Global functional assessment, 339
Glomerular filtration rate, 321
Glossectomy, 325
Glossopharyngeal breathing, 236
Glossopharyngeal nerve, function of, 25, 28
α-Glucosidase inhibitors, 500
Gluteus maximus, in gait cycle, 50
Gluteus medius, right, testing of, 50
Godfrey test, 291
Golfer's elbow. *See* Epicondylitis, medial
Graft-versus-host disease, chronic, 319–320
Grants, administrative and financial management of, 19
Grasp of test situation, in metabolic or toxic
    encephalopathies, 103
Gravity
  center of, during ambulation, 113
  line of, in erect body position, 115
Gravity traction, 529
Groin pain, in dancers, 394
Growth factors, as pressure ulcer treatment, 465

Gullain-Barré syndrome, 436
Guyon's canal
  anatomy of, 145, 146
  as ulnar nerve entrapment site, 145, 389
Guyon's canal syndrome, 144
Gymnasts, low back pain in, 389

Haglund's deformity, 297
Hallux limitus, 301
Hallux rigidus, 297, 301, 347
Hallux valgus, 347
Haloperidol
  as Gilles de la Tourette syndrome treatment, 188
  as traumatic brain injury treatment, 228
Halo vest orthosis, 586, 587
Hammertoe, 297, 300
Hand
  as acupuncture site, 546
  anatomy of, 272–273
  dorsum of, 273
  "no man's land" of, 273
  orthoses for, 564, 565
  rehabilitation of, **276–279**
  rheumatoid arthritis-related deformities of, 275
  segmental weight of, 560
  splinting of, 564
Hand dominance, 416
Hand grasp, 562
  of infants, 416
Hand grasp system, functional electrical stimulation
    implantable, 525
Hand grips, 274
Handicap
  definition of, 5
  differentiated from impairment and disability, 11, 121
  in organ transplant recipients, 320
HANDS Tremor mnemonic, for clinical features of
    cerebellar disease, 108
Headaches
  cervicogenic, 253
  "computer," 253
  greater occipital neuralgia-related, 253
  renal disease-related, 322
  translaminar epidural injection-related, 534
  trauma-related, 313
Head injury. *See also* Brain injury
  in children, 414
  hypertension associated with, 437
  multiple, as parkinsonism cause, 183
Head tilt, determination of cause of, 27
Healing, acupuncture-induced, 543
Health, definition of, 4
Health Care Financing Administration, 13, 92
Health care workers, AIDS risk of, 334
Health insurance. *See also* Medicaid; Medicare
  for disabled persons, 92
Hearing aid dispensers, 71
Hearing aids, 68–69, 70–71, 72
  for children, 73–74
Hearing aid-wearing patients, 58–59
Hearing-impaired patients, **68–75**
  assistive technology devices for, 68–69, 70–71, 72, 506
  communication with, 58, 59
  environmental adaptations for, 87–88
  interpreters for, 59, 87
  telecommunications access by, 92

Hearing loss
  definition of, 68
  types of, 69
Hearing tests, 70
Heart disease, effect on sexual activity, 79
Heart transplantation patients, cardiac rehabilitation of, 246
Heating, of tissue
  mechanisms of, 513
  ultrasound-related, 517
Heat lamps, 513, 514, 515
Heat therapy, 513–515
  for rheumatic disease, 340
  for vertebral compression fractures, 452
Heberden's nodes, 275
Heel
  beveled, 303
  flared, 303
  painful, 297
  soft, 303
  solid ankle cushioned (SACH), 303, 577
Heel rise, 112
  uneven, 583
Heel spurs, 300
Heel-to-shin test, 108
Hellebrand technique, 490
HelpMate mobile cart, 505
Hematoma
  acupuncture-related, 544
  epidural injection-related, 534
Hematomyelia, 206–207
Hemianopsia
  bitemporal, 27
  cerebral palsy-related, 420
  left homonymous, 27
  stroke-related, 168
Hemiarthroplasty, of the hip, 283–284, 287
Hemiballismus, 191
Hemifacial spasm, 190
Hemiparesis, stroke-related, 220–223
Hemiplegia, 168–169
  cerebral palsy-related, 419
  treatment of, 171–172
Hemispatial neglect, 104, 174
Hemodialysis, 321–322
  exercise during, 323–324
Hemorrhoids, as bowel care complication, 469
Henneman size principle, of muscle strength, 487
Heparin, anticoagulant activity of, 498
Hepatitis B, transmission by acupuncture needles, 544
Herbal preparations, 496
Herbicide exposure, as Parkinson's disease risk factor, 183
Herniated discs. See Intervertebral discs, herniated
H (Hoffman)-reflex, 135
  differentiated from F-wave, 129
Hip, 283–289
  anatomy of, 280
  arthritis of, 110, 281, 284
  arthrodesis of, effects on adjacent joints, 288
  avascular necrosis of, 280, 284, 289
  blood supply to, 280
  contractures of, 280–281, 287
  dislocation of, 180, 420
  effusions of, 342
  examination of, in children, 418

Hip (cont.)
  flexion of, 110
  fractures of, 282–283, 455
    in the elderly, 119, 311
  hemiarthroplasty of, 283
  innervation of, 280
  pain in, 549
  "snapping," 281
  stability of, 49, 280
  total arthroplasty of, 283–284, 285–286, 287, 343
    avascular necrosis-related, 289
    in elderly patients, 120
Hip extensors, weakness of, 114
Hip joint capsule, anatomy of, 49
Hip-knee-ankle-foot orthoses, 575
Hip pointer, 282, 387
Hip surgery. See also Hip, total arthroplasty of
  resisted concentric exercises after, 287
Histamine receptor2 antagonists, 431
Holding reflex, 472
Home cervical traction, 529
Home environment
  assessment of, 82–83, 84–85
  environmental adaptations in, 83, 85–87, 119
    for prevention of falls, 451–452
  sources of assistance for patients in, 99
Honeymoon palsy, 145
Hook of the hamate, 145, 146
Hook prehension, 562
Horner's syndrome, 26, 146, 328, 382
Horseback-riding programs, for cerebral palsy patients, 423
Hospitalization, as depersonalization cause, 81
Hospitals, rehabilitation, diagnosis-related group (DRG)-exempt status of, 13
Hot packs, 513, 514
Housemaid's knee, 292
Human immunodeficiency virus (HIV) infection, **333–337**
  transmission by acupuncture needles, 544
Humeral head, replacement of, 262–263
Humerus, fractures of, axillary nerve involvement in, 21
Humor, as aid to sexual satisfaction, 80
Huntington's disease, 189, 192
Hyaline G-F 20, 550–551
Hydrocephalus, 30, 199, 425
Hydrocollator packs, 514
Hydromyelia, meningomyelocele-related, 425–426
Hydrotherapy, 516
Hyperalgesia, 373
Hypercalcemia, 433
  cancer-related, 326
  immobilization, 209
Hypercapnia, exercise reconditioning in, 240
Hypercholesterolemia, as stroke risk factor, 167
Hyperextension overload syndrome, 268
Hyperglycemia, diabetic, as limb amputation risk factor, 554
Hypernatremia, 433
Hyperpolarization, 366
Hypersensitivity, in amputees, 559
Hypertension
  as atherosclerotic peripheral vascular disease risk factor, 247
  as coronary artery disease risk factor, 244, 245

Hypertension (*cont.*)
　in inpatient rehabilitation unit patients, 436, 437
　pulmonary, in organ transplant patients, 318
Hypertensive emergencies, 437
Hyperthermia, central, traumatic brain injury-related, 197
Hypnotics, soporific effect of, 497
Hypogastric nerve, 465
　as penile innervation, 76–77
Hypoglossal nerve
　function of, 26
　injuries to, 28
Hypogonadism, bone loss in, 454
Hypometria, Parkinson's disease-related, 183
Hyponatremia, 432
Hypophonia, Parkinson's disease-related, 183
Hypotension
　in inpatient rehabilitation unit patients, 436–437
　orthostatic, 153, 499
　postural, 184, 436
Hypotheses, 14, 17
Hypoventilation, oxygen therapy for, 236–237
Hysteria, visual field defects associated with, 105

Ice packs, 515, 516
Ideal body weight (IBW), 494
Ideational apraxia, 174
Ideomotor apraxia, 174, 229
Iliofemoral ligament, 280
Iliohypogastric nerve, 24
Iliopsoas maximus muscle, in gait cycle, 50
Iliopsoas muscle, "snapping" of, as groin pain cause, 394
Iliotibial band, contracture of, 281
Iliotibial band friction syndrome, 291, 388
Ilizarov, Gavriil, 410
Illness
　biomedical and biopsychosocial models of, 6
　definition of, 4
Immersion, in paraffin baths, 515
Immobilization. *See also* Bed rest
　delayed, 277
　methods of, 307
　of organ transplant patients, 318
　as osteoporosis cause, 450
Immunosuppressive drugs, side effects of, 318
Impairment
　definition of, 6, 11
　differentiated from disability and handicap, 11, 121
　evaluation of, **121–124**
　in organ transplant recipients, 320
Impedance audiometry, 70
Income assistance, for disabled persons, 93–94
Incontinence
　in multiple sclerosis patients, 180
　in stroke patients, 168, 171
Independent living, by spinal cord injury patients, 206
Independent living movement, 53
Independent living trial apartments, 82
Independent medical examinations, 123
Individual Education Plan (IEP), 95
Individual Family Service Plan, 420
Individuals with Disabilities Education Act (IDEA), 94–95
Infantile spinal muscular atrophy, 213, 214

Infants
　hearing loss in, 73, 74
　muscle tone of, 415
　premature, 412, 415
　spinal muscular atrophy in, 409
　upper-limb prostheses for, 567
Infection
　acupuncture-related, 544
　spinal, 135
Inferential statistics, 17
Informatics, medical, 503
Informed consent, for research studies, 14–15
Infraspinatus muscle, 47–48
Injured workers, **403–407**
　recidivism among, 405
Injury prevention, for pediatric patients, 413–414
Inpatient rehabilitation unit patients, common medical problems of, **429–438**
　blood pressure abnormalities, 436–438
　dyspnea, 434–436
　electrolyte disorders, 432–433
　fever, 429–430
　gastrointestinal disorders, 430–432
　mental status changes, 434
Insole, multidensity, 302
Inspiratory muscle aids, 235
Instantaneous axis of rotation, of joints, 110
Institutional review boards (IRBs), 20
Insulin therapy, 500
Interdisciplinary rehabilitation teams, 6–7
Interferential current, 521
Interferon-b1, as multiple sclerosis treatment, 181
Interleukin-6, as bone loss risk factor, 454
Intermediolateral cell columns, 208
Intermittent abdominal-pressure ventilator, 235
Intermittent positive pressure ventilation, 235–236
Internal validity, of functional assessment scales, 11
International Classification of Impairments, Disabilities, and Handicaps, 5, 11
Interossei muscles, key actions of, 272
Interosseous membrane, 48
Interpreters, for hearing-impaired persons, 59, 87
Interrater validity, of functional assessment scales, 11
Interval measurement, 16
Interval scales, for functional assessment, 12
Intervertebral discs
　anatomy of, 45
　disruption of, as low back pain cause, 535
　herniated, 45–46
　　cervical,136
　　lumbosacral, 136
　　pain caused by, 330
　　sports-related, 389
　lumbar, innervation of, 533
　posterolateral protrusion of, 45–46
In-toeing, 575
Intradiscal electrothermal (IDET) annuloplasty, 535
Intrathecal pumps, 368, 422, 445, 502
Intrinsic tightness test, 278
Invalidating statements, 62–63
Ion channels, voltage-dependent, 32–33
Iontophoresis, 520–521
Iron deficiency, 431
Iron supplementation, 431

Ischemia
cardiac, cardiac stress test evaluation of, 244
coronary, in spinal cord injury patients, 210
as cryotherapy contraindication, 516
Ischemic index, 557
Ischiofemoral ligament, 280

Jejunostomy, percutaneous endoscopic (PEJ), 495
Jewett orthosis, 587
Joint movement, muscular basis of, 44
Joint replacement. *See also* Arthroplasty
in arthritic patients, 343
Joint rest, as heterotopic ossification treatment, 458
Jointritis, 501
Joints
corticosteroid injections in, 547–551
protection techniques for, 343
Joint stretching, contraindication in rheumatic disease,
342
Judgment, physician's suspension of, 5
Jumper's knee, 291

Katz Index of ADL (activities of daily living), 12
Kenny Self-Care Evaluation, 12
Ketorolac, 500
Kidney transplantation, 319, 321, 322
Kienböck's disease, 276
Kinematics, differentiated from kinetics, 113
Kinesiology, **111–116**
Kinetics, differentiated from kinematics, 113
Kitchen, environmental adaptations for, 86–87
Kleinert rehabilitation, 277
Klenzack joint, 574
Klumpke's palsy, 410
Klüver-Bucy syndrome, 79
Knee, **293–296**
anatomy of, 289
anterior pain in, 292
contractures of, 115
effusions of, 110, 290, 342
flexion of, 112
excessive, 578–579
housemaid's, 292
meniscal injuries to, 290, 387
osteoarthritis of, 115, 293, 550–551
sodium hyaluronate and hyaline treatment for,
550–551
preservation of, in transfemoral amputation,
120
range-of-motion of, 294
stability of, in extension, 50
stabilization of, in polymyositis patients, 347–348
total arthroplasty of, 119–120, 293–296
vicar's, 292
Knee-ankle-foot orthoses, 575
Knee surgery, resisted concentric exercises after,
287
Krusen, Frank, 2
Kugelberg-Welander disease, 214
Kyphosis, 252, 426

Lacertus fibrosis, as median nerve compression site,
142
Lachman's test, 289, 292
reverse, 291
Lambert-Eaton myasthenic syndrome, 157, 159

Language
of confusion, 480
disorders of, evaluation of, 482
of generalized intellectual impairment, 480
Language development, 415
delayed, 416
Laser therapy, 522
Lateral collateral ligament, injuries to, 291
Lateral femoral nerve entrapment, 144
Lateral recesses, 46
"Lateral thrust," 580
Latex hypersensitivity, meningomyelocele-related, 425
Lathyrism, 211, 212
Latissimus dorsi muscle, 48
Laughing, pathologic, 218
"Law of the intestine," 466
Laxatives, 469, 503
"Learned nonuse," 221
Leg. *See also* Lower extremity
ataxia testing of, 108
muscle weakness in, 106
segmental weight of, 560
Legg-Calvé-Perthes disease, 280, 574
Legislative issues, in physical medicine and
rehabilitation, **90–96**
Leg-length discrepancy
intertrochanteric osteotomy-related, 288
during running, 115
shoes for correction of, 575–576
Leg pain, sacroiliac joint dysfunction-related, 534–535
Leigh's disease, dystonia associated with, 189
Leisure, definition of, 508
Leisure education, 509
Lhermitte's sign, 209
Lhermitte's syndrome, 327–328
Lidocaine, topical, 501
Life years, disability-adjusted, 63
Lifting, safety limits for, 404
Ligament of Struthers, as median nerve compression
site, 142
Light-headedness, 436
Lighting
for kitchens, 86
for visually-impaired persons, 87
Limb apraxia, 229–230
Limb loss, incidence and prevalence of, 553
Limbs. *See also* Lower extremity; Upper extremity
dysvascular, prognosis for, 557
motor pathways to, 24–25
segmental weights of, 560
synergy patterns of, 169–170
Limb salvage, 328, 555–556
Lipid storage diseases, 189
Lip-reading (speech reading), 59, 72
Literature searches, 14
Little leaguer's elbow, 268, 389
Living arrangements
accessibility of, 85–86
for disabled persons, 61
for the elderly, 119
Living room, environmental adaptations in, 87
Locked-in syndrome, 168
Locks, keyless, 86
Locomotor training, 230–231
Locus coeruleus, 26
Logorrhea, 481

Long thoracic nerve, 21
  injury to, 22, 149
  palsy of, differentiated from C5–6 cervical
    radiculopathy, 148
Lordosis, 420, 426
Low back pain, **254–258**
  chronic, lumbar facet joint radiofrequency treatment
    for, 535–536
  as disability cause, 123
  discogenic, 535
  epidural steroid injection treatment for, 533, 534
  facet block therapy for, 367
  functional capacity evaluation of, 122
  in gymnasts, 389
  lumbosacral orthoses for, 587–588
  non-specific, 254
  sacroiliac joint pain-associated, 534
  vocational rehabilitation in, 401
  in workers, 403, 404
Low dye taping, 301
Lower extremity
  amputation of, 553–561
    levels of, 554–555
    postoperative dressings for, 556
  anatomy and kinesiology of, 49–50
  orthoses for, **572–576**
  peripheral nerves of
    injuries to, 24
    routes of, 23
  segmental weights of, 560
  synergy patterns of, 170
Lower-motor neuron bowel, 466–467
Low-vision aids, 66–67
Lumbar facet syndrome, 534
Lumbar sympathetic block, 382–383
Lumbar traction, 529
Lumbosacral junction, in L5 spondylolysis and
  spondylolisthesis, 47
Lumbosacral orthoses, 585, 587–588
Lumbosacral plexus
  anatomy of, 24
  injuries to, 22–23
Lumbosacral spicas, 588
Lumbosacral supports, workers' dependency on,
  405–406
Lumbrical muscles, anatomy and function of, 273
Lumbrical plus deformity, 277
"Lump syndrome," 56
Lunate bone, dislocations of, 48
Lung cancer, 154, 331
Lung transplantation, 319
Luschka's joints, 46
Lymphatic system, 247, 249
Lymphedema, 249–250
  postmastectomy, 332–333

Magnetic field stimulation, 522
Magnetic resonance imaging
  for cerebral palsy evaluation, 412
  cochlear implants as contraindication to, 59
  of fractures, 307
  for multiple sclerosis evaluation, 178
Magnification disorders, 406
Mainstreaming, of disabled children, 94–95
Maissoneuve fractures, 300
Malabsorption, HIV infection-related, 334

Malingering, 105, 406
Mallet finger, 275, 278, 345
Mallet toe, 297
Malnutrition
  cancer-related, 325
  definition of, 494
  effect on lower-limb amputation healing, 560
  as pressure ulcer risk factor, 461
  in rehabilitation patients, 494
  in stroke patients, 171
  weight loss in, 495
Manipulation, 530–531
  as heterotopic ossification treatment, 459
  as low back pain treatment, 256
Manual dexterity impairment, Parkinson's disease-
  related, 185
Manual muscle testing, **109–111**
Map, clinical care, 101
Martin-Gruber anastomosis, 129–130, 141
"Masked facies," Parkinson's disease-related, 183
Massage, therapeutic, 531–532
  contraindications to, 532
  as fibromyalgia treatment, 351
  with ice, 515, 516
  as vertebral compression fracture treatment, 452
"Massed practice," 221
Mastectomy, 332
  as lymphedema cause, 332–333
Maximum aerobic capacity (VO₂max), 243
Maximum heart rate, 243
Maximum rate of oxygen consumption (VO₂max), 491
McMurray's test, 290, 292
Measurements, types of, 16
Measurement scales, for functional assessment, 11–13
Mechanical ventilation, 235–237
Medial branch nerve block, 534
Medial collateral ligament
  injuries to, 290
  strains of, 291
Medial cord entrapment, in musicians, 392
Medial femoral circumflex artery, 49
Medial longitudinal fasciculus, 26
Median nerve
  branch nerves of
    palmar cutaneous, 48
    radiofrequency neurotomy of, 536
  injuries to, 22
Median nerve blocks, as spasticity treatment, 445
Median nerve branch nerves, radiofrequency
  neurotomy of, 536
Median nerve neuropathy, 142, 144
  electromyographic evaluation of, 141
  at the wrist, 405
    differentiated from carpal tunnel syndrome, 139,
      140–141
    electrodiagnosis of, 140–141
    nerve conduction studies of, 140–141
Median nerve palsy, 279
Median plantar nerve, 51
Medicaid, 92, 93, 400
Medical continuum, 97
Medical core teams, 399
Medical examinations, independent, 123
Medicare, 92–93, 116, 400
Medulla, 25
  as cranial nerve exit site, 26

Megestrol acetate, as pressure ulcer risk factor, 501
Meissner's plexus, 466
Melodic Intonation Therapy (MIT), 173–174, 483
Memories, procedural, 41
Meninges, of spinal cord, 24
Meningocele, 424
Meningomyelocele, 424, 425
Meniscus, injuries to, 290, 387
Menopause
    hormone replacement therapy during, 450, 454–455
    peak bone mass decline during, 447
Menstruation, following central nervous system trauma, 76
Mental functioning, assessment of, 10
Mental retardation, cerebral palsy-related, 419
Mental status changes
    in inpatient rehabilitation unit patients, 434
    as pressure ulcer risk factor, 461
Mental status testing, bedside, 102
Meperidine, side effects of, 499
Meralgia paresthetica, 24, 144, 148
Meta-analysis, 19
Metabolic bone disease, **447–456**
Metastases
    to bone, 306, 327, 329–330
    as brachial plexopathy cause, 154
    spinal, 330–331
Metatarsal pad, 301
Methadone, as cancer pain treatment, 327
Methotrexate, long-term use of, adverse effects of, 338
Methylphenidate, 226, 227
    interaction with norepinephrine, 35
Metronidazole, 431
Mexiletine, as neuropathic pain treatment, 154
Micrographia, Parkinson's disease-related, 183
Microstomia, 360
Microwave diathermy, 517, 519
Micturition, physiology of, 472
Midbrain, 25
    acupuncture-related stimulation of, 543
    as cranial nerve exit site, 26
Midodrine, 499
Milwaukee bracing, 587
Minimus medius muscle, testing of, 50
Minspeak system, 506
Mirtazapine, 497
Mixed nerve study, 128
Mobility. *See also* Ambulation
    forms of, 10
Mobility assistance, for visually-impaired patients, 57, 67
Möbius syndrome, 27
Mononeuritis multiplex, 152
Mononeuropathies, cranial, diabetes-related, 151
Mononeuropathy multiplex, 152
Moro reflex, 417
Morphine
    as cancer pain treatment, 327
    intrathecal administration of, 368
Morton's neuroma, 149–150
Motor cortex, 40
Motorcycle helmet use, effect on traumatic brain injury risk, 194
Motor evoked potentials, transcranial, 164
Motor facilitation approach, in physical therapy with stroke patients, 171–172

Motor function
    developmental milestones of, 415
    evaluation of, 105–107
Motor learning, 41
Motor nerve conduction velocities, in children, 409
Motor neuron disease, **211–219**
    classification of, 211–212
    upper distinguished from lower, 25
Motor pathways, to the extremities, 24–25
Motor point blocks, as spasticity treatment, in cerebral palsy patients, 421
Motor relearning program, 172
Motor system, 40–41
Motor unit action potentials (MUAPs), 127
Motor unit recruitment, size principle of, 127
Mouthpiece intermittent positive pressure ventilation, 235
Movement disorders, **182–193**
    HIV infection-related, 335
    hyperkinetic, 182, 187–192
    hypokinetic (Parkinson's disease), 182, 183–187, 189, 191
    psychogenic, 192–193
    traumatic brain injury-related, 199
Movies, use in community reintegration programs, 511
Mucolytic agents, 502
Mucositis, cancer-related, 327
Mucous plugs, as dyspnea cause, 435
Multidisciplinary practice, of patient care, 6
Multiple sclerosis, **177–181**
    brainstem auditory evoked potential/auditory brainstem response diagnosis of, 162
    clinical outcome measures for, 178
    new pharmacologic therapies for, 181
    pseudoexacerbation of, 177
Multiple Sclerosis Functional Composite, 178
Multisystem atrophy, 183
Multitrauma patients, fracture rehabilitation in, 307
Muscle
    agonistic, 44
    anatomy of, 36
    antagonistic, 44
    atrophy of, 214, 338, 440
    shapes of, 488
    spinal, 47
    synergistic, 44
Muscle co-contraction, 35–36
Muscle contraction, 35–38, 488
    concentric, 44, 489
    eccentric, 45, 489
    isokinetic, 489
    isometric, 45
    isotonic, 44, 488–489
    as joint movement cause, 44
    shortening, 44
    sliding filament theory of, 37
    types of, 488–489
Muscle fibers, types of, 487
    exercise-induced change of, 491
Muscle spasm, 370
Muscle strength, 440
    effect of aging on, 492
    determinants of, 488
    electrical stimulation-induced increase of, 521
    grading of, 45
    Henneman size principle of, 487

Muscle strength (*cont.*)
  relationship with muscle hypertrophy, 488
  relationship with osteoporosis, 450
  in women, 492
Muscle tone
  effect of cerebral descending tracts on, 39
  of infants, 415
Muscle weakness, 106
  amyotrophic lateral sclerosis-related, 213
  focal, 110
  poliomyelitis-related, 212
  post-polio syndrome-related, 214, 215
Muscular dystrophy
  progressive, 213
  spinal curvature in, 410
Musculocutaneous blocks, as spasticity treatment, 445
Musculocutaneous nerve
  entrapment of, in athletes, 387
  injuries to, 22
Musculoskeletal examination, 386
Musculoskeletal injuries and disorders, **312–315**
  acupuncture treatment for, 546
Musculoskeletal system, anatomy and kinesiology of,
    44–51
Musicians
  nerve entrapments in, 392
  physical examination of, 391–392
Myasthenia gravis, 156–157, 159
Myasthenic syndrome, 156
Myelodysplasia, 424
Myeloma, 329
Myelomeningocele, 412
Myelopathy
  delayed, 328
  transient, 327–328
  vacuolar, HIV infection-related, 336
Myocardial infarction, effect on sexual activity, 79
Myoclonus, 192
  psychogenic, 192
Myodesis, 556
Myoelectric-type prostheses, 571
Myofascial pain, 314, 366, **369–378**
  acupuncture treatment for, 544
  differentiated from fibromyalgia, 371–372
  relationship with joint dysfunction, 313
  relationship with spinal segmentation sensitization,
    375
Myofascial release, 532
Myokymic discharges, 127
Myometric evaluation, of upper-limb amputees, 572
Myopathies, 106
  HIV infection-related, 335
Myoplasty, 556
Myosin, 37
Myositis ossification, 267
Myotonia, cold-induced, 128

Narcotics, for pain control, in burn patients, 356
National Institute of Occupational Safety and Health
    (NIOSH), 404
Naturalistic studies, 16
Nausea, Parkinson's disease therapy-related, 184
Neck dissection, radical, 325, 331
Neck pain, **251–253**
Necrosis, avascular, 276, 280, 284, 288–289
"Needle shock," acupuncture-related, 544

Needling, 375
Neglect
  hemispatial, 104, 174
  unilateral, 104, 231–232
Neologism, 481
Neonatal reflexes, 411
Nephrolithiasis, in spinal cord injury patients, 432
Nerve blocks, 366, 534
  as muscle spasticity treatment, 421, **537–541**
Nerve conduction studies, 125, 128
  of carpal tunnel syndrome, 140–141
  of radiculopathies, 135
Nerve injuries. *See also specific nerves*
  classification of, 130, 144
Nerve roots, nerve fibers of, 21
Nervi erigentes, 76–77, 465
Nervous system, anatomy of, **20–30**
Neuralgia, greater occipital, as headache cause, 253
Neural network, 33–34
Neural tube defects, **424–427**
Neurapraxia, 144
Neuritis
  Morton's, 301, 302
  optic, multiple sclerosis-related, 181
Neuroablative procedures, for cancer pain management,
    327
Neuroarthropathy, 299
Neurodevelopmental therapy
  for cerebral palsy, 422
  for hemiplegia, 171
Neuroendocrine disorders, traumatic brain injury-
    related, 197
Neurolemma, 32
Neuroleptics
  as chemical restraint, 502–503
  as Gilles de la Tourette syndrome treatment, 188
  as tardive dyskinesia cause, 190–191
Neurologic disorders
  HIV infection-related, 335
  neonatal, 411
Neurologic evaluation, of the rehabilitation patient,
    102–109
Neuroma
  acoustic, 162
  in amputees, 559
  Morton's, 149–150
Neuroma pad, 301
Neuromuscular disease
  electrophysiology of, **156–160**
  fatigability associated with, 106
  respiratory monitoring in, 234–235
Neuromuscular junction, definition of, 156
Neuromuscular stimulation, functional, 521
Neuromuscular transmission, "safety factor" in, 157
Neuromyokymic discharges, 127
Neuronopathy, subacute sensory, 152
Neurons
  elements and function of, 31, 32
  polymodal wide dynamic range, 366
  regeneration of, in central nervous system, 223–224
Neuropathies
  in burn patients, 356
  diabetic, truncal, 151
  entrapment, **144–150**
    mixed, sensory conduction studies of, 145
    in musicians, 392

Neuropathies (*cont.*)
  entrapment (*cont.*)
    sports-related, 386–387
  focal, traumatic brain injury-related, 199
  HIV infection-related, 336
  peripheral, 106, **150–155**
Neurophysiology, **30–44**
Neuroplasticity, 221
Neuropraxia, 130
Neurorehabilitation, frontiers and fundamentals of, **220–232**
Neurostimulatory procedures, for cancer pain management, 327
Neurotmesis, 130, 144
Neurotomy
  lumbar facet joint radiofrequency, 535–536
  lumbar medial branch, 368
  percutaneous radiofrequency, 368
Neurotransmitters, 32
  extrathalamic systems of, 34–35
  of neuromuscular junction, 156
Nifedipine, side effects of, 499
NIOSH (National Institute of Occupational Safety and Health), 404
Nitrate-containing medication, interaction with Viagra, 501
Nodules, rheumatoid, 345
Nominal scales, for functional assessment, 12
Non-nucleoside analogue reverse transcriptase inhibitors, 334
Nonsteroidal anti-inflammatory drugs
  action mechanisms of, 338
  as cancer pain treatment, 327
  as low back pain treatment, 256
  new, 500
  as vertebral compression fracture treatment, 452
"No pain, no gain," 360, 390
Norepinephrine, 35
Norepinephrine reuptake inhibitors, 497
Nortriptyline, interaction with norepinephrine, 35
Nuclear stress testing, 244
Nucleoside analogue reverse transcriptase inhibitors, 334
Nucleus ambiguus, 27
Nucleus pulposus, 45
Nucleus solitarius, 27
Null hypothesis, 17
Nutrition, **494–496**
  of cancer patients, 325–326
  of cardiac rehabilitation patients, 245
  of cerebral palsy patients, 423
  of the elderly, 119
Nutritional assessment, bedside, 494
Nutritional support, 495

Ober test, 281
Obesity
  meningomyelocele-related, 425
  as peripheral vascular disease risk factor, 247
  as stroke risk factor, 167
  total knee arthroplasty in, 296
Obturator artery, 280
Obturator nerve, 280
  injuries to, 24
Obturator nerve blocks, as spasticity treatment, 445
Occipital lobe, lesions of, 28

Occupational Safety and Health Administration (OSHA), 404
Occupational therapy
  for Parkinson's disease patients, 186–187
  for total hip arthroplasty patients, 286
  for total knee arthroplasty patients, 295
Oculomotor nerve
  diabetic palsy of, 161
  function of, 25
O'Donoghue's triad, 290
Okay sign, absence of, 274
Olecranon impingement syndrome, 268
Olfactory nerve, function of, 25
Olfactory system, 34
Olivoponto-cerebellar degeneration, 183
Operant conditioning therapy, for pain, 364–365
Ophthalmic artery, 29
Ophthalmoplegia, diabetic, 151
Opioids, as pain treatment, 367
Optical character recognition, 506
Optic nerve, function of, 25
Optic nerve fibers, of vision pathway, 26
Ordinal measurement, 15
Ordinal scales, for functional assessment, 12
Organ transplant patients, rehabilitation of, **317–320**
Orgasm
  in men, 77
  in spinal cord injury patients, 80
  in women, 76
Orientation, in metabolic or toxic encephalopathies, 103
Orthographic symbols, 506
Orthopedic deficits, meningomyelocele-related, 426
Orthopedic surgery, as spasticity treatment, 422, 446
Orthoses. *See also* Orthotics
  ankle-foot, 113, 422–423, 572–573, 574
  definition of, 562
  lower-limb, **572–576**
  reciprocating gait, 525
  spinal, **584–588**
  thoracolumbar, 451
  transparent face, 360
  upper-limb, **562–566**
Orthostatic reflex, 440
Orthotics
  for meningomyelocele patients, 426–427
  for rheumatic disease patients, 343
Osgood-Schlatter disease, 291
OSHA (Occupational Safety and Health Administration), 404
Ossification, heterotopic, 283, 286, **456–460**
  in burn patients, 355–356
  definition of, 456
  spinal cord injury-related, 198
  synonyms of, 457
  traumatic brain injury-related, 198
Osteitis fibrosa, 322
Osteoarthritis, 337, 347
  of the hip, 281, 284
  of the knee, 293, 550–551
  treatment for, 119–120, 550–551
Osteoblasts
  origins of, 453
  stimulants of, 453, 454
Osteochondritis dissecans, 268–269, 291

Osteoclasts
inhibitors of, 452
origins of, 453
stimulants of, 454
Osteodystrophy, renal, 322
Osteomalacia, 322, 447
Osteomyelitis, pressure ulcer-related, 464
Osteonecrosis. *See* Necrosis, avascular
Osteopenia, definition of, 447
Osteoporosis, 447–456
bed rest (immobilization)-related, 440
classification of, 448–449
"codfish vertebrae" deformity associated with, 453
definition of, 447
diagnosis of, 449–450
as fracture risk factor, 305
prevention of, 287, 440
in spinal cord injury patients, 456
treatment for, 450–456
Osteotomy
intertrochanteric, effect on leg length, 288
in osteoarthritis, 293
Otoacoustic auditory emission peaks, 163
Otoacoustic auditory emission testing, 73
Outcome, functional, 9
Outcome analysis, functional assessment in, **9–14**
Outpatient rehabilitation
of burn patients, 360
of multiple sclerosis patients, 178
Overload principle, 490
Overuse, in performing artists, 392–393
Oxford technique, 490
Oximetry, in noninvasive intermittent positive-pressure
ventilation, 235–236
Oxycodone, as cancer pain treatment, 327
Oxygenation impairment, respiratory disease-related,
233, 237–240
Oxygen consumption rate (VO_2), 491
Oxygen therapy
for chronic obstructive pulmonary disease, 239–240
for hypoventilation, 236–237
Oxyhemoglobin saturation (SaO_2), 235, 236

Paget's disease, 286, 447
Pain
acromioclavicular, 261
anterior knee, 292
arterial occlusion-related, 554
cancer-related, 327
cervical, **251–253**
chronic, 363–367
complex regional pain syndrome-related, 380
definition of, 363
differentiated from suffering, 5
epidural tumor-related, 330
gate theory of, 379, 519, 526
in hip, 549
surgery-related, 284, 288
as Trendelenburg gait cause, 114
HIV infection-related, 336
motor neuron disease-related, 217
multiple sclerosis-related, 180–181
musculoskeletal, 314, 518
neuropathic
acupuncture treatment for, 544
differentiated from nociceptive pain, 153

Pain (*cont.*)
neuropathic (*cont.*)
treatment for, 153–154
nociceptive, differentiated from neuropathic pain,
153
patellofemoral, 290, 388
post-stroke, 173
radicular, 252
rheumatoid disease-related, 343
scoliosis-related, 410
in shoulder, 258–260, 261
sympathetically-maintained, 379–380
thromboembolism-related, 248
Pain assessment, 407
in children, 357
Pain management, **363–369**
with acupuncture, 542, 543, 544, 545, 546
in elderly patients, 121
with transcutaneous electrical stimulation, 526–527
Pain sensation, 107
Palilalia, 481
Pallor, 248, 554
Pancoast's syndrome, 327
Pancreatitis, in spinal cord injury patients, 432
Panner disease, 268
Papaverine, as erectile dysfunction treatment, 77
"Paper bag test," 496
Parachute response, 418
Paraffin baths, 514, 515
Paralysis
arterial occlusion-related, 554
poliomyelitis-related, 212
thromboembolism-related, 248
women's sexual adjustment to, 79–80
Paraneoplastic syndromes, 152–153, 326
Paraphrasias, 481
Paraplegia
respiratory dysfunction in, pharmacologic
management of, 502
rotator cuff tears associated with, 210
Paraspinous block, 375
Parastep System, 525
Parasympathetic nerves, 20–21
Parasympathetic nervous system, functions of, 34
Parathyroid hormone, as osteoporosis treatment,
453
Paravertebral lumbar spinal nerve blocks, as spasticity
treatment, 445
Paresthesia
arterial occlusion-related, 554
thromboembolism-related, 248
Parietal cortex, 40
Parietal lobe, function of, 28
Parietal region, lateral, 42
Parking spaces, accessibility of, 85
Parkinsonism
drug-induced, 183
psychogenic, 192, 193
Parkinsonism pugilistica, 183
Parkinson's disease, 182, 183–187
dystonia associated with, 189
on-off syndrome of, 185
pharmacologic treatment for, 183–184
side effects of, 191
physical therapy for, 185–186
surgical treatment for, 184

Participation
    dimensions of, 512
    relationship to handicap, 5
Passive modalities, use in sports medicine, 389
PASSOR (Physiatric Association for Spine, Sports, and
        Occupational Rehabilitation), 385
PASS (Plan for Achieving Self-Support), 401
Past-pointing, 41
Patella, subluxed, 289
Patella alta, 290
Patellofemoral angle (Q angle), 289–290
Patellofemoral pain syndrome, 290, 388
Patient-controlled analgesia, for burn patients, 356
Patient Evaluation and Conference System (PECS), 13
Patient history-taking, 98–99
Patients
    definition of, 4
    disabled persons as, 53–54
Payment, by patients, 5
PE. See Embolism, pulmonary
Peabody Developmental Test of Motor Proficiency, 417
Peak bone mass, 447
Pectoralis major muscle, 48
Pectoralis minor syndrome, 147
Pectoralis muscles, involvement in torso injuries, 313
Pediatric rehabilitation. See Children
PEDS-Pediatric Evaluation of Development, 417
PEG (percutaneous endoscopic gastrostomy), 495
PEJ (percutaneous endoscopic jejunostomy), 495
Pelvic floor, innervation of, 465–466
Pelvic-girdle dysfunction, 313
Pelvic rotation, 112
Pelvic tilt, 112
Pelvis, lateral displacement of, 113
Pemoline, 226
Pendulum exercises, 259
Penile implants, 77
Penis, innervation of, 76–77
Percutaneous endoscopic gastrostomy (PEG), 495
Percutaneous endoscopic jejunostomy (PEJ), 495
Performing artists, rehabilitation of, 391–395
Perianal area, in spinal cord injury, 204
Perianal sensation, 472
Perineum, innervation of, 24
Peripheral nerves, 20
    anatomy of, 21–24
    of lower extremity, 23–24
Peripheral nervous system
    anatomy of, 20
    components of, 34
    functions of, 34
Peripheral neuropathy, 150–155
    cancer-related, 327
    differentiated from central nervous system lesions,
        21
    traumatic brain injury-related, 199
    upper-extremity, 22
Peripheral vascular disease, 247–250
    as limb loss risk factor, 553
    as pressure ulcer risk factor, 461
Peristalsis, intestinal, 465–466
Peritoneal dialysis, 321–322
Peroneal nerve
    common, injuries to, 24
    entrapment of, 144
    palsy of, 149, 296

Person, concept of, 4
Personhood
    concept of, 4
    relationship with physical environment, 81
Pes anserinus, 549
Pes anserinus syndrome, 292
Pes cavus, 297
Pes planus, 297, 298
Pesticide exposure, as Parkinson's disease risk factor,
        183
Petrissage, 531
Phalen wrist flexion test, 139
    reverse, 140
Phantom limb pain, 557–558
Phantom sensation, 557
Phenobarbital, as traumatic brain injury treatment, 198
Phenol injections, as spasticity treatment, 421, 445,
        537, 538, 539–540
Phenol motor point blocks, 538
Phenytoin
    as cancer pain treatment, 327
    as traumatic brain injury treatment, 198
Philadelphia collars, 586
Phonophoresis, 517–518
Phrenic nerve, electrical pacemaker for, 526
Physiatric Association for Spine, Sports, and
        Occupational Rehabilitation (PASSOR), 385
Physiatrists
    certification of, 2
    role of, 3
    training of, 2–3
Physiatry, 1–4
    definition of, 1
    history of, 2
    interventional, 533
    mission and motto of, 1
Physiatry procedures, invasiveness of, 546
Physical agents, 513–522
    alternative and new agents, 522
    definition of, 513
    electricity, 513, 519–521
    heat and cold, 513–516
    pressure, 521–522
    shortwaves and microwaves, 513, 518–519
    ultrasound, 513, 517–518
    water, 516
Physical assistance, to disabled patients, 55
Physical environment, of handicapped persons, 5
Physical examination
    of dancers, 392
    of musicians, 391–392
    preparticipation in sports, 385–386
    of visually-impaired patients, 57–58
    of wheelchair users, 55–56
Physical medicine, definition of, 1
Physical therapy
    for cerebral palsy patients, 422
    for heterotopic ossification patients, 458
    for osteoporosis patients, 450–451
    for stroke patients, 171–172
Physician-patient relationship
    communication in, 53
    countertransference and transference in, 54
    patient's and physician's responsibilities in, 5
Pia, 24
Pilates, Joseph, 394

Pillows, abduction, 286
Pimozide, as Gilles de la Tourette syndrome treatment, 188
Pirouette turn, 395
Pisiform bone, 145, 146
Plantar fasciitis, 300, 301
Plastic body jacket, as vertebral compression fracture treatment, 451
Play audiometry, 73
Play therapy, 510
Plexopathies
   differentiated from carpal tunnel syndrome, 142
   traumatic brain injury-related, 199
Plica, 291
PLISSIT model, of sex therapy, 78
Pneumatic pumps, 521, 522
Pneumonia
   in inpatient rehabilitation unit patients, 435–436
   Pneumocystis carinii, 334
   in spinal cord injury patients, 435
   in stroke patients, 171
Pneumothorax, acupuncture-related, 544
Poliomyelitis, 212
   post-polio syndrome of, 214–215
Political environment, of handicapped persons, 5
Polymyositis, 348–349
Polyneuropathy
   chronic inflammatory demyelinating, 152–153
   differentiated from carpal tunnel syndrome, 142
   diffuse, 155
   HIV infection-related, 336
   traumatic brain injury-related, 199
Polypharmacy, 118–119, 496
Pons, 25
   as cranial nerve exit point, 26
Pontomedullary junction, as cranial nerve exit point, 27
Positioning, therapeutic, of burn patients, 358–359
Positive end-expiratory pressure (PEEP), 237
Positive sharp waves, 126
Posterior cord syndrome, 206
Posterior cruciate ligament, injuries to, 291
Posterior interosseous nerve syndrome, 268
Posterior tibial tendon insufficiency, 301
Post-polio syndrome, 214–215
Post-stroke pain syndrome, 173
Posture
   as neck pain cause, 252
   of Parkinson's disease patients, 183, 185, 186
Posture-training supports, as vertebral compression fracture treatment, 451
Postvoid residual, 473
Potassium channels, voltage-dependent, 32–33
PQRST mnemonic, for clinical evaluations, 252
Preganglionic lesions, 131
Pregnancy
   in meralgia paresthetica patients, 283
   in multiple sclerosis patients, 181
   in spinal cord injury patients, 76
Preinjection blocks, 375–376
Premotor systems, medial and lateral, 43
Preparticipation history and examination, 385–386
Prescriptions, physiatric, 101
Pressure, therapeutic use of, 521–522
Pressure garments, 521–522
   for burn patients, 358
Pressure support ventilation, 237

Preventive medicine, 97, 98
PRICE mnemonic, for meniscal injury treatment, 290
Primidone, as essential tremor treatment, 188
Primitive reflexes, 419
Probability, 18
Product waveforms, 521
Progressive bulbar paralysis, 213
   of childhood, 214
Progressive muscular dystrophy, 213
Progressive supranuclear palsy, 183
Prolotherapy, 551
Promoting Aphasics' Communicative Competence (PACE), 483
Pronation, biomechanical effect of, 303
Pronator syndrome, 268
Pronator teres, as median nerve compression site, 142
Propranolol, as essential tremor treatment, 187–188
Proprioception, 107
Proprioception-stereognosis pathway, 25
Proprioceptive neuromuscular facilitation, 172
Propulsion, Parkinson's disease-related, 185
Prospective payment system, for rehabilitation, 13, 92–93
Prostaglandin E_1, as erectile dysfunction treatment, 77
Prostheses
   immediate postoperative fitting, 556
   lower-limb
      for elderly patients, 120
      as gait deviation cause, **577–584**
   upper-limb, **567–572**
Prosthesis-assisted ambulation, energy expenditure during, 559–560
Protease inhibitors, 334
Protein, dietary intake, for pressure ulcer prevention, 501
Provocative lumbar discography, 535
Pruritus, in burn patients, 357
Pseudobulbar affect, 218
Pseudobulbar palsy, 168
Pseudoeschar, 358
Pseudoexacerbation, of multiple sclerosis, 177
Pseudofacilitation, 159
Pseudomembranous colitis, 431
Psychoactive medications, neurotransmitter-based, 35
Psychological environment, of handicapped persons, 5
Psychotherapy, for Gilles de la Tourette syndrome patients, 188
Public accommodations, accessibility of, 91–92
Public Law 100–407, 504
Public transportation, accessibility of, 91
Pudendal nerve, 24, 466, 471
Pulleys, effect on range of motion, 490
Pulmonary rehabilitation, **233–241**
   in oxygenation impairment, 233, 237–240
   in ventilatory impairment, 233, 234–237
Pulse, tibial, 435
Pulselessness
   arterial occlusion-related, 554
   thromboembolism-related, 248
PULSES Profile, 11, 12
"Pump bumps," 549
p-value, 18
Pyramidal tract, 204

Q (quadriceps) angle, 289–290
Quadrantanopsia, superior, 27

Quadratus femoris, innervation of, 280
Quadriceps muscle
  malalignment of, 289
  polymyositis-related weakness of, 347–348
Quadriplegia
  C6 complete, independent living in, 206
  cerebral palsy-related, 419
  complete traumatic, 206–207
  differentiated from tetraplegia, 205
  hand grasp restoration in, 525
  respiratory dysfunction in, pharmacologic
    management of, 502
Quality of daily living, assessment of, 10
Quasi-experiments, 16

Radial nerve, 49
  injuries to, 22
Radial nerve palsy, 147, 148, 279
Radiation burns, 353
Radiation therapy
  for heterotopic ossification, 458–459
  side effects of, 154, 325, 327–328
Radicular artery, lumbar, 205
Radicular pain, epidural steroid injection treatment for,
    533
Radiculopathies, **132–137**
  cervical, 133, 134
    differentiated diagnosis of, 142, 147–148
    C8–T1, differentiated from ulnar neuropathy at the
      elbow, 131
  diabetic truncal, 151
  lumbar L3, differentiated from femoral neuropathy,
    149
  lumbar L5, differentiated from peroneal nerve palsy,
    149
  lumbosacral, 133–134
    differentiated from meralgia paresthetica, 148
  nondiscogenic, 132
  steroid therapy for, 367
  traumatic brain injury-related, 199
Radiofrequency neuroablation, 368
Radionuclide renal perfusion imaging, 475
Radius bone
  distal fractures of, 277, 278
  load transfer across, 48
Raloxifen, 453
Ramps, 85
Rancho Los Amigos Scale scores, in traumatic brain
    injury, 197
Randomized control trials, 17
Range of motion
  active, 110
  active-assisted, 111
  effect of cam varied resistance on, 490
  effect of free weights on, 490
  of knee, 294
  passive, 110
  effect of pulleys on, 490
  self, 111
Range-of-motion exercises, 110–111
Range-of-motion testing, 99
Ratio measurements, 16
Ratio scales, for functional assessment, 12
Raynaud's syndrome, as cryotherapy contraindication,
    516
Reciprocating gait orthosis, 575

Recombinant human DNA-ase, 502
Reconditioning exercises, for pulmonary disease
    patients, 240
Recreation therapists, 508, 509, 510
Recreation therapy, 508–509
  for cerebral palsy patients, 423
Rectal examination, for urologic management, 472–473
Rectoanal inhibitory reflex, 467
Rectus femoris muscle, tightness assessment of, 281
Red nucleus, 26, 39
Re-entrant loop, cerebellar, 40
Reference pain zones, 370
Reflexes, grading system for, 106–107
Reflex sympathetic dystrophy, 278, 379, 381, 382
Refractory period, 33
Regression, statistical, 19
Rehabilitation
  cost-effectiveness of, 9
  definition of, 1, 6
  goal of, 9
  patient-centered, 6
  person-centered, **4–9**
  as phase of medical continuum, 97–98
  phases of, 7
  prospective payment reimbursement for, 13, 92–93
Rehabilitation Act of 1973, 85, 90, 91, 94
"Rehabilitation beyond the resolution of symptoms,"
    390
Reintegration to Normal Living Index (RNLI), 512
Reiter's syndrome, 335, 346
Relaxation exercises, as Gilles de la Tourette syndrome
    treatment, 188
Reliability, of functional assessment scales, 11
Renal disease, end-stage, **321–324**
Renal failure
  chronic, **321–324**
  meningomyelocele-related, 425
Renal transplantation, 319, 321, 322
Repetitive nerve stimulation, 157, 158–159, 160
Repetitive trauma syndromes, in workers, 403–405
Reporting, as physician's responsibility, 5
Research, basic differentiated from applied, 15
Research concepts, in physical medicine and
    rehabilitation medicine, 14–20
Reserpine, as tardive dyskinesia treatment, 191
Residency training programs, in physiatry, 2, 3
Respiratory assistance, with functional electrical
    stimulation, 526
Respiratory difficulty, motor neuron disease-related,
    219
Respiratory diseases, categories of, 233
Respiratory dysfunction
  as endotracheal intubation or tracheostomy
    indication, 236
  paraplegia/tetraplegia-related, 502
Respiratory muscle aids, 235
Respiratory muscles, exercise training of, 240
Resting membrane potential, 32
Rest pain, 247
Reticulospinal tract, 25, 38, 39
Retinopathy, diabetic, 65
Retropulsion, Parkinson's disease-related, 185
Retrospective sociobehavioral mapping, 82
Return to work
  effect on disability benefits, 400
  by injured workers, 400, 405

Return to work (*cont.*)
  by low back pain patients, 122
  by traumatic brain injury patients, 202
Rheumatic diseases, **337–351**
  diagnosis of, 337–338
  functional assessment of, 339–340
  treatment of, 338
Rheumatoid arthritis, 343–346
  flexor pollicis longus tendon ruptures associated
    with, 275
  of foot and ankle, 297–298
  functional assessment of, 339–340
  hand deformities associated with, 275
  juvenile, 351
Rheumatoid factor, 344
Rheumatoid nodules, 345
Rhizotomy, dorsal, as cerebral palsy-related spasticity
    treatment, 421, 422, 446
Rib, involvement in torso injuries, 313
RICE (rest, ice, compression, elevation) treatment, 515
Rigidity
  decerebrate, 39
  definition of, 105
  lead pipe, 105
  Parkinson's disease-related, 183
Risperidone, as tardive dyskinesia-related psychosis
    treatment, 191
Roberts, Ed, 63
Robots, 505
Role changes, of disabled patients, 84
Romberg sign, positive, 107–108
Rood method, of motor facilitation, 172
Rotationplasty, tibial, 328–329
Rotator cuff
  anatomy of, 258
  muscles of, 47–48
  tears/injuries to, 259, 388
    differentiated from tendinitis, 258
    in paraplegic patients, 210
  tendinitis of, 262
Rotator cuff repair, rehabilitation after, 262
Rubrospinal tract, 25, 38
  effect on muscle tone, 39
Running
  differentiated from walking, 112
  by infants, 114
  injuries associated with, 387

Sacral evoked potential, 474
Sacroiliac joint
  dysfunction of, 534–535, 550
  in low back pain, 368
  pain in, 534–535
Sacroiliitis, 346
Salivatory nucleus, 27
Salt tablets, as orthostatic hypotension treatment, 499
Sample size, 18
Sand-pivot-sit transfers, 10
Sarcoma, osteogenic, of the hip, in children, 282
Saturday night palsy, 145
Scalene, involvement in torso injuries, 313
Scalenus anticus syndrome, 146
Scalp, as acupuncture site, 546
Scaphoid bone, fractures of, 48, 275–276, 307
Scapula, winging of, 48, 149
Scapulohumeral rhythm, 260

Scarring
  gliotic, 223
  hypertrophic, prevention of, with silicone inserts,
    360
SCFE (slipped capital femoral epiphysis), 282, 284
Sciatic nerve
  entrapment of, 148–149
  injuries to, 24
SCIWORA (spinal cord injury without radiologic
    abnormality), 203, 412
Scoliosis, 218–219
  cerebral palsy-related, 420
  idiopathic, 410
  meningomyelocele-related, 426
Seizures
  cerebral palsy-related, 420
  traumatic brain injury-related, 199, 503
Selective estrogen receptor modulators, 453
Selective serotonin reuptake inhibitors, 497
Selegiline, as Parkinson's disease treatment, 184
Self-care devices, for visually-impaired patients, 67
Self-care skills, 10
Sensitization
  peripheral, 373
  spinal segmental, 373–375, 377
Sensory conduction studies, of mixed nerve
    entrapment, 145
Sensory deficits, stroke-related, 168
Sensory examination, 107–108
Sensory modalities, primary and secondary, 107
Sensory nerve action potentials, effect of temperature
    on, 128
Sensory nerve conduction studies, 125
Sensory Stimulation Assessment Scale, 197
Sensory systems, of central nervous system, 34
Sepsis, brain injury-associated, 430
Sepsis syndrome, 430
Serotonin, 35
Serratus anterior muscle, 48
Sertraline, interaction with serotonin, 35
Service animals, for disabled patients, 61
SEWHO (shoulder-elbow-wrist-hand orthosis), 564
Sex therapists, consultations with, 79
Sex therapy, PLISSIT model of, 78
Sexual history-taking, 78
Sexuality, **75–80**
  of cancer patients, 326
  definition of, 75
  of hip replacement patients, 287
  of total knee arthroplasty patients, 295
Sexual literacy, 75
Sexual orientation, 75
Sexual response
  in men, 77, 78
  physiologic stages of, 76
  in women, 76
SGA (Substantial Gainful Activity), 401
Shelving, accessible, 86–87
Shin splints, 387
Shober test, 110
"Shock response," 62
Shock wave therapy, 522
Shoes
  high-heeled, as knee osteoarthritis risk factor, 115
  impact on orthotics, 576
  effect on knee, foot, and ankle motions, 576

Shoes (*cont.*)
  for leg-length discrepancy correction, 575–576
  for lower-limb prostheses wearers, 583
  pointe, 394
  for rheumatoid arthritis patients, 345
Shortwave diathermy, 517, 518–519
Shoulder
  abduction in, range of motion of, 110
  anatomy of, 258
  arthritis of, 262–263
  "crutch-walking" muscles of, 48
  dislocation of, 21, 260–261
  fractures of, 263–264
  "frozen," 259, 263
  impingement syndrome of, 260
  instability of, 264–265
  involvement in torso injuries, 313
  pain in, 258–260, 261
  stiff, 261–262
  stroke-related disorders of, 172–173
  subluxation of, 260
  total replacement of, 262–263
Shoulder-elbow-wrist-hand orthosis (SEWHO), 564
Shoulder joint. *See* Glenohumeral joint
Shoulder prosthesis, 572
Shoulder surgery, rehabilitation after, 261
Shy-Drager syndrome, 183
Sialorrhea, 217–218
Sick role, 53–54
Side-slide transfers, 10
Significance level, 18
Sign language, 59, 74, 231
Silicone inserts, as hypertrophic scarring prophylaxis, 360
Simulated community environments, 82
Sinding-Larsen-Johannson disease, 291
Sinus tarsi syndrome, 302
Sinuvertebral nerve, 533
Sip-and-puff switch systems, 504
Skier's thumb, 276
Skin, capillary filling pressure of, 441
Skin grafting, for burn wound coverage, 354–355
Sleep aids, 497
Sleep disturbances
  fibromyalgia-related, 350
  renal disease-related, 322
"Sleep palsies," 145
Slipped capital femoral epiphysis (SCFE), 282, 284
Slocum test, 291
Slow-acting antirheumatic drugs, 338
Smith, Eleanor, 87
Smoke alarms, for hearing-impaired persons, 87
Smoking
  as atherosclerotic peripheral vascular disease risk factor, 247
  as coronary artery disease risk factor, 244, 245
  as pressure ulcer risk factor, 461
  as stroke risk factor, 167
  vascular complications of, 557
"Snapping hip," 281
Sneakers, fit of, 302
Social environment, of handicapped persons, 5
Social functioning, assessment of, 10
Social Security Act, 92, 93
Social Security Administration, disability definition of, 122

Social Security Disability Insurance (SSDI), 93, 94, 399, 400
Social Security Insurance (SSI), 93
Social skills, developmental milestones of, 415–416
Sodium channels, voltage-dependent, 32
Sodium fluoride, as osteoporosis treatment, 453
Sodium hyaluronate, 550–551
Soft tissue, definition of, 312
Soft-tissue injuries, **312–315**
Soft-tissue mobilization, 531–532
Soleus muscle, during standing, 50
Somatization disorders, 406
Somatosensory evoked potential (SEP) studies, 160–162
Somatosensory system, 34
Somogyi effect, 493
Soporific agents, 497
Spasms, hemifacial, 190
Spasticity, **442–446**
  amyotrophic lateral sclerosis-related, 213
  cerebral palsy-related, 419, 420, 421, 422, 423
  clasp-knife, 105
  cryotherapy for, 516
  definition of, 38, 105, 442
  mechanism of, 442
  multiple sclerosis-related, 179
  muscle tone in, 110
  nerve block treatment for, **537–541**
  neurophysiologic basis of, 38
  pharmacologic treatment for, 443–445
  severity grading of, 443
  spinal cord injury-related, 198
  stroke-related, 172
  traumatic brain injury-related, 198
Speaking valve, unidirectional, 485
Special Olympics, 423
Speech. *See also* Aphasia; Communication
  gesture-facilitated, in nonfluent aphasia, 231
  natural, communication alternatives to, 483
Speech disorders
  of cerebral palsy patients, 423
  of Parkinson's disease patients, 185
  telegraphic speech, 481
Speech-impaired persons, telecommunications access by, 92
Speech interpreters, for hearing-impaired patients, 59, 87
Speech-language pathology evaluation, 478
Speech production, assessment of, 482–483
Speech reading (lip-reading), 59, 72
Speech reception threshold, 70
Speech recognition testing, 70
Speech synthesis devices, 506
Speech therapy, for Parkinson's disease patients, 187
Spina bifida, 424, 575
Spinal accessory nerve, injury to, as scapular winging cause, 149
Spinal arteries, 205
Spinal blocks, diagnostic, 368
Spinal canal, lateral recesses of, 46
Spinal cancer, magnetic resonance imaging of, 134
Spinal cord
  anatomy of, 24
  blood supply of, 29, 205
  HIV infection-related disorders of, 336
  innervation of, 24

Spinal cord (*cont.*)
  lesions of
    cervical, 107
      differentiated from peripheral neuropathies, 106
    long tracts in, 204
    sensory pathways in, 25
Spinal cord injury, **203–211**
  aerobic exercise in, 246
  ambulation rehabilitation in, 230–231
  antihypertensive therapy in, 499
  bladder dysfunction associated with, 472, 474–475
  in children, 412
  colostomy in, 469
  drug-attenuated orthostatic hypotension in, 499
  erogenous zone relocation in, 80
  effect on female sexual response, 76
  effect on fertility, 76, 77–78
  functional electrical stimulation therapy for, 524–526
  functional group classifications of, 206
  gastrointestinal disorders associated with, 432
  hypercalcemia associated with, 433
  motor levels of, 203
  motor recovery after, 207
  neurologic levels of, 204
  pneumonia associated with, 435
  radiation-induced, 327–328
  as reduced cardiovascular capacity cause, 246
  sensory levels of, 203
  syndromes of, 205–206
  traumatic brain injury associated with, 194
  upper-extremity contractures associated with, 207
  upper-neuron lesions associated with, 474
  urinary tract infections associated with, 476
  vocational rehabilitation in, 401–402
Spinal cord injury without radiologic abnormality
    (SCIWORA), 203, 412
Spinal cord stimulator, 368
Spinal cord tumors, 330–331
Spinal curvature, in cerebral palsy, muscular dystrophy
    and idiopathic scoliosis, 410
Spinal flexion exercises, contraindication in
    postmenopausal spinal osteoporosis, 451
Spinal nerves
  course of, 46
  dorsal rami of, 47
Spinal tap, 30
Spine
  anatomy of, 45–46
  innervation of, 46, 47
  metastases to, 330–331
  motions of, 47
  muscles of, 47
Spinocerebellar tract, 204
Spinothalamic system, 34
Spinothalamic tracts, 25, 204, 208–209
Spiritual dimension, of rehabilitation, 5–6
SPLATT (slit anterior tibial transfer) procedure, as
    spasticity treatment, 446
Splinting
  in median nerve palsy, 279
  opponens, 565
  in radial nerve palsy, 279
  transparent, in burn patients, 360
  in ulnar nerve palsy, 279
  upper-limb, 562, 565–566
  of wrist or hand, 564

Splinting (*cont.*)
  in burn patients, 359
Spondylitis, 346–347
Spondyloarthropathies, 346
Spondylolisthesis, 47, 409–410
Spondylolysis, 47, 395
Spondylosis, as neuropathic pain cause, 544
Sports medicine, **385–390**
Sports participation
  after hip replacement surgery, 284–285
  after medial collateral ligament injury, 291
  after total knee arthroplasty, 295
  as osteoarthritis risk factor, 347
Sprains
  adductor, in ballet dancers, 395
  cervical, 312–313
  differentiated from strains, 312
  inversion, sports-related, 386
  lumbar, 313
  of rib cage, 313
Spurling test, 111, 252
Stair ambulation
  after total knee replacement, 295
  by children, 416
Staphylococcus epidermidis infections, as discitis
    cause, 535
Static shoulder orthosis, 563, 564
Statistical power, 18
Statistics, 17–19
Steinmann's test, 290
Stellate ganglion block, 382
Stem cells, as central nervous system injury treatment,
    223
Stenosis, spinal, 46, 135
Stereognasia, 107
Stereotactic-guided surgery, for Parkinson's disease,
    184
Steroids. *See also* Corticosteroids
  as avascular necrosis cause, 280, 288
  epidural injections of, 533–534
Stimulants, use in neurorehabilitation, 225–227
"Stingers," 253, 387
Stoma, continent appendicocecostomy, 470
"Stones, bones, and abdominal groans" mnemonic, for
    hypercalcemia, 209, 433
Stool softeners, 469, 503
Strabismus, cerebral palsy-related, 420
Straight-leg-raising test, 110
Strains
  cervical muscle, 586
  differentiated from sprains, 312
"Stranger anxiety," 417–418
Strength testing, 99
Stress tests, cardiac, 244
Stroke, **167–177**
  benzodiazepine-inhibited recovery from, 228
  cerebral artery, 100–101
  constraint-induced movement therapy (CIMT) for,
    221–222
  definition of, 167
  in elderly patients, 120
  as foot and ankle deformity cause, 299
  functional outcomes of, 175
  hemispheric, weakness associated with, 106
  hypertension associated with, 437
  "learned nonuse" in, 221

Stroke (*cont.*)
    mortality causes in, 170
    neuroprotective therapy for, 220
    risk factors for, 167
    effect on sexual activity, 79
    subsequent, prevention of, 167
    types of, 167–168
Stroke volume, 243
Stump care, upper-extremity, 568
Stump pain, 557
Stump syndrome, choked, 559
Subluxation, 311
    atlantoaxial, rheumatoid arthritis-related, 345
    differentiated from dislocation, 313
Submission, by patients, 5
Subscapularis muscle, 47–48
Subspecialty training, in physiatry, 3
Substance P, 366
Substantial Gainful Activity (SGA), 401
Substantia nigra, 26
Subtalar-midtarsal joint complex, 302
Sudden unexpected death, in hospitalized patients, 441
Suffering, 5
Suicide, assisted, 63
Sulfonylureas, oral, 500
Superior gluteal artery, 280
Superior gluteal nerve, 280
Supination, biomechanical effect of, 303
Supplemental Security Income (SSI), 399, 400
Suppositories, chronic use of, 469
Suprapubic tapping, 473
Suprascapular nerve
    entrapment of, in athletes, 386–387
    lesions of, differentiated from C5–6 cervical
        radiculopathy, 147–148
Supraspinatus muscle, 47–48
Swallowing. *See also* Dysphagia
    evaluations of, 483–484
        in cerebral palsy patients, 423
        in Parkinson's disease patients, 187
    HIV infection-related disorders of, 334
    stages of, 483
"Swan neck" deformity, 275, 345
Switch, 504
Sympathectomy, surgical paravertebral, 383
Sympathetic nerves, 20–21
Sympathetic nervous system, functions of, 34
Symptom magnification, 406
Synapses, 32
Synchronized intermittent mandatory ventilation, 237
Syndrome of inappropriate secretion of antidiuretic
        hormone, 432–433
Synergy patterns, of the limbs, 169–170
Synovectomy, in rheumatoid arthritis patients, 346
Syringomyelia, 208–209, 425
Systemic lupus erythematosus, 349–350

Tabes dorsalis, 209
Tachycardia, immobilization, 318
Tamoxifen, 453
Taping, low dye, 301
Tapotement, 531
Tap water, use in iontophoresis, 520
Tardive dyskinesia, 190–191
Tardy ulnar nerve palsy, 144
Tarsal tunnel syndrome, 144, 149

TART mnemonic, for somatic dysfunction diagnosis,
        530
Task, definition of, 6
Task reacquisition, as phase of rehabilitation process, 7
Taut bands, 369
    needling and infiltration of, 375
Tax Equity and Fiscal Responsibility Act of 1982, 92
Taylor brace, 587
TDD (telephone devices for the deaf), 87, 506
Technology Related Assistance for Individuals with
        Disabilities Act, 94
Tectospinal tract, 25, 38
Telecommunications, accessibility of, 92
Telephone amplifiers, 71
Telephone devices for the deaf (TDD), 87, 506
Television, closed captioning on, 71, 92
Temperature, effect on electrodiagnostic measurements,
        128
Temperature perception, 107
    in spinal cord injury patients, 208–209
Temporal lobe, lesions of, 28
Tenants, disabled, rights of, 85
Tender points, 369, 370, 371, 378
Tendinitis, 549
    bicipital, 260
    differentiated from partial rotator cuff tear, 258
    rotator cuff, 262
    ultrasound therapy for, 518
Tendons, rheumatoid disease-related rupture of, 343
Tendon stretching, contraindication in rheumatic
        disease, 341
Tendon transfers, 277
Tennis elbow. *See* Epicondylitis, lateral
Tenosynovitis, deQuervain's, 278–279
TENS. *See* Transcutaneous electrical nerve stimulation
        (TENS)
Tensor fasciae latae muscle, contracture of, 281
Teres major muscle, 47–48
Teres minor muscle, 47–48
Testosterone
    as osteoporosis treatment, 453
    as pressure ulcer prophylaxis, 501
Test-retest validity, of functional assessment scales, 11
Tethered cord, meningomyelocele-related, 425
Tethered median nerve stress test, 140
Tetrapelgia. *See also* Quadriplegia
    definition of, 205
Thalamic pain, 173
Thalamus, blood supply of, 29
Theater sign, 290
Thecal sac, epidural injection-related puncture of, 534
Theories, scientific, 15
Thermal burns, 352, 354
Thiamine deficiency, chemotherapy-related, 326
Thiazilodinediones, 500
Third nerve palsy, 151
Thomas test, 111, 280–281
Thoracic compression fractures, 587
Thoracic orthoses, 586
Thoracic outlet syndrome, 22
    in athletes, 386
    definition of, 253
    in musicians, 392
    neurogenic, 146
    neurovascular bundle entrapment sites in, 146–147
    torso injury-related, 313

Thoracolumbar sacral orthosis, 586
Thrombocytopenia, cancer-related, 328
Thromboembolism
  diabetes-related, 554
  "6 Ps" of, 248
  total hip replacement-related, 283
Thrombosis
  arterial, diabetes-related, 554
  deep venous
    heparin treatment for, 434–435
    hip replacement-related, 286
    prophylaxis against, 249, 294
    as pulmonary embolism cause, 249
    spinal cord injury-related, 208
    stroke-related, 170
    total hip arthroplasty-related, 283
    total knee arthroplasty-related, 294
Thrust techniques, in manipulation, 530–531
Thumb
  motion of, 49
  opposable, 562
Tibial nerve
  entrapment of, 144, 148–149
  injuries to, 24
Tibial nerve blocks, as spasticity treatment, 445
Tibial torsion, cerebral palsy-related, 419
Ticket to Work program, 400–401
Tics, 188
Tikhoff-Lindberg procedure, 329
Tinel's sign, 139
Tinnitus, 69, 72
Tissue healing, acupuncture-related, 543
Tissue plasminogen activator, as stroke treatment, 220
Tizanidine, as spasticity treatment, 444, 445, 501–502
Toes, deformities of, 297
Toe walking, by cerebral palsy patients, 419
Toilets, accessibility of, 86
Toilet training, 416
Tolcapone, as Parkinson's disease treatment, 184
Tongue, hypoglossal nerve injury-related deviation of, 28
Tonic neck reflexes, asymmetric and symmetric, 411
Topical agents, analgesic, 501
  as neuropathic pain treatment, 154
Topical analgesics, 501
Topiramate, as neuropathic pain treatment, 154
Topognosia, 107
Torso, injuries to, 313
Torticollis, 188
  spasmodic, 189
Total body surface area, of burn patients, 352, 354
Touch, sense of, 107
Tourette's syndrome, 188
Tracheostomy
  in respiratory distress, 236
  in ventilatory failure rehabilitation, 237
Tracheostomy patients, unidirectional speaking valve
    use by, 485
Traction, 307, 528–530
  cervical, 253
  intermittent, 529–530
Tramadol, as neuropathic pain treatment, 153, 154
Transcortical motor aphasia, 173
Transcortical sensory aphasia, 173
Transcutaneous electrical stimulation, 382, 519–521,
    526–527
  contraindications to, 527

Transdisciplinary rehabilitation teams, 7
Transference, in physician-patient relationship, 54
Transfers, 10
Transforaminal epidural injections, 533, 534
Translaminar epidural injections, 533, 534
Transplant patients, rehabilitation of, **317–320**
Trapezius muscle, 48
Trauma
  as brachial plexopathy cause, 154
  as limb loss cause, 553
  as neck pain cause, 252
Trazodone, soporific effect of, 497
Tremor
  classification of, 187–188
  definition of, 187
  drug-induced parkinsonism-related, 183
  Parkinson's disease-related, 183
  psychogenic, 192, 193
Trendelenburg sign, 581
Tricyclic antidepressants, 497
  antiarrhythmic activity of, 437
  as cancer pain treatment, 327
  as fibromyalgia treatment, 351
  as pain treatment, 366
  side effects of, 436
Trigeminal nerve
  function of, 25
  sensory branches of, 27
Trigger finger, 274–275
Trigger point injections, 351, 375
Trigger points, 350, 366, 369, 370, 371, 375, 376, 378
Trochanter
  bursitis of, 281–282
  sitting-related pressure on, 461
Trochlear nerve
  brain stem exit point of, 27
  function of, 25
  palsy of, 27
Tub lifts, 86
Tuning forks, 107
Tunnel vision, 105
"Turf toe," 388
Turning "en bloc," by Parkinson's disease patients, 183
"Turn-offs," in communication with disabled patients,
    62–63
Turnout, in dancers, 393–394, 395
Twins, multiple sclerosis in, 177
Type I and type II errors, 17–18

Uhthoff's phenomenon, 179
Ulcers
  in amputees, 559
  nonhealing, 249
  pressure, **460–465**
    adjuvant therapies for, 464–465
    debridement of, 462–463
    healing of, 441
    meningomyelocele-related, 425
    repetitive or poorly healing, 501
Ulnar artery, passage through Guyon's canal, 145
Ulnar deviation, of the fingers, 275
Ulnar nerve
  entrapment of, 144
    along the cubital tunnel, 268, 272
    at the elbow, 131, 271, 272
    at Guyon's canal, 145, 389

Ulnar nerve (*cont.*)
   entrapment of (*cont.*)
      at the wrist, 145
   injuries to, 22
   palsy of, 146, 279
   passage through Guyon's canal, 145, 146
Ultrasound
   broadband, for osteoporosis diagnosis, 449
   characteristics of, 517
   as reflex sympathetic dystrophy treatment, 382
   renal, 475
Ultrasound diathermy, 517–518
Uncovertebral joints, 46
Unified Parkinson's Disease Rating Scale, 185
United States Department of Health and Human
      Services, 241
University of Pennsylvania classification, for
      osteonecrosis management, 288
Unna paste dressing, 556
Unna's boot, 301
Upper extremity
   anatomy and kinesiology of, 47–48
   congenital deficiency of, 567
   orthoses for, **562–566**
   peripheral nerve injuries in, 22
   peripheral nerves of, 22
   prostheses for, **567–572**
   segmental weights of, 560
   spinal cord injury-related contractures of, 207
   synergy patterns of, 169–170
Upper-motor neuron bowel, 466, 467–468
Upper-motor neuron syndrome, 39–40, 443
Uremia, 322
Urethral pressure profile, 473
Urethritis, 346
Urinary incontinence, in stroke patients, 168, 171
Urinary tract infections, 440, 476
Urination, in bed-confined patients, 440
Urodynamic evaluation, 473
Urogram, intravenous, 475
Urologic disorders, **471–478**

Vacuum tumescence constriction therapy, 77
Vagus nerve, 465, 466
   function of, 26
Validity, of functional assessment scales, 11
Valium, as spasticity treatment, 502
Valproate, as traumatic brain injury treatment,
      198
Valsalva maneuver, 473
Vancomycin, 431
Van Nes procedure, 328–329
Vapocoolant sprays, 515
Variables, 15–16
   latent, 12
Varus deformities, 298, 299
Vascular disease, systemic, 436
Vasodilation, acupuncture-induced, 543
Vaso-occlusion, diabetes-related, 554
Vegetative state, traumatic brain injury-related,
      200–201
Venlafaxine, 497
Venous insufficiency, chronic, 249
Ventilator weaning, 237
Ventilatory impairment, respiratory disease-related,
      233, 234–237

Vertebral bodies, polymethylmethacrylate injections
      into, 536
Vertebral compression fractures, 120, 305, 451–452
Vertebroplasty, 536
Vesicoureteral dysfunction, spinal cord injury-related,
      474
Vestibular system, 34
Vestibulocochlear nerve, function of, 25
Vestibulospinal tract, 25, 38
   effect on muscle tone, 39
Viagra, interaction with nitrate-containing medications,
      501
Vibrating devices, for hearing-impaired persons, 87
Vibration sense, 107
Vibration testing, 107
Vicar's knee, 292
Videofluoroscopic swallowing study, 484
Video urodynamics, 473
Vigilance network, 42
Virchow's triad, 208, 248–249
Vision, neural pathway for, 26
Visitability, 87
Visual Action Therapy (VAT), 483
Visual Communication Therapy (VIC), 483
Visual evoked potential (VEP) study, 162
Visual fields, evaluation of, 104–105
Visual impairment
   classification of, 65–66
   common causes of, 65
   HIV infection-related, 335
Visually impaired patients, 57–58, **65–68**
   assistive technology devices for, 506
   environmental adaptations for, 87
   mobility assistance for, 57, 67
   physical examination of, 57–58
Visual system, 34
Vitamin B_{12} deficiency, 503
Vitamin K deficiency, chemotherapy-related, 326
Vocation, definition of, 397
Vocational rehabilitation, 94, **397–403**
   of HIV-infected patients, 337
Voice control (voice recognition) switches, 504
Voiding cystourethrogram, 475
Voluntary movement, neural control of, 40–41
VO_2max (maximum rate of oxygen consumption),
      491
von Monakow, Constantin, 224
VO_2 (oxygen consumption rate), 491

Waddell's signs, 256
Walkers
   use by multiple sclerosis patients, 180
   use by Parkinson's disease patients, 186
Walking
   as developmental milestone, 416
   differentiated from running, 112
   energy consumption during, 578
   by geriatric stroke patients, 120
   by infants, 114
   by paraplegics, functional electrical stimulation-
      assisted, 525
   by Parkinson's disease patients, 185
   speed of, 113
Wallerian degeneration, 144
Warfarin, anticoagulant activity of, 498
War injuries, phantom pain associated with, 558

Warm-up periods, prior to exercise
  in cardiac rehabilitation, 245, 246
Warm-up periods, prior to exercise, 491
Warts, differentiated from plantar callus, 304
Weaver's bottom bursitis, 549
Wedge resection, as heterotopic ossification treatment, 459
Wedges, for the foot, 301
Wee-FIM (functional independence measure), 413
Weight-bearing, 283
  by fracture patients, 308–310
Weight loss, in malnourished patients, 495
Werdnig-Hoffmann disease, 213, 409
Wernicke's aphasia, 103, 173
Western Neuro Sensory Stimulation Profile, 197
Wheelchair mobility, 10
Wheelchairs
  for cerebral palsy patients, 420, 423
  electric, for children, 411
  environmental accessibility of, 54
  manual, **589–593**
  for Parkinson's disease patients, 186
  safety of, 589
  for scoliosis patients, 218–219
Wheelchair users
  communication with, 55
  physical examination of, 55–56
Whiplash injury, 253, 312
Whirlpools, 514, 515, 516
  use by burn patients, 357
Wilson's disease, 189
"Within-subjects" research design, 16–17
Wolff, Julius, 450

Wolff's law, 450, 492
Workers' compensation, 92
  disability definition of, 121–122
  for performing artists, 393
Workplace adaptations, for Parkinson's disease
  patients, 186–187
Work simplification, for reduction of vertebral
  compressive forces, 452
World Health Organization, 447, 511, 512
Wound healing
  ankle-brachial index level of, 298
  in controlled environment, 556
Wounds, hydrotherapy treatment for, 516
Wright-Schöber test, 346
Wrist disorders, **276–279**
  orthoses for, 564, 565
  primary and secondary repair of, 276
  splinting of, 564
Writer's cramp, 188, 189

X-rays
  of cervical spine, 252
  for complex regional pain syndrome evaluation, 381
  of foot and ankle disorders, 304
  of fractures, 306
  for heterotopic ossification evaluation, 458

Yohimbine, as erectile dysfunction treatment, 77
Young adults, stroke rehabilitation in, 176

Zalepon, soporific effect of, 497
Zolpidem, soporific effect of, 497